Immunotherapies for Neurological Disorders

Immunotherapies for Neurological Disorders

Unlocking the Brain's Defenses

Edited by

Akash Gautam

Centre for Neural and Cognitive Sciences, School of Medical Sciences, University of Hyderabad, India

Micaela Morelli

University of Cagliari, Italy

ELSEVIER

ACADEMIC PRESS

An imprint of Elsevier

Academic Press is an imprint of Elsevier
125 London Wall, London EC2Y 5AS, United Kingdom
50 Hampshire Street, 5th Floor, Cambridge, MA 02139, United States

For accessibility purposes, images in electronic versions of this book are accompanied by alt text descriptions independently provided by Elsevier, generated with the aid of AI. For more information, see https://www.elsevier.com/about/accessibility or Radarweg 29, 1043 NX Amsterdam, Netherlands.

Books and Journals published by Elsevier comply with applicable product safety requirements. For any product safety concerns or queries, please contact our authorised representative, Elsevier B.V., at productsafety@elsevier.com.

Publisher's note: Elsevier takes a neutral position with respect to territorial disputes or jurisdictional claims in its published content, including in maps and institutional affiliations.

Notices
Knowledge and best practice in this field are constantly changing. As new research and experience broaden our understanding, changes in research methods, professional practices, or medical treatment may become necessary.

Practitioners and researchers must always rely on their own experience and knowledge in evaluating and using any information, methods, compounds, or experiments described herein. In using such information or methods they should be mindful of their own safety and the safety of others, including parties for whom they have a professional responsibility.

To the fullest extent of the law, neither the Publisher nor the authors, contributors, or editors, assume any liability for any injury and/or damage to persons or property as a matter of products liability, negligence or otherwise, or from any use or operation of any methods, products, instructions, or ideas contained in the material herein.

ISBN: 978-0-443-44631-3

For information on all Academic Press publications visit our website at https://www.elsevier.com/books-and-journals

Publisher: Megan Ball
Acquisitions Editor: Simonetta Harrison
Editorial Project Manager: Himanshi Yadav
Production Project Manager: Sathyavani Deiva Sigamani
Cover Designer: Arumugam Kothandan

Typeset by TNQ Tech

Contents

Contributors

Sagar Acharya
Department of Zoology, Vidyasagar University, Midnapore, West Bengal, India

Sahin Ali
Department of Zoology, Vidyasagar University, Midnapore, West Bengal, India

Clement Arava
Université de Rouen Normandie, Laboratoire Sciences et Méthodes Séparatives, Rouen, France

Vineet Arora
Department of Behavioral Health, Children's Hospital of Philadelphia, Philadelphia, PA, United States

J. Deepa Arul Priya
Department of Biotechnology, Sri Paramakalyani College, Alwarkurichi, Tamil Nadu, India

Santhra Segaran Balan
Faculty of Health and Life Sciences, Management and Science University, Shah Alam, Selangor, Malaysia

Victor Bushlyar
Department of Neurology, Yale School of Medicine, New Haven, CT, United States

Atri Chatterjee
Department of Neurology, Varshman Mahavir Medical College & Safdarjung Hospital, New Delhi, Delhi, India

Yanying Chen
Center for Life Sciences, Shaoxing Institute, Zhejiang University, Shaoxing, China

Anisha David
Department of Biology, St. Joseph's University, Bengaluru, Karnataka, India

Pamela David
Department of Anatomy, Faculty of Medicine, Universiti Malaya, Kuala Lumpur, Malaysia

Mohd Farhan
Lombardi Comprehensive Cancer Center, Georgetown University Medical Center, Washington, DC, United States

Anirban Ghosh
Department of Zoology, Cell Development and Immunobiology Laboratory (CDIL), School of Sciences, Netaji Subhas Open University, Kolkata, West Bengal, India

Shariff Halim
Universiti Teknologi MARA (UiTM), Penang Branch Bertam Campus, Kepala Batas, Pulau Pinang, Malaysia

Md Sahidul Islam
Roswell Park Comprehensive Cancer Center, Buffalo, NY, United States

Hamda Khan
Department of Biochemistry, Jawaharlal Nehru Medical College, Aligarh Muslim University, Aligarh, Uttar Pradesh, India

Akhilesh Kumar
Division of Medicine, ICAR-Indian Veterinary Research Institute, Bareilly, Uttar Pradesh, India

Diji Kuriakose
Department of Anatomy and Developmental Biology, Monash University, Clayton, VIC, Australia

Ruth Naomi
Institute of Ocean and Earth Sciences, Universiti Malaya, Kuala Lumpur, Malaysia

Spoorthy Pathikonda
City University of Hong Kong, Department of Chemistry, Hong Kong, China

Pooja Solanki Pooja
Division of Medicine, ICAR-Indian Veterinary Research Institute, Bareilly, Uttar Pradesh, India

Uday Pratap
Department of Obstetrics and Gynecology, University of Texas Health San Antonio, San Antonio, TX, United States

Roslee Rajikan
Centre for Healthy Aging and Wellness, Faculty of Health Sciences, Universiti Kebangsaan Malaysia, Kuala Lumpur, Malaysia

Amala Reddy D.
Department of Biotechnology, School of Bioengineering, SRM Institute of Science and Technology (Deemed to be University), Chennai, Tamil Nadu, India

Rohit Kumar Rohit
Division of Medicine, ICAR-Indian Veterinary Research Institute, Bareilly, Uttar Pradesh, India

Bhaskar Roy
Department of Neurology, Yale School of Medicine, New Haven, CT, United States

S. Winkins Santosh
PG & Research Department of Advanced Zoology & Biotechnology, Toxicology Research on Endocrine Disruptors (TRENDS) Laboratory, Government Arts College, Chennai, Tamil Nadu, India

Harshit Saxena
ICAR-IVRI, Izatnagar, Division of Medicine, Bareilly, Uttar Pradesh, India

Akshat Sharma
Department of Cancer Genetics and Genomics, Roswell Park Comprehensive Cancer Centre, Buffalo, NY, United States

Jyotsana Singh
Department of Hematopoietic Biology and Malignancy, The University of Texas MD Anderson Cancer Center, Houston, TX, United States

Pardeep Kumar Singh
Department of Neuroimaging and Interventional Radiology, National Institute of Mental Health and Neurosciences, Bangalore, Karnataka, India

Yogesh Srivastava
Department of Genetics, The University of Texas MD Anderson Cancer Center, Houston, TX, United States; Center for Precision Health, McWilliams School of Biomedical Informatics, The University of Texas Health Science Center, Houston, TX, United States

Ramasamy Vasantharekha
Department of Biotechnology, School of Bioengineering, SRM Institute of Science and Technology (Deemed to be University), Chennai, Tamil Nadu, India

Zhicheng Xiao
Center for Life Sciences, Shaoxing Institute, Zhejiang University, Shaoxing, China; Department of Anatomy and Developmental Biology, Monash University, Clayton, VIC, Australia

Qingyu Zhang
Guangdong Medical University, Zhanjiang, Guangdong, China

Saiful Irwan Zubairi
Department of Food Sciences, Faculty of Science and Technology, Universiti Kebangsaan Malaysia, Bangi, Selangor, Malaysia

Preface

Rationale of the title

In the last 30 years, neuroscience has changed its ideas more than ever before. For a large part of the 20th century, people thought of the brain as an immunologically privileged organ. The blood–brain barricr kcpt the systemic immune system from getting to the brain, and the brain was mostly protected from inflammation events in the rest of the body. This doctrine influenced numerous generations of research, diagnostics, and therapeutics. Neurological disorders were approached predominantly through neuronal, synaptic, and electrophysiological frameworks, while immune processes were often considered secondary, reactive, or even irrelevant. That perspective is no longer sustainable.

We now understand that the central nervous system (CNS) is not immunologically inert but is dynamically integrated with the immune system. Microglia, astrocytes, infiltrating lymphocytes, meningeal immunity, cytokine networks, complement cascades, and peripheral immune–brain interactions collectively orchestrate the processes essential for development, plasticity, repair, and disease. Immune dysfunction is not simply an observer in neurological disorders; it often serves as a catalyst, enhancer, or regulator of pathology. This paradigm shift has sparked one of the most thrilling frontiers in translational neuroscience: immunotherapy for neurological disorders.

Immunotherapies for Neurological Disorders: Unlocking the Brain's Defenses is a book that was written at this important time in biomedical science. It aims to combine the basic immunological principles with the newest treatment methods to give a full picture of how immune systems can be changed, redirected, or used to treat nervous system diseases. The goal is not just to make a list of new treatments, but also to help researchers, doctors, and advanced trainees understand the concepts, mechanisms, and real-world applications of these treatments in this quickly changing field.

Neurological disorders, including multiple sclerosis, autoimmune encephalitis, Alzheimer's disease, Parkinson's disease, stroke, epilepsy, glioblastoma, and neuropsychiatric conditions, exhibit a common theme of immune dysregulation. In some conditions, such as multiple sclerosis, immune-mediated damage is overt and primary. In certain conditions, like Alzheimer's disease, immune responses can be maladaptive, inadequate, or persistently inflammatory. There is a growing trend to look at conditions that were thought to be "noninflammatory" in a new way, through the lens of neuro-immune interactions. Immunotherapy has also changed oncology, rheumatology, and the way autoimmune diseases are treated. Monoclonal antibodies, checkpoint inhibitors, recombinant cytokines, gene therapies, cell-based immunotherapies, RNA interference, and nanotechnology-driven delivery systems have transitioned from experimental concepts to clinical applications.

It is only natural to ask if these advances can be used in the field of neurology. The answer is complex. The CNS has its own unique anatomical and physiological problems. The blood–brain barrier keeps drugs from getting into the brain. Immune responses in neural tissue must be tightly regulated to avoid collateral neuronal damage. Neuroinflammation may serve dual functions—protective in acute injury and detrimental in chronic conditions. Therapeutic timing, specificity, and safety become of utmost importance. But even with these problems, progress is speeding up. Targeted antibodies are being used in real life to treat neuroinflammatory diseases. Nucleic acid-based therapies are gaining approval for genetic CNS disorders. Strategies for gene editing are being worked on. Cell-based immunotherapies are being explored for neurodegeneration and brain tumors. Vaccines are being made to not only stop neurological problems caused by infections, but also to attack harmful proteins in neurodegenerative diseases. This book was written because there is a need to put these new ideas into a clear framework.

Structure of the book

The structure of this volume is intentional, moving from understanding how the immune system works in brain disorders to looking at treatment options that use or block these mechanisms.

Chapter 1: A meaningful therapeutic strategy must start with a clear understanding of how things work. The first chapter sets the stage for the immunological aspects of neurological disorders. It examines innate and adaptive immune components in the CNS, encompassing microglial activation states, astrocytic responses, T- and B-cell infiltration, cytokine networks, complement pathways, and systemic immune influences. This important chapter of the book makes a point that immunotherapy must be disease-specific and aware of the situation. Neuroinflammation is not uniform; it differs in timing, intensity, cellular composition, and functional outcome. To be successful in therapy, you need to be able to tell the difference between protective immune surveillance and harmful inflammation.

Chapter 2: Monoclonal antibodies represent one of the most mature immunotherapeutic platforms. In the field of neurology, antibodies have shown effectiveness in autoimmune disorders and are being increasingly investigated in neurodegeneration. This chapter looks at how antibodies work, such as neutralization, opsonization, complement activation, and receptor blockade. It also talks about problems that are unique to delivering antibodies to the CNS. It also considers engineering strategies to enhance blood–brain barrier penetration and specificity. The clinical achievements and constraints of antibody-based therapies provide essential insights for future advancement.

Chapter 3: Some conditions call for immune activation, while others necessitate exact suppression. Overactive immune responses can make demyelination, neuronal death, synaptic dysfunction, and chronic degeneration worse. This chapter examines immunosuppressive strategies designed explicitly for CNS disorders, encompassing cytokine blockade, modulation of T-cell responses, inhibition of microglial hyperactivation, and targeted intervention in inflammatory pathways. The focus is on finding a balance—reducing harmful inflammation without hurting the body's natural defenses.

Chapter 4: Recombinant cytokines, growth factors, and immune modulators provide precise methods for adjusting immune responses. This chapter delves into therapeutic proteins designed to promote neuroprotection, regulate immune signaling, or enhance repair processes. The conversation also includes pharmacokinetics, problems with delivery, and protein engineering methods that make proteins more stable and better at targeting the CNS.

Chapter 5: Peptide-based therapies are in a class of their own because they are both specific and easy to make and change. This chapter discusses new ways to precisely change immune pathways, from immune-modulating peptides to ligand–receptor targeting strategies. The therapeutic promise of peptides lies in their adaptability; however, their clinical translation requires overcoming issues of stability and bioavailability, topics explored in depth.

Chapter 6: Vaccination, which has long been linked to infections, is now being looked into for autoimmune and neurodegenerative diseases. This chapter looks at both preventive and therapeutic vaccines that are meant to change how the immune system responds to disease-related antigens or pathological proteins. The ethical, mechanistic, and translational aspects of CNS-targeted vaccines are examined in detail.

Chapter 7: Nucleic acid therapeutics have changed very quickly in a few areas. Antisense oligonucleotides, mRNA therapies, and gene-silencing strategies are transforming the therapeutic paradigm for genetic neurological disorders. This chapter gives a full picture of the delivery platforms, safety issues, how long the response lasts, and regulatory milestones. It also talks about where immunomodulation through nucleic acids might go in the future.

Chapter 8: Cell-based immunotherapies signify a frontier with transformative potential. Regulatory T cells, engineered T cells, dendritic cells, and various immune populations can be altered to target pathological processes specifically. This chapter looks at the reasons for, early clinical studies, and preclinical evidence of immune cell therapies in neurological settings, including both their potential and their risks.

Chapter 9: Gene therapy presents the potential for enduring or even permanent alterations of immune pathways within the central nervous system (CNS). This chapter talks about viral vectors, gene-editing tools, and ways to change the immune system using genetic engineering. It is also important to think about how the immune system reacts to the vectors themselves, which is a key issue for the safe use of gene therapies.

Chapter 10: RNA interference (RNAi) is a strong way to turn off genes that are involved in neuroinflammation. This chapter examines siRNA, shRNA, and the associated platforms designed to mitigate pathological immune signaling in the brain. Precision, specificity, and delivery challenges are examined alongside the emerging therapeutic successes.

Chapter 11: Nanotechnology connects biology and engineering, making it possible to send immunomodulatory agents directly to the brain through the blood–brain barrier. Nanocarriers, nanoparticles, and hybrid systems are revolutionizing how immune-targeted therapies reach neural tissue. This last chapter shows how modern immunotherapy brings together materials science, immunology, and neuroscience.

Ethical and clinical factors

As immunotherapies are used more widely in clinical settings, ethical issues become more important. Changing how the immune system works in the brain can be dangerous because it can cause autoimmune diseases, make you more likely to get infections, have effects that are not what you want, and have long-term effects that may not show up for a long time. It is important to carefully choose patients, design clinical trials carefully, and be open about the risks and benefits. Also, getting fair access to advanced biologics and gene therapies is still a problem around the world. This book does not shy away from these problems. Instead, it encourages people to think critically about both the benefits and drawbacks of the current strategies.

This book is meant for scholars from multidisciplinary fields. For example, neuroscientists who want to include immunological points of view in their work, immunologists examining CNS applications of immune-targeted therapies, medical doctors and neurologists who are interested in new ways to treat diseases, graduate students and postdoctoral researchers who are new to the field of neuroimmunology, and translational scientists working at the interface of laboratory discovery and clinical implementation. The volume aspires to function as both a reference and a conceptual guide by integrating mechanistic depth with therapeutic breadth.

The central theme of this book relies on precision and equilibrium, moving away from broad immunosuppression toward targeted treatments that balance the central nervous system's complex immune responses. Overcoming the physical hurdle of the blood–brain barrier is essential, necessitating innovations in nanotechnology and specialized delivery methods to ensure that the drugs reach their destination. Furthermore, the path from basic research to clinical success requires a rigorous translational framework—utilizing biomarkers and accurate patient stratification—and a deeply interdisciplinary approach that unites experts from immunology to computational biology to turn scientific potential into viable patient care.

Acknowledgments

The authors who contributed to this volume's creation were very knowledgeable and committed. Each chapter shows that the author has done careful research, critical thinking, and is dedicated to spreading knowledge. The contributors come from a wide range of fields and points of view, which is similar to how the field itself is interdisciplinary. We hope that the resource they all worked on together will help with research, spark new ideas, and, ultimately, lead to better patient outcomes.

Final note

The brain's defenses are very strong, complicated, and always changing. For many years, people thought of them as things that kept people from getting therapy. We are starting to see them as possible friends more and more. To unlock the brain's defenses, you do not have to take them apart; you just have to understand them and guide them. It takes humility to understand how complicated biology is and bravery to look for new ways to solve problems. It needs strict science, careful translation, and moral responsibility.

As the editors of this book, we both hope that *Immunotherapies for Neurological Disorders: Unlocking the Brain's Defenses* will be both a scholarly resource and a catalyst that encourages more research, collaboration, and faster development of therapies that restore neurological health. The field is at a very important crossroads. Immunotherapy could change the field of neurological medicine in ways that were once thought impossible if scientists keep being strict and work together. We encourage the readers to think critically about the ideas presented here, to add to them, and to help shape the ongoing story of neuroimmunology and new treatments. How well we learn to use and balance the immune system inside our bodies may have a significant effect on the health of our brains in the future.

Micaela Morelli
Akash Gautam

CHAPTER

1 Understanding the immunological components of brain disorders

Sahin Ali[1], **Sagar Acharya**[1] and **Anirban Ghosh**[2]

[1]*Department of Zoology, Vidyasagar University, Midnapore, West Bengal, India;* [2]*Department of Zoology, Cell Development and Immunobiology Laboratory (CDIL), School of Sciences, Netaji Subhas Open University, Kolkata, West Bengal, India*

Abbreviations

BDNF Brain-Derived Neurotrophic Factor
CCL2 C–C Motif Chemokine Ligand 2
CD Cluster of Differentiation
CLR C-type Lectin Receptor
CX3CR1 C-X3-C Motif Chemokine Receptor 1
FADD Fas-Associated Death Domain Protein
FcγR Fc Gamma Receptor
FGF Fibroblast Growth Factor
GLAST Glutamate Aspartate Transporter
HMGB1 High Mobility Group Box 1
Iba1 Ionized Calcium-Binding Adapter Molecule 1
ICAM1 Intercellular Adhesion Molecule 1
IFN Interferon
IL Interleukin
Ly6C Lymphocyte Antigen 6 Complex, Locus C
LYVE1 Lymphatic Vessel Endothelial Hyaluronan Receptor 1
MCP1 Monocyte Chemoattractant Protein-1
MerTK MER Proto-Oncogene Tyrosine Kinase
MMP Matrix Metalloproteinase
NGF Nerve Growth Factor
NLRP3 NOD-Like Receptor Pyrin Domain Containing 3
P2X7 Purinergic Receptor P2X, Ligand-Gated Ion Channel 7
P2Y G Protein-Coupled, 12
P2Y12 Purinergic Receptor
PDL Programmed Death Ligand
PNS Peripheral Nervous System
PRR Pattern Recognition Receptor
RNS Reactive Nitrogen Species
ROS Reactive Oxygen Species
S100B S100 Calcium-Binding Protein B

Immunotherapies for Neurological Disorders. https://doi.org/10.1016/B978-0-443-44631-3.00005-6

SALL1 Spalt Like Transcription Factor 1
TGF Transforming Growth Factor
TLR Toll-Like Receptor
TMEM119 Transmembrane Protein 119
TNF Tumor Necrosis Factor
TNFRs Tumor Necrosis Factor Receptors
VCAM1 Vascular Cell Adhesion Molecule 1
VEGF Vascular Endothelial Growth Factor

1. Introduction

The brain is recognized as a singularly unique and critical organ, centrally involved in the regulation and homeostasis of virtually all physiological activities. It is the anatomical substrate for both fundamental and higher-order behavioral and cognitive functions, supported by diverse and complex neuronal and non-neuronal cellular interactions. The organisation and performance of the brain's immune system are substantially different from those of systemic immunity, and the conceptualization of this system has undergone tremendous revision over the past century. Specifically, the last three - decades have yielded an immense and expanding volume of scientific data exploring brain immune functions across contexts ranging from development and behavior to various neurological disorders (Kumar et al., 2024). Consequently, to effectively advance the use of immunity as a therapeutic strategy for neurological pathology, a prerequisite is the detailed comprehension of the components of brain immunity and their general functional mechanisms within this specialized, cranially restricted compartment. The present chapter will be the primer to understand the present immunotherapeutic approaches against neurological disorders.

2. CNS immunity is specialized

In contrast to peripheral organs, the central nervous system (CNS) is not subject to circulating peripheral immune monitoring. CNS was once considered an immune-privileged site due to the apparent restriction on the entry of blood-borne factors and immune cells (Bechmann et al., 2007). However, the idea has changed over time with the admission that the brain has a specialized immune environment delicately protected and communicated with the peripheral immunity, which may be massively disrupted in different neuropathogenic conditions (Kettenmann et al., 2011; Zhu et al., 2022). CNS immunity is marked by notable complexity, and the processes regulating its involvement in neurological pathology continue to be clarified (Höftberger & Lassmann, 2017).

Distinct from other organs or tissues, the brain CNS have resident immune components that are mainly distributed through the brain parenchyma and interfaces between the CNS and periphery (Matejuk et al., 2021). Brain CNS harbors diverse types of resident immune cells like microglia, astrocytes that are located in brain parenchyma, along with at the CNS border-the perivascular space, choroid plexus and meninges—particular border-associated macrophages, dendritic cells, mast cells and lymphocytes cells (T cells and B cells) dwell in cerebrospinal niches (Muzio & Perego, 2024). After getting immune responses, the native immune cells, microglia and astrocytes, regulate metabolic supports, synaptic coordination, remove apoptotic residue, cytokine signaling, and modulate neuronal plasticity to create a neuroprotective environment. At the CNS border, specialized immune cell types provide antigen presentation to lymphocyte cells, maintain blood-brain barrier (BBB) integrity, and produce antibodies. Within this arrangement, the brain CNS is protected from possible threats and maintains brain homeostasis.

This chapter focuses exclusively on these immunological components of the CNS. By outlining their origin, markers, niches, and core functions. We will provide a clear framework for understanding how immune cells define the brain's unique immune micro-environment.

3. Immunological components in the CNS

The central nervous system (CNS) has a very specialized and tightly controlled immune system, which is often called neuroimmunity. This system protects the CNS while maintaining its neural function. The CNS is protected by structural barriers, such as the BBB, which is composed of endothelial cells, pericytes, and astrocytic end-feet. These barriers prevent immune cells from entering when the body is in a state of homeostasis. Microglia are the main immune cells that live in the CNS. They are macrophage-like cells derived from the yolk sac that continuously monitor the parenchyma. They also help with synaptic pruning, clearing away debris, and quickly responding to injury or infection. Astrocytes, while primarily glial support cells, actively engage in immune signaling by producing cytokines, chemokines, and complement components, and by regulating BBB integrity. Perivascular macrophages, meningeal immune cells, and infiltrating lymphocytes during pathological states are other immune system factors that play a role.

The newly identified meningeal lymphatic vessels enhance CNS immunity by promoting antigen drainage to cervical lymph nodes, thereby integrating central and systemic immune surveillance. Cytokines (such as IL-1β and TNF-α), interferons, chemokines, and complement proteins are all molecular mediators that help the innate and adaptive immune systems work together in the CNS. This tightly controlled immune environment is necessary for protecting the host and repairing tissue, but when CNS immune components are not functioning properly, it can lead to neuroinflammatory and neurodegenerative diseases such as multiple sclerosis, Alzheimer's disease, and Parkinson's disease (Gilani & Gautam, 2025). So, the immune system in the CNS is always changing between being immune privileged and immune competent.

Some of the important immunological components in the brain are mentioned in Table 1.1.

4. Resident immune cells in brain parenchyma

4.1 Microglia

The microglia are an innate, primary, and resident immune cell in the brain. Microglia originate from erythro-myeloid progenitor cells in the yolk sac during embryonic development (Schetters et al., 2018). Microglia comprise about 10%-15% of all glial cells in the CNS. They are the main antigen-presenting cells (APCs) in the CNS, liable for immune monitoring (Block & Hong, 2005; Ghosh, 2010). Primarily, microglia reside in the brain parenchyma at the resting, or inactive, stage. Uniformly distributed microglia are mainly located in the hippocampus, olfactory bulb, basal ganglia, and substantia nigra, and are less distributed in fiber tracts, the cerebellum, and most of the brainstem.

During brain development, a myeloid cell-specific gene, Trem2, is expressed only by microglia and contributes to microglia-mediated synaptic refinement. Under homeostatic conditions, the microglia

Table 1.1 Immunological components of the CNS.

Immune components							
Resident immune cells in brain parenchyma	**Border-associated immune cells**				**Adaptive immune cells**		**Structural unit**
Microglia Astrocytes	Macrophages	DCs	NK cells	Mast Cells	T cells	B Cells	NVU
	PVM SDM DM CPM $CP^{epi}M$	–			MT CSFT	–	Pericytes ECs Glial cells BBB

BBB, *Blood-brain barrier;* CPM, *Choroid plexus macrophage;* CSFT, *Cerebrospinal Fluid T cells;* $CP^{epi}M$, *Choroid epiplexus macrophages;* DCs, *Dendritic Cells;* DM, *Dural macrophages;* ECs, *Endothelial cells;* MT, *Meningeal T cells;* NVU, *Neurovascular Unit;* NK, *Natural Killer;* PVM, *Perivascular macrophage;* SDM, *Subdural macrophages.*

appear with a highly branched ramified morphology. The key phenotypic markers expressed by these resting cells are TMEM119, SALL1, CX3CR1, P2Y12, MerTK, and Iba1 (Kierdorf & Prinz, 2017).

Activation of microglia is initiated through cell surface receptors TLR, TNFRs, and P2X7, which are associated with the NF-κB signaling pathway. This signaling pathway involves multiple factors in both homeostatic and reactive conditions (Baidya et al., 2021). Moreover, the central player of the immune system in the brain, CNS- microglia, constantly surveys the CNS environment, maintains synapse plasticity, and has Fas ligand, which can induce programmed cell death, modulate and regulate the activity of neurons and astrocytes. Conversely, disease-associated microglia have the potential to produce cytotoxic superoxide molecules that can harm neurons and cause the death of immune cells (Simpson & Oliver, 2020). Thus, microglial activation in response to inflammation has self-limitation.

In neuroinflammation, microglia undergo activation and cellular morphology shifts from ramified to ameboid due to shortening and thickening of cellular processes and are presently subdivided into several other morphological and functional subtypes (Paolicelli et al., 2022) (Fig. 1.1). This phenotypical alteration from homeostatic to disease-associated microglia is sometimes called microgliosis (Streit et al., 1999). Apart from the activation of microglia, the phenotypical alteration provides both neuroprotective and neurotoxic attributes (Kempuraj et al., 2024). Conventionally, activated microglia are classified as the M1-M2 dichotomy. The classical M1 phenotype is considered disease-associated microglia. In an inflammation-rich environment, stimuli like IFN-γ and LPS promote the polarisation of resting microglia into an M1 phenotype. The neurotoxic, pro-inflammatory microglia secrete IL-6, IL-1β, TNF-α, MMP, and CCL2, and increase the production of ROS and NO, associated with markers such as CD86, CD80, CD11b, and CD11c. On the other hand, a neuroinflammatory environment rich in anti-inflammatory IL-4 or IL-13 promotes the development of an M2 phenotype. Now, these neuroprotective anti-inflammatory microglia secrete IL-4, IL-10, IL-13, TGF-β, FGF, NGF, BDNF, and VEGF-like factors that are associated with key markers like CD163, CD204 and CD206 (Kempuraj et al., 2024; Shao et al., 2022).

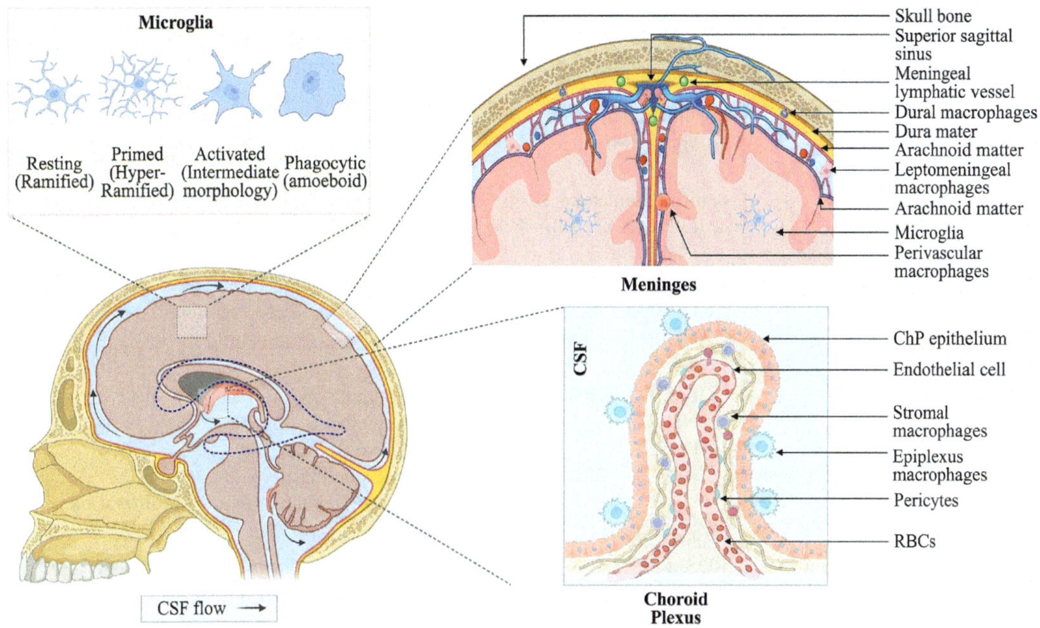

FIGURE 1.1 Anatomical Compartments and Niches of Brain and their Immune Connections.

The sagittal section of brain shows the outer meningeal layers, then the brain parenchyma and the ventricular region. Different forms of microglia, as the resident immune cell of brain, are found in the CNS parenchyma. The second anatomically important position is the meningeal structures between the skull and brain parenchyma, which have a complex layered structure with various compartments, lymphatic venules, and blood-borne cells that form specific niches. The third important anatomical location relevant for the blood-brain communication is the choroid plexus region at the interface of brain tissue and ventricular spaces. *(created in www.biorender.com).*

However, recent findings and single-cell omics studies reveal that resident microglia may have a wide variety of morphological and functional heterogeneity across developmental phases, ages, neurophysiological conditions and according to the layers of complexity and contexts (Ghosh et al., 2021; Paolicelli et al., 2022; Stratoulias et al., 2019). A community approach by the prominent neuroimmunologists reached no consensus to formalize the heterogeneous subgrouping and admitted a wide spectrum of immune-functional categories (Healy et al., 2022; Paolicelli et al., 2022). This actually reiterated the significance of microglia again and again as the most sensitive and omni-responsive cell population within CNS parenchyma. Table 1.2 represents only a few of the prominent factors derived from microglia and their functions. It is to be kept in mind that microglial functions are delicately balanced within the CNS parenchyma, and all these functions vary according to the situations, microenvironmental combination of cues and contexts.

Table 1.2 Microglial products and their role.

Microglial products			Role
Cytokines	**M1**	Pro-inflammatory- IL-6, IL-1β, TNF-α	Neuroprotective (delicately balanced, overexpression leads to inflammatory damage)
	M2	Anti-inflammatory- IL-4, IL-10, IL-13, TGF- β	Neurotoxic (situation and context dependent, in other forms—helping tissue repair or promoting immune-quiescence)
Chemokines		CCL2, CCL2, CCL3, CCL5, CXCL8, CXCL10, CXCL12 and MCP1	**i.** Immune cells (monocytes, lymphocytes, dendritic cells, neutrophils) recruitment. **ii.** Neuroinflammation
Growth factors		TGF-β, FGF, NGF, BDNF, VEGF, M-CSF, GM-CSF	Neuronal growth Angiogenic growth Neurogenesis Synaptic plasticity Microglial activation and proliferation
Complement proteins		C1q, C3, C4	Synaptic pruning
Reactive species		ROS, RNS	Mediators of neuroinflammation
Proteases		Elastase, plasminogen	It may be important in microglial migration or the breakdown of the BBB by acting as an adhesion molecule.

4.2 Astrocytes

Astrocytes are a major glial cell type in the CNS, comprising about 20%–40% of total cells (Khakh & Sofroniew, 2015). The term "astrocyte," derived from the Greek word astro, meaning "star," was first introduced by Mihaly von Lenhossek in 1895, reflecting their star-like morphology (Sofroniew & Vinters, 2010). Morphologically, they are classified as protoplasmic astrocytes (star-shaped, fine projections, mainly in gray matter) and fibrous astrocytes (long filamentous processes, mainly in white matter). Other specialized forms include velate, radial, and interlaminar astrocytes, found in regions such as the cerebellum, olfactory bulb, and cortex. They are commonly identified by GFAP (Glial Fibrillary Acidic Protein), a reliable immunocytochemical marker expressed specifically in these cells, which can vary under homeostatic and disease conditions (Hamby & Sofroniew, 2010). Additional markers used for astrocyte identification include GLAST, S100B, and aquaporin-4 (Gradisnik & Velnar, 2023).

With regard to astroglial functions in the brain CNS environment, they performed at both innate and adaptive immunity, both in the normal and inflamed CNS. Astrocytes play essential roles in regulating synapse formation and function Table 1.3. The fibrous astrocytes anchor themselves with their long filamentous projections to the nodes of Ranvier for neuronal communication, and protoplasmic astrocytes wrap the synapses (López-Hidalgo & Schummers, 2014). Astrocytes have been shown to act as APCs to $CD4^+$ T cells, to express MHC-I and MHC-II molecules, to upregulate costimulatory molecules CD80 and CD86, and to activate $CD4^+$ and $CD8^+$ T cells. Astrocytes also express PRRs, TLRs, dsRNA-dependent protein kinase, complement receptors, mannose receptors,

Table 1.3 Major functions of astrocytes maintaining CNS homeostasis.

1. Maintain neuronal communication
2. Neurotransmission by taking up the transmitters and providing support to the neurons.
3. Maintains the integrity of BBB
4. Antigen presentation
5. In a pathological condition astrocyte communicates with lymphocytes
6. Protect the brain from oxidative damage
7. Participate in angiogenesis for CNS development and repair

and scavenger receptors (Nair et al., 2008). Under pathological states, astrocytes become reactive and facilitate immune responses in the CNS environment through astrocyte-lymphocyte interaction, following this manner: firstly, loosening the integrity of the BBB, secondly, by expression of adhesion molecules such as ICAM-1 and VCAM-1, and thirdly, release of chemokines such as CCL5, CCL2, CXCL8, and CXCL10. Astrocytes also secrete a variety of cytokines, such as IL-1, IL-6, and IL-10, and TNFα and TGFβ, which correlate with T cell responses (Nair et al., 2008).

Incidentally, in immunological insults to the brain, the resident immune cell microglia play a leading role, where astrocytes interact with microglia to maintain brain homeostasis. To shape the inflammatory landscape, microglia-derived mediators influence astrocyte activation and sometimes reciprocally. But evidence showed that activated microglia secrete cytokines such as IL-1β and TNF-α, which induce astrocytic reactivity (Müller et al., 2025). Hence, it states that astrocytes are only playing a supportive role in brain immunity, but the major player is microglia.

5. Border-associated immune cells

5.1 Macrophages

Non-parenchymal border-associated macrophages (BAMs) are part of the innate immune system in the brain CNS. The phagocytic nature of these cells originates from the erythro-myeloid progenitor cells (EMPCs) during embryogenesis. In 2020, Utz et al. confirmed that BAMs originate from EMPCs, not definitive hematopoiesis. They prepared a tamoxifen-inducible Runx1^{CreER}R26^{YFP}fate-mapping mouse model in the yolk sac, which gave rise to two different macrophage populations: one is CD206^{+} (BAM progenitors), and the other is CD206^{-} marked as microglial progenitor. As they are non-parenchymal, they are found in the meninges, choroid plexus and perivascular spaces of the brain (Muzio & Perego, 2024; Utz et al., 2020).

BAMs are classified into several subtypes depending on their anatomical site Table 1.4. They are grouped as subdural/leptomeningeal macrophages (sdMΦ), dural macrophages (dmMΦ), stromal choroid plexus macrophages (cpMΦ), choroid epiplexus macrophages (cp^{epi}MΦ), and peri-vascular macrophages (PvMΦ). To distinguish the BAM subtypes, several surface proteins have been pointed out. Approximately 75% of BAM subtypes are CD38^{+} or LYVE 1^{+} MHC-II^{-} subset. The CD38^{+} (or LYVE1^{+}) MHCII^{+} BAMs mainly make up subpopulations of sdMΦ and PVMs. The dmMΦ predominantly contain single-positive MHC-II^{+} BAMs and a smallerfewer CD38^{+} (or LYVE1^{+}) MHC-II^{+} subset. Choroid plexus macrophages consist of three BAM subsets, each with a

Table 1.4 Subtypes of BAMs and their location, markers and role in the CNS.

BAM	Subset	Location	Cell-specific markers	Role
	sdMΦ	Pia mater of the meninges	CCR2,CD36,CD163, CD169,CD206 and LYVE1	They both play a crucial role in viral infection.
	dmMΦ	Dura mater of the meninges		
	cpMΦ	Stromal space between the epithelial and endothelial layers		Involved in lipid metabolism, phagocytosis, antigen presentation and regulates CSF homeostasis.
	cp^{epi}MΦ	Epical epithelial surface		
	PvMΦ	Cerebral vessels		Maintaining BBB integrity and patrolling the entry of macromolecules into the brain

similar frequency: MHC-II^{-}, LYVE1^{+}MHC-II^{+}, and single-positive MHC-II^{+}. Furthermore, MHC-II^{+} BAMs, located in the choroid plexus and dura mater, uniquely express CCR2 (Mrdjen et al., 2018; Silvin et al., 2023). Overall, BAM consists of a significant populations of blood-borne monocytic lineage cells which lines the CNS parenchymal boundaries from meninges to choroid plexus in different forms and positions, occupying the immune-niches surrounding the brain as potential candidates to infiltrate these boundaries in any inflammatory or barrier disruption scenario.

5.2 Dendritic cells

Linking innate and adaptive immunity, Dendritic cells (DCs) are considered potent antigen-presenting cells. They are the only cell types that can activate naïve T cells (Steinman, 1991). DCs arise from precursors in the bone marrow and take up residence in somatic tissues and organs, serving as sentinels with an immature phenotype (Banchereau & Steinman, 1998). The study found that DCs are mostly located in all three layers of the meninges (dura mater, arachnoid, and pia mater), the choroid plexus and some are scattered in the perivascular space in the healthy CNS, while they invade the parenchyma in response to CNS disturbance (Ludewig et al., 2016).

CNS-DCs subpopulation is mainly categorized into three main classes, cDCs1, cDC2, and pDCs, which can be identified by the differential expression of several markers, such as CD11b, CD172, and CD24 Table 1.5. Normally, in the brain CNS cDC2 subset is slightly more abundant than the cDC1 subset (Butovsky & Weiner, 2018). Plasmacytoid DCs (pDCs) are atypical DCs that do not present antigens but produce interferon type 1 cytokines in response to pathogen-specific disturbance (Hornero & Idoyaga, 2023). The immune functions of DCs are initiated upon capturing an antigen, which triggers the activation of naïve T cells. At the same time, DCs are highly expressed PRRs, such as CLRs, TLRs, and Fc receptors, to recognize and engulf diverse antigens, including bacteria, viruses, apoptotic debris, and soluble inflammatory proteins (Jin et al., 2025). As their position suggests, these DCs are in the use of sampling and representing CNS-derived factors or else from systemic circulation and provoking mostly the T cells at the CNS boundary to become activated with molecular drive to enter the CNS parenchyma crossing the barriers.

Table 1.5 Subset of DCs.

DCs	Subset	Specific markers	Role
	cDCs1	$CD11b^{low}$ $CD172^{low}$ $CD24^{+}$ $CD135^{high}$ $CD117^{+}$	Antigen presentation to T cells
	cDCs2	$CD11b^{high}$ $CD172^{high}$ $CD135^{high}$ $PDL1^{+}$	
	pDCs	$Ly6C^{+}$ $B220^{+}$ Siglec-H^{+}	Produce type-I interferon in response to viral infection.

5.3 Natural killer cells

Natural killer cells (NK cells) are innate immune cells that belong to the innate lymphoid cell (ILC) family. Mass cytometry and single-cell transcriptomic analysis suggested that the NK cell population in the healthy brain make up a small fraction ($1.1 \pm 0.14\%$) of the total immune cells in the CNS. In the CNS environment, instead of the brain parenchyma, they are located at the boundaries, like the meninges and the choroid plexus (Ning et al., 2023). In humans, CNS NK cells differ from the blood NK cells in their molecular expression. Most NK cells in the blood are $CD56^{dim,}$ while the $CD56^{bright}$ population represents the majority in cerebrospinal fluid (Schafflick et al., 2020). In terms of different molecular marker expression of CD56 and lack of CD3 ($CD56^{+}CD3^{-}$) are typical features of human NK cells (Abel et al., 2018). NK cells usually don't get much attention from other such immune cells, but they play an important role in the crosstalk between the immune system and the CNS in the context of normal aging and many neurological diseases. They also play a role as a gatekeeper in the CNS, allowing immune cell infiltration and initiating inflammation. Thus, NK cells maintain CNS homeostasis, and they are mostly associated with the immunological niches surrounding the CNS boundaries with the systemic circulatory interfaces (Ning et al., 2023).

5.4 Mast cells

Among all immune cells, Mast Cell (MC) is the most prevalent. Their nature is pro-inflammatory. MCs originate from multipotent hematopoietic progenitor cells and can be easily identified through expression of the tyrosine kinase receptor c-kit and the Fc receptor for IgE. In the CNS environment, they are mainly located in the thalamus, but also present in circumventricular organs, in the meninges, hypophysis, pineal gland, area postrema, the median eminence and hypothalamus (Hendrix et al., 2013). Furthermore, MCs are located abluminal side of the BBB (Mittal et al., 2019). In the absence of pathological stimuli, MCs release some mediators that promote neuroprotection and repair. Although MCs are among the "first responders" at the blood-brain interfaces surrounding the brain, it is provocative to predict that their mediators have the ability to modulate the brain-associated macrophages (BAM) in the neurovasculatures and barriers surrounding the brain Table 1.6. Oppositely, if the inflammatory stimuli increase in the brain, MCs contribute to the disruption of the BBB (Huang et al., 2024).

Table 1.6 MCs Mediators and their role in CNS.

MCs mediators	Role
Histamin	Regulate sleep-wake cycles, neuroendocrine responses, suppress food intake, increase water intake, and increase antinociception.
NGF	Regulate neuron development and functional characteristics.
Serotonin	Neurogenesis
Angiogenin	Neuron survival and formation.

6. Adaptive immune cells

6.1 T cells

Thymus-derived T lymphocytes, or T cells, belong to the cell-mediated adaptive immune system. They develop, differentiate, and mature primarily in the thymus, where they undergo positive and negative selection to ensure MHC restriction and autoimmune tolerance. Once mature, naive T cells migrate to peripheral immune organs (Shen et al., 2024). In a controlled environment, generally naïve T cells are absent in the brain parenchyma. Mature T cells are found in dural lymphatic vessels. Under pathological circumstances, T cells usually gain entry into the CNS through the CNS meningeal layer, the choroid plexus and the BBB (Engelhardt et al., 2016). T cells from the meningeal layer directly bind APCs to induce a local inflammatory response, promoting them to enter the brain parenchyma. Whereas CSF T cells can not bind APCs directly, instead CSF serves as the main route driving meningeal T cells' cytokines to the neural cells within different CNS regions through paravascular influx toward the glial limitans (Abbaoui et al., 2023).

T cells are activated upon encounter of CNS injury, and based on their functions, these cells are categorized into T regulatory (T_{reg}), T helper (T_h) and T cytotoxic (T_c). Among them, T_{reg} suppress the immune response and prevent its overexpression. T_h cells support other immune cells by secreting cytokines, but do not directly kill target cells. While T_c cells can specifically target and kill infected cells (Braun, 2021).

Activation achieved by antigen-peptide-MHC complexes on APCs or target cells. Generally, T cells cannot directly recognize the epitope of the antigen; thus, they need co-stimulatory molecules to activate (Dustin, 2009). Upon activation, based on surface marker, T cells are further divided into $CD4^+$ helper T cells (T_h cells), Foxp3+ regulatory T cells (T_{reg} cells) and $CD8^+$ cytotoxic T cells (T_c). Biding upon the APCs with antigen complex differentiated $CD4^+$ T_h cells into different subtypes like T_h1, Th2, Th17 and Foxp3+ regulatory cells. Among these subtypes, Th1 and Th17 cells play essential pro-inflammatory roles, secreting IFN-γ, TNF-α, IL-17, and IL-22 cytokines. Conversely, Tregs and Th2 cells have major anti-inflammatory functions, secreting IL-4, IL-5, IL-9, IL-10, and TGF-β cytokines (Li et al., 2024). Following $CD8^+$ T_c cell activation, these cells release cytotoxic substances like perforin and granzyme. The action of perforin causes target cell membrane pore formation and creates a transmembrane channel where granzyme enters the target cell and inducing programmed cell death of the target cell (Andersen et al., 2006).

Thus, T cells represent a dynamic link between peripheral immunity and the CNS, ensuring both protective vigilance and regulatory equilibrium, and the circum ventricular organs, leptomeninges,

Table 1.7 B cell subsets and their functions in the CNS.

B cell	Subset	Marker	Role
	B1B	CD5, CD11b	Clear myelin debris Regulator of IL-10 production Oligodendrogenesis
	B2B	CD23	Immunomodulatory effects
	Marginal B	CD1d	Clear self-antigens to reduce autoimmunity
	Memory B cell	CD27	Powerful APCs
	Plasma B cell	CD138	Produce protective antibodies

choroid plexus and associated marginal interfaces of brain play the crucial role in the "in and out" interaction to pave the way of T cells to the brain tissue (Hsiao et al., 2025; Smolders et al., 2022).

6.2 B cells

Antibody-producing, humoral immune cells originating from the skull cap bone marrow are a lifelong source of continuous B cell generation from pluripotent hematopoietic stem cells. After leaving the bone marrow, immature B cells express IgM BCR(B Cell Receptor) and these cells are populated into secondary lymphoid organs, where they undergo further development (Cardani-Boulton et al., 2022). Single-cell RNAseq analysis exposed that B cells make up to 30% of the total immune cells in the dura mater (Brioschi et al., 2021). More in-depth analysis showed that in humans, B cells in a healthy CNS environment are rarely found in the parenchyma, although small numbers are stated (Machado-Santos et al., 2018), but they are more frequent in the meninges, particularly in the dura mater regions (Fitzpatrick et al., 2020). Though the understanding of B cell involvement and their contribution to brain immunity and diseases is limited, Table 1.7 summarizes different B cell subsets and their involvement in brain health, as evident so far.

7. Structural unit

7.1 NVU (Neurovascular unit)

The structural and functional network of the brain that maintains integration, protection and adaptability in brain health and disease. This network, shortly termed as NVU (Neurovascular Unit), is composed of glial cells, pericytes, endothelial cells, vascular basement membrane and BBB (Kempuraj et al., 2024). Different components of this NVU are shown in Table 1.8.

Together, these components regulate blood flow and metabolism in the brain's CNS environment. In addition, NVU components are essential for cerebral protection and equilibrium, as endothelial cells constitute the BBB, while glial wrapping of blood vessels functions as a secondary defense. Under immunological conditions, dysregulation of NVU is characterized by neuron death, activation of glial cells, immune cell infiltration, vascular leakage, and BBB disruption (Kugler et al., 2021).

Table 1.8 Summary of NVU components location and functional role in CNS.

NVU components	Location	Role
Endothelial Cells (ECs)	Single-layer lining of tubular blood vessels situated on the vascular bed.	Reduced pinocytosis/transcytosis. Increased expression of tight junction molecules, such as claudins, occludin, or zonula occludens 1 Exclude free transport of substances over 400 kDa
Pericytes	Positioned in the basement membrane shared with ECs	Vasodilation, contraction, vascular stability, and gives structural support to the blood vessels.
Glial cells	Enwrap blood vessels with their end feet.	Connect to the neurons for neuro-communication. Also plays a role in phagocytosis in inflammatory conditions.
Vascular basement membrane	Abluminal side of the endothelial cells	Acts as a passage for fluid transport and gives mechanical support.
Blood-brain barrier (BBB)	Cerebral microvasculature specifically in the capillaries formed by endothelial cells.	Acts as a selective barrier. Limits immune cell entry. Prevents entry of toxic substances into brain tissue Homeostatic maintenance
Perivascular macrophages	Position between the vascular endothelium and the brain parenchyma	Monitoring, regulating, and responding to changes in BBB integrity

7.2 BBB (Blood-brain barrier)

BBB is the most dynamic, complex and selective barrier that regulates limited transportation between the peripheral blood and the brain parenchyma and is the most studied structure of NVUs. Capillaries are the major site of the BBB. From the physiological point of view, endothelial cells (ECs), astroglia, pericytes, and junctional complexes, including tight junctions (TJs) and adherens junctions (AJs), are the main structural components of the BBB (Wu et al., 2023). Fig. 1.2 shows the structure of the BBB in healthy and diseased conditions Fig. 1.2.

In a steady-state environment, the BBB provides a controlled microenvironment by regulating the exchange of ions and molecules between the bloodstream and brain tissues. Maintains internal equilibrium through limited transportation, facilitating the transport of the essential molecules (Banks, 2015). During immune challenges, the BBB is disrupted and permeability increases, allowing the influx of inflammatory mediators and toxins from peripheral blood (Musafargani et al., 2020). An increased neuroinflammatory response leads to the breakdown of paracellular multiprotein complexes, such as tight junctions (TJs) and AJs, resulting in a loss of BBB permeability (Bhowmick et al., 2019). BBB plays a crucial role in different neuropathological states, mostly by acting as a leaky barrier with transverse movements of factors and blood-borne immune cells, and participates in influencing the immune reactivity within the brain parenchyma. Table 1.9 will elaborate on the BBB function in homeostasis and disease.

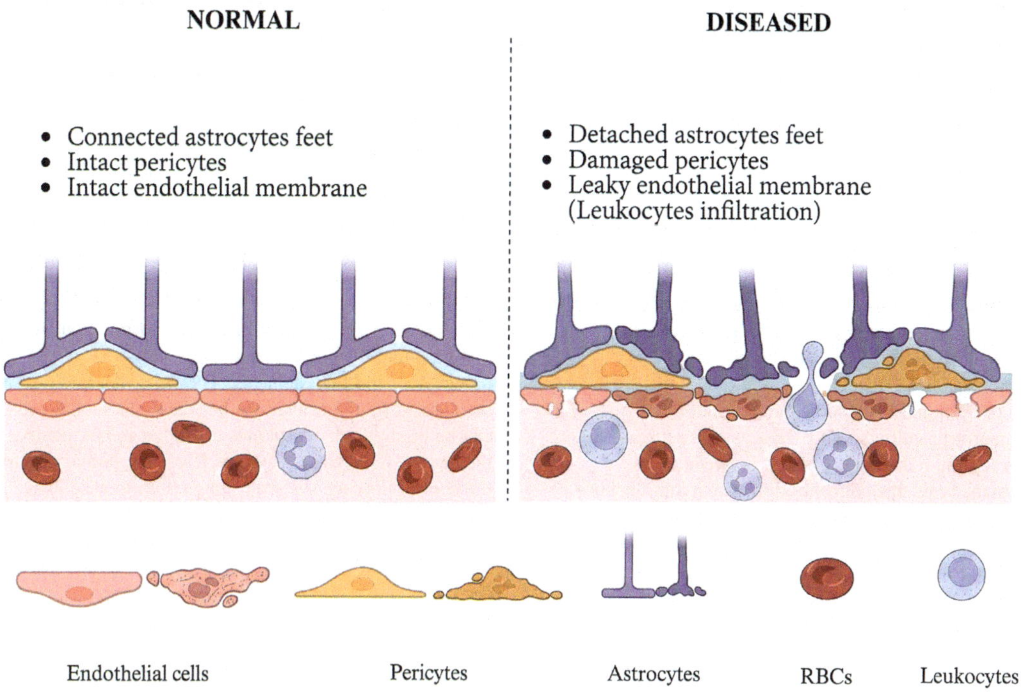

FIGURE 1.2 BBB in Normal and Diseased Brain.

The structure and components of blood-brain barrier (BBB) in normal homeostatic and diseased conditions showing disrupted structural components and organization allowing infiltration of leukocytes in brain parenchyma in later condition.

(created in www.biorender.com).

7.3 Perivascular macrophages (PVMs)

Associated with the above-mentioned BBB function in health and disease, it is essential to consider the role of perivascular macrophages (PVMs). Perivascular macrophages occupy a strategic position between the vascular endothelium and the brain parenchyma, where they play a crucial role in monitoring, regulating, and responding to changes in BBB integrity. Under pathological conditions, their activity becomes particularly significant, as they influence the entry and behavior of circulating leukocytes, monocytes, and macrophages within the CNS.

As an innate, non-parenchymal type of immune cell in the brain that has also been shown to contribute to maintaining brain stability (Goldmann et al., 2016). Less than 5% of all CNS macrophages are derived from early erythro-myeloid progenitors in the yolk sac, which migrate into the brain in the early stage of the embryo. They are located in the boundary region of fluid fluid-filled compartment known as Virchow Robin Space, meninges and choroid plexus (Zheng et al., 2022). There are several marker proteins associated with PVMs identification, including CD45, CD11b, CX3CR1, CD64, etc. Distinctively, CD206 is a crucial marker to distinguish PVMs from microglia (Wen et al., 2024).

Table 1.9 BBB in homeostatic conditions and disease conditions.

BBB in homeostatic conditions (Adopted from (Abbott *et al.*, 2010)	BBB in disease conditions
BBB not only acts as a protective barrier, but also maintains the pH and ion balance that is optimal for synaptic signaling function, which makes a stable environment for neuronal function. Neurotoxins such as endogenous metabolites or proteins, or xenobiotics ingested in the diet or otherwise acquired from the environment, could harm the healthy brain. BBB minimizes this issue, preventing the entry of such toxin molecules. As CNS and PNS both share common neurotransmitters, the BBB acts as a separator to keep the reducing cross-talk between them. In the brain, the concentration of macromolecules in the CSF is normally much lower than in plasma. When macromolecular substances gain entry into the CSF, they can trigger pathological processes such as seizures, glial activation, abnormal glial proliferation, and ultimately cell death. To prevent such neurotoxic events, the BBB plays a critical protective role by restricting the passage of potentially nerve-damaging macromolecules, including albumin, prothrombin, and plasminogen. BBB have some transporter systems, which allow essential water-soluble nutrients and metabolites that promote nervous tissue development. Thus, BBB also act as a nutritive function. The multiprotein junctional complex (TJs, AJs) in the BBB, which is situated between ECs, is responsible for the restriction of diffusion and blocks the penetration of macromolecules by this route.	BBB dysfunction is associated with many pathological conditions, including neurodegenerative diseases. These circumstances promote increased BBB permeability, immune cell and blood-borne cells infiltration into the brain parenchyma (Patabendige & Janigro, 2023). At sites of BBB inflammation, circulating neutrophils and mononuclear cells penetrate the barrier and accumulate in the perivascular space, forming patches that facilitate the entry of additional leukocytes, monocytes, and macrophages. The BBB, normally maintained by tight junctions between endothelial cells, can be disrupted by cytokines and other inflammatory mediators. As a result, mononuclear cells gain access to the central nervous system through both transcellular and paracellular routes (Abbott et al., 2010). A series of factors during immune responses in the brain leads to loss of integrity, disruption and dysfunction of the BBB. In combination with such immunological factors, including reactive oxygen species (ROS), pro-inflammatory cytokines (TNF α, IL-6, IL-1α, IL-1β and IFN γ) and matrix metalloproteinases that can activate microglia, astrocytes and endothelial cells, promoting the expression of molecules that can contribute to the destruction of the BBB (Patabendige & Janigro, 2023). Thus, BBB dysfunction not only permits the infiltration of circulating immune and blood-borne cells into the brain parenchyma but also amplifies local inflammatory cascades through cytokines, reactive oxygen species, and matrix metalloproteinases. The resulting activation of microglia, astrocytes, and endothelial cells perpetuates a cycle of barrier breakdown and neuronal injury.

Physiological functions played by PVMs are accompanied by antigen presentation, removing waste materials and apoptotic debris by the process of phagocytosis, and maintaining BBB integrity for normal brain homeostasis (Zhan et al., 2025). As we already know, in maintaining BBB integrity, the main key players are brain capillary endothelial cells and their tight junctions. Coexistently, PVMs are also recognised as maintaining BBB permeability. Under immune stimulation, the area postrema (AP) of the microvasculature is more permissive than the BBB due to the absence of tight junctions. In this setting, PVMs play a protective role. They capture serum protein (10–70 kDa) and, combined with the laminin layer, provide further restriction of entry of solutes above 10 kDa into the parenchyma (Zheng et al., 2022). Viewed in sum, PVMs also play a vital role in regulating BBB integrity.

8. Mechanism of work of the neuroimmune system in the diseased brain

Contrary to the previous belief, the brain is now considered a highly immunocompetent site, and the scientific literature is now flooded with evidence and documentation of immune activity of the brain from development to disease, homeostasis to inflammation and even in behavioral anomalies. It is now evident that CNS immune components and compartments play the key role in both physiological and pathophysiological situations (Toader et al., 2024).

In diseased tissue environments, the principal resident neuroimmune cells, microglia, interact with astrocytes and other immune cell types, including border-associated macrophages, adaptive T cells, and B cells. Together, these cells secrete many of the chemical signaling factors typically associated with neuroprotection. However, under severe adverse conditions—such as traumatic brain injury, epilepsy, HIV-1 infection, alcohol abuse, gliomas, or processes involved in neurodegenerative diseases (e.g., multiple sclerosis, Alzheimer's disease) and psychiatric disorders (e.g., depression)—their phenotypes can shift. These alterations lead to dysregulated expression of immune mediators (Gruol, 2021). Commonly, in these inflamed situations, many neuroimmune factors are produced, and many of these have overlapping actions. The action of these factors can cause microglial polarisation, astrocytic reactivity, disruption of the BBB, infiltration of peripheral immune cells, and malfunction of inflammatory signaling. Thus, the inflammatory products have the ability to upregulate the neurotoxic substance and downregulate the neuroprotective mediators (Gruol, 2021; Hours et al., 2025).

In the context of traumatic brain injury (TBI), where the state of consciousness alters due to endogenous molecules such as purines, heat shock proteins, and ligands of pathogen-associated molecular patterns (PAMPs) and damage-associated molecular patterns (DAMPs) are released, which activate immune receptors and promote neuroinflammation. In combination with these factors, easily triggered neuroinflammation in the brain that infiltrates microglia, astrocytes and other cell populations, and produces proinflammatory stimuli (Xu et al., 2022). In this situation, the immediate induction of the apoptotic signal causes cell death, which releases DAMPs that activate microglia, astrocytes and then recruit peripheral immune cells to pass through the damaged BBB (Loane & Kumar, 2016). Now, these activated immune cells produce neurotoxic substances that lead to neuronal dysfunctions (David & Kroner, 2011). In a study, it was suggested that TNF-α is an important factor in TBI pathophysiology (Liberman et al., 2018). In general, a low level of TNF-α is considered neuroprotective; a high level of this cytokine in TBI, TNF-α bind with TNF-R1, which initiates a cascade pathway. It activates FADD/Caspase-8 and classical NF-κB signaling pathways. That induces cell-dependent apoptosis or necroptosis (Zhan et al., 2025).

Similarly, degenerative neurological diseases trigger immune mechanisms in the brain through immune modulatory factors. Neurodegeneration occurs along with the aggregation of malfunctioning proteins and genetic variations that share hallmark neuroinflammation (Zhang et al., 2023). This diseased state provokes immune cells to become active and produce disease-promoting mediators like cytokines (IL-1β, IL-6, TNF-α), chemokines, reactive oxygen species (ROS), and nitric oxide (NO), which amplify immune responses that ultimately cause neurotoxicity. In AD (Alzheimer's disease), active glial cells promote the aggregation of amyloid beta and tau proteins, aiding the formation of neurofibrillary tangles (NFTs). These tangles can further activate BAMs via the TLR4 receptor and also lead to the loss of neuronal function (Dani et al., 2018). In addition to dead neurons, products such as ATP, HMGB1, S100B, DNA, etc., can further activate glial cells to create a more inflammatory environment (Venegas & Heneka, 2017). Another neurodegenerative condition, PD (Parkinson's disease), is associated with the accumulation of α-synuclein aggregates. These complexes interact with glial cells through binding to specific surface receptors (e.g., TLRs, FcγR) or intracellular receptors (e. g., NLRP3) (Tansey et al., 2022). After activation, glial cells secrete pro-inflammatory mediators that dysregulate neuronal functions (Pajares et al., 2020). Along with the adaptive immune cells, $CD4^+$ T cells recruit IFN-γ and granzymes, which weaken the endothelial tight junctions, promoting immune cell infiltration into the CNS. Ultimately, this suggests that in degenerative disease conditions, immune cells fail to protect the CNS; instead, in adverse conditions, they play a neurodestructive role through infiltration of peripheral immune cells, BBB disruption, and neuronal death, thus facilitating disease progression.

An autoimmune condition in the central nervous system (CNS), characterized by MS (Multiple Sclerosis), involves dysregulation of adaptive immune cells, including T and B cell activity within the CNS, leading to recurrent demyelination and neuronal injury (Lovett-Racke et al., 2019). The accumulation of autoreactive T cells and B cells, which are major drivers of tissue-damage mediators, enters the brain parenchyma through disruption of the BBB from the periphery. This aggregation provokes resident glial cells to become active, although infiltrating cells also stimulate them to secrete pro-inflammatory cytokines (i.e., IL-12, IFN-γ, and TNF), nitric oxide, and free radicals. These settings are enough to play a critical role in demyelination, contributing to oligodendrocyte loss and degenerative axonal pathology (Giallongo et al., 2022).

The fascinating paradox of immunology is manifested in CNS neoplasms. In glioblastoma (GBM), immune cells are recruited with the intent to mount an antitumor response, yet the tumor microenvironment reprograms them into an immunosuppressive state that ultimately supports, rather than opposes, tumor growth (Zhu et al., 2023). This transformation affects the resident immune cells and tumor-associated macrophages to secrete immunosuppressive cytokines such as IL-10 and TGFβ. These cytokines also play a crucial role in suppressing the broader immune response, shielding the tumor from immune monitoring (Toader et al., 2024). GBM cells-derived IL-10 predominantly induces the immunosuppressive role. In the GBM environment, increasing the production of these cytokines enhances the downregulation of the expression of antigen-presenting molecules, thereby impairing $CD4^+$ T cell activation (Rocha Pinheiro et al., 2023). For a tumor protective environment, glioma altered the regulatory T cell functions and made them immune-tolerant (Wang et al., 2024). Recent evidence shows that tiny extracellular vesicles originated from glioma cells, called exosomes, which are loaded with miRNAs, namely miR-21 and miR-146a. These exosomal miRNAs can dampen immune cells, preparing them to support the tumour (Hermann et al., 2022; Xia et al., 2019). Taken together, it is found that immune cells are recruited into the tumor microenvironment but are reprogrammed into immunosuppressive facilitators. Through cytokine secretion, regulatory T cell modulation, and exosomal-derived miRNAs, GBM reshapes the immune landscape to protect rather than eliminate malignant cells from immune cell arrest.

9. Conclusion

Presently, it has been accepted that in any neurological disorder or pathological condition, the brain's immune system actively engages its components and acts through layered communication with the peripheral immune system. While in normal development and homeostatic maintenance of the brain, this immune system acts in a well-regulated and specific manner, with controlled exchange of materials and cells between the brain and the peripheral system. Neuronal disorders or pathogenic conditions disrupt this balance. Researchers are now engaged in mapping such alterations and changes in different forms and through various strategies. The present era of single-cell genomic and proteomic analysis is making these efforts more robust and detailed, with obvious heterogeneity and cross-presentation of data that need to be analyzed properly. Also, the communication routes, barriers, interfaces and immune niches surrounding the brain have now come into the spotlight like never before. We are realising that there is an active process of communication and passage between systemic and neuronal compartments capable of shaping the brain's immune functions. Now, depending on the understanding sketched in this chapter, we will proceed to explore the contemporary development and delivery of immunotherapeutic strategies in neurological disorders in the chapters to come.

Acknowledgment

The authors are thankful to Amartya Saha of the Cell Development and Immunobiology Lab (CDIL) of Netaji Subhas Open University and to Dr Krishnendu Ghosh, Department of Pathology, Carver College of Medicine, Iowa University, USA, for the diagrams. The authors express their sincere thanks to the authorities of the Vidyasagar University and Netaji Subhas Open University for overall institutional support in this work.

References

Abbaoui, A., Fatoba, O., & Yamashita, T. (2023). Meningeal T cells function in the central nervous system homeostasis and neurodegenerative diseases. *Frontiers in Cellular Neuroscience, 17*. https://doi.org/10.3389/fncel.2023.1181071

Abbott, N. J., Patabendige, A. A. K., Dolman, D. E. M., Yusof, S. R., & Begley, D. J. (2010). Structure and function of the blood-brain barrier. *Neurobiology of Disease, 37*(1), 13–25. https://doi.org/10.1016/j.nbd.2009.07.030

Abel, A. M., Yang, C., Thakar, M. S., & Malarkannan, S. (2018). Natural killer cells: Development, maturation, and clinical utilization. *Frontiers in Immunology, 9*. https://doi.org/10.3389/fimmu.2018.01869. Frontiers Media S.A., United States.

Andersen, M. H., Schrama, D., Straten, P. T., & Becker, J. C. (2006). Cytotoxic T cells. *Journal of Investigative Dermatology, 126*(1), 32–41.

Baidya, F., Bohra, M., Datta, A., Sarmah, D., Shah, B., Jagtap, P., Raut, S., Sarkar, A., Singh, U., Kalia, K., Borah, A., Wang, X., Dave, K. R., Yavagal, D. R., & Bhattacharya, P. (2021). Neuroimmune crosstalk and evolving pharmacotherapies in neurodegenerative diseases. *Immunology, 162*(2), 160–178. https://doi.org/10.1111/imm.13264. Blackwell Publishing Ltd, India.

Banchereau, J., & Steinman, R. M. (1998). Dendritic cells and the control of immunity. *Nature, 392*(6673), 245–252.

Banks, W. A. (2015). The blood-brain barrier in neuroimmunology: Tales of separation and assimilation. *Brain, Behavior, and Immunity, 44*, 1–8. https://doi.org/10.1016/j.bbi.2014.08.007

Bechmann, I., Galea, I., & Perry, V. H. (2007). What is the blood-brain barrier (not)? *Trends in Immunology, 28*(1), 5–11. https://doi.org/10.1016/j.it.2006.11.007

Bhowmick, S., D'Mello, V., Caruso, D., Wallerstein, A., & Abdul-Muneer, P. M. (2019). Impairment of pericyte-endothelium crosstalk leads to blood-brain barrier dysfunction following traumatic brain injury. *Experimental Neurology, 317*, 260–270. https://doi.org/10.1016/j.expneurol.2019.03.014

Block, M. L., & Hong, J. S. (2005). Microglia and inflammation mediated neurodegeneration: Multiple triggers with a common mechanism. *Progress in Neurobiology, 76*(2), 77–98.

Braun, M. Y. (2021). The natural history of T cell metabolism. *International Journal of Molecular Sciences, 22* (13), 6779. https://doi.org/10.3390/ijms22136779

Brioschi, S., Wang, W.-L., Peng, V., Wang, M., Shchukina, I., Greenberg, Z. J., Bando, J. K., Jaeger, N., Czepielewski, R. S., Swain, A., Mogilenko, D. A., Beatty, W. L., Bayguinov, P., Fitzpatrick, J. A. J., Schuettpelz, L. G., Fronick, C. C., Smirnov, I., Kipnis, J., Shapiro, V. S., … Colonna, M. (2021). Heterogeneity of meningeal B cells reveals a lymphopoietic niche at the CNS borders. *Science., 373*(6553). https://doi.org/10.1126/science.abf9277

Butovsky, O., & Weiner, H. L. (2018). Microglial signatures and their role in health and disease. *Nature Reviews Neuroscience, 19*(10), 622–635.

Cardani-Boulton, A., Boylan, B. T., Stetsenko, V., & Bergmann, C. C. (2022). B cells going viral in the CNS: Dynamics, complexities, and functions of B cells responding to viral encephalitis. *Immunological Reviews, 311*(1), 75–89. https://doi.org/10.1111/imr.13124. John Wiley and Sons Inc, United States.

Dani, M., Wood, M., Mizoguchi, R., Fan, Z., Walker, Z., Morgan, R., Hinz, R., Biju, M., Kuruvilla, T., Brooks, D. J., & Edison, P. (2018). Microglial activation correlates in vivo with both tau and amyloid in alzheimer's disease. *Brain, 141*(9), 2740–2754. https://doi.org/10.1093/brain/awy188

David, S., & Kroner, A. (2011). Repertoire of microglial and macrophage responses after spinal cord injury. *Nature Reviews Neuroscience, 12*(7), 388–399. https://doi.org/10.1038/nrn3053

Dustin, M. L. (2009). The cellular context of T cell signaling. *Immunity, 30*(4), 482–492. https://doi.org/10.1016/j.immuni.2009.03.010

Engelhardt, B., Carare, R. O., Bechmann, I., Flügel, A., Laman, J. D., & Weller, R. O. (2016). Vascular, glial, and lymphatic immune gateways of the central nervous system. *Acta Neuropathologica, 132*(3), 317–338. https://doi.org/10.1007/s00401-016-1606-5. Springer Verlag, Switzerland.

Fitzpatrick, Z., Frazer, G., Ferro, A., Clare, S., Bouladoux, N., Ferdinand, J., Tuong, Z. K., Negro-Demontel, M. L., Kumar, N., Suchanek, O., Tajsic, T., Harcourt, K., Scott, K., Bashford-Rogers, R., Helmy, A., Reich, D. S., Belkaid, Y., Lawley, T. D., McGavern, D. B., & Clatworthy, M. R. (2020). Gut-educated IgA plasma cells defend the meningeal venous sinuses. *Nature, 587*(7834), 472–476. https://doi.org/10.1038/s41586-020-2886-4

Ghosh, A. (2010). Brain APCs including microglia are only differential and positional polymorphs. *Annals of Neurosciences, 17*(4). https://doi.org/10.5214/ans.0972.7531.1017410

Ghosh, A., Ghosh, P., Deb, I., & Bandyopadhyay, S. (2021). Morpho-functional variation and response pattern of microglia through rodent ontogeny showing infant microglia as stable and adaptive than matured. *Brain and Behavior, 11*(8). https://doi.org/10.1002/brb3.2315. John Wiley and Sons Ltd, India.

Giallongo, S., Longhitano, L., Denaro, S., D'Aprile, S., Torrisi, F., Spina, E. La, Giallongo, C., Mannino, G., Lo Furno, D., Zappalà, A., Giuffrida, R., Parenti, R., Volti, G. L., Tibullo, D., & Vicario, N. (2022). The role of epigenetics in neuroinflammatory-driven diseases. *International Journal of Molecular Sciences, 23*(23), Article 15218. https://doi.org/10.3390/ijms232315218

Gilani, F., & Gautam, A. (2025). Regulation of RNA transcriptomics during ageing-and neurodegeneration-associated cognitive changes. In *Decoding aging and neurodegeneration: The role of nucleic acid epigenetics* (pp. 69–93). Cham: Springer Nature. Switzerland.

Goldmann, T., Wieghofer, P., Jordão, M. J. C., Prutek, F., Hagemeyer, N., Frenzel, K., Amann, L., Staszewski, O., Kierdorf, K., Krueger, M., Locatelli, G., Hochgerner, H., Zeiser, R., Epelman, S., Geissmann, F., Priller, J., Rossi, F. M. V., Bechmann, I., Kerschensteiner, M., … Prinz, M. (2016). Origin, fate and dynamics of macrophages at central nervous system interfaces. *Nature Immunology, 17*(7), 797–805. https://doi.org/10.1038/ni.3423. Nature Publishing Group, Germany.

Gradisnik, L., & Velnar, T. (2023). Astrocytes in the central nervous system and their functions in health and disease: A review. *World Journal of Clinical Cases, 11*(15), 3385–3394.

Gruol, D. L. (2021). Neuroimmune actions in the brain and interactions with the effects of alcohol. *Neural Regeneration Research, 16*(9), 1791–1792. https://doi.org/10.4103/1673-5374.306079. Wolters Kluwer Medknow Publications, United States.

Hamby, M. E., & Sofroniew, M. V. (2010). Reactive astrocytes as therapeutic targets for CNS disorders. *Neurotherapeutics, 7*(4), 494–506.

Healy, L. M., Zia, S., & Plemel, J. R. (2022). Towards a definition of microglia heterogeneity. *Communications Biology, 5*(1). https://doi.org/10.1038/s42003-022-04081-6. Nature Research, Canada.

Hendrix, S., Kramer, P., Pehl, D., Warnke, K., Boato, F., Nelissen, S., Lemmens, E., Pejler, G., Metz, M., Siebenhaar, F., & Maurer, M. (2013). Mast cells protect from post-traumatic brain inflammation by the mast cell-specific chymase mouse mast cell protease-4. *FASEB Journal, 27*(3), 920–929. https://doi.org/10.1096/fj.12-204800

Hermann, D. M., Xin, W., Bähr, M., Giebel, B., & Doeppner, T. R. (2022). Emerging roles of extracellular vesicle-associated non-coding RNAs in hypoxia: Insights from cancer, myocardial infarction and ischemic stroke. *Theranostics, 12*(13), 5776–5802.

Höftberger, R., & Lassmann, H. (2017). Immune-mediated disorders. *Handbook of Clinical Neurology, 145*, 285–299. https://doi.org/10.1016/B978-0-12-802395-2.00020-1

Hornero, R. A., & Idoyaga, J. (2023). Plasmacytoid dendritic cells: A dendritic cell in disguise. *Molecular Immunology, 159*, 38–45.

Hours, C., Vayssière, P., Gressens, P., & Laforge, M. (2025). Immunity in neuromodulation: Probing neural and immune pathways in brain disorders. *Journal of Neuroinflammation, 22*(1). https://doi.org/10.1186/s12974-025-03440-4

Hsiao, C. C., Engelenburg, H. J., Rip, J., Wierenga-Wolf, A. F., van Puijfelik, F., van Luijn, M. M., Huitinga, I., Hamann, J., & Smolders, J. (2025). Acquisition of residency programs by T cells entering the human brain. *Cell Reports, 44*(7). https://doi.org/10.1016/j.celrep.2025.115960. Elsevier B.V., Netherlands.

Huang, X., Lan, Z., & Hu, Z. (2024). Role and mechanisms of mast cells in brain disorders. *Frontiers in Immunology, 15*. https://doi.org/10.3389/fimmu.2024.1445867

Jin, F., Xie, L., Zhang, H., Fan, X., Tian, J., Liu, W., Xiao, Y., & Fan, X. (2025). Dendritic cells: Origin, classification, development, biological functions, and therapeutic potential. *MedComm, 6*(11). https://doi.org/10.1002/mco2.70455

Kempuraj, D., Dourvetakis, K. D., Cohen, J., Valladares, D. S., Joshi, R. S., Kothuru, S. P., Anderson, T., Chinnappan, B., Cheema, A. K., Klimas, N. G., & Theoharides, T. C. (2024). Neurovascular unit, neuroinflammation and neurodegeneration markers in brain disorders. *Frontiers in Cellular Neuroscience, 18*. https://doi.org/10.3389/fncel.2024.1491952. Frontiers Media SA, United States.

Kettenmann, H., Hanisch, U.-K., Noda, M., & Verkhratsky, A. (2011). Physiology of microglia. *Physiological Reviews, 91*(2), 461–553. https://doi.org/10.1152/physrev.00011.2010

Khakh, B. S., & Sofroniew, M. V. (2015). Diversity of astrocyte functions and phenotypes in neural circuits. *Nature Neuroscience, 18*(7), 942–952. https://doi.org/10.1038/nn.4043. Nature Publishing Group, United States.

Kierdorf, K., & Prinz, M. (2017). Microglia in steady state. *The Journal of Clinical Investigation, 127*(9), 3201–3209. https://doi.org/10.1172/JCI90602

Kugler, E. C., Greenwood, J., & MacDonald, R. B. (2021). The "neuro-glial-vascular" unit: The role of glia in neurovascular unit formation and dysfunction. *Frontiers in Cell and Developmental Biology, 9*. https://doi.org/10.3389/fcell.2021.732820. Frontiers Media S.A., United Kingdom.

Kumar, P., Zelena, D., & Gautam, A. (2024). Neurological disorders and challenges in their theranostics. In *Theranostic applications of nanotechnology in neurological disorders* (pp. 1–29). Hungary: Springer. https://doi.org/10.1007/978-981-99-9510-3_1. Springer, Hungary.

Li, K., Chen, R., Wang, R., Fan, W., Zhao, N., Yang, Z., & Yan, J. (2024). Neuroinflammation in neurodegenerative diseases: Focusing on the mediation of T lymphocytes. *Neural Regeneration Research, 21*(5), 1864–1889.

Liberman, A. C., Trias, E., da Silva Chagas, L., Trindade, P., Dos Santos Pereira, M., Refojo, D., Hedin-Pereira, C., & Serfaty, C. A. (2018). Neuroimmune and inflammatory signals in complex disorders of the central nervous system. *Neuroimmunomodulation, 25*(5–6), 246–270. https://doi.org/10.1159/000494761

Loane, D. J., & Kumar, A. (2016). Microglia in the TBI brain: The good, the bad, and the dysregulated. *Experimental Neurology, 275*, 316–327. https://doi.org/10.1016/j.expneurol.2015.08.018. Academic Press Inc., United States.

López-Hidalgo, M., & Schummers, J. (2014). Cortical maps: A role for astrocytes? *Current Opinion in Neurobiology, 24*, 176–189.

Lovett-Racke, A. E., Gormley, M., Liu, Y., Yang, Y., Graham, C., Wray, S., Racke, M. K., Shubin, R., Twyman, C., Alvarez, E., Bass, A., Eubanks, J. L., & Fox, E. (2019). B cell depletion with ublituximab reshapes the T cell profile in multiple sclerosis patients. *Journal of Neuroimmunology, 332*, 187–197. https://doi.org/10.1016/j.jneuroim.2019.04.017. Elsevier B.V., United States.

Ludewig, P., Gallizioli, M., Urra, X., Behr, S., Brait, V. H., Gelderblom, M., Magnus, T., & Planas, A. M. (2016). Dendritic cells in brain diseases. *Biochimica et Biophysica Acta - Molecular Basis of Disease, 1862*(3), 352–367. https://doi.org/10.1016/j.bbadis.2015.11.003. Elsevier B.V., Germany.

Müller, L., Di Benedetto, S., & Müller, V. (2025). The dual nature of neuroinflammation in networked brain. *Frontiers in Immunology, 16*. https://doi.org/10.3389/fimmu.2025.1659947

Machado-Santos, J., Saji, E., Tröscher, A. R., Paunovic, M., Liblau, R., Gabriely, G., Bien, C. G., Bauer, J., & Lassmann, H. (2018). The compartmentalized inflammatory response in the multiple sclerosis brain is composed of tissue-resident CD8+ T lymphocytes and B cells. *Brain, 141*(7), 2066–2082. https://doi.org/10.1093/brain/awy151. Oxford University Press, Austria.

Matejuk, A., Vandenbark, A. A., & Offner, H. (2021). Cross-talk of the CNS with immune cells and functions in health and disease. *Frontiers in Neurology, 12*. https://doi.org/10.3389/fneur.2021.672455. Frontiers Media S. A., Poland.

Mittal, A., Sagi, V., Gupta, M., & Gupta, K. (2019). Mast cell neural interactions in health and disease. *Frontiers in Cellular Neuroscience, 13*. https://doi.org/10.3389/fncel.2019.00110

Mrdjen, D., Pavlovic, A., Hartmann, F. J., Schreiner, B., Utz, S. G., Leung, B. P., Lelios, I., Heppner, F. L., Kipnis, J., Merkler, D., Greter, M., & Becher, B. (2018). High-dimensional single-cell mapping of central nervous system immune cells reveals distinct myeloid subsets in health, aging, and disease. *Immunity, 48*(2), 380. https://doi.org/10.1016/j.immuni.2018.01.011. Cell Press, Switzerland.

Musafargani, S., Mishra, S., Gulyás, M., Mahalakshmi, P., Archunan, G., Padmanabhan, P., & Gulyás, B. (2020). Blood brain barrier: A tissue engineered microfluidic chip. *Journal of Neuroscience Methods, 331*, Article 108525. https://doi.org/10.1016/j.jneumeth.2019.108525

Muzio, L., & Perego, J. (2024). CNS resident innate immune cells: Guardians of CNS homeostasis. *International Journal of Molecular Sciences, 25*(9), 4865. https://doi.org/10.3390/ijms25094865

Nair, A., Frederick, T. J., & Miller, S. D. (2008). Astrocytes in multiple sclerosis: A product of their environment. *Cellular and Molecular Life Sciences, 65*(17), 2702–2720.

Ning, Z., Liu, Y., Guo, D., Lin, W. J., & Tang, Y. (2023). Natural killer cells in the central nervous system. *Cell Communication and Signaling, 21*(1). https://doi.org/10.1186/s12964-023-01324-9. BioMed Central Ltd, China.

Pajares, M., Rojo, A. I., Manda, G., Boscá, L., & Cuadrado, A. (2020). Inflammation in parkinson's disease: Mechanisms and therapeutic implications. *Cells, 9*(7), 1687. https://doi.org/10.3390/cells9071687

Paolicelli, R. C., Sierra, A., Stevens, B., Tremblay, M. E., Aguzzi, A., Ajami, B., Amit, I., Audinat, E., Bechmann, I., Bennett, M., Bennett, F., Bessis, A., Biber, K., Bilbo, S., Blurton-Jones, M., Boddeke, E., Brites, D., Brône, B., Brown, G. C., … Wyss-Coray, T. (2022). Microglia states and nomenclature: A field at its crossroads. *Neuron, 110*(21), 3458–3483. https://doi.org/10.1016/j.neuron.2022.10.020. Cell Press, Switzerland.

Patabendige, A., & Janigro, D. (2023). The role of the blood-brain barrier during neurological disease and infection. *Biochemical Society Transactions, 51*(2), 613–626. https://doi.org/10.1042/BST20220830. PMID: 36929707; PMICID: PMC10212550.

Rocha Pinheiro, S. L., Bueno Lemos, F. F., Santos Marques, H., Silva Luz, M., de Oliveira Silva, L. G., dos Santos, C. F. S. M., Evangelista, K.da C., Santos Calmon, M., Matheus, S. L., & Fabrício, F.de M. (2023). Immunotherapy in glioblastoma treatment: Current state and future prospects. *World Journal of Clinical Oncology, 14*(4), 138–159. https://doi.org/10.5306/wjco.v14.i4.138

Schafflick, D., Xu, C. A., Hartlehnert, M., Cole, M., Schulte-Mecklenbeck, A., Lautwein, T., Wolbert, J., Heming, M., Meuth, S. G., Kuhlmann, T., Gross, C. C., Wiendl, H., Yosef, N., & Meyer zu Horste, G. (2020). Integrated single cell analysis of blood and cerebrospinal fluid leukocytes in multiple sclerosis. *Nature Communications, 11*(1). https://doi.org/10.1038/s41467-019-14118-w. Nature Research, Germany.

Schetters, S. T. T., Gomez-Nicola, D., Garcia-Vallejo, J. J., & Van Kooyk, Y. (2018). Neuroinflammation: Microglia and T cells get ready to tango. *Frontiers in Immunology, 8.* https://doi.org/10.3389/fimmu.2017.01905. Frontiers Media S.A., Netherlands.

Shao, F., Wang, X., Wu, H., Wu, Q., & Zhang, J. (2022). Microglia and neuroinflammation: Crucial pathological mechanisms in traumatic brain injury-induced neurodegeneration. *Frontiers in Aging Neuroscience, 14.* https://doi.org/10.3389/fnagi.2022.825086

Shen, J., Bian, N., Lu, Z., & Wei, J. (2024). The role of T-lymphocytes in central nervous system diseases. *Brain Research Bulletin, 209*, Article 110904. https://doi.org/10.1016/j.brainresbull.2024.110904

Silvin, A., Qian, J., & Ginhoux, F. (2023). Brain macrophage development, diversity and dysregulation in health and disease. *Cellular and Molecular Immunology, 20*(11), 1277–1289. https://doi.org/10.1038/s41423-023-01053-6

Simpson, D. S. A., & Oliver, P. L. (2020). Ros generation in microglia: Understanding oxidative stress and inflammation in neurodegenerative disease. *Antioxidants, 9*(8), 1–27. https://doi.org/10.3390/antiox9080743. MDPI, United Kingdom.

Smolders, J., van Luijn, M. M., Hsiao, C. C., & Hamann, J. (2022). T-cell surveillance of the human brain in health and multiple sclerosis. *Seminars in Immunopathology, 44*(6), 855–867. https://doi.org/10.1007/s00281-022-00926-8

Sofroniew, M. V., & Vinters, H. V. (2010). Astrocytes: Biology and pathology. *Acta Neuropathologica, 119*(1), 7–35.

Steinman, R. (1991). The dendritic cell system and its role in immunogenicity. *Annual Review of Immunology, 9* (1), 271–296. https://doi.org/10.1146/annurev.immunol.9.1.271

Stratoulias, V., Luis Venero, J., Ève Tremblay, M.-, & Joseph, B. (2019). Microglial subtypes: Diversity within the microglial community. *The EMBO Journal, 38*(17). https://doi.org/10.15252/embj.2019101997

Streit, W. J., Walter, S. A., & Pennell, N. A. (1999). Reactive microgliosis. *Progress in Neurobiology, 57*(6), 563–581. https://doi.org/10.1016/S0301-0082(98)00069-0

Tansey, M. G., Wallings, R. L., Houser, M. C., Herrick, M. K., Keating, C. E., & Joers, V. (2022). Inflammation and immune dysfunction in parkinson disease. *Nature Reviews Immunology, 22*(11), 657–673. https://doi.org/10.1038/s41577-022-00684-6. Nature Research, United States.

Toader, C., Tataru, C. P., Munteanu, O., Covache-Busuioc, R. A., Serban, M., Ciurea, A. V., & Enyedi, M. (2024). Revolutionizing neuroimmunology: Unraveling immune dynamics and therapeutic innovations in CNS disorders. *International Journal of Molecular Sciences, 25*(24). https://doi.org/10.3390/ijms252413614. Multidisciplinary Digital Publishing Institute (MDPI), Romania.

Utz, S. G., See, P., Mildenberger, W., Thion, M. S., Silvin, A., Lutz, M., Ingelfinger, F., Rayan, N. A., Lelios, I., Buttgereit, A., Asano, K., Prabhakar, S., Garel, S., Becher, B., Ginhoux, F., & Greter, M. (2020). Early fate defines microglia and non-parenchymal brain macrophage development. *Cell, 181*(3), 557. https://doi.org/10.1016/j.cell.2020.03.021. Cell Press, Switzerland.

Venegas, C., & Heneka, M. T. (2017). Danger-associated molecular patterns in Alzheimer's disease. *Journal of Leukocyte Biology, 101*(1), 87–98.

Wang, Y., Li, J., Nakahata, S., & Iha, H. (2024). Complex role of regulatory T cells (tregs) in the tumor microenvironment: Their molecular mechanisms and bidirectional effects on cancer progression. *International Journal of Molecular Sciences, 25*(13), 7346. https://doi.org/10.3390/ijms25137346

Wen, W., Cheng, J., & Tang, Y. (2024). Brain perivascular macrophages: Current understanding and future prospects. *Brain, 147*(1), 39–55. https://doi.org/10.1093/brain/awad304

Wu, Di, Chen, Q., Chen, X., Han, F., Zhong, C., & Wang, Y. (2023). The blood–brain barrier: Structure, regulation and drug delivery. *Signal Transduction and Targeted Therapy, 8*(1). https://doi.org/10.1038/s41392-023-01481-w

Xia, X., Wang, Y., Huang, Y., Zhang, H., Lu, H., & Zheng, J. C. (2019). Exosomal miRNAs in central nervous system diseases: Biomarkers, pathological mediators, protective factors and therapeutic agents. *Progress in Neurobiology, 183*, Article 101694. https://doi.org/10.1016/j.pneurobio.2019.101694

Xu, J., Ma, C., Hua, M., Li, J., Xiang, Z., & Wu, J. (2022). CNS and CNS diseases in relation to their immune system. *Frontiers in Immunology, 13*. https://doi.org/10.3389/fimmu.2022.1063928

Zhan, X., Wang, S., Bèchet, N., Gouras, G., & Wen, G. (2025). Perivascular macrophages in the central nervous system: Insights into their roles in health and disease. *Cell Death and Disease, 16*(1). https://doi.org/10.1038/s41419-025-07592-2. Springer Nature, China.

Zhang, W., Xiao, D., Mao, Q., & Xia, H. (2023). Role of neuroinflammation in neurodegeneration development. *Signal Transduction and Targeted Therapy, 8*(1), 267. https://doi.org/10.1038/s41392-023-01486-5

Zheng, L., Guo, Y., Zhai, X., Zhang, Y., Chen, W., Zhu, Z., Xuan, W., & Li, P. (2022). Perivascular macrophages in the CNS: From health to neurovascular diseases. *CNS Neuroscience and Therapeutics, 28*(12), 1908–1920. https://doi.org/10.1111/cns.13954

Zhu, X., Fang, Y., Chen, Y., Chen, Y., Hong, W., Wei, W., & Tu, J. (2023). Interaction of tumor-associated microglia/macrophages and cancer stem cells in glioma. *Life Sciences, 320*. https://doi.org/10.1016/j.lfs.2023.121558. Elsevier Inc., China.

Zhu, Y., Duan, S., Wang, M., Deng, Z., & Li, J. (2022). Neuroimmune interaction: A widespread mutual regulation and the weapons for barrier organs. *Frontiers in Cell and Developmental Biology, 10*, Article 906755. https://doi.org/10.3389/fcell.2022.906755

CHAPTER

Harnessing antibodies for treating neurological disorders

2

Akshat Sharma

Department of Cancer Genetics and Genomics, Roswell Park Comprehensive Cancer Centre, Buffalo, NY, United States

1. Introduction

Immunology and neuroscience are akin to the Romance Languages. Much like speakers of Italian and Spanish, the immunologist and the neuroscientist can understand each other, but not perfectly. However, as inflammatory mechanisms are increasingly implicated in neurologic diseases, the opportunity to apply immunotherapy—once considered the domain of cancer treatment—also becomes more apparent. Thus, the mutual intelligibility between the two fields must also be refined.

In this chapter, I have focused on monoclonal antibody treatment for four "models" whose sequelae result from strong cooperation between the nervous and immune systems. Migraine, where neuroinflammation results in neuropathic pain. Myasthenia gravis, where innate inflammatory processes at the neuromuscular junctions harm motor functions. Multiple sclerosis, where adaptive or lymphocyte-driven inflammation causes neurodegeneration. Finally, Attention Deficit Hyperactivity Disorder, as an example of a neuropsychiatric condition where pathogenesis is a developing story, but where neuroinflammatory machinations are undeniable.

For three of these four disorders, antibody therapies have come a long way. However, ADHD serves as a model for neuropsychiatric disorders where antibody targets worth pursuit are found in the CNS, and strategies for traversing the blood-brain barrier are discussed.

2. A brief history of antibody treatments for neurological disorders

While predating monoclonal antibody (mAb) therapies by ~30 years, intravenous immunoglobulin (IVIG) transfer have relatively parallel histories in the management of neurological disorders. IVIG is an immunotherapy made up of antibodies pooled from healthy donors and was initially used for the treatment of primary immune deficiencies such as agammaglobulinemia (Bruton, 1952). Its first recorded use for a neurological disorder was in the 1980s to manage autoimmune neuromuscular diseases such as myasthenia gravis (MG). An autoimmune subtype of MG is characterized by pathological autoimmune antibodies against acetylcholine receptors (AChRs) at the neuromuscular junction (NMJ). The NMJ sustains damage by autoantibody-mediated degradation of AChRs and complement activation, whose membrane attack complexes lead to simplified postsynaptic folds in the muscle membrane. Damage to the NMJ results in impaired muscle contraction, which manifests as

Immunotherapies for Neurological Disorders. https://doi.org/10.1016/B978-0-443-44631-3.00010-X

extreme generalized muscle weakness and fatigue, which can prove fatal if muscles that support ventilation are involved (Berrih-Aknin & Le Panse, 2014; Patrick & Lindstrom, 1973; Phillips & Vincent, 2016).

IVIG for MG works by immunomodulating pathogenic autoantibodies by neutralizing the anti-AChR antibodies themselves (Cavill et al., 2003) and blocking B-cell activating factor (BAFF), thus nipping the production of autoantibodies at its very source (Ragheb et al., 2008). Relatedly, the first mAb therapy for MG was the anti-CD20, i.e., B-cell depleting antibody rituximab, which showed great efficacy in a single patient in 1999 (Zaja et al., 2000) and launched clinical trials in 2004 and beyond (Dodd et al., 2023).

Historically, MG, which will be discussed in greater detail later, highlights the importance of considering the immune system in the treatment or management of neurological disorders, many of which may have an autoimmune component or are characterized by inflammatory pathways gone awry.

3. Migraine

3.1 Introduction

Migraine refers to a cluster of chronic symptoms of neurological origin which affects ~15% of people worldwide (Jensen & Stovner, 2008). Migraine manifests as a debilitating headache accompanied by nausea, vomiting, extreme photo- or phonophobia lasting anywhere from 4 to 72 h (Goadsby et al., 2002). Migraine has been classified as the third most disabling disease in the world by the Global Burden of Disease Study, and, in the United States, the total indirect economic burden of migraine is estimated to exceed $19.3 billion. The economic burden is attributable to absenteeism (either due to active migraine or the premonitory phase of migraine) and impaired productivity (Yucel et al., 2020).

Migraine can manifest at any age, though initial attacks are more common in adolescence and decline around age 50 (Jensen & Stovner, 2008). There is also a significant sex difference associated with the disease: women experience migraines 3–4 times more frequently than men, and the duration and severity of these migraines is also significantly greater, likely due to variability in ovarian steroids (estrogen, progesterone) notably known to affect the autonomic and peripheral nervous systems and driving neuroinflammation (Godley et al., 2024; van Oosterhout et al., 2018). Yet, the relationship between sex hormones and migraines is abstruse: oral contraceptives, for example, may increase (Calhoun & Batur, 2017) or decrease (Lyall et al., 2023) the risk and severity of migraines, and the mechanisms behind these phenomena remain understudied.

From a genetic standpoint, migraine is 42%–64% heritable via polygenic inheritance (though rare monogenic variants exist), thereby implicating a cluster of genes whose small additive or synergistic effects give rise to migraine (Bron et al., 2021). GWAS studies have identified several gene candidates involved in migraine pathophysiology, but few have been rigorously tested to highlight their roles (if any) in disease origin or progression (Gormley et al., 2016; Hautakangas et al., 2022). Putative gene candidates largely include genes associated with ion channel functioning, neurotransmission and vascular biology (Bron et al., 2021; Grangeon et al., 2023).

3.2 Pathogenesis

Migraine is a heterogeneous disease and thus one mechanism of disease pathogenesis cannot be singled out as a sole cause. Once thought of as exclusively a vascular disease, it is becoming clear that migraines have strong neurologic and inflammatory underpinnings as well. To be clear, this section is not an exhaustive exegesis on the mechanisms of migraine induction and progression but, rather, focuses more on mAb targets.

Now, the trigeminal nerve is the largest and most complex of the cranial nerves, supplying sensory information to the head and face via three main tributaries (Laine & Smoker, 1998). It stands to reason, then, that the trigeminal nerve and, by extension, the trigeminovascular system (Ashina et al., 2019) be our cynosure in this section.

Investigations in the 1940s showing that mechanical stimulation of trigeminal blood vessels evoked pain was one of the initial "smoking guns" drawing attention to the trigeminal nexus as a source of nociception (Ray & Wolff, 1940). The link between migraine and the trigeminovascular system was solidified with the identification of Calcitonin-related Peptide (CGRP) as a conduit of pain signals and neuroinflammation (Goadsby and Edvinsson, 1994). CGRP is abundantly expressed in trigeminal ganglia, and its release is a consequence of trigeminovascular activation (Eftekhari et al., 2010). Trigeminovascular activation is initiated in nociceptive C-fibers in the trigeminal ganglia as they sense pro-inflammatory cytokines or migraine-triggering stimuli in the meninges, and subsequently promote CGRP release in an antidromic fashion (Edvinsson & Ho, 2010). CGRP drives vasodilation of meningeal vessels and promotes neurogenic inflammation (Edvinsson & Ho, 2010; Wattiez et al., 2020). The orthodromic delivery of CGRP to the trigeminal nucleus caudalis exacerbates pain and promulgates more CGRP release (Edvinsson & Ho, 2010). CGRP further uses two main mechanisms to perpetuate its release: via neuroinflammation and via peripheral and central sensitization where even seemingly innocuous gestures like moving one's head can contribute to CGRP release (Cady et al., 2011; Iyengar et al., 2019).

The role of cation channels of the Transient Receptor Potential (TRP) family, notably TRP Vanilloid 1 (TRPV1) and TRP Ankyrin 1 (TRPA1) must not be discounted in trigeminovascular activation and CGRP modulation. TRPV1 and TRPA1 are located in the nerve terminals of nociceptive neurons and share signaling pathways, thus enabling the potential for cross-regulation. TRPV1 and TRPA1 sense noxious chemical, and mechanical stimuli; their activation also drives CGRP release (Benemei et al., 2013, 2014; Staruschenko et al., 2010).

Other neuropeptides involved in migraine pathogenesis include Pituitary Adenylate Cyclase Activating Polypeptide (PACAP) and Vasoactive Intestinal Peptide (VIP). PACAP, like CGRP is vasodilatory and neuroinflammatory (Amin et al., 2014; Guo et al., 2023), and there is evidence to suggest that, despite occupying different receptors, both neuropeptides activate similar downstream signaling suites (Kuburas & Russo, 2023). Unlike CGRP, PACAP is found in sphenopalatine ganglia (Hensley et al., 2019), and this differential anatomic distribution is seemingly the only major difference between both neuropeptides, given that they also mediate largely the same symptoms in migraine. Vasoactive Intestinal Peptide (VIP) also has overlapping functions with CGRP and PACAP, yet less is known about its mechanism(s) of action in migraine (Goadsby et al., 1990; Hamelink et al., 2002; Pellesi et al., 2020).

Finally, extracellular ATP (eATP) is released from neuronal cells, endothelial cells, astrocytes and immune cells during the course of migraine. Its origin is thought to be cortical spreading depression (Charles & Baca, 2013), a wave of electrical activity altering the physiology of neurons, glia and the vasculature. eATP has direct nociceptive functions by binding to purinergic receptors like P2X3 and P2Y13 on trigeminal neurons (Cieślak et al., 2015; Giniatullin & Nistri, 2023; Zimmermann et al.,

2002). It is also worth noting that CGRP-mediated vasodilation enhances P2X and P2Y receptor levels on the trigeminal nerve (Fabbretti et al., 2006; Zimmermann et al., 2002).

The multifariousness of pro-migraine pathways may prove overwhelming in a didactic sense, but the involvement of so many mediators creates opportunities for more directed therapeutics, as we shall explore below.

3.3 Interventions

From a pharmacological standpoint, migraine is treated with vasoconstrictive agents like triptans—typically the first line of defense against acute migraine attacks (Tepper & Rapoport, 1999). Similar to the triptans, Lasmiditan also targets serotonin receptors like the triptans, but brings pain relief without vasoconstriction via a yet unclear mechanism (Berger et al., 2020). Botulinum toxin (Botox) is also a popular choice given its blockade of pain-inductive neuropeptides and a pleasing esthetic effect as an added bonus (Burstein et al., 2020). Pain management is aided by off-the-shelf non-steroidal anti-inflammatory drugs (NSAIDs) (Pardutz & Schoenen, 2010) as well as simple modulation of one's environment, such as occupying a dark room and using cold compresses to relieve pain (Sprouse-Blum et al., 2013).

The agents highlighted above are largely broad-spectrum players focused on "calming down" the neuroinflammation and pain associated with migraine. They are highly effective for acute migraine attacks but have limited use as preventative drugs. Monoclonal antibody (mAb) infusions are becoming increasingly popular to treat migraineurs, given their highly specific mode of action, such as targeting neuropeptides like CGRP and PACAP, and cation channels like TRPV1 (Fig. 2.1).

Perhaps the most successful of the mAb interventions in migraine involves targeting CGRP. This choice of target makes sense given the prominent role that CGRP plays in orchestrating migraine attacks and the ubiquity of CGRP receptors in the trigeminovascular system. Before mAb therapy, however, small-molecule CGRP receptor antagonists known as the gepants were developed. Gepants proved effective in treating migraine both prophylactically and acutely for both episodic and chronic migraine cases (Chiang & VanderPluym, 2021; Croop et al., 2021; Lipton et al., 2019). However, gepants' pharmacokinetics show short half-lives (hours to days) (Moreno-Ajona et al., 2022), liver toxicity and suboptimal bioavailability (Argyriou et al., 2022), and potential for medication-overuse headache (MOH)—a common syndrome seen in migraineurs (Vandenbussche et al., 2018).

In a way, gepants proved to be precursors to mAb therapies for migraine, acting as a sort of proof-of-concept showing that targeting CGRP and CGRP receptors is a highly effective strategy in treating migraines. As often happens in science, early discoveries, damned with faint praise at first, become the therapeutics of tomorrow. In that vein, the first documented use of an anti-CGRP mAb was in a 2008 paper where Zeller et al. used the antibody as an experimental tool and not therapeutically (Zeller et al., 2008). With increasing confidence in CGRP as a target in migraine and advances in the mAb development, notably improved humanization (Yamashita et al., 2007) and affinity maturation(Goydel et al., 2020), anti-CGRP ligand and receptor antibodies were developed and went into clinical trials in the early 2010s. Clinical trials of CGRPR-targeting Erenumab (Goadsby et al., 2017; Tepper et al., 2017) and CGRP ligand-targeting Fremanezumab (Silberstein et al., 2017), Galcanezumab (Detke et al., 2018; Stauffer et al., 2018) and Eptinezumab (Ashina et al., 2020; Lipton et al., 2020) were all well-tolerated with low adverse effects (barring minor injection site reactions), reduced monthly

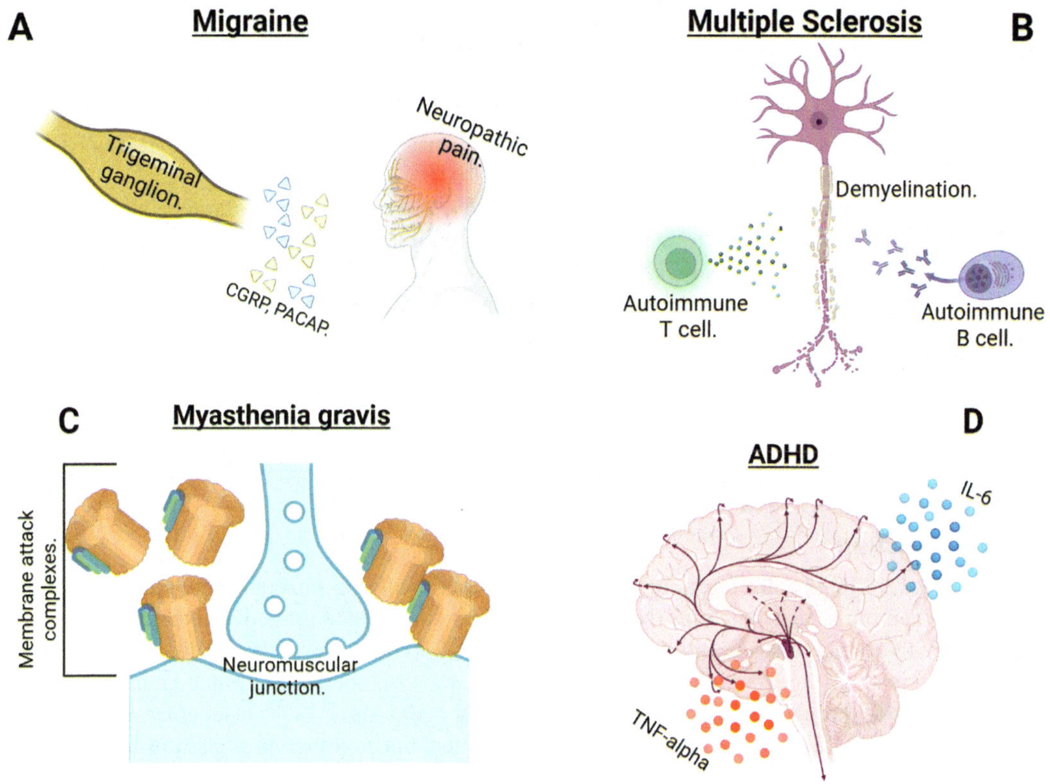

FIGURE 2.1 Mechanisms of neurologic diseases with viable mAb targets highlighted.

In migraine, neuropathic pain results from the binding of pain-associated neuropeptides like CGRP, PACAP and VIP-1 with their receptors (A) Thus antibody blockade of that receptor ligand interaction brings relief and is also preventative. In multiple sclerosis, lymphocyte-driven autoimmunity at the level of T cell and B cell effector functions (B) Presents several avenues of mAb therapy. Antibody-mediated disruption of the innate immune complement system (C) Is one efficacious strategy to treat myasthenia gravis, though autoimmune lymphocytes, like in MS, are also implicated in the disease. Comparatively less is known about ADHD pathogenesis, but observed neuroinflammation (D) makes a case for anti-pro-inflammatory cytokine mAbs for treatment.

migraine days (MMDs) by 43%–59% and were particularly effective in treating drug-resistant migraine.

The success of anti-CGRP(R) mAbs has prompted the development of mAbs focused on other mediators of trigeminovascular activation, though many of these are still in their infancy or haven't lived up to the promise shown by targeting CGRP. PACAP ligand is a tempting mAb target. Raising antibodies against PACAP ligands made the most sense since neutralizing the ligands allows one to bypass their complex receptor occupancy (PAC1, and VPACs 1 and 2). However, a Phase II clinical trial of Lu AG09222 has shown a statistically significant reduction in MMDs, yet Phase III data will serve to solidify whether antibody-mediated capture of PACAP is a reliable strategy in migraine management (Ashina et al., 2024). AM301, a mAb raised against the high-affinity PACAP receptor PAC1, did not demonstrate clinical benefit (Ashina et al., 2021). It is likely that inhibiting PAC1 alone has limited efficacy since PACAP can also functionally engage VPACs 1 and 2 (Waschek et al., 2018). Relatedly, there are no mAb treatments developed against VIP yet, though VIP infusions show intriguing, if inconclusive results (Pellesi et al., 2020, 2021).

Apart from neuropeptides, moieties like TRP-V1 and A1 are viable mAb targets. However, anti-TRP antibodies have challenges to overcome, i.e., inaccessible epitopes given the small TRP extracellular domains and the ubiquity of TRPs in human tissue, which creates the risk of off-target effects. Yet, preclinical work exploring the TRPs as mAb targets is ongoing (Koivisto et al., 2024).

Finally, while not a standard treatment for migraine, neutralizing pro-inflammatory cytokines like IL-6 (Jiao & Guo, 2022) and TNFα (Sudershan et al., 2024) could also help manage migraine, perhaps adjunctively, by rendering key players in neuroinflammation out of commission.

4. Myasthenia gravis (MG)

4.1 Introduction

As noted above, MG is a disease of numerically and functionally diminished acetylcholine receptors (AChRs) at neuromuscular junctions (NMJ) and is emblematic of autoantibody-mediated pathologies. MG is a relatively rare disease with a prevalence of 150–200 cases per million (Phillips, 2003). MG onset can occur at any age, but it is commonly seen in women in their 20–30s and men in their 70–80s (Carr et al., 2010), though late-onset MG (at ~50 years of age) (Aarli, 1997) is an emerging variant of the disease as well. MG can and does affect all ethnicities, but is over-represented in individuals of African descent (Oh et al., 2009). Some of the first signs of MG include drooping eyelids or double vision (Wong, 2022). Other symptoms include chronic muscular fatigue (Torpy et al., 2005), bulbar muscle dysregulation impacting speech and mastication, facial weakness (Basiri et al., 2015) and, at its very worst, myasthenic crises, which are the result of the wasting away of breathing apparatus, i.e., the diaphragm and the intercostal muscles leading to respiratory failure (Stetefeld & Schroeter, 2019).

Autoimmune MG (as opposed to congenital MGs) is not inherited, though, intriguingly, ~5% of MG sufferers show a familial history of autoimmunity (Renton et al., 2015). The etiologic mechanisms of MG remain shrouded in the same mists of esoteric gene-environment interactions that obscure why self-reactive T cells demyelinate axons in multiple sclerosis (discussed later) or what triggers anti-nucleic acid antibodies in lupus. Indeed, why the immune system attacks AChRs in MG is unknown, but certain genes are suspected. As is often the case in autoimmunity, specific Human Leukocyte Antigen (HLA) alleles, critical for antigen presentation and the immune system's acuity vis-à-vis distinguishing self from non-self, are strongly associated with MG. These include both Class I and Class II HLAs, and some notable alleles implicated in MG susceptibility include HLA-DRB1*03, HLA-DRB1*07 and HLA-DQB1*02 in Europeans (Creary et al., 2021) and HLA-DRB1*08, HLA-DQB1*06 and HLA-DQB1*13 in people of African descent (Badi et al., 2013). Otherwise, fairly comprehensive lists of other MG-associated HLA haplotypes are documented in several superlative reviews (Alahgholi-Hajibehzad et al., 2013; Kurian & Khera, 2024; Muñiz-Castrillo et al., 2020; Xie et al., 2011). Non-HLA genetic risk factors include genetic variants of *PTPN22* gene which encodes lymphoid-specific phosphatase (LYP)—a negative regulator of T cell receptor (TCR) signaling—which are major risk factors for not only MG, but also lupus, type 1 diabetes, rheumatoid arthritis and vitiligo (Armitage et al., 2021; Tizaoui et al., 2021; Xiong et al., 2015). Relatedly, variants of the *CTLA4* gene, which encodes another negative regulator of T-cell function (Chikuma, 2017), are also associated with MG development (Li et al., 2018; Renton et al., 2015; Sun et al., 2014). Taken together, variants of genes with such critical roles in initiating and leading immune responses point to breakdown in immune tolerance, which is in line with the autoimmune nature of MG.

To be sure, the multifactorial nature of MG also includes underlying infections (Gilhus et al., 2018), certain medications (Sheikh et al., 2021), stress (Bogdan et al., 2020), and environmental factors like seasonal changes (Falso et al., 2025). Moreover, lifestyle factors like smoking (Petersson et al., 2025) or obesity (Chang et al., 2021) may trigger or exacerbate symptoms.

4.2 Pathogenesis

MG pathogenesis involves autoantibody-mediated attacks on primarily nicotinic AChRs speckled on NMJs (Lindstrom, 2000). An explanation of healthy neuromuscular transmission is likely useful to fully contextualize the pathogenesis of MG. In brief, the arrival of an action potential at an axon terminus triggers Ca^{2+} influx. This initiates a series of events mediated by multiple proteins (especially the SNARE system) which shepherd the fusion of acetylcholine-containing vesicles to the presynaptic membrane of the motor neuron in question and, ultimately, the release of acetylcholine into the synaptic cleft (Giraudo et al., 2006; Ramakrishnan et al., 2012). ACh binding to nicotinic AChRs initiates a depolarization of the muscle fiber membrane, or an endplate potential (EPP). If the EPP so generated achieves a level of depolarization enough to initiate an action potential, muscular contraction occurs (Gollapudi et al., 2014). In MG, autoimmune destruction of AChRs means that EPPs are diminished and, thus, action potentials are diminished, leading to the severe muscular weakness seen in the disease (Phillips & Vincent, 2016).

Anti-AChR autoantibodies are typically of the IgG1 and IgG3 isotypes (Tzartos et al., 1998). Mechanistically, these function by binding to AChRs and recruiting proteins of the complement system and initiating the classic complement pathway, which culminates in membrane attack complex (MAC) formation. MACs bore pores into cell membranes and cause large-scale damage to the postsynaptic membrane as a whole (Behan & Behan, 1979; Michailidou et al., 2025; Sahashi et al., 1980). Loss of voltage-gated ion channels is also collateral damage caused by MACs (Ruff & Lennon, 2008). Apart from MAC formation, anti-AChR IgG may also cross-link AChRs and enhance the rate of internalization (Loutrari et al., 1992). Taken together, these mechanisms greatly reduce EPP amplitude.

Apart from AChR, autoantibodies to Muscle Specific Kinase (MuSK) are the source of MG in some patients (Oh, 2009). Anti-MuSK antibodies are typically IgG4 (Koneczny et al., 2017)—this is important because IgG4, unlike IgG1, can only poorly fix complement (Schumaker et al., 1976), which suggests that MuSK dysfunction-driven MG is not purely an immunopathology. At a healthy NMJ, the proteoglycan, agrin, involved in the development and maintenance of NMJs, binds low-density lipoprotein receptor 4 (LRP4). The agrin-LRP4 complex dimerizes and activates MuSK. Active MuSK phosphorylates downstream proteins like Dok7 while also recruiting scaffold proteins like rapsyn, ultimately leading to the anchoring of AChRs and successful neuromuscular transmission (Barik et al., 2014; Burden et al., 2013; DeChiara et al., 1996; Xie et al., 2023). Anti-MuSK antibodies, therefore, interfere with the MuSK pathway and prevent the successful arrangement of postsynaptic AChR clusters. Consequently, impaired EPPs do not rise to the threshold of initiating action potentials in muscle. Of course, the MuSK "flavor" of MG doesn't always mean that autoantibodies are specifically anti-MuSK. Anti-agrin and LRP4 antibodies have also been observed in a proportion of patients (Yan et al., 2018).

It is notable that in AChR-mediated MG, there is a compensatory increase in AChR turnover or increase in ACh-containing vesicles. Such compensatory mechanisms do not seem to exist for MuSK-related MG. This difference may explain why cachexia in the latter form of MG appears more severe (Vincent, 2002).

4.3 Interventions

The first hints that inhibition of ACh degradation relieves MG symptoms were observed in the 1930s when physostigmine—an antidote to the poison curare, a competitive inhibitor of ACh—was used to treat MG (McCarter et al., 2019). Mechanistically, physostigmine functions as an acetyl cholinesterase (AChE) inhibitor by reversibly introducing a carbamyl group to the enzyme's active site (Arens & Kearney, 2019). Since AChE's function is to break down ACh, its inhibition results in higher concentrations of ACh in the synapse for a longer duration. ACh molecules can then bind the AChRs currently unaffected by the pathologic antibodies, and thus provide relief from MG symptoms. Physostigmine, however, is a short-acting agent (Hartvig et al., 1986); thus, its longer-acting structural analogs—pyridostigmine and neostigmine—are the preferred options for MG treatments (Alhaidar et al., 2022).

The agents above are certainly useful for tackling the AChR-MG, they are not likely to be salubrious (and perhaps deleterious) in addressing the agonies of MuSK-MG (Ricciardi et al., 2024). So far, steroidal immunosuppressants like prednisone and non-steroidal options like azathioprine, tacrolimus, cyclosporine, methotrexate and mycophenolate mofetil are commonly relied upon to relieve the symptoms of MuSK-MG, but patient responses to these vary, and steroids do not engender long-term remission (Bae et al., 2006; Tan et al., 2022).

Advanced immunotherapies for MuSK-MG and generalized MG (gMG), particularly antibody-based therapies, have shown great promise. IVIG, mentioned above, certainly provides relief from MG symptoms. However, strategies using precise mAbs targeting different autoimmune effectors in MG have either shown great potential or are currently in clinical trials. Rituximab, an anti-CD20, i.e., B-cell depleting mAb, has shown more utility in treating MuSK-MG specifically compared to gMG (Chayanopparat et al., 2025; Vesperinas-Castro & Cortés-Vicente, 2023). Meanwhile, inebilizumab, whose specificity is CD19 and thus vacates pro-B cells, plasmablasts and plasma cells, has been useful in treating both gMG and MuSK-MG (Chen et al., 2016). Some notable features that distinguish it from rituximab include its comparatively selective and longer-lasting depletion of B cells and not complement proteins (Gallagher et al., 2016). More indirect ways of targeting B cells include belimumab, which neutralizes the B-cell survival factor BlyS (B lymphocyte Stimulator) and curtails the survival of B-cells, including the autoreactive ones. However, its efficacy in MG is still unclear (Hewett et al., 2018). Iscalimab targets, not B cells, but CD40L/CD154 on T cells. The CD40:CD40L axis is critical to B cell: T cell congress which results in antibody production. To interfere in this process is a clever idea, but results for MG have been modest (GomezMancilla et al., 2024).

The complement system in MG is also targeted by a host of mAbs (Fig. 2.1). In 2017, the first complement inhibitor, eculizumab, was approved by the FDA for MG treatment (Howard et al., 2017), and 2018 saw the approval of ravulizumab (Vu et al., 2022). Both of these mAbs are inhibitors of the complement protein C5, but ravulizumab has a longer half-life, thus maintenance dosing only needs to performed every 8 weeks compared to eculizumab's fortnightly infusions (Lee et al., 2019). As noted, the classical pathway of complement activation is active in AChR-MG, and the cleavage of C5 into C5a and C5b is a critical step for MAC formation; thus, inhibition of C5 (and subsequently its cleavage) has been an important and efficacious strategy to treat MG. Polezimab also targets C5, but by blocking the enzyme that cleaves C5, i.e., C5 convertase. Polezimab, when used in conjunction with the siRNA cemdisiran, has a two-pronged effect of inhibiting C5 convertase but also mitigating C5 synthesis in the liver (Kelly et al., 2023).

The neonatal Fc receptor (FcRn) or, eponymously, the Brambell receptor binds the CH2 and CH3 domains of IgG. It is critical for the transport of maternal antibodies to the fetus and its retrieval of IgG from endosomes, ultimately preventing IgG degradation in lysosomal compartments, significantly increases the half-life of circulating IgG (which is typically 21 days) (Zhu et al., 2023). Antagonism of FcRn by rozanolixizumab has been shown to significantly improve MG symptoms by reducing the half-life of pathogenic IgGs seen in MG (Bril et al., 2021; Hoy, 2023).

5. Multiple sclerosis (MS)

5.1 Introduction

MS has been known since antiquity: St. Lidwina of Schiedam's account of what we now know as MS dates back to the 14th century (Murray, 2009) while Sir Augustus d'Este's diaries from the 1700–1800s describe a quarter century's worth of visual impairment and progressively worsening motor issues that led to his demise in the 1840s (Landtblom et al., 2010). It was in 1868 when Jean-Martin Charcot gave us the term "sclerose en plaques" and defined the disease as falling within the ambit of three early clinical signs: involuntary eye movements, tremors while performing motor tasks and irregularities in speech (Poser & Brinar, 2001). Late symptoms of MS include muscular spasms, incontinence, gait instability, cognitive deterioration and worsening ocular disturbances (Ghasemi et al., 2017).

Today, MS affects nearly 2.8 million people worldwide (Walton et al., 2020), of which about 1 million cases are seen in the USA (Nelson et al., 2019). MS affects women more than men, with the current sex ratio being 3:1 (Coyle, 2021), and while it is often a young or new adult disease (Romero-Pinel et al., 2022), it has also been seen in pediatric patients (Gadoth, 2003). Interestingly (but tragically), the incidence of MS appears to be increasing worldwide. The extent of the increase (nearly double) is greater in women compared to men. The causes behind the increase remain unknown, and while increased awareness, superior diagnostic tools certainly contribute (Koch-Henriksen & Magyari, 2021), environmental/epigenetic (Olsson et al., 2017) and genetic factors (Hafler et al., 2007), as well as certain viral infections (Bjornevik et al., 2023) also play a significant role (Tarlinton et al., 2020).

MS is another example of a debilitating neurological autoimmune disease, and thus it is unsurprising that allelic variations in HLA genes are implicated in the development of the disease (Bertrams et al., 1972). Of these, *HLA-DRB1*15:10* is a common allele which spells high risk of developing MS (Alcina et al., 2012). MS inheritance is non-Mendelian (Patsopoulos, 2018), and it does, like the disorders covered here, subscribe to a polygenic model of risk (Khan et al., 2025). Some of the other implicated genes include cytokine receptors like *IL2Rα* (Maier et al., 2009) and *IL7Rα* (Gregory et al., 2007; Hafler et al., 2007). It is estimated, however, that genetic factors account for about 30% of MS risk (Barrie et al., 2024). Thus, the contribution of environmental and lifestyle factors cannot be ignored. Epstein–Barr Virus (EBV) infections are an emerging risk factor for MS (Bjornevik et al., 2023; Tarlinton et al., 2020): this is also true of obesity (Wu et al., 2025), smoking (Nishanth et al., 2020), and diet, or more, specifically diet-induced changes in the gut microbiome (Chen et al., 2016; Wang & Kasper, 2014) which are known to affect tolerance mechanisms in mucosal T cells (Hebbandi Nanjundappa et al., 2022; Kim, 2022).

5.2 Pathogenesis

An exhaustive account of all known cellular mechanisms resulting in the sequelae of MS goes beyond the scope of this chapter, given its focus on antibody therapies. However there are several excellent, compendious reviews on detailed molecular mechanisms of MS (Filippi et al., 2018; Gupta et al., 2025; Lyu et al., 2025; Woo et al., 2024). This chapter provides a precise context to understand and underscore the impact of the therapies used to manage it. There are four major subtypes of MS: Clinically Isolated Syndrome (CIS) (Makhani & Tremlett, 2021), relapsing-remitting (RRMS), primary progressive (PPMS), and active or non-active secondary progressive MS (SPMS) (Klineova & Lublin, 2018). All four subtypes involve autoimmune attack, which results in neurological sequelae (Weiner, 2008).

CIS is driven by autoimmune $CD4^+$ and $CD8^+$ T cells with specificity for myelin antigens like myelin basic protein (MBP) and myelin oligodendrocyte glycoprotein (MOG) (Kerlero de Rosbo et al., 1993). Inflammation is initiated when autoimmune T cells cross the blood-brain barrier (BBB) (Alvarez et al., 2011; Poser, 1986). CIS is an early event in MS, resulting in acute and often reversible symptoms like ocular neuritis.

CIS may transition to RRMS. The pathogenesis of RRMS is predominated by Th1 (Voskuhl et al., 1993) and Th17 (Volpe et al., 2015). T cells which activates cytotoxic cells and unfettered production of pro-inflammatory cytokines (IL-17, IFNγ, GM-CSF) all contribute to cellular damage vis-à-vis demyelination, axonal injury and general and microglia activation (Kunkl et al., 2020). B cells are also important in RRMS: they present myelin-based antigens to T cells, form ectopic lymphoid structures (ELS), often containing germinal-center-like structures where B cells receive T cell help to produce more autoimmune antibodies (Salomonsson et al., 2003; Zhan et al., 2021). All three pathways of the complement system are also major contributors to cellular damage in RRMS (Cao et al., 2025; Hong et al., 2016; Pekna & Pekny, 2021).

Where RRMS is the most inflammatory form of MS, PPMS and SPMS appear to be driven by cytokines associated with chronic inflammatory molecules (IL-6, IL-21, TNFα, TGFβ) (Albelo-Martínez & Rizvi, 2025; Pasquali et al., 2015; Romme Christensen et al., 2013), promoting deleterious architectural changes in the CNS and thus exacerbating disease. Unlike RRMS, T cell activation appears to occur to a lower degree (Nielsen et al., 2017; Pender et al., 2014; Zastepa et al., 2014): there are fewer brain lesions in SPMS and PPMS compared to RRMS, but these lesions are "smoldering" i.e., bearing the signs of chronic inflammation (Oladosu et al., 2022; Siger, 2022). PPMS and SPMS are more concentrated in the spinal cord (Siger, 2022).

Meningeal ELS are more common in PPMS and SPMS (compared to CIS or RRMS) (Magliozzi et al., 2007) and their maintenance is under the purview of IL-21—a cytokine increased in PP- and SPMS (Gharibi et al., 2019)—and likely contributing to isotype switching by autoimmune pathogenic B cells (Negron et al., 2020; Tangye & Ma, 2020). Axonal loss (Tallantyre et al., 2009) and demyelination (Bramow et al., 2010) are chronic, progressive features in PPMS and SPMS. Atrophy of white and gray matter (Ladopoulos et al., 2025; Sepulcre et al., 2009) has also been observed and is associated with exacerbated disabling symptoms. Coeval neurological damage is caused by metabolic changes like mitochondrial dysfunction (Atkinson et al., 2025), increased production of reactive oxygen species (ROS) (Gray et al., 2008) and glutamate excitotoxicity (Matute et al., 2007).

5.3 Interventions

DMTs or Disease-Modifying Therapies are a common recourse for MS. Orally administered DMTs are typically small molecules that exert immunomodulatory effects. Fingolimod, for example, binds with sphingosine-1-phosphate receptors (S1PRs) found on the lymphocyte cell surface. S1P–S1PR signaling is critical for lymphocyte trafficking (Graeler & Goetzl, 2002), and fingolimod essentially sequesters autoimmune T cells in lymph nodes, limiting immune attack in MS (Chun & Hartung, 2010). Other S1P modulators include Siponimod, Ozanimod and Ponesimod (Coyle et al., 2024). Oral DMTs are not limited to presiding over T cell trafficking: teriflunomide inhibits dihydroorotate dehydrogenase (DHOD), an enzyme required for pyrimidine synthesis, and ultimately the nucleic acid metabolism. Given how pivotal DHOD is for T cell proliferation and effector functions, its inhibition is an effective treatment for MS (Bar-Or et al., 2014) and other autoimmune inflammatory diseases (Zewail et al., 2022). Teriflunomide also reduces absolute B cell counts (Gandoglia et al., 2017), and a notable lesson from graft-versus-host disease (GVHD) models shows that the selective inhibition of T cells by DHOD inhibitors reduces GVHD while preserving the Graft-vs-leukemia (GVL) effect (Kumar et al., 2025).

Additionally, there is a classical MS therapy which entails infusions of interferon-beta (IFNβ) 1a and 1b. IFNβ works at the crossroads of neurological and immunological features of MS. While it downregulates anti-inflammatory cytokine production (Šega et al., 2004), modifies T cell trafficking by downregulating adhesion molecules like Very Late Antigen-4 (VLA-4) thus preventing BBB breach (Calabresi et al., 1997) and concurrently upregulating CXCR3, ICAM-1 and CXCL10 in the spleen thereby sequestering pathogenic T cells there (Wang et al., 2019), it also stabilizes the BBB (Kraus & Oschmann, 2006) and promotes Nerve Growth Factor (NGF) production by astrocytes (Boutros et al., 1997). Finally, IFNβ has a complex relationship with remyelination: the evidence so far suggests that acute treatment with IFNβ can promote remyelination (at least in murine models) while long-term treatment aggravates demyelination (Njenga et al., 2000). Relatedly, IFNβ-deficient mice showed increased recruitment of oligodendrocytes and remyelination (Trebst et al., 2007).

Of treatments harnessing antibodies, IVIG has been shown to provide relief to RRMS patients but has limited utility for PP- and SSMS (Sorensen, 2003). In terms of mAb therapy, rituximab is used off-label in RRMS patients. Given rituximab's target antigen of CD20, the mAb depletes pathogenic B cells (Cross et al., 2006) as well as a pro-inflammatory subset of $CD20^{+}$ T cells (Wilk et al., 2009), which accumulate in the CNS of MS patients and their CNS frequency correlates with disease severity (von Essen et al., 2019). Other anti-CD20 mAbs used include ofatumumab (Awada et al., 2024) and ublitixumab (Martin et al., 2024). Ocrelizumab (Montalban et al., 2017) also targets CD20, but the phosphorylated form is often seen on highly activated B and T cells (Valentine et al., 1987).

Why do we have so many CD20 abs at all? For one, each anti-CD20 mAb binds a different epitope (Binder et al., 2006; Le Garff-Tavernier et al., 2014; Pawluczkowycz et al., 2009; Sorensen & Blinkenberg, 2016) or region of CD20, thus creating options for patients who grow refractory to rituximab treatment (Czuczman et al., 2008; Popa et al., 2024). Each generation of anti-CD20 mAb comes with improved pharmacokinetics, immunogenicity and enhancements inducing complement-dependent or antibody-dependent cellular cytotoxicity (CDC or ADCC) (Cree, 2022; Dabkowska et al., 2024; Delgado et al., 2024). They also differ in their mechanism of recruiting CD20, with some translocating the molecule via lipid raft (Cragg et al., 2003; Mariam et al., 2012). Finally, anti-CD20 mAbs do not deplete as wide a portfolio of B cell subsets as anti-CD19 mAbs. Therefore, humoral immunity is spared: there are minimal perturbations in serum immunoglobulin levels, and vaccine-induced memory also remains upon anti-CD20 treatment, though new immune responses are transiently impaired (Vijenthira et al., 2021) (Fig. 2.2).

Alemtuzumab is another typically anti-tumor mAb repurposed for neuroimmune therapy (Li et al., 2018): CD52 is a glycoprotein found on activated B cells, T cells and NK cells (Hu et al., 2009). By targeting CD52, alemtuzumab depletes autoimmune lymphocytes while also breaking up lymphocyte aggregates in the CNS (Simon et al., 2018). Natalizumab's target is the α4 integrin (O'Leary et al., 2023), which can heterodimerize with CD29 to form VLA-4 or with integrin β7to form lymphocyte Peyer's patch Adhesion Molecule-1 (LPAM-1) (DeNucci et al., 2010). VLA-4 binding to the adhesion ligand Vascular Cell Adhesion Molecule-1 (VCAM-1) is a common mechanism by which lymphocytes traverse the BBB, especially given inflammation-driven elevation in VCAM-1 levels in the CNS. Given that the α4 integrin is required for LPAM-1 formation, natalizumab also prevents lymphocytic influx into the CNS by blocking this port of entry as well (Yu et al., 2013) (Fig. 2.2).

mAbs against more MS-specific targets are also under investigation. Repulsive Guidance Molecule-a (RGMa) provides axonal guidance (Hata et al., 2006) in the developing visual system (Monnier et al., 2002). Its ligand, neogenin, is expressed on $CD4^+$ T cells and DCs in MS patients (Muramatsu et al., 2011). Neogenin-RGMa binding increases $CD4^+$ adhesion to CNS Intercellular Cell Adhesion Molecule-1 (ICAM-1) likely by "opening" signals given to dormant Leukocyte Function-associated Antigen-1 molecules on the T cell surface (Sharma et al., 2018). Neogenin-RGMa binding in DCs acts as a maturation signal by increasing co-stimulatory molecules and pro-inflammatory cytokine production, thus making DCs more efficient and potent in their activation of T cells (Fujita & Yamashita, 2017). Elazanumab is an anti-RGMa mAb which targets two immunological mechanisms by preventing the union of neogenin and RGMa: T cell trafficking and autoimmune antigen presentation (Jacobson et al., 2021), and perhaps even promoting ant-inflammatory immune programs, seeing as RGMa-silenced (Xu, Gao, Shan, et al., 2016) or antibody-blocked DCs show a more tolerogenic phenotype (Xu, Gao, Zhai, et al., 2016) (Fig. 2.2).

Relatedly, GNbAC1 is a mAb that also targets an MS-associated target: the envelope protein of the Human Endogenous Retrovirus (HERV)-W endogenous to the human genome (Blond et al., 1999; Diebold & Derfuss, 2019). The HERV hypothesis of MS is controversial, but remains an intriguing and active area of investigation (Censi et al., 2024). GNbAC1 is currently under investigation for remyelinating activity since no immunomodulatory activity was detected (Hartung et al., 2022).

A concise summary of FDA-approved mAbs for the treatment of these neurological disorders has been provided at Table 2.1.

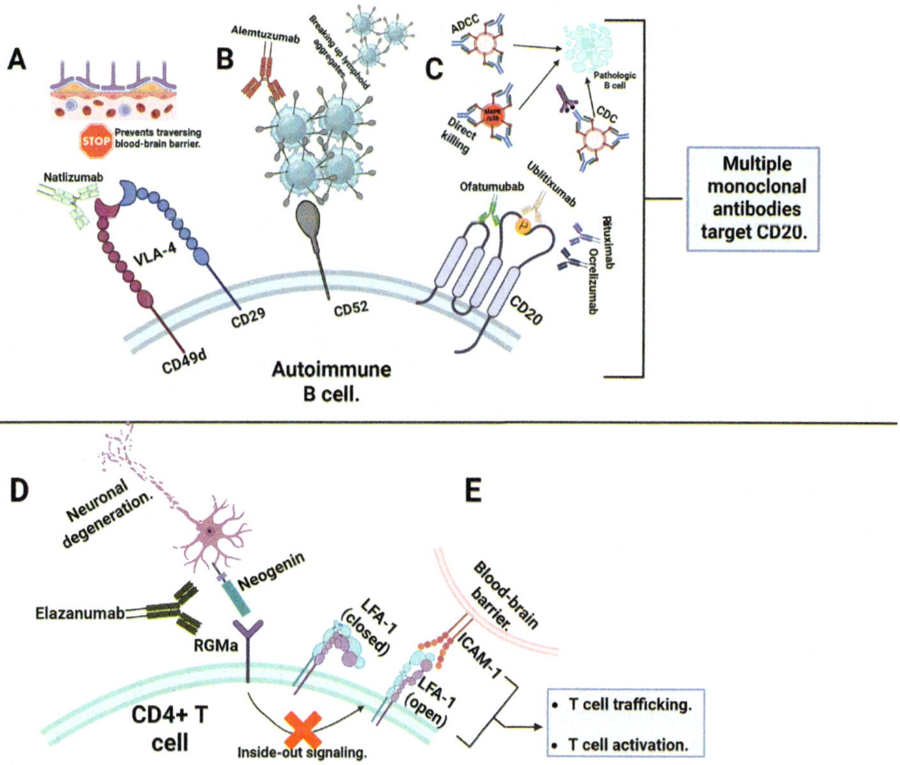

FIGURE 2.2 mAb-directed immunomodulation in multiple sclerosis.

MS is an autoimmune neurodegenerative disease and mAb therapies, understandably, are deployed against targets on pathogenic immune cells and their effector functions. Natalizumab (A) Binds the CD49d/α4 subunit of the integrin VLA-4. The blood-brain barrier is enriched in VLA-4's cognate ligand, vascular cell adhesion Molecule-1 (VCAM-1). By preventing VLA-4:VCAM-1 binding, natalizumab prevents autoimmune B and T cells from traversing the blood-brain barrier (A). Alemtuzumab CD52, which is highly elevated on pathogenic B and T cells in MS and thus depletes them. Alemtuzumab also breaks up lymphoid aggregates associated with disease progression and tissue damage (B). B cells may also be depleted by targeting CD20 which is expressed on activated B cells. The range of anti-CD20 mAbs all promote similar mechanisms of cell death, but target different epitopes (C). Elazanumab targets a more CNS-specific target, neogenin. Neogenin engagement with its receptor RGMa (expressed on pathogenic $CD4^+$ T cells) activates pathways culminating in neuronal degeneration (D). RGMa also activates inside-out signaling leading to the unfolding of the integrin and costimulatory molecule Leukocyte function-associated Antigen-1 (LFA-1). LFA-1 facilitates blood-brain barrier breach while also supporting Th1 polarization of T cells (E). Neogenin blockade, thus, has multifaceted protective effects at the level of neuron protection and abrogation of T cell trafficking and activation.

Table 2.1 A summary of FDA-approved mAbs showing efficacy in the treatment of the cited neurological disorders.

Therapeutic area	Name (brand)	FDA approval date	Target antigen	Brief mechanism of action
Migraine	Erenumab (Aimovig)	May 17, 2018	CGRP receptor	Blockade of CGRP-R to prevent CGRP-driven vasodilation and neuropathic pain.
	Fremanezumab (Ajovy)	September 14, 2018	CGRP ligand (α and β)	Blockade CGRP ligand: CGRP-R binding, and subsequent receptor activation.
	Galcanezumab (Emgality)	September 27, 2018	CGRP ligand	
	Eptinezumab (Vyepti)	February 2020	CGRP ligand (α and β)	
Myasthenia gravis	Efgartigimod (VYVGART)		Neonatal FcRn	FcRn blockade and subsequent reduction of autoimmune pathogenic IgG.
	Nipocalimab (IMAAVY)	April 30, 2025	Neonatal FcRn	
	Eculizumab (Soliris)	2018	Complement C5	Prevention of complement-mediated damage to neuromuscular junctions.
	Ravulizumab (Ultomiris)	April 2022	Complement C5	
	Zilucoplan (ZILBRYSQ)	17-Oct-23	Complement C5 (macrocyclic)	
Multiple sclerosis	Natalizumab (Tysabri)	June 2004, (re-;approved 2006)	α4-integrin	Prevention of lymphocyte trafficking to CNS via VLA-4 blockade.
	Alemtuzumab	November 2014	CD52	Depletion of activated lymphocytes and disruption of lymphoid aggregates.
	Ocrelizumab (Ocrevus)	28-Mar-17	CD20	B Cell depletion in RR and PPMS.
	Ofatumumab (Kesimpta)	Late 2019	CD20	B Cell depletion in RRMS.
	Ublituximab (Briumvi)	Late 2022	CD20	B Cell cytolysis in RRMS.

Table 2.1 A summary of FDA-approved mAbs showing efficacy in the treatment of the cited neurological disorders.—cont'd

Therapeutic area	Name (brand)	FDA approval date	Target antigen	Brief mechanism of action
Attention deficit hyperactivity disorder	None approved to date.			Promising CNS like DAT, NET and NDMA receptors have been identified but are hindered by poor BBB penetration by antibodies. Anti-inflammatory cytokine antibodies may be useful given the neuroinflammatory component of ADHD.

6. Attention-deficit/hyperactivity disorder (ADHD)

6.1 Introduction

ADHD is characterized by inattention, difficulty focusing on tasks, forgetfulness, and hyperactivity, such as excessive physical activity or general restlessness. ADHD is a cluster of disorders and presents differently in individual patients (Administration, 2016). ADHD prevalence is high and increasing: approximately 7 million children in the US have received ADHD diagnoses (Danielson et al., 2024). However, what was once called "a defect of moral control" (Lange et al., 2010) is now treated more compassionately. The recent increase in ADHD diagnoses (Xu et al., 2018) is a result of more accurate diagnostic criteria (Posner et al., 2020), increased access to care (Kataoka, 2016) and social media presence (Karasavva et al., 2025), though concerns about overdiagnosis have been voiced (Abdelnour et al., 2022).

Individuals with ADHD live with great stigma, given stereotypical views of individuals with ADHD as unreliable, unfocused or untrustworthy (Godfrey et al., 2021; Hosseinnia et al., 2020; Metzger & Hamilton, 2021; Mueller et al., 2012). The emotional stress of the stereotypes, coupled to cognitive impairment, leads to a lower quality of life (Agarwal et al., 2012; Danckaerts et al., 2010) and poor health outcomes for sufferers of ADHD (Jennum et al., 2025; Nigg, 2013; Schoenfelder & Kollins, 2016).

6.2 Pathogenesis

There is a case to be made for ADHD as a neurological disorder. Several genes associated with neurodevelopmental pathways appear to be associated with neurodevelopmental processes and dopamine pathway regulation (Demontis et al., 2019; Faraone et al., 2021; Hess et al., 2021). For example, *FOXP2* (Schreiweis et al., 2014) and *SORCS3* (Breiderhoff et al., 2013) are genetic risk loci that govern neuronal pathways of learning. *DUSP6* regulates dopamine, a pleasure-inducing neurotransmitter involved in reward pathways is also a key gene linked to ADHD susceptibility (Namipashaki et al., 2024). Like other disorders covered here, ADHD also appears to follow a polygenic model of disease. Notably, these ADHD risk loci are also associated with the risk of developing bipolar disorder and schizophrenia (O'Connell et al., 2021).

Morphological and physiological changes observed in the brains of ADHD-afflicted individuals also support a neurological mechanism for ADHD development and progression. These changes include smaller volumes in all four lobes of the brain (Gehricke et al., 2017) and volumetric abnormalities in gray matter and basal ganglia, especially in the right putamen (Max et al., 2002). Admittedly, studies document that brain volumes in ADHD largely normalize in adulthood and are associated with ADHD remission (Hoogman et al., 2017; Onnink et al., 2014; Zhang-James et al., 2021).

Taken together, these pieces of evidence inform the striatal hypothesis of ADHD. The striatum is a triumvirate of three interconnected nuclei—the caudate nucleus, the nucleus accumbens and the putamen. The striatum controls voluntary movement, executive function, reward processing and habit formation/addiction (Báez-Mendoza & Schultz, 2013; Bamford & Bamford, 2019; Yager et al., 2015). The striatum is also innervated by the basal ganglia (Báez-Mendoza & Schultz, 2013) and is enriched for dopamine receptors (Meador-Woodruff et al., 1996). The striatal hypothesis holds that dysfunction in striatal physiology is a cause of ADHD (Oldehinkel et al., 2016; von Rhein et al., 2016). Yet, other hypotheses can co-exist with the striatal: neuroinflammation (Dunn et al., 2019; Vázquez-González et al., 2023) is being increasingly observed in ADHD, as are gut dysbioses (which inform immune tolerance) (Cickovski et al., 2023; Lewis et al., 2025), and so, as our understanding of ADHD improves, we are likely to observe a more multitudinous neuroinflammatory model of the disease emerge.

Again, like other diseases cited here, environmental factors appear important to ADHD pathogenesis as well. Putative environmental exposures for ADHD include prenatal drug or alcohol use, exposure to heavy metals or chemicals and food additives (Froehlich et al., 2011), and video game addiction (Masi et al., 2021).

6.3 Interventions

Currently, the first line of treatment includes methylphenidate-based stimulants like Ritalin or Daytrana, which are administered as a transdermal patch. Methylphenidate stimulants elevate norepinephrine and dopamine levels in the synaptic cleft, thereby promoting increased neurotransmission and improvement in executive function (Stevens et al., 2019). Amphetamine-based stimulants are also a popular choice. These include Adderall or Vyvanse. Amphetamine-based stimulants function at the level of preventing dopamine and norepinephrine reuptake and stimulating the release of both neurotransmitters from synaptic vesicles (Denzer et al., 2019). Stimulant therapy has been successful for 70%–80% who've been prescribed the drugs (Spencer et al., 2005).

Ideally, the paragraph above should be enough for us to close the book on ADHD management, but stimulant therapy, over time, shows diminishing returns. One critical reason is poor adherence to the drug regimen, with the majority of adults and adolescents reporting discontinuation of therapy, citing side effects like personality changes and mood volatility, decreasing quality of life (Advokat & Scheithauer, 2013). Furthermore, a striking result highlighted in a study by Lensing et al. (2013) showed that pharmacotherapy with stimulants was less effective after 2 years of use. At the 4-year time point, self-reported symptoms and impairment were similar between patients still adhering to therapy and those who had stopped. There is much more to be said about stimulant therapy, treating acute symptoms, not necessarily improving cognitive function long-term, as well as the abuse potential of these drugs.

To my knowledge, there are no current mAbs on the market or in human trials for ADHD. Given the neuroinflammatory nature of ADHD, a case for treatment with anti-cytokine mAbs targeting IL-6 or TNFα can be made; however, studies show that not all cases of ADHD consistently show elevated cytokine levels. Therefore, mAbs for more ADHD-specific targets are required (Corominas-Roso et al., 2017).

The dopamine transporter, DAT, presents as a cardinal target not just for ADHD but for other neuropsychiatric diseases like addiction, schizophrenia and bipolar disorder (Yatham et al., 2022; Zhu & Reith, 2008). That is to say, an effective DAT-targeting mAb could help a vast swathe of the population living with often deeply incumbering disorders. Similarly, the norepinephrine transporter, NET (Zhou, 2004), is a viable target worth exploring for mAb therapy. That the selective norepinephrine reuptake inhibitor (SNRI) atomoxetine dramatically attenuates ADHD symptoms in adults and children (Garnock-Jones & Keating, 2009; Rezaei et al., 2016) singles out NET as an intriguing mAb prospect for ADHD, certainly, and other studies also highlight NET dysfunction in depression and post-traumatic stress (Zhang et al., 2024).

7. Current challenges and future prospects

A significant challenge for mAb therapy for CNS-located targets is BBB penetration. BBB architecture, with its tight junctions, efflux transporters and paucity of influx mechanisms like receptor-mediated transcytosis (RMT), makes it hostile to the transport of mAbs, which are relatively large (~150 kDa) hydrophilic molecules. Indeed, an estimated 0.1% of peripherally administered mAbs can make it across the BBB (Bajracharya et al., 2021). In fact, the targets highlighted for ADHD are all expressed on neuronal membranes, so high BBB penetration is a critical requirement for mAbs meant to treat ADHD and other neuropsychiatric disorders, as well as broadening the range of targets for the diseases mentioned herein. However, strategies like RMT (Haqqani et al., 2024) and Brainshuttle (Grimm et al., 2023), osmotic opening (Rapoport, 2000), and the use of camelid (Vandesquille et al., 2017) or selachian (Pornnoppadol et al., 2024) antibodies (Table 2.2) are intriguing and promising avenues to help mAbs and drugs transcytose across the BBB.

Table 2.2 A summary of current and emerging technologies facilitating BBB breach and drug delivery.

Strategy	Mechanism of action in brief
Receptor-mediated transcytosis (RMT)	Bispecific mAb targetting BBB transsporter proteins (e.g., transferrin receptor, insulin receptor) and target (e.g., DAT) can "hitch a ride" with the transport protein to traverse the BBB and reach the target.
Brainshuttle (Roche)	Next-generation RMT using single fragment anti-transferrin receptor antibody to facilitate trancytosis across the BBB for therapeutic mAb delivery.
Osmotic opening	Use of hypertonic solutions to temporarily permeabilize the BBB and create a literal window of opportunity for mAb delivery.
Camelid antibodies	Single domain antibodies smaller than multimeric conventional antibodies engineered for high affinity to target can transcytose across the BBB via RMT.
Selachian antibodies	Shark antibodies, much smaller in size compared to conventional antibodies are made up of heavy chains only and, like camelid antibodies, are small enough to contact hard-to-reach targets in the CNS.

References

Aarli, J. (1997). Late onset myasthenia gravis. *European Journal of Neurology, 4*(3), 203–209.

Abdelnour, E., Jansen, M. O., & Gold, J. A. (2022). ADHD diagnostic trends: Increased recognition or overdiagnosis? *Missouri Medicine, 119*(5), 467–473.

SubstanceAbuse and MentalHealthServices Administration. (2016). *DSM-5 changes: Implications for child serious emotional disturbance*. Rockville (MD).

Advokat, C., & Scheithauer, M. (2013). Attention-deficit hyperactivity disorder (ADHD) stimulant medications as cognitive enhancers. *Frontiers in Neuroscience, 7*, 82. https://doi.org/10.3389/fnins.2013.00082

Agarwal, R., et al. (2012). The quality of life of adults with attention deficit hyperactivity disorder: A systematic review. *Innovations in clinical neuroscience., 9*(5–6), 10–21.

Alahgholi-Hajibehzad, M., et al. (2013). Association of HLA-DRB1*14, -DRB1*16 and -DQB1*05 with MuSK-myasthenia gravis in patients from Turkey. *Human Immunology, 74*(12), 1633–1635. https://doi.org/10.1016/j.humimm.2013.08.271

Albelo-Martínez, M., & Rizvi, S. (2025). Progressive multiple sclerosis: Evaluating current therapies and exploring future treatment strategies. *Neurotherapeutics*, Article e00601. https://doi.org/10.1016/j.neurot.2025.e00601

Alcina, A., et al. (2012). Multiple sclerosis risk variant HLA-DRB1*1501 associates with high expression of DRB1 gene in different human populations. *PLoS One, 7*(1), Article e29819. https://doi.org/10.1371/journal.pone.0029819

Alhaidar, M. K., et al. (2022). Current treatment of myasthenia gravis. *Journal of Clinical Medicine, 11*(6), 1597.

Alvarez, J. I., Cayrol, R., & Prat, A. (2011). Disruption of central nervous system barriers in multiple sclerosis. *Biochimica et Biophysica Acta, 1812*(2), 252–264. https://doi.org/10.1016/j.bbadis.2010.06.017

Amin, F. M., et al. (2014). Investigation of the pathophysiological mechanisms of migraine attacks induced by pituitary adenylate cyclase-activating polypeptide-38. *Brain, 137*(Pt 3), 779–794. https://doi.org/10.1093/brain/awt369

Arens, A. M., & Kearney, T. (2019). Adverse effects of physostigmine. *Journal of Medical Toxicology, 15*(3), 184–191. https://doi.org/10.1007/s13181-019-00697-z

Argyriou, A. A., et al. (2022). A systematic review with expert opinion on the role of gepants for the preventive and abortive treatment of migraine. *Expert Review of Neurotherapeutics, 22*(6), 469–488. https://doi.org/10.1080/14737175.2022.2091435

Armitage, L. H., Wallet, M. A., & Mathews, C. E. (2021). Influence of PTPN22 allotypes on innate and adaptive immune function in health and disease. *Frontiers in Immunology, 12–2021*. https://doi.org/10.3389/fimmu.2021.636618

Ashina, M., et al. (2019). Migraine and the trigeminovascular system—40 years and counting. *The Lancet Neurology, 18*(8), 795–804. https://doi.org/10.1016/S1474-4422(19)30185-1

Ashina, M., et al. (2020). Eptinezumab in episodic migraine: A randomized, double-blind, placebo-controlled study (PROMISE-1). *Cephalalgia, 40*(3), 241–254. https://doi.org/10.1177/0333102420905132

Ashina, M., et al. (2021). A phase 2, randomized, double-blind, placebo-controlled trial of AMG 301, a pituitary adenylate cyclase-activating polypeptide PAC1 receptor monoclonal antibody for migraine prevention. *Cephalalgia, 41*(1), 33–44. https://doi.org/10.1177/0333102420970889

Ashina, M., et al. (2024). A monoclonal antibody to PACAP for migraine prevention. *New England Journal of Medicine, 391*(9), 800–809. https://doi.org/10.1056/NEJMoa2314577

Atkinson, K. C., et al. (2025). Decreased mitochondrial activity in the demyelinating cerebellum of progressive multiple sclerosis and chronic EAE contributes to Purkinje cell loss. *Proceedings of the National Academy of Sciences, 122*(25), Article e2421806122. https://doi.org/10.1073/pnas.2421806122

Awada, Z., Hameed, N., & Harel, A. (2024). Profile of ofatumumab in the treatment of multiple sclerosis: Design, development and place in therapy. *Drug design, development and therapy, 18*, 5985–5996. https://doi.org/10.2147/dddt.S315174

Bae, J. S., Go, S. M., & Kim, B. J. (2006). Clinical predictors of steroid-induced exacerbation in myasthenia gravis. *Journal of Clinical Neuroscience, 13*(10), 1006–1010. https://doi.org/10.1016/j.jocn.2005.12.041

Báez-Mendoza, R., & Schultz, W. (2013). The role of the striatum in social behavior. *Frontiers in Neuroscience, 7*, 233. https://doi.org/10.3389/fnins.2013.00233

Bajracharya, R., et al. (2021). Current and emerging strategies for enhancing antibody delivery to the brain. *Pharmaceutics, 13*(12). https://doi.org/10.3390/pharmaceutics13122014

Bamford, I. J., & Bamford, N. S. (2019). The striatum's role in executing rational and irrational economic behaviors. *The Neuroscientist, 25*(5), 475–490. https://doi.org/10.1177/1073858418824256

Bar-Or, A., et al. (2014). Teriflunomide and its mechanism of action in multiple sclerosis. *Drugs, 74*(6), 659–674. https://doi.org/10.1007/s40265-014-0212-x

Barik, A., et al. (2014). LRP4 is critical for neuromuscular junction maintenance. *Journal of Neuroscience, 34*(42), 13892–13905. https://doi.org/10.1523/jneurosci.1733-14.2014

Barrie, W., et al. (2024). Elevated genetic risk for multiple sclerosis emerged in steppe pastoralist populations. *Nature, 625*(7994), 321–328. https://doi.org/10.1038/s41586-023-06618-z

Basiri, K., Ansari, B., & Okhovat, A. A. (2015). Life-threatening misdiagnosis of bulbar onset myasthenia gravis as a motor neuron disease: How much can one rely on exaggerated deep tendon reflexes. *Advanced Biomedical Research, 4*, 58. https://doi.org/10.4103/2277-9175.151874

Behan, W. M., & Behan, P. O. (1979). Immune complexes in myasthenia gravis. *Journal of Neurology Neurosurgery and Psychiatry, 42*(7), 595–599. https://doi.org/10.1136/jnnp.42.7.595

Benemei, S., et al. (2013). TRPA1 and other TRP channels in migraine. *The Journal of Headache and Pain, 14*(1), 71. https://doi.org/10.1186/1129-2377-14-71

Benemei, S., et al. (2014). The TRPA1 channel in migraine mechanism and treatment. *British Journal of Pharmacology, 171*(10), 2552–2567. https://doi.org/10.1111/bph.12512

Berger, A. A., et al. (2020). Lasmiditan for the treatment of migraines with or without aura in adults. *Psychopharmacology Bulletin, 50*(4 Suppl. 1), 163–188.

Berrih-Aknin, S., & Le Panse, R. (2014). Myasthenia gravis: A comprehensive review of immune dysregulation and etiological mechanisms. *Journal of Autoimmunity, 52*, 90–100. https://doi.org/10.1016/j.jaut.2013.12.011

Bertrams, J., Kuwert, E., & Liedtke, U. (1972). HL-A antigens and multiple sclerosis. *Tissue Antigens, 2*(6), 405–408. https://doi.org/10.1111/j.1399-0039.1972.tb00060.x

Binder, M., et al. (2006). The epitope recognized by rituximab. *Blood, 108*(6), 1975–1978. https://doi.org/10.1182/blood-2006-04-014639

Bjornevik, K., et al. (2023). Epstein–Barr virus as a leading cause of multiple sclerosis: Mechanisms and implications. *Nature Reviews Neurology, 19*(3), 160–171. https://doi.org/10.1038/s41582-023-00775-5

Blond, J. L., et al. (1999). Molecular characterization and placental expression of HERV-W, a new human endogenous retrovirus family. *Journal of Virology, 73*(2), 1175–1185. https://doi.org/10.1128/jvi.73.2.1175-1185.1999

Bogdan, A., et al. (2020). Prospective study of stress, depression and personality in myasthenia gravis relapses. *BMC Neurology, 20*(1), 261. https://doi.org/10.1186/s12883-020-01802-4

Boutros, T., Croze, E., & Yong, V. W. (1997). Interferon-beta is a potent promoter of nerve growth factor production by astrocytes. *Journal of Neurochemistry, 69*(3), 939–946. https://doi.org/10.1046/j.1471-4159.1997.69030939.x

Bramow, S., et al. (2010). Demyelination versus remyelination in progressive multiple sclerosis. *Brain, 133*(10), 2983–2998. https://doi.org/10.1093/brain/awq250

Breiderhoff, T., et al. (2013). Sortilin-related receptor SORCS3 is a postsynaptic modulator of synaptic depression and fear extinction. *PLoS One, 8*(9), Article e75006. https://doi.org/10.1371/journal.pone.0075006

Bril, V., et al. (2021). Efficacy and safety of rozanolixizumab in moderate to severe generalized myasthenia gravis: A phase 2 randomized control trial. *Neurology, 96*(6), e853–e865. https://doi.org/10.1212/wnl.0000000000011108

Bron, C., Sutherland, H. G., & Griffiths, L. R. (2021). Exploring the hereditary nature of migraine. *Neuropsychiatric Disease and Treatment, 17*, 1183–1194. https://doi.org/10.2147/ndt.S282562

Bruton, O. C. (1952). Agammaglobulinemia. *Pediatrics, 9*(6), 722–728. https://doi.org/10.1542/peds.9.6.722

Burden, S. J., Yumoto, N., & Zhang, W. (2013). The role of MuSK in synapse formation and neuromuscular disease. *Cold Spring Harbor Perspectives in Biology, 5*(5), Article a009167. https://doi.org/10.1101/cshperspect.a009167

Burstein, R., et al. (2020). Mechanism of action of onabotulinumtoxinA in chronic migraine: A narrative review. *Headache, 60*(7), 1259–1272. https://doi.org/10.1111/head.13849

Cady, R. J., et al. (2011). Calcitonin gene-related peptide promotes cellular changes in trigeminal neurons and glia implicated in peripheral and central sensitization. *Molecular Pain, 7*, 94. https://doi.org/10.1186/1744-8069-7-94

Calabresi, P. A., et al. (1997). VLA-4 expression on peripheral blood lymphocytes is downregulated after treatment of multiple sclerosis with interferon beta. *Neurology, 49*(4), 1111–1116. https://doi.org/10.1212/wnl.49.4.1111

Calhoun, A. H., & Batur, P. (2017). Combined hormonal contraceptives and migraine: An update on the evidence. *Cleveland Clinic Journal of Medicine, 84*(8), 631–638. https://doi.org/10.3949/ccjm.84a.16033

Cao, R., et al. (2025). The contribution of complement system in multiple sclerosis: Mechanisms and therapeutic potentials. *Immunology, 175*(3), 263–279. https://doi.org/10.1111/imm.13929

Carr, A. S., et al. (2010). A systematic review of population based epidemiological studies in myasthenia gravis. *BMC Neurology, 10*, 46. https://doi.org/10.1186/1471-2377-10-46

Cavill, D., Waterman, S. A., & Gordon, T. P. (2003). Antiidiotypic antibodies neutralize autoantibodies that inhibit cholinergic neurotransmission. *Arthritis & Rheumatism, 48*(12), 3597–3602. https://doi.org/10.1002/art.11343

Censi, S. T., Mariani-Costantini, R., Granzotto, A., Tomassini, V., & Sensi, S. L. (2024). Endogenous retroviruses in multiple sclerosis: A network-based etiopathogenic model. *Ageing Research Reviews, 99*. https://doi.org/10.1016/j.arr.2024.102392

Chang, C. C., et al. (2021). Assessment of sarcopenia and obesity in patients with myasthenia gravis using dual-energy X-ray absorptiometry: A cross-sectional study. *Journal of personalized medicine, 11*(11). https://doi.org/10.3390/jpm11111139

Charles, A. C., & Baca, S. M. (2013). Cortical spreading depression and migraine. *Nature Reviews Neurology, 9* (11), 637–644. https://doi.org/10.1038/nrneurol.2013.192

Chayanopparat, S., et al. (2025). Efficacy and safety of rituximab in anti-MuSK myasthenia gravis: A systematic review and meta-analysis. *Scientific Reports, 15*(1), 7219. https://doi.org/10.1038/s41598-025-90937-w

Chen, D., et al. (2016). Inebilizumab, a B cell-depleting Anti-CD19 antibody for the treatment of autoimmune neurological diseases: Insights from preclinical studies. *Journal of Clinical Medicine, 5*(12). https://doi.org/10.3390/jcm5120107

Chen, J., et al. (2016). Multiple sclerosis patients have a distinct gut microbiota compared to healthy controls. *Scientific Reports, 6*, Article 28484. https://doi.org/10.1038/srep28484

Chiang, C. C., & VanderPluym, J. H. (2021). Ubrogepant in the acute management of migraine: A narrative review. *Journal of Pain Research, 14*, 1185–1192. https://doi.org/10.2147/jpr.S244249

Chikuma, S. (2017). CTLA-4, an essential immune-checkpoint for T-Cell activation. *Current Topics in Microbiology and Immunology, 410*, 99–126. https://doi.org/10.1007/82_2017_61

Chun, J., & Hartung, H. P. (2010). Mechanism of action of oral fingolimod (FTY720) in multiple sclerosis. *Clinical Neuropharmacology, 33*(2), 91–101. https://doi.org/10.1097/WNF.0b013e3181cbf825

Cickovski, T., et al. (2023). Attention deficit hyperactivity disorder (ADHD) and the gut microbiome: An ecological perspective. *PLoS One, 18*(8), e0273890. https://doi.org/10.1371/journal.pone.0273890

Cieślak, M., et al. (2015). The role of purinergic signaling in the etiology of migraine and novel antimigraine treatment. *Purinergic Signalling, 11*(3), 307–316. https://doi.org/10.1007/s11302-015-9453-8

Corominas-Roso, M., et al. (2017). IL-6 and TNF-α in unmedicated adults with ADHD: Relationship to cortisol awakening response. *Psychoneuroendocrinology, 79*, 67–73. https://doi.org/10.1016/j.psyneuen.2017.02.017

Coyle, P. K. (2021). What can we learn from sex differences in MS? *Journal of Personalized Medicine, 11*(10). https://doi.org/10.3390/jpm11101006

Coyle, P. K., et al. (2024). Sphingosine 1-phosphate receptor modulators in multiple sclerosis treatment: A practical review. *Annals of Clinical and Translational Neurology, 11*(4), 842–855. https://doi.org/10.1002/acn3.52017

Cragg, M. S., et al. (2003). Complement-mediated lysis by anti-CD20 mAb correlates with segregation into lipid rafts. *Blood, 101*(3), 1045–1052. https://doi.org/10.1182/blood-2002-06-1761

Creary, L. E., et al. (2021). Next-generation sequencing identifies extended HLA class I and II haplotypes associated with early-onset and late-onset myasthenia gravis in Italian, Norwegian, and Swedish populations. *Frontiers in Immunology, 12–2021*. https://doi.org/10.3389/fimmu.2021.667336

Cree, B. A. (2022). All anti-CD20 monoclonal antibodies have similar efficacy and safety risks: Yes. *Multiple Sclerosis, 28*(12), 1843–1844. https://doi.org/10.1177/13524585221108294

Croop, R., et al. (2021). Oral rimegepant for preventive treatment of migraine: A phase 2/3, randomised, double-blind, placebo-controlled trial. *Lancet, 397*(10268), 51–60. https://doi.org/10.1016/s0140-6736(20)32544-7

Cross, A. H., et al. (2006). Rituximab reduces B cells and T cells in cerebrospinal fluid of multiple sclerosis patients. *Journal of Neuroimmunology, 180*(1), 63–70. https://doi.org/10.1016/j.jneuroim.2006.06.029

Czuczman, M. S., et al. (2008). Acquirement of rituximab resistance in lymphoma cell lines is associated with both global CD20 gene and protein down-regulation regulated at the pretranscriptional and posttranscriptional levels. *Clinical Cancer Research, 14*(5), 1561–1570. https://doi.org/10.1158/1078-0432.Ccr-07-1254

Dabkowska, A., Domka, K., & Firczuk, M. (2024). Advancements in cancer immunotherapies targeting CD20: From pioneering monoclonal antibodies to chimeric antigen receptor-modified T cells. *Frontiers in Immunology, 15–2024*. https://doi.org/10.3389/fimmu.2024.1363102

Danckaerts, M., et al. (2010). The quality of life of children with attention deficit/hyperactivity disorder: A systematic review. *European Child & Adolescent Psychiatry, 19*(2), 83–105. https://doi.org/10.1007/s00787-009-0046-3

Danielson, M. L., et al. (2024). ADHD prevalence among U.S. children and adolescents in 2022: Diagnosis, severity, co-occurring disorders, and treatment. *Journal of Clinical Child and Adolescent Psychology, 53*(3), 343–360. https://doi.org/10.1080/15374416.2024.2335625

DeChiara, T. M., et al. (1996). The receptor tyrosine kinase MuSK is required for neuromuscular junction formation in vivo. *Cell, 85*(4), 501–512. https://doi.org/10.1016/S0092-8674(00)81251-9

Delgado, S. R., et al. (2024). Key characteristics of anti-CD20 monoclonal antibodies and clinical implications for multiple sclerosis treatment. *Journal of Neurology, 271*(4), 1515–1535. https://doi.org/10.1007/s00415-023-12007-3

Demontis, D., et al. (2019). Discovery of the first genome-wide significant risk loci for attention deficit/hyperactivity disorder. *Nature Genetics, 51*(1), 63–75. https://doi.org/10.1038/s41588-018-0269-7

DeNucci, C. C., et al. (2010). Control of α4β7 integrin expression and CD4 T cell homing by the β1 integrin subunit. *The Journal of Immunology, 184*(5), 2458–2467. https://doi.org/10.4049/jimmunol.0902407

Denzer, C., et al. (2019). Treatment of hypothalamic obesity with dextroamphetamine: A case series. *Obesity Facts, 12*(1), 91–102. https://doi.org/10.1159/000495851

Detke, H. C., et al. (2018). Galcanezumab in chronic migraine: The randomized, double-blind, placebo-controlled REGAIN study. *Neurology, 91*(24), e2211–e2221. https://doi.org/10.1212/wnl.0000000000006640

Diebold, M., & Derfuss, T. (2019). The monoclonal antibody GNbAC1: Targeting human endogenous retroviruses in multiple sclerosis. *Therapeutic advances in neurological disorders, 12*, Article 1756286419833574. https://doi.org/10.1177/1756286419833574

Dodd, K. C., et al. (2023). Rituximab for myasthenia gravis. *Cochrane Database of Systematic Reviews*, (4)https://doi.org/10.1002/14651858.CD014574

Dunn, G. A., Nigg, J. T., & Sullivan, E. L. (2019). Neuroinflammation as a risk factor for attention deficit hyperactivity disorder. *Pharmacology, biochemistry, and behavior, 182*, 22–34. https://doi.org/10.1016/j.pbb.2019.05.005

Edvinsson, L., & Ho, T. W. (2010). CGRP receptor antagonism and migraine. *Neurotherapeutics, 7*(2), 164–175. https://doi.org/10.1016/j.nurt.2010.02.004

Eftekhari, S., et al. (2010). Differential distribution of calcitonin gene-related peptide and its receptor components in the human trigeminal ganglion. *Neuroscience, 169*(2), 683–696. https://doi.org/10.1016/j.neuroscience.2010.05.016

Fabbretti, E., et al. (2006). Delayed upregulation of ATP P2X3 receptors of trigeminal sensory neurons by calcitonin gene-related peptide. *Journal of Neuroscience, 26*(23), 6163–6171. https://doi.org/10.1523/jneurosci.0647-06.2006

Falso, S., et al. (2025). Seasonal variation in myasthenia gravis incidence. *Journal of Neuroimmunology, 399*, Article 578524. https://doi.org/10.1016/j.jneuroim.2025.578524

Faraone, S. V., et al. (2021). The World Federation of ADHD International Consensus Statement: 208 evidence-based conclusions about the disorder. *Neuroscience & Biobehavioral Reviews, 128*, 789–818. https://doi.org/10.1016/j.neubiorev.2021.01.022

Filippi, M., et al. (2018). Multiple sclerosis. *Nature Reviews Disease Primers, 4*(1), 43. https://doi.org/10.1038/s41572-018-0041-4

Froehlich, T. E., et al. (2011). Update on environmental risk factors for attention-deficit/hyperactivity disorder. *Current Psychiatry Reports, 13*(5), 333–344. https://doi.org/10.1007/s11920-011-0221-3

Fujita, Y., & Yamashita, T. (2017). The roles of RGMa-neogenin signaling in inflammation and angiogenesis. *Inflammation and Regeneration, 37*(1), 6. https://doi.org/10.1186/s41232-017-0037-6

Gadoth, N. (2003). Multiple sclerosis in children. *Brain & Development, 25*(4), 229–232. https://doi.org/10.1016/s0387-7604(03)00035-4

Gallagher, S., et al. (2016). Pharmacological profile of MEDI-551, a novel anti-CD19 antibody, in human CD19 transgenic mice. *International Immunopharmacology, 36*, 205–212. https://doi.org/10.1016/j.intimp.2016.04.035

Gandoglia, I., et al. (2017). Teriflunomide treatment reduces B cells in patients with MS. *Neurol Neuroimmunol Neuroinflamm, 4*(6), Article e403. https://doi.org/10.1212/nxi.0000000000000403

Garnock-Jones, K. P., & Keating, G. M. (2009). Atomoxetine: A review of its use in attention-deficit hyperactivity disorder in children and adolescents. *Paediatric drugs, 11*(3), 203–226. https://doi.org/10.2165/00148581-200911030-00005

Gehricke, J. G., et al. (2017). The brain anatomy of attention-deficit/hyperactivity disorder in young adults - A magnetic resonance imaging study. *PLoS One, 12*(4), e0175433. https://doi.org/10.1371/journal.pone.0175433

Gharibi, T., et al. (2019). IL-21 and IL-21-producing T cells are involved in multiple sclerosis severity and progression. *Immunology Letters, 216*, 12–20. https://doi.org/10.1016/j.imlet.2019.09.003

Ghasemi, N., Razavi, S., & Nikzad, E. (2017). Multiple sclerosis: Pathogenesis, symptoms, diagnoses and cell-based therapy. *Cell Journal, 19*(1), 1–10. https://doi.org/10.22074/cellj.2016.4867

Gilhus, N. E., et al. (2018). Myasthenia gravis and infectious disease. *Journal of Neurology, 265*(6), 1251–1258. https://doi.org/10.1007/s00415-018-8751-9

Giniatullin, R., & Nistri, A. (2023). Role of ATP in migraine mechanisms: Focus on P2X3 receptors. *The Journal of Headache and Pain, 24*(1), 1. https://doi.org/10.1186/s10194-022-01535-4

Giraudo, C. G., et al. (2006). A clamping mechanism involved in SNARE-dependent exocytosis. *Science, 313* (5787), 676–680. https://doi.org/10.1126/science.1129450

Goadsby, P. J., & Edvinsson, L. (1994). Human in vivo evidence for trigeminovascular activation in cluster headache. neuropeptide changes and effects of acute attacks therapies. *Brain, 117*(Pt 3), 427–434. https://doi.org/10.1093/brain/117.3.427

Goadsby, P. J., Edvinsson, L., & Ekman, R. (1990). Vasoactive peptide release in the extracerebral circulation of humans during migraine headache. *Annals of Neurology, 28*(2), 183–187. https://doi.org/10.1002/ana.410280213

Goadsby, P. J., et al. (2017). A controlled trial of erenumab for episodic migraine. *New England Journal of Medicine, 377*(22), 2123–2132. https://doi.org/10.1056/NEJMoa1705848

Goadsby, P. J., Lipton, R. B., & Ferrari, M. D. (2002). Migraine—Current understanding and treatment. *New England Journal of Medicine, 346*(4), 257–270. https://doi.org/10.1056/NEJMra010917

Godfrey, E., et al. (2021). Public perceptions of adult ADHD: Indications of stigma? *Journal of Neural Transmission, 128*(7), 993–1008. https://doi.org/10.1007/s00702-020-02279-8

Godley, F., 3rd, et al. (2024). How sex hormones affect migraine: An interdisciplinary preclinical research panel review. *Journal of Personalized Medicine, 14*(2). https://doi.org/10.3390/jpm14020184

Gollapudi, S. K., Michael, J. J., & Chandra, M. (2014). Striated muscle dynamics. In *Reference module in biomedical sciences*. https://doi.org/10.1016/B978-0-12-801238-3.00251-8

GomezMancilla, B., et al. (2024). Efficacy and safety of iscalimab, a novel anti-CD40 monoclonal antibody, in moderate-to-severe myasthenia gravis: A phase 2 randomized study. *Journal of Clinical Neuroscience, 119*, 76–84. https://doi.org/10.1016/j.jocn.2023.11.013

Gormley, P., et al. (2016). Meta-analysis of 375,000 individuals identifies 38 susceptibility loci for migraine. *Nature Genetics, 48*(8), 856–866. https://doi.org/10.1038/ng.3598

Goydel, R. S., et al. (2020). Affinity maturation, humanization, and co-crystallization of a rabbit anti-human ROR2 monoclonal antibody for therapeutic applications. *Journal of Biological Chemistry, 295*(18), 5995–6006. https://doi.org/10.1074/jbc.RA120.012791

Graeler, M., & Goetzl, E. J. (2002). Activation-regulated expression and chemotactic function of sphingosine 1-phosphate receptors in mouse splenic T cells. *Faseb Journal, 16*(14), 1874–1878. https://doi.org/10.1096/fj.02-0548com

Grangeon, L., et al. (2023). Genetics of migraine: Where are we now? *The Journal of Headache and Pain, 24*(1), 12. https://doi.org/10.1186/s10194-023-01547-8

Gray, E., et al. (2008). Elevated activity and microglial expression of myeloperoxidase in demyelinated cerebral cortex in multiple sclerosis. *Brain Pathology, 18*(1), 86–95. https://doi.org/10.1111/j.1750-3639.2007.00110.x

Gregory, S. G., et al. (2007). Interleukin 7 receptor alpha chain (IL7R) shows allelic and functional association with multiple sclerosis. *Nature Genetics, 39*(9), 1083–1091. https://doi.org/10.1038/ng2103

Grimm, H. P., et al. (2023). Delivery of the Brainshuttle™ amyloid-beta antibody fusion trontinemab to non-human primate brain and projected efficacious dose regimens in humans. *mAbs, 15*(1), Article 2261509. https://doi.org/10.1080/19420862.2023.2261509

Guo, S., et al. (2023). Role of PACAP in migraine: An alternative to CGRP? *Neurobiology of Disease, 176*, Article 105946. https://doi.org/10.1016/j.nbd.2022.105946

Gupta, N. S., et al. (2025). Decoding the molecular and cellular aspects of multiple sclerosis: From diagnosis to therapeutic strategies. *Brain Research, 1863*, Article 149844. https://doi.org/10.1016/j.brainres.2025.149844

Hafler, D. A., et al. (2007). Risk alleles for multiple sclerosis identified by a genomewide study. *New England Journal of Medicine, 357*(9), 851–862. https://doi.org/10.1056/NEJMoa073493

Hamelink, C., et al. (2002). Coincident elevation of cAMP and calcium influx by PACAP-27 synergistically regulates vasoactive intestinal polypeptide gene transcription through a novel PKA-independent signaling pathway. *Journal of Neuroscience, 22*(13), 5310–5320. https://doi.org/10.1523/jneurosci.22-13-05310.2002

Haqqani, A. S., Bélanger, K., & Stanimirovic, D. B. (2024). Receptor-mediated transcytosis for brain delivery of therapeutics: Receptor classes and criteria. *Frontiers in Drug Delivery, 4–2024*. https://doi.org/10.3389/fddev.2024.1360302

Hartung, H. P., et al. (2022). Efficacy and safety of temelimab in multiple sclerosis: Results of a randomized phase 2b and extension study. *Multiple Sclerosis, 28*(3), 429–440. https://doi.org/10.1177/13524585211024997

Hartvig, P., Wiklund, L., & Lindström, B. (1986). Pharmacokinetics of physostigmine after intravenous, intramuscular and subcutaneous administration in surgical patients. *Acta Anaesthesiologica Scandinavica, 30*(2), 177–182. https://doi.org/10.1111/j.1399-6576.1986.tb02392.x

Hata, K., et al. (2006). RGMa inhibition promotes axonal growth and recovery after spinal cord injury. *Journal of Cell Biology, 173*(1), 47–58. https://doi.org/10.1083/jcb.200508143

Hautakangas, H., et al. (2022). Genome-wide analysis of 102,084 migraine cases identifies 123 risk loci and subtype-specific risk alleles. *Nature Genetics, 54*(2), 152–160. https://doi.org/10.1038/s41588-021-00990-0

Hebbandi Nanjundappa, R., Sokke Umeshappa, C., & Geuking, M. B. (2022). The impact of the gut microbiota on T cell ontogeny in the thymus. *Cellular and Molecular Life Sciences, 79*(4). https://doi.org/10.1007/s00018-022-04252-y

Hensley, K., et al. (2019). PAC1 receptor mRNA and protein distribution in rat and human trigeminal and sphenopalatine ganglia, spinal trigeminal nucleus and in dura mater. *Cephalalgia, 39*(7), 827–840. https://doi.org/10.1177/0333102418821621

Hess, J. L., et al. (2021). Autophagy, apoptosis, and neurodevelopmental genes might underlie selective brain region vulnerability in attention-deficit/hyperactivity disorder. *Molecular Psychiatry, 26*(11), 6643–6654. https://doi.org/10.1038/s41380-020-00974-2

Hewett, K., et al. (2018). Randomized study of adjunctive belimumab in participants with generalized myasthenia gravis. *Neurology, 90*(16), e1425–e1434. https://doi.org/10.1212/wnl.0000000000005323

Hong, S., et al. (2016). Complement and microglia mediate early synapse loss in Alzheimer mouse models. *Science, 352*(6286), 712–716. https://doi.org/10.1126/science.aad8373

Hoogman, M., et al. (2017). Subcortical brain volume differences in participants with attention deficit hyperactivity disorder in children and adults: A cross-sectional mega-analysis. *The Lancet Psychiatry, 4*(4), 310–319. https://doi.org/10.1016/s2215-0366(17)30049-4

Hosseinnia, M., Mazaheri, M. A., & Heidari, Z. (2020). Knowledge, attitude, and behavior of elementary teachers regarding attention deficit hyperactivity disorder. *Journal of Education and Health Promotion, 9*(1).

Howard, J. F., Jr., et al. (2017). Safety and efficacy of eculizumab in anti-acetylcholine receptor antibody-positive refractory generalised myasthenia gravis (REGAIN): A phase 3, randomised, double-blind, placebo-controlled, multicentre study. *The Lancet Neurology, 16*(12), 976–986. https://doi.org/10.1016/S1474-4422(17)30369-1

Hoy, S. M. (2023). Rozanolixizumab: First approval. *Drugs, 83*(14), 1341–1347. https://doi.org/10.1007/s40265-023-01933-1

Hu, Y., et al. (2009). Investigation of the mechanism of action of alemtuzumab in a human CD52 transgenic mouse model. *Immunology, 128*(2), 260–270. https://doi.org/10.1111/j.1365-2567.2009.03115.x

Iyengar, S., et al. (2019). CGRP and the trigeminal system in migraine. *Headache, 59*(5), 659–681. https://doi.org/10.1111/head.13529

Jacobson, P. B., et al. (2021). Elezanumab, a human anti-RGMa monoclonal antibody, promotes neuroprotection, neuroplasticity, and neurorecovery following a thoracic hemicompression spinal cord injury in non-human primates. *Neurobiology of Disease, 155*, Article 105385. https://doi.org/10.1016/j.nbd.2021.105385

Jennum, P., et al. (2025). Long-term effects of attention deficit hyperactivity disorder (ADHD) on social functioning and health care outcomes. *Journal of Psychiatric Research, 182*, 212–220. https://doi.org/10.1016/j.jpsychires.2025.01.016

Jensen, R., & Stovner, L. J. (2008). Epidemiology and comorbidity of headache. *The Lancet Neurology, 7*(4), 354–361. https://doi.org/10.1016/s1474-4422(08)70062-0

Jiao, L., & Guo, S. (2022). Anti-IL-6 therapies in central nervous system inflammatory demyelinating diseases. *Frontiers in Immunology, 13*, Article 966766. https://doi.org/10.3389/fimmu.2022.966766

Karasavva, V., et al. (2025). A double-edged hashtag: Evaluation of #ADHD-related TikTok content and its associations with perceptions of ADHD. *PLoS One, 20*(3), e0319335. https://doi.org/10.1371/journal.pone.0319335

Kataoka, S. H. (2016). ADHD among U.S. children and adults: Increasing access to care. *Psychiatric Services, 67* (9). https://doi.org/10.1176/appi.ps.670902, 937.

Kelly, R., et al. (2023). P797: A phase 2, open-labelstudy evaluatingthesafetyandefficacy of combination pozelimab andcemdisirantherapy in patientswith paroxysmal nocturnal hemoglobinuria who switch fromeculizumab. *HemaSphere, 7*(S3), e6873083. https://doi.org/10.1097/01.Hs9.0000970092.68730.83

Kerlero de Rosbo, N., et al. (1993). Reactivity to myelin antigens in multiple sclerosis. Peripheral blood lymphocytes respond predominantly to myelin oligodendrocyte glycoprotein. *Journal of Clinical Investigation, 92* (6), 2602–2608. https://doi.org/10.1172/jci116875

Khan, Z., et al. (2025). The polygenic nature of multiple sclerosis: Genetic variants, immunological modulation, and environmental connections. *Endocrine Metabolic & Immune Disorders Drug Targets, 25*(7), 527–559. https://doi.org/10.2174/0118715303325979241206115417

Kim, K. S. (2022). Regulation of T cell repertoires by commensal microbiota. *Frontiers in Cellular and Infection Microbiology, 12–2022*. https://doi.org/10.3389/fcimb.2022.1004339

Klineova, S., & Lublin, F. D. (2018). Clinical course of multiple sclerosis. *Cold Spring Harbor Perspectives in Medicine, 8*(9). https://doi.org/10.1101/cshperspect.a028928

Koch-Henriksen, N., & Magyari, M. (2021). Apparent changes in the epidemiology and severity of multiple sclerosis. *Nature Reviews Neurology, 17*(11), 676–688. https://doi.org/10.1038/s41582-021-00556-y

Koivisto, A.-P., et al. (2024). Targeting TRP channels for pain relief: A review of current evidence from bench to bedside. *Current Opinion in Pharmacology, 75*, Article 102447. https://doi.org/10.1016/j.coph.2024.102447

Koneczny, I., et al. (2017). IgG4 autoantibodies against muscle-specific kinase undergo Fab-arm exchange in myasthenia gravis patients. *Journal of Autoimmunity, 77*, 104–115. https://doi.org/10.1016/j.jaut.2016.11.005

Kraus, J., & Oschmann, P. (2006). The impact of interferon-beta treatment on the blood-brain barrier. *Drug Discovery Today, 11*(15–16), 755–762. https://doi.org/10.1016/j.drudis.2006.06.008

Kuburas, A., & Russo, A. F. (2023). Shared and independent roles of CGRP and PACAP in migraine pathophysiology. *The Journal of Headache and Pain, 24*(1), 34. https://doi.org/10.1186/s10194-023-01569-2

Kumar, R., et al. (2025). DHODH inhibition alters T cell metabolism limiting acute graft-versus-host disease while retaining graft-versus-leukemia response. *The Journal of Immunology, 214*(4), 818–827. https://doi.org/10.1093/jimmun/vkaf023

Kunkl, M., et al. (2020). T helper cells: The modulators of inflammation in multiple sclerosis. *Cells, 9*(2). https://doi.org/10.3390/cells9020482

Kurian, M., & Khera, N. (2024). Correlation between the prevalence of myasthenia gravis and the frequency of class II human leucocyte antigen alleles in various geographical locations around the world. *Cureus, 16*(9), Article e69791. https://doi.org/10.7759/cureus.69791

Ladopoulos, T., et al. (2025). Neurological disability and brain grey matter atrophy in primary progressive multiple sclerosis are determined by microstructural lesional changes, but not by lesion load. *Journal of Neurology, 272*(4), 302. https://doi.org/10.1007/s00415-025-13043-x

Laine, F. J., & Smoker, W. R. K. (1998). Anatomy of thecranialnerves. *Neuroimaging Clinics of North America, 8* (1), 69–100. https://doi.org/10.1016/S1052-5149(25)00502-7

Landtblom, A. M., et al. (2010). The first case history of multiple sclerosis: Augustus d'Esté (1794-1848). *Neurological Sciences, 31*(1), 29–33. https://doi.org/10.1007/s10072-009-0161-4

Lange, K. W., et al. (2010). The history of attention deficit hyperactivity disorder. *Attention Deficit and Hyperactivity Disorders, 2*(4), 241–255. https://doi.org/10.1007/s12402-010-0045-8

Le Garff-Tavernier, M., et al. (2014). Antibody-dependent cellular cytotoxicity of the optimized anti-CD20 monoclonal antibody ublituximab on chronic lymphocytic leukemia cells with the 17p deletion. *Leukemia, 28*(1), 230–233. https://doi.org/10.1038/leu.2013.240

Lee, J. W., et al. (2019). Ravulizumab (ALXN1210) vs eculizumab in adult patients with PNH naive to complement inhibitors: The 301 study. *Blood, 133*(6), 530–539. https://doi.org/10.1182/blood-2018-09-876136

Lensing, M. B., et al. (2013). Four-year outcome in psychopharmacologically treated adults with attention-deficit/hyperactivity disorder: A questionnaire survey. *The Journal of Clinical Psychiatry, 74*(1), e87–e93. https://doi.org/10.4088/JCP.12m07714

Lewis, N., Villani, A., & Lagopoulos, J. (2025). Gut dysbiosis as a driver of neuroinflammation in attention-deficit/hyperactivity disorder: A review of current evidence. *Neuroscience, 569*, 298–321. https://doi.org/10.1016/j.neuroscience.2025.01.031

Li, Z., et al. (2018). Clinical pharmacology of alemtuzumab, an anti-CD52 immunomodulator, in multiple sclerosis. *Clinical and Experimental Immunology, 194*(3), 295–314. https://doi.org/10.1111/cei.13208

Lindstrom, J. M. (2000). Acetylcholine receptors and myasthenia. *Muscle & Nerve, 23*(4), 453–477. https://doi.org/10.1002/(sici)1097-4598(200004)23:4<453::aid-mus3>3.0.co;2-o

Lipton, R. B., et al. (2019). Effect of ubrogepant vs placebo on pain and the Most bothersome associated symptom in the acute treatment of migraine: The ACHIEVE II randomized clinical trial. *JAMA, 322*(19), 1887–1898. https://doi.org/10.1001/jama.2019.16711

Lipton, R. B., et al. (2020). Efficacy and safety of eptinezumab in patients with chronic migraine. *Neurology, 94*(13), e1365–e1377. https://doi.org/10.1212/WNL.0000000000009169

Loutrari, H., Kokla, A., & Tzartos, S. J. (1992). Passive transfer of experimental myasthenia gravis via antigenic modulation of acetylcholine receptor. *European Journal of Immunology, 22*(9), 2449–2452. https://doi.org/10.1002/eji.1830220939

Lyall, M., de Oliveira, B. R., & Mody, S. K. (2023). Considerations for contraceptive use among patients with migraines. *Current Obstetrics and Gynecology Reports, 12*(2), 57–63. https://doi.org/10.1007/s13669-023-00349-8

Lyu, L., Li, Q., & Wang, C. (2025). EBV latency programs: Molecular and epigenetic regulation and its role in disease pathogenesis. *Journal of Medical Virology, 97*(7), Article e70501. https://doi.org/10.1002/jmv.70501

Magliozzi, R., et al. (2007). Meningeal B-cell follicles in secondary progressive multiple sclerosis associate with early onset of disease and severe cortical pathology. *Brain, 130*(Pt 4), 1089–1104. https://doi.org/10.1093/brain/awm038

Maier, L. M., et al. (2009). Soluble IL-2RA levels in multiple sclerosis subjects and the effect of soluble IL-2RA on immune responses. *Journal of Immunology., 182*(3), 1541–1547. https://doi.org/10.4049/jimmunol.182.3.1541

Makhani, N., & Tremlett, H. (2021). The multiple sclerosis prodrome. *Nature Reviews Neurology, 17*(8), 515–521. https://doi.org/10.1038/s41582-021-00519-3

Mariam, H., et al. (2012). Membrane microdomain sphingolipids are required for anti-CD20-induced death of chronic lymphocytic leukemia B cells. *Haematologica, 97*(2), 288–296. https://doi.org/10.3324/haematol.2011.051938

Martin, S. J., Guenette, M., & Oh, J. (2024). Evaluating the therapeutic potential of ublituximab in the treatment of MS: Design, development and place in therapy. *Drug Design, Development and Therapy, 18*, 3025–3042. https://doi.org/10.2147/dddt.S388410

Masi, L., et al. (2021). Video games in ADHD and Non-ADHD children: Modalities of use and association with ADHD symptoms. *Frontiers in Pediatrics, 9*, Article 632272. https://doi.org/10.3389/fped.2021.632272

Matute, C., et al. (2007). Excitotoxic damage to white matter. *Journal of Anatomy, 210*(6), 693–702. https://doi.org/10.1111/j.1469-7580.2007.00733.x

Max, J. E., et al. (2002). Putamen lesions and the development of attention-deficit/hyperactivity symptomatology. *Journal of the American Academy of Child & Adolescent Psychiatry, 41*(5), 563–571. https://doi.org/10.1097/00004583-200205000-00014

McCarter, S. J., et al. (2019). The Mary Walker effect: Mary Broadfoot Walker. *Journal of the Royal College of Physicians of Edinburgh, 49*(3), 255–259. https://doi.org/10.4997/jrcpe.2019.317

Meador-Woodruff, J. H., et al. (1996). Dopamine receptor mRNA expression in human striatum and neocortex. *Neuropsychopharmacology, 15*(1), 17–29. https://doi.org/10.1016/0893-133x(95)00150-c

Metzger, A. N., & Hamilton, L. T. (2021). The stigma of ADHD: Teacher ratings of labeled students. *Sociological Perspectives, 64*(2), 258–279.

Michailidou, I., et al. (2025). The role of complement in the immunopathogenesis of acetylcholine receptor antibody-positive generalized myasthenia gravis: Bystander or key player? *Frontiers in Immunology, 16*, Article 1526317. https://doi.org/10.3389/fimmu.2025.1526317

Monnier, P. P., et al. (2002). RGM is a repulsive guidance molecule for retinal axons. *Nature, 419*(6905), 392–395. https://doi.org/10.1038/nature01041

Montalban, X., et al. (2017). Ocrelizumab versus placebo in primary progressive multiple sclerosis. *New England Journal of Medicine, 376*(3), 209–220. https://doi.org/10.1056/NEJMoa1606468

Moreno-Ajona, D., Villar-Martínez, M. D., & Goadsby, P. J. (2022). New generation gepants: Migraine acute and preventive medications. *Journal of Clinical Medicine, 11*(6). https://doi.org/10.3390/jcm11061656

Mueller, A. K., Fuermaier, A. B., Koerts, J., & Tucha, L. (2012). Stigma in attention deficit hyperactivity disorder. *Attention Deficit and Hyperactivity Disorders, 4*(3), 101–114. https://doi.org/10.1007/s12402-012-0085-3

Muñiz-Castrillo, S., Vogrig, A., & Honnorat, J. (2020). Associations between HLA and autoimmune neurological diseases with autoantibodies. *Autoimmunity Highlights, 11*(1), 2. https://doi.org/10.1186/s13317-019-0124-6

Muramatsu, R., et al. (2011). RGMa modulates T cell responses and is involved in autoimmune encephalomyelitis. *Nature Medicine, 17*(4), 488–494. https://doi.org/10.1038/nm.2321

Murray, T. J. (2009). The history of multiple sclerosis: The changing frame of the disease over the centuries. *Journal of the Neurological Sciences, 277*(Suppl. 1), S3–S8. https://doi.org/10.1016/s0022-510x(09)70003-6

Namipashaki, A., et al. (2024). Mapping the impact of <em>DUSP6</em> in an ADHD iPSC derived-dopaminergic neuronal model. *bioRxiv*. https://doi.org/10.1101/2024.11.18.624053

Negron, A., Stüve, O., & Forsthuber, T. G. (2020). Ectopic lymphoid follicles in multiple sclerosis: Centers for disease control? *Frontiers in Neurology, 11*, Article 607766. https://doi.org/10.3389/fneur.2020.607766

Nelson, L. M., et al. (2019). A new way to estimate neurologic disease prevalence in the United States. *Neurology, 92*(10), 469–480. https://doi.org/10.1212/WNL.0000000000007044

Nielsen, B. R., et al. (2017). Characterization of naïve, memory and effector T cells in progressive multiple sclerosis. *Journal of Neuroimmunology, 310*, 17–25. https://doi.org/10.1016/j.jneuroim.2017.06.001

Nigg, J. T. (2013). Attention-deficit/hyperactivity disorder and adverse health outcomes. *Clinical Psychology Review, 33*(2), 215–228. https://doi.org/10.1016/j.cpr.2012.11.005

Nishanth, K., et al. (2020). Role of smoking in the pathogenesis of multiple sclerosis: A review article. *Cureus, 12*(8), Article e9564. https://doi.org/10.7759/cureus.9564

Njenga, M. K., et al. (2000). Short-term treatment with interferon-alpha/beta promotes remyelination, whereas long-term treatment aggravates demyelination in a murine model of multiple sclerosis. *Journal of Neuroscience Research, 59*(5), 661–670. https://doi.org/10.1002/(sici)1097-4547(20000301)59:5<661::Aid-jnr9>3.0.Co;2-e

O'Connell, K. S., Shadrin, A., Bahrami, S., Smeland, O. B., Bettella, F., Frei, O., Krull, F., et al. (2021). Identification of genetic overlap and novel risk loci for attention-deficit/hyperactivity disorder and bipolar disorder. *Molecular Psychiatry, 26*(8), 4055–4065. https://doi.org/10.1038/s41380-019-0613-z

O'Leary, S., et al. (2023). Practical clinical guidelines for Natalizumab treatment in patients with relapsing multiple sclerosis. *Journal of Infusion Nursing, 46*(6), 347–359. https://doi.org/10.1097/nan.0000000000000519

Oh, S. J. (2009). Muscle-specific receptor tyrosine kinase antibody positive myasthenia gravis current status. *Journal of Clinical Neurology, 5*(2), 53–64. https://doi.org/10.3988/jcn.2009.5.2.53

Oh, S. J., et al. (2009). Racial differences in myasthenia gravis in Alabama. *Muscle & Nerve, 39*(3), 328–332. https://doi.org/10.1002/mus.21191

Oladosu, O., et al. (2022). Advanced diffusion MRI and image texture analysis detect widespread brain structural differences between relapsing-remitting and secondary progressive multiple sclerosis. *Frontiers in Human Neuroscience, 16–2022*. https://doi.org/10.3389/fnhum.2022.944908

Oldehinkel, M., et al. (2016). Attention-deficit/hyperactivity disorder symptoms coincide with altered striatal connectivity. *Biological Psychiatry: Cognitive Neuroscience and Neuroimaging, 1*(4), 353–363. https://doi.org/10.1016/j.bpsc.2016.03.008

Olsson, T., Barcellos, L. F., & Alfredsson, L. (2017). Interactions between genetic, lifestyle and environmental risk factors for multiple sclerosis. *Nature Reviews Neurology, 13*(1), 25–36. https://doi.org/10.1038/nrneurol.2016.187

Onnink, A. M. H., et al. (2014). Brain alterations in adult ADHD: Effects of gender, treatment and comorbid depression. *European Neuropsychopharmacology, 24*(3), 397–409. https://doi.org/10.1016/j.euroneuro.2013.11.011

Pardutz, A., & Schoenen, J. (2010). NSAIDs in the acute treatment of migraine: A review of clinical and experimental data. *Pharmaceuticals, 3*(6), 1966–1987. https://doi.org/10.3390/ph3061966

Pasquali, L., et al. (2015). A clinical and laboratory study evaluating the profile of cytokine levels in relapsing remitting and secondary progressive multiple sclerosis. *Journal of Neuroimmunology, 278*, 53–59. https://doi.org/10.1016/j.jneuroim.2014.12.005

Patrick, J., & Lindstrom, J. (1973). Autoimmune response to acetylcholine receptor. *Science, 180*(4088), 871–872. https://doi.org/10.1126/science.180.4088.871

Patsopoulos, N. A. (2018). Genetics of multiple sclerosis: An overview and new directions. *Cold Spring Harbor Perspectives in Medicine, 8*(7). https://doi.org/10.1101/cshperspect.a028951

Pawluczkowycz, A. W., et al. (2009). Binding of submaximal C1q promotes complement-dependent cytotoxicity (CDC) of B cells opsonized with Anti-CD20 mAbs ofatumumab (OFA) or rituximab (RTX): Considerably higher levels of CDC are induced by OFA than by RTX1. *The Journal of Immunology, 183*(1), 749–758. https://doi.org/10.4049/jimmunol.0900632

Pekna, M., & Pekny, M. (2021). The complement system: A powerful modulator and effector of astrocyte function in the healthy and diseased central nervous system. *Cells, 10*(7). https://doi.org/10.3390/cells10071812

Pellesi, L., et al. (2020). Two-hour infusion of vasoactive intestinal polypeptide induces delayed headache and extracranial vasodilation in healthy volunteers. *Cephalalgia, 40*(11), 1212–1223. https://doi.org/10.1177/0333102420937655

Pellesi, L., et al. (2021). Effect of vasoactive intestinal polypeptide on development of migraine headaches: A randomized clinical trial. *JAMA Network Open, 4*(8), e2118543. https://doi.org/10.1001/jamanetworkopen.2021.18543

Pender, M. P., et al. (2014). Deficiency of CD8+ effector memory T cells is an early and persistent feature of multiple sclerosis. *Multiple Sclerosis, 20*(14), 1825–1832. https://doi.org/10.1177/1352458514536252

Petersson, M., et al. (2025). Nicotine, alcohol consumption, and risk of myasthenia gravis. *Neurology, 105*(1), Article e213771. https://doi.org/10.1212/WNL.0000000000213771

Phillips, L. H., 2nd (2003). The epidemiology of myasthenia gravis. *Annals of the New York Academy of Sciences, 998*, 407–412. https://doi.org/10.1196/annals.1254.053

Phillips, W. D., & Vincent, A. (2016). Pathogenesis of myasthenia gravis: Update on disease types, models, and mechanisms. *F1000Research, 5*. https://doi.org/10.12688/f1000research.8206.1

Popa, L. G., et al. (2024). Mechanisms of resistance to rituximab used for the treatment of autoimmune blistering diseases. *Life (Basel)., 14*(10). https://doi.org/10.3390/life14101223

Pornnoppadol, G., et al. (2024). Bispecific antibody shuttles targeting CD98hc mediate efficient and long-lived brain delivery of IgGs. *Cell Chemical Biology, 31*(2), 361–372.e8. https://doi.org/10.1016/j.chembiol.2023.09.008

Poser, C. M. (1986). Pathogenesis of multiple sclerosis. A critical reappraisal. *Acta Neuropathologica, 71*(1–2), 1–10. https://doi.org/10.1007/bf00687954

Poser, C. M., & Brinar, V. V. (2001). Diagnostic criteria for multiple sclerosis. *Clinical Neurology and Neurosurgery, 103*(1), 1–11. https://doi.org/10.1016/S0303-8467(00)00125-6

Posner, J., Polanczyk, G. V., & Sonuga-Barke, E. (2020). Attention-deficit hyperactivity disorder. *Lancet, 395* (10222), 450–462. https://doi.org/10.1016/s0140-6736(19)33004-1

Ragheb, S., et al. (2008). A potential role for B-cell activating factor in the pathogenesis of autoimmune myasthenia gravis. *Archives of Neurology, 65*(10), 1358–1362. https://doi.org/10.1001/archneur.65.10.1358

Ramakrishnan, N. A., Drescher, M. J., & Drescher, D. G. (2012). The SNARE complex in neuronal and sensory cells. *Molecular and Cellular Neuroscience, 50*(1), 58–69. https://doi.org/10.1016/j.mcn.2012.03.009

Rapoport, S. I. (2000). Osmotic opening of the blood–brain barrier: Principles, mechanism, and therapeutic applications. *Cellular and Molecular Neurobiology, 20*(2), 217–230. https://doi.org/10.1023/A:1007049806660

Ray, B. S., & Wolff, H. G. (1940). Experimental studies on headache: Pain-sensitive structures of the head and their significance in headache. *Archives of Surgery, 41*(4), 813–856.

Renton, A. E., et al. (2015). A genome-wide association study of myasthenia gravis. *JAMA Neurology, 72*(4), 396–404. https://doi.org/10.1001/jamaneurol.2014.4103

Rezaei, G., et al. (2016). Comparative efficacy of methylphenidate and atomoxetine in the treatment of attention deficit hyperactivity disorder in children and adolescents: A systematic review and meta-analysis. *Medical Journal of the Islamic Republic of Iran, 30*, 325.

Ricciardi, R., et al. (2024). Acetylcholinesterase inhibitors are ineffective in MuSK-antibody positive myasthenia gravis: Results of a study on 202 patients. *Journal of the Neurological Sciences, 461*, Article 123047. https://doi.org/10.1016/j.jns.2024.123047

Romero-Pinel, L., et al. (2022). The age at onset of relapsing-remitting multiple sclerosis has increased over the last five decades. *Multiple Sclerosis and Related Disorders, 68*, Article 104103. https://doi.org/10.1016/j.msard.2022.104103

Romme Christensen, J., et al. (2013). Systemic inflammation in progressive multiple sclerosis involves follicular T-helper, Th17- and activated B-cells and correlates with progression. *PLoS One, 8*(3), Article e57820. https://doi.org/10.1371/journal.pone.0057820

Ruff, R. L., & Lennon, V. A. (2008). How myasthenia gravis alters the safety factor for neuromuscular transmission. *Journal of Neuroimmunology, 201–202*, 13–20. https://doi.org/10.1016/j.jneuroim.2008.04.038

Šega, S., et al. (2004). IFN-β1a and IFN-β1b have different patterns of influence on cytokines. *Clinical Neurology and Neurosurgery, 106*(3), 255–258. https://doi.org/10.1016/j.clineuro.2004.02.010

Sahashi, K., et al. (1980). Ultrastructural localization of the terminal and lytic ninth complement component (C9) at the motor end-plate in myasthenia gravis. *Journal of Neuropathology & Experimental Neurology, 39*(2), 160–172. https://doi.org/10.1097/00005072-198003000-00005

Salomonsson, S., et al. (2003). Cellular basis of ectopic germinal center formation and autoantibody production in the target organ of patients with sjögren's syndrome. *Arthritis & Rheumatism, 48*(11), 3187–3201. https://doi.org/10.1002/art.11311

Schoenfelder, E. N., & Kollins, S. H. (2016). Topical review: ADHD and health-risk behaviors: Toward prevention and health promotion. *Journal of Pediatric Psychology, 41*(7), 735–740. https://doi.org/10.1093/jpepsy/jsv162

Schreiweis, C., et al. (2014). Humanized Foxp2 accelerates learning by enhancing transitions from declarative to procedural performance. *Proceedings of the National Academy of Sciences of the United States of America, 111*(39), 14253–14258. https://doi.org/10.1073/pnas.1414542111

Schumaker, V. N., et al. (1976). Ultracentifuge studies of the binding of IgG of different subclasses to the Clq subunit of the first component of complement. *Biochemistry, 15*(23), 5175–5181. https://doi.org/10.1021/bi00668a035

Sepulcre, J., et al. (2009). Contribution of white matter lesions to gray matter atrophy in multiple sclerosis: Evidence from voxel-based analysis of T1 lesions in the visual pathway. *Archives of Neurology, 66*(2), 173–179. https://doi.org/10.1001/archneurol.2008.562

Sharma, A., et al. (2018). LFA-1 ligation by high-density ICAM-1 is sufficient to activate IFN-γrelease by innate T lymphocytes. *Journal of Immunology, 201*(8), 2452–2461. https://doi.org/10.4049/jimmunol.1800537

Sheikh, S., et al. (2021). Drugs that induce or cause deterioration of myasthenia gravis: An update. *Journal of Clinical Medicine, 10*(7). https://doi.org/10.3390/jcm10071537

Siger, M. (2022). Magnetic resonance imaging in primary progressive multiple sclerosis patients : Review. *Clinical Neuroradiology, 32*(3), 625–641. https://doi.org/10.1007/s00062-022-01144-3

Silberstein, S. D., et al. (2017). Fremanezumab for the preventive treatment of chronic migraine. *New England Journal of Medicine, 377*(22), 2113–2122. https://doi.org/10.1056/NEJMoa1709038

Simon, M., et al. (2018). Anti-CD52 antibody treatment depletes B cell aggregates in the central nervous system in a mouse model of multiple sclerosis. *Journal of Neuroinflammation, 15*(1), 225. https://doi.org/10.1186/s12974-018-1263-9

Sorensen, P. S. (2003). The role of intravenous immunoglobulin in the treatment of multiple sclerosis. *Journal of the Neurological Sciences, 206*(2), 123–130. https://doi.org/10.1016/S0022-510X(02)00343-X

Sorensen, P. S., & Blinkenberg, M. (2016). The potential role for ocrelizumab in the treatment of multiple sclerosis: Current evidence and future prospects. *Therapeutic Advances in Neurological Disorders, 9*(1), 44–52. https://doi.org/10.1177/1756285615601933

Spencer, T., Biederman, J., Wilens, T., Doyle, R., Surman, C., Prince, J., Mick, E., et al. (2005). A large, double-blind, randomized clinical trial of methylphenidate in the treatment of adults with attention-deficit/hyperactivity disorder. *Biological Psychiatry, 57*(5), 456–463. https://doi.org/10.1016/j.biopsych.2004.11.043

Sprouse-Blum, A. S., et al. (2013). Randomized controlled trial: Targeted neck cooling in the treatment of the migraine patient. *Hawaii Journal of Medicine & Public Health, 72*(7), 237–241.

Staruschenko, A., Jeske, N. A., & Akopian, A. N. (2010). Contribution of TRPV1-TRPA1 interaction to the single channel properties of the TRPA1 channel. *Journal of Biological Chemistry, 285*(20), 15167–15177. https://doi.org/10.1074/jbc.M110.106153

Stauffer, V. L., et al. (2018). Evaluation of galcanezumab for the prevention of episodic migraine: The EVOLVE-1 randomized clinical trial. *JAMA Neurology, 75*(9), 1080–1088. https://doi.org/10.1001/jamaneurol.2018.1212

Stetefeld, H., & Schroeter, M. (2019). SOP myasthenic crisis. *Neurological Research and Practice, 1*(1), 19. https://doi.org/10.1186/s42466-019-0023-3

Stevens, T., et al. (2019). PharmGKB summary: Methylphenidate pathway, pharmacokinetics/pharmacodynamics. *Pharmacogenet Genomics, 29*(6), 136–154. https://doi.org/10.1097/fpc.0000000000000376

Sudershan, A., et al. (2024). Role of TNF-α in the pathogenesis of migraine. *Pain Research and Management, 2024*, Article 1377143. https://doi.org/10.1155/2024/1377143

Sun, L., et al. (2014). CTLA4 variants and haplotype contribute genetic susceptibility to myasthenia gravis in northern Chinese population. *PLoS One, 9*(7), Article e101986. https://doi.org/10.1371/journal.pone.0101986

Tallantyre, E. C., et al. (2009). Greater loss of axons in primary progressive multiple sclerosis plaques compared to secondary progressive disease. *Brain, 132*(Pt 5), 1190–1199. https://doi.org/10.1093/brain/awp106

Tan, Y., et al. (2022). Long-term efficacy of non-steroid immunosuppressive agents in anti-muscle-specific kinase positive myasthenia gravis patients: A prospective study. *Frontiers in Neurology, 13*, Article 877895. https://doi.org/10.3389/fneur.2022.877895

Tangye, S. G., & Ma, C. S. (2020). Regulation of the germinal center and humoral immunity by interleukin-21. *Journal of Experimental Medicine, 217*(1). https://doi.org/10.1084/jem.20191638

Tarlinton, R. E., et al. (2020). Role of viruses in the pathogenesis of multiple sclerosis. *Viruses, 12*(6). https://doi.org/10.3390/v12060643

Tepper, S., et al. (2017). Safety and efficacy of erenumab for preventive treatment of chronic migraine: A randomised, double-blind, placebo-controlled phase 2 trial. *The Lancet Neurology, 16*(6), 425–434. https://doi.org/10.1016/S1474-4422(17)30083-2

Tepper, S. J., & Rapoport, A. M. (1999). The triptans. *CNS Drugs, 12*(5), 403–417. https://doi.org/10.2165/00023210-199912050-00007

Tizaoui, K., et al. (2021). The role of PTPN22 in the pathogenesis of autoimmune diseases: A comprehensive review. *Seminars in Arthritis and Rheumatism, 51*(3), 513–522. https://doi.org/10.1016/j.semarthrit.2021.03.004

Torpy, J. M., Glass, T. J., & Glass, R. M. (2005). Myasthenia gravis. *JAMA, 293*(15). https://doi.org/10.1001/jama.293.15.1940, 1940–1940.

Trebst, C., et al. (2007). Lack of interferon-beta leads to accelerated remyelination in a toxic model of central nervous system demyelination. *Acta Neuropathologica, 114*(6), 587–596. https://doi.org/10.1007/s00401-007-0300-z

Tzartos, S. J., et al. (1998). Anatomy of the antigenic structure of a large membrane autoantigen, the muscle-type nicotinic acetylcholine receptor. *Immunological Reviews, 163*, 89–120. https://doi.org/10.1111/j.1600-065x.1998.tb01190.x

Vázquez-González, D., et al. (2023). A potential role for neuroinflammation in ADHD. *Advances inExperimental Medicine and Biology., 1411*, 327–356. https://doi.org/10.1007/978-981-19-7376-5_15

Valentine, M. A., et al. (1987). Expression of the human B-cell surface protein CD20: Alteration by phorbol 12-myristate 13-acetate. *Proceedings of the National Academy of Sciences of the United States of America, 84*(22), 8085–8089. https://doi.org/10.1073/pnas.84.22.8085

van Oosterhout, W. P. J., et al. (2018). Female sex hormones in men with migraine. *Neurology, 91*(4), e374–e381. https://doi.org/10.1212/WNL.0000000000005855

Vandenbussche, N., et al. (2018). Medication-overuse headache: A widely recognized entity amidst ongoing debate. *The Journal of Headache and Pain, 19*(1), 50. https://doi.org/10.1186/s10194-018-0875-x

Vandesquille, M., et al. (2017). Chemically-defined camelid antibody bioconjugate for the magnetic resonance imaging of Alzheimer's disease. *mAbs, 9*(6), 1016–1027. https://doi.org/10.1080/19420862.2017.1342914

Vesperinas-Castro, A., & Cortés-Vicente, E. (2023). Rituximab treatment in myasthenia gravis. *Frontiers in Neurology, 14*, Article 1275533. https://doi.org/10.3389/fneur.2023.1275533

Vijenthira, A., et al. (2021). Vaccine response following anti-CD20 therapy: A systematic review and meta-analysis of 905 patients. *Blood Advances, 5*(12), 2624–2643. https://doi.org/10.1182/bloodadvances.2021004629

Vincent, A. (2002). Unravelling the pathogenesis of myasthenia gravis. *Nature Reviews Immunology, 2*(10), 797–804. https://doi.org/10.1038/nri916

Volpe, E., Battistini, L., & Borsellino, G. (2015). Advances in T helper 17 cell biology: Pathogenic role and potential therapy in multiple sclerosis. *Mediators of Inflammation, 2015*, Article 475158. https://doi.org/10.1155/2015/475158

von Essen, M. R., et al. (2019). Proinflammatory CD20+ T cells in the pathogenesis of multiple sclerosis. *Brain, 142*(1), 120–132. https://doi.org/10.1093/brain/awy301

von Rhein, D., et al. (2016). Aberrant local striatal functional connectivity in attention-deficit/hyperactivity disorder. *Journal of Child Psychology and Psychiatry, 57*(6), 697–705. https://doi.org/10.1111/jcpp.12529

Voskuhl, R. R., et al. (1993). T helper 1 (Th1) functional phenotype of human myelin basic protein-specific T lymphocytes. *Autoimmunity, 15*(2), 137–143. https://doi.org/10.3109/08916939309043888

Vu, T., et al. (2022). Terminal complement inhibitor ravulizumab in generalized myasthenia gravis. *NEJM Evidence, 1*(5), Article EVIDoa2100066. https://doi.org/10.1056/EVIDoa2100066

Walton, C., et al. (2020). Rising prevalence of multiple sclerosis worldwide: Insights from the atlas of MS, third edition. *Multiple Sclerosis, 26*(14), 1816–1821. https://doi.org/10.1177/1352458520970841

Wang, W., et al. (2019). Type I interferon therapy limits CNS autoimmunity by inhibiting CXCR3-Mediated trafficking of pathogenic effector T cells. *Cell Reports, 28*(2), 486–497.e4. https://doi.org/10.1016/j.celrep.2019.06.021

Wang, Y., & Kasper, L. H. (2014). The role of microbiome in central nervous system disorders. *Brain, Behavior, and Immunity, 38*, 1–12. https://doi.org/10.1016/j.bbi.2013.12.015

Waschek, J. A., Baca, S. M., & Akerman, S. (2018). PACAP and migraine headache: Immunomodulation of neural circuits in autonomic ganglia and brain parenchyma. *Journal of Headache and Pain, 19*(1), 23. https://doi.org/10.1186/s10194-018-0850-6

Wattiez, A. S., Sowers, L. P., & Russo, A. F. (2020). Calcitonin gene-related peptide (CGRP): Role in migraine pathophysiology and therapeutic targeting. *Expert Opinion on Therapeutic Targets, 24*(2), 91–100. https://doi.org/10.1080/14728222.2020.1724285

Weiner, H. L. (2008). A shift from adaptive to innate immunity: A potential mechanism of disease progression in multiple sclerosis. *Journal of Neurology, 255*(Suppl. 1), 3–11. https://doi.org/10.1007/s00415-008-1002-8

Wilk, E., et al. (2009). Depletion of functionally active CD20+ T cells by rituximab treatment. *Arthritis & Rheumatism, 60*(12), 3563–3571. https://doi.org/10.1002/art.24998

Wong, S. H. (2022). Clinical signs in neuro-ophthalmology: Eye signs in myasthenia gravis. *Annals of Indian Academy of Neurology, 25*(Suppl. 2), S91–s93. https://doi.org/10.4103/aian.aian_163_22

Woo, M. S., Engler, J. B., & Friese, M. A. (2024). The neuropathobiology of multiple sclerosis. *Nature Reviews Neuroscience, 25*(7), 493–513. https://doi.org/10.1038/s41583-024-00823-z

Wu, J., et al. (2025). Obesity affects disease activity and progression, cognitive functioning, and quality of life in people with multiple sclerosis. *Neurology Neuroimmunology & Neuroinflammation, 12*(1), Article e200334. https://doi.org/10.1212/NXI.0000000000200334

Xie, Y., et al. (2011). Association between HLA-DRB1 and myasthenia gravis in a northern han Chinese population. *Journal of Clinical Neuroscience, 18*(11), 1524–1527. https://doi.org/10.1016/j.jocn.2011.05.002

Xie, T., et al. (2023). Structural insights into the assembly of the agrin/LRP4/MuSK signaling complex. *Proceedings of the National Academy of Sciences, 120*(23), Article e2300453120. https://doi.org/10.1073/pnas.2300453120

Xiong, X., et al. (2015). PTPN22 R620W polymorphism is associated with myasthenia gravis risk: A systematic review and meta-analysis. *Medical Science Monitor, 21*, 2567–2571. https://doi.org/10.12659/msm.894307

Xu, G., et al. (2018). Twenty-year trends in diagnosed attention-deficit/hyperactivity disorder among US children and adolescents, 1997–2016. *JAMA Network Open, 1*(4), Article e181471. https://doi.org/10.1001/jamanetworkopen.2018.1471

Xu, X., Gao, Y., Shan, F., et al. (2016a). A novel role for RGMa in modulation of bone marrow-derived dendritic cells maturation induced by lipopolysaccharide. *International Immunopharmacology, 33*, 99–107. https://doi.org/10.1016/j.intimp.2016.02.008

Xu, X., Gao, Y., Zhai, Z., et al. (2016b). Repulsive guidance molecule a blockade exerts the immunoregulatory function in DCs stimulated with ABP and LPS. *Human Vaccines &Immunotherapeutics, 12*(8), 2169–2180. https://doi.org/10.1080/21645515.2016.1164361

Yager, L. M., et al. (2015). The ins and outs of the striatum: Role in drug addiction. *Neuroscience, 301*, 529–541. https://doi.org/10.1016/j.neuroscience.2015.06.033

Yamashita, M., Katakura, Y., & Shirahata, S. (2007). Recent advances in the generation of human monoclonal antibody. *Cytotechnology, 55*(2–3), 55–60. https://doi.org/10.1007/s10616-007-9072-5

Yan, M., et al. (2018). Agrin and LRP4 antibodies as new biomarkers of myasthenia gravis. *Annals of the New York Academy of Sciences, 1413*(1), 126–135. https://doi.org/10.1111/nyas.13573

Yatham, L. N., et al. (2022). A positron emission tomography study of dopamine transporter density in patients with bipolar disorder with current mania and those with recently remitted mania. *JAMA Psychiatry, 79*(12), 1217–1224. https://doi.org/10.1001/jamapsychiatry.2022.3541

Yu, Y., Schürpf, T., & Springer, T. A. (2013). How natalizumab binds and antagonizes α4 integrins. *Journal of Biological Chemistry, 288*(45), 32314–32325. https://doi.org/10.1074/jbc.M113.501668

Yucel, A., et al. (2020). Estimating the economic burden of migraine on US employers. *American Journal of Managed Care, 26*(12), e403–e408. https://doi.org/10.37765/ajmc.2020.88547

Zaja, F., et al. (2000). Rituximab for myasthenia gravis developing after bone marrow transplant. *Neurology, 55*(7), 1062–1063. https://doi.org/10.1212/wnl.55.7.1062-a

Zastepa, E., et al. (2014). Naive CD4 T-cell activation identifies MS patients having rapid transition to progressive MS. *Neurology, 82*(8), 681 690. https://doi.org/10.1212/wnl.0000000000000146

Zeller, J., et al. (2008). CGRP function-blocking antibodies inhibit neurogenic vasodilatation without affecting heart rate or arterial blood pressure in the rat. *British Journal of Pharmacology, 155*(7), 1093–1103. https://doi.org/10.1038/bjp.2008.334

Zewail, M., et al. (2022). Hyaluronic acid coated teriflunomide (A771726) loaded lipid carriers for the oral management of rheumatoid arthritis. *International Journal of Pharmaceutics, 623*, Article 121939. https://doi.org/10.1016/j.ijpharm.2022.121939

Zhan, J., et al. (2021). Ectopic lymphoid follicles in progressive multiple sclerosis: From patients to animal models. *Immunology, 164*(3), 450–466. https://doi.org/10.1111/imm.13395

Zhang, H., et al. (2024a). Dimerization and antidepressant recognition at noradrenaline transporter. *Nature, 630*(8015), 247–254. https://doi.org/10.1038/s41586-024-07437-6

Zhang, H.-R., et al. (2024b). The GFPT2-O-GlcNAcylation-YBX1 axis promotes IL-18 secretion to regulate the tumor immune microenvironment in pancreatic cancer. *Cell Death & Disease, 15*(4), 244. https://doi.org/10.1038/s41419-024-06589-7

Zhang-James, Y., et al. (2021). Evidence for similar structural brain anomalies in youth and adult attention-deficit/hyperactivity disorder: A machine learning analysis. *Translational Psychiatry, 11*(1), 82. https://doi.org/10.1038/s41398-021-01201-4

Zhou, J. (2004). Norepinephrine transporter inhibitors and their therapeutic potential. *Drugs of the Future, 29*(12), 1235–1244. https://doi.org/10.1358/dof.2004.029.12.855246

Zhu, L. N., et al. (2023). FcRn inhibitors: A novel option for the treatment of myasthenia gravis. *Neural Regeneration Research, 18*(8), 1637–1644. https://doi.org/10.4103/1673-5374.363824

Zhu, J., & Reith, M. E. (2008). Role of the dopamine transporter in the action of psychostimulants, nicotine, and other drugs of abuse. *CNS & Neurological Disorders: Drug Targets, 7*(5), 393–409. https://doi.org/10.2174/187152708786927877

Zimmermann, K., Reeh, P. W., & Averbeck, B. (2002). ATP can enhance the proton-induced CGRP release through P2Y receptors and secondary PGE(2) release in isolated rat dura mater. *Pain, 97*(3), 259–265. https://doi.org/10.1016/s0304-3959(02)00027-1

Further reading

Abraham, C., Griffith, J., & Miller, J. (1999). The dependence for leukocyte function-associated antigen-1/ICAM-1 interactions in T cell activation cannot be overcome by expression of high density TCR ligand. *Journal of Immunology, 162*(8), 4399–4405. Retrieved from.

Afkarian, M., et al. (2002). T-bet is a STATI-induced regulator for IL-12R expression in naïve CD4+ T cells. *Nature Immunology, 3*(6), 549–557. https://doi.org/10.1038/ni794

Aguirre, A., et al. (2013). FasL-triggered death of Jurkat cells requires caspase 8-induced, ATP-dependent cross-talk between Fas and the purinergic receptor P2X(7). *Journal of Cellular Physiology, 228*(2), 485–493. https://doi.org/10.1002/jcp.24159

Akita, K., et al. (1997). Involvement of caspase-1 and caspase-3 in the production and processing of mature human interleukin 18 in monocytic THP.1 cells. *Journal of Biological Chemistry, 272*(42), 26595–26603. https://doi.org/10.1074/jbc.272.42.26595

Alsaleh, G., et al. (2009). Bruton's tyrosine Kinase is involved in miR-346-Related regulation of IL-18 release by lipopolysaccharide-activated rheumatoid fibroblast-like synoviocytes 1. *The Journal of Immunology, 182*(8), 5088–5097. https://doi.org/10.4049/jimmunol.0801613

Banda, N. K., et al. (2003). Mechanisms of inhibition of collagen-induced arthritis by Murine IL-18 binding protein 1. *The Journal of Immunology, 170*(4), 2100–2105. https://doi.org/10.4049/jimmunol.170.4.2100

Barnett, K. K., et al. (2025). FDA approval summary: Afamitresgeneautoleucel for adults with HLA-restricted MAGE-A4 positive unresectable or metastatic synovial sarcoma after prior chemotherapy. *Clinical Cancer Research.* https://doi.org/10.1158/1078-0432.Ccr-25-0595

Barr, T., et al. (2024). Recent advances and remaining challenges in lung cancer therapy. *Chinese Medical Journal, 137*(05), 533–546. https://doi.org/10.1097/CM9.0000000000002991

Bazan, J. F., Timans, J. C., & Kastelein, R. A. (1996). A newly defined interleukin-1? *Nature, 379*(6566). https://doi.org/10.1038/379591a0, 591.

Bedard, M., et al. (2019). Sterile activation of invariant natural killer T cells by ER-stressed antigen-presenting cells. *Proceedings of the National Academy of Sciences, 116*(47), 23671–23681. https://doi.org/10.1073/pnas.1910097116

Black, R. A., et al. (1988). Generation of biologically active interleukin-1 beta by proteolytic cleavage of the inactive precursor. *Journal of Biological Chemistry, 263*(19), 9437–9442.

Boes, C. J., & Capobianco, D. J. (2005). Chronic migraine and medication-overuse headache through the ages. *Cephalalgia, 25*(5), 378–390. https://doi.org/10.1111/j.1468-2982.2005.00868.x

Boldt, C. (2023). MD Anderson and replay announce FDA clearance of IND application for first-in-class TCR NK cell therapy for multiple myeloma. *MD Anderson Newsroom.* https://www.mdanderson.org/newsroom/novel-tcr-nk-cell-therapy-multiple-myeloma-receives-ind-clearance-fda.h00-159620223.html.

Bufler, P., et al. (2002). A complex of the IL-1 homologue IL-1F7b and IL-18-binding protein reduces IL-18 activity. *Proceedings of the National Academy of Sciences, 99*(21), 13723–13728. https://doi.org/10.1073/pnas.212519099

Bytnar, J. A., et al. (2025). Incidence rates of soft tissue sarcoma among U.S. military servicemen: Comparison with the rates in the general U.S. population. *Cancer, 131*(1), Article e35607. https://doi.org/10.1002/cncr.35607

Chakir, H., et al. (2003). Bystander polarization' of CD4+ T cells: Activation with high-dose IL-2 renders naive T cells responsive to IL-12 and/or IL-18 in the absence of TCR ligation. *European Journal of Immunology, 33*(7), 1788–1798. https://doi.org/10.1002/eji.200323398

Chandrasekar, B., et al. (2004). Activation of intrinsic and extrinsic proapoptotic signaling pathways in interleukin-18-mediated human cardiac endothelial cell death. *Journal of Biological Chemistry, 279*, 20221–20233. https://doi.org/10.1074/jbc.M313980200

Chen, C. S., & Aylett, C. H. S. (2025). New insights into tuberous sclerosis complex: From structure to pathogenesis. *Frontiers in Cell and Developmental Biology, 13*, Article 1595867. https://doi.org/10.3389/fcell.2025.1595867

Chen, Q., & Massagué, J. (2012). Molecular pathways: VCAM-1 as a potential therapeutic target in metastasis. *Clinical Cancer Research, 18*(20), 5520–5525. https://doi.org/10.1158/1078-0432.Ccr-11-2904

Coindre, J. M., et al. (1996). Prognostic factors in adult patients with locally controlled soft tissue sarcoma. A study of 546 patients from the French Federation of Cancer Centers Sarcoma Group. *Journal of Clinical Oncology, 14*(3), 869–877. https://doi.org/10.1200/jco.1996.14.3.869

Dalakas, M. C. (2020). Progress in the therapy of myasthenia gravis: Getting closer to effective targeted immunotherapies. *Current Opinion in Neurology, 33*(5), 545–552. https://doi.org/10.1097/wco.0000000000000858

Deng, J., Yu, X. Q., & Wang, P. H. (2019). Inflammasome activation and Th17 responses. *Molecular Immunology, 107*, 142–164. https://doi.org/10.1016/j.molimm.2018.12.024

Devant, P., et al. (2023). Structural insights into cytokine cleavage by inflammatory caspase-4. *Nature, 624*(7991), 451–459. https://doi.org/10.1038/s41586-023-06751-9

Dransfield, I., et al. (1992). Divalent cation regulation of the function of the leukocyte integrin LFA-1. *The Journal of Cell Biology, 116*(1), 219–226. https://doi.org/10.1083/jcb.116.1.219

Dudley, M. E., et al. (2002). Cancer regression and autoimmunity in patients after clonal repopulation with antitumor lymphocytes. *Science, 298*(5594), 850–854. https://doi.org/10.1126/science.1076514

Eberhard, J. M., et al. (2014). CD161+ MAIT cells are severely reduced in peripheral blood and lymph nodes of HIV-infected individuals independently of disease progression. *PLoS One, 9*(11), Article e111323. https://doi.org/10.1371/journal.pone.0111323

Ellison-Wright, I., Ellison-Wright, Z., & Bullmore, E. (2008). Structural brain change in attention deficit hyperactivity disorder identified by meta-analysis. *BMC Psychiatry, 8*(1), 51. https://doi.org/10.1186/1471-244X-8-51

Elsadek, A. E., et al. (2020). Serum levels of Interleukin-6 and tumor necrosis factor alpha in children with attention-deficit hyperactivity disorder. *Journal of Pediatric Neurosciences, 15*(4), 402–408. https://doi.org/10.4103/jpn.JPN_1_20

Felley, L. E., et al. (2016). Human invariant NKT cells induce IL-1β secretion by peripheral blood monocytes via a P2X7-independent pathway. *The Journal of Immunology, 197*(6), 2455–2464.

Gajdos, P., et al. (1984). High-dose intravenous gammaglobulin for myasthenia gravis. *Lancet, 1*(8373), 406–407. https://doi.org/10.1016/s0140-6736(84)90469-0

Gajdos, P., et al. (1997). Clinical trial of plasma exchange and high-dose intravenous immunoglobulin in myasthenia gravis. Myasthenia Gravis Clinical Study Group. *Annals of Neurology, 41*(6), 789–796. https://doi.org/10.1002/ana.410410615

Huppa, J. B., & Davis, M. M. (2003). T-cell-antigen recognition and the immunological synapse. *Nature Reviews Immunology, 3*(12), 973–983. https://doi.org/10.1038/nri1245

Kim, S., et al. (2024). Interleukin-18 binding protein (IL-18BP): A long journey from discovery to clinical application. *Immune Network, 24*(1), e1. https://doi.org/10.4110/in.2024.24.e1

Latour, S., & Aguilar, C. (2015). XIAP deficiency syndrome in humans. *Seminars in Cell & Developmental Biology, 39*, 115–123. https://doi.org/10.1016/j.semcdb.2015.01.015

Lee, H.-G., Cho, M.-J., & Choi, J.-M. (2020). Bystander CD4+ T cells: Crossroads between innate and adaptive immunity. *Experimental & Molecular Medicine, 52*(8), 1255–1263. https://doi.org/10.1038/s12276-020-00486-7

Lub, M., van Kooyk, Y., & Figdor, C. G. (1995). Ins and outs of LFA-1. *Immunology Today, 16*(10), 479–483. https://doi.org/10.1016/0167-5699(95)80031-x

Ma, S.-D., et al. (2016). PD-1/CTLA-4 blockade inhibits Epstein-Barr virus-induced lymphoma growth in a cord blood humanized-mouse model. *PLoS Pathogens, 12*(5), e1005642.

Mandala, S., et al. (2002). Alteration of lymphocyte trafficking by sphingosine-1-phosphate receptor agonists. *Science, 296*(5566), 346–349. https://doi.org/10.1126/science.1070238

Meisel, A., et al. (2023). Long-term efficacy and safety of ravulizumab in adults with anti-acetylcholine receptor antibody-positive generalized myasthenia gravis: Results from the phase 3 CHAMPION MG open-label extension. *Journal of Neurology, 270*(8), 3862–3875. https://doi.org/10.1007/s00415-023-11699-x

Miller, S. A., et al. (2008). Coordinated but physically separable interaction with H3K27-demethylase and H3K4-methyltransferase activities are required for T-box protein-mediated activation of developmental gene expression. *Genes & Development, 22*(21), 2980–2993. https://doi.org/10.1101/gad.1689708

Paprckova, D., et al. (2023). Bystander activation in memory and antigen-inexperienced memory-like CD8 T cells. *Current Opinion in Immunology, 82*, Article 102299. https://doi.org/10.1016/j.coi.2023.102299

Patel, M. N., et al. (2017). Inflammasome priming in sterile inflammatory disease. *Trends in Molecular Medicine, 23*(2), 165–180. https://doi.org/10.1016/j.molmed.2016.12.007

Pomary, P. K., et al. (2023). Multifaceted analysis of cerebrospinal fluid and serum from progressive multiple sclerosis patients: Potential role of vitamin C and metal ion imbalance in the divergence of primary progressive multiple sclerosis and secondary progressive multiple sclerosis. *Journal of Proteome Research, 22*(3), 743–757. https://doi.org/10.1021/acs.jproteome.2c00460

Ricardo-Gonzalez, R. R., et al. (2018). Tissue signals imprint ILC2 identity with anticipatory function. *Nature Immunology, 19*(10), 1093–1099. https://doi.org/10.1038/s41590-018-0201-4

Sada-Ovalle, I., et al. (2008). Innate invariant NKT cells recognize mycobacterium tuberculosis-infected macrophages, produce interferon-gamma, and kill intracellular bacteria. *PLoS Pathogens, 4*(12), e1000239. https://doi.org/10.1371/journal.ppat.1000239

Shimizu, Y. (2003). LFA-1: More than just T cell velcro. *Nature Immunology, 4*(11), 1052–1054. https://doi.org/10.1038/ni1103-1052

Silva-Santos, B., Mensurado, S., & Coffelt, S. B. (2019). γδ T cells: Pleiotropic immune effectors with therapeutic potential in cancer. *Nature Reviews Cancer, 19*(7), 392–404. https://doi.org/10.1038/s41568-019-0153-5

Smits, H. H., et al. (2002). Intercellular adhesion molecule-1/LFA-1 ligation favors human Th1 development1. *The Journal of Immunology, 168*(4), 1710–1716. https://doi.org/10.4049/jimmunol.168.4.1710

Somaiah, N., et al. (2024). Malignant peripheral nerve sheath tumor, a heterogeneous, aggressive cancer with diverse biomarkers and no targeted standard of care: Review of the literature and ongoing investigational agents. *Targeted Oncology, 19*(5), 665–678. https://doi.org/10.1007/s11523-024-01078-5

Sudre, G., Mangalmurti, A., & Shaw, P. (2018). Growing out of attention deficit hyperactivity disorder: Insights from the 'remitted' brain. *Neuroscience & Biobehavioral Reviews, 94*, 198–209. https://doi.org/10.1016/j.neubiorev.2018.08.010

Uhlén, M., et al. (2015). Tissue-based map of the human proteome. *Science, 347*(6220), Article 1260419. https://doi.org/10.1126/science.1260419

Vandiedonck, C., Giraud, M., & Garchon, H.-J. (2005). Genetics of autoimmune myasthenia gravis: The multifaceted contribution of the HLA complex. *Journal of Autoimmunity, 25*, 6–11. https://doi.org/10.1016/j.jaut.2005.09.010

Verma, N. K., et al. (2012). Leukocyte function-associated antigen-1/intercellular adhesion molecule-1 interaction induces a novel genetic signature resulting in T-cells refractory to transforming growth factor-β signaling. *Journal of Biological Chemistry, 287*(32), 27204–27216. https://doi.org/10.1074/jbc.M112.376616

Wang, Y., et al. (2008). LFA-1 decreases the antigen dose for T cell activation in vivo. *International Immunology, 20*(9), 1119–1127. https://doi.org/10.1093/intimm/dxn070

Wang, Z., et al. (2018). TRAF6 interacts with and ubiquitinates PIK3CA to enhance PI3K activation. *FEBS Letters, 592*(11), 1882–1892. https://doi.org/10.1002/1873-3468.13080

Xu, X., et al. (2016c). Human iNKT cells promote protective inflammation by inducing oscillating purinergic signaling in monocyte-derived DCs. *Cell Reports, 16*(12), 3273–3285.

Yang, Y., & Cao, Y. (2022). The impact of VEGF on cancer metastasis and systemic disease. *Seminars in Cancer Biology, 86*, 251–261. https://doi.org/10.1016/j.semcancer.2022.03.011

Yang, W., et al. (2004). Activation of integrin beta-subunit I-like domains by one-turn C-terminal alpha-helix deletions. *Proceedings of the National Academy of Sciences U S A, 101*(8), 2333–2338. https://doi.org/10.1073/pnas.0307291101

Yoshimoto, T., et al. (1992). High serum IL-6 level reflects susceptible status of the host to endotoxin and IL-1/tumor necrosis factor. *The Journal of Immunology, 148*(11), 3596–3603. https://doi.org/10.4049/jimmunol.148.11.3596

Zenewicz, L. A., & Flavell, R. A. (2011). Recent advances in IL-22 biology. *International Immunology, 23*(3), 159–163. https://doi.org/10.1093/intimm/dxr001

Zhang, D., et al. (2020). VCAM1 promotes tumor cell invasion and metastasis by inducing EMT and transendothelial migration in colorectal cancer. *Frontiers in Oncology, 10*, 1066. https://doi.org/10.3389/fonc.2020.01066

CHAPTER

Strategies for suppressing immune responses in the brain

3

Ramasamy Vasantharekha[1], S. Winkins Santosh[2], Uday Pratap[3] and Amala Reddy D.[1]

[1]*Department of Biotechnology, School of Bioengineering, SRM Institute of Science and Technology (Deemed to be University), Chennai, Tamil Nadu, India;* [2]*PG & Research Department of Advanced Zoology & Biotechnology, Toxicology Research on Endocrine Disruptors (TRENDS) Laboratory, Government Arts College, Chennai, Tamil Nadu, India;* [3]*Department of Obstetrics and Gynecology, University of Texas Health San Antonio, San Antonio, TX, United States*

1. Introduction

The brain is considered an immunologically restricted organ due to the blood-brain barrier (BBB), which is highly efficient at inhibiting the entry of cellular and humoral components from the blood into the brain. The primary immune cells of the brain are astrocytes, microglia, and oligodendrocytes, which are essential for neural homeostasis and repair. In pathological conditions associated with neurodegenerative diseases, these immune cells are chronically activated. Any injury/infection in the brain disrupts the BBB, permitting the entry of immune cells from the periphery (Smith et al., 1992). Brain damage results in neuronal injury and inflammation, which ultimately leads to immunosuppression. Catecholamines were released when the sympathetic nervous system (SNS) was activated during trauma, injury, lesion, stroke, tumors, and infections in the brain. Catecholamines trigger the release of preformed IL-10, an anti-inflammatory molecule, and inhibit immunosuppression (Plata-Salaman, 1998). Injury to the central nervous system (CNS) disrupts the delicate balance between cellular and molecular integrity, leading to damage to blood vessels and neurons. The key molecular events include impairment of the BBB, cytotoxicity, tissue damage, ionic imbalance, and mitochondrial dysfunction, leading to the generation of reactive oxygen species (ROS), loss of neuronal integrity, glial cell activation, and neuroinflammation (Jassam et al., 2017).

The primary event in CNS damage occurs at the cell membrane, disrupting cellular homeostasis, molecular signaling, ion homeostasis, lipid peroxidation, and cell communication. The abundant glial cells in the brain are microglia and astrocytes. Microglia survey the brain for toxic substances, physiological disturbance, and any injuries. It is activated in pathological conditions such as Alzheimer's disease (AD), Parkinson's disease (PD), and Multiple sclerosis (MS) through the release of proinflammatory cytokines, neurotransmitter imbalance, ionic imbalance, and loss of inhibitory molecules in the brain (Hanisch & Kettenmann, 2007).

Immunotherapies for Neurological Disorders. https://doi.org/10.1016/B978-0-443-44631-3.00003-2

Astrocytes regulate neuronal activity, maintain BBB integrity, and reduce peripheral immune infiltration. It serves as a minor regulator of adaptive and innate immune responses in the brain, maintains neural homeostasis, and protects neural tissue and neurological function following CNS infections and injuries (Rodgers et al., 2020). The brain, considered an immunologically privileged site, is characterized by the concomitant transfer of cells and molecules from the periphery, a process regulated by the neurovascular unit. Studies have reported that T cells, B cells, dendritic cells, and natural killer cells (NK cells) are present in the brain, and that alterations in the neurovascular unit may induce a pathological state in the CNS (Zou et al., 2022).

In Alzheimer's disease [AD], the infiltrated T cells are found surrounding the amyloid β (Aβ) protein aggregates and tau proteins. Amyloid aggregates increase peripheral T-cell migration in the brain (Zou et al., 2022). BBB disruption facilitates the entry of NK cells and the infiltration of other immune cells through the expression of cytokines and chemokines. The mobilization of immune cells is driven by central nervous system inflammation, and astrocytes express proteins that further exacerbate neuroinflammation by triggering advanced glycation end products (RAGE) and sustaining the inflammatory response (Zou et al., 2022). Immune cells in the CNS are activated by infection, neurotoxicity, trauma, autoimmune disorders, and neurodegeneration, thereby triggering neuroinflammation. Long-term activation of immune cells dysregulates oxidative stress, synaptic dysfunction, oncogenic process, glioma, and tumor microenvironment (TME).

Aging and neurodegenerative disease are associated with a decline in immune function, primarily due to thymic involution, changes in the ratio of regulatory and cytotoxic T cells, lymphopenia, and ultimately, immunosenescence. Increased levels of astrocytes were observed in the aged brain due to senescence, which in turn triggers the release of excessive pro-inflammatory cytokines (Ladomersky et al., 2020). Immunosuppression is a critical barrier to neurological disorders, patient health outcomes, and survival, as well as the effectiveness of immune-modulating therapies. In neuroinflammation and neurological disorders, the immune system's functions and the underlying mechanisms of autoimmune disorders and immunosuppression remain largely unknown. The activation and infiltration of immune cells have been central areas of research in neuropathology and neuroimmunology. The primary and secondary lymphoid organs were affected during immunosuppression (Bao et al., 2025).

Systemic immunosuppression in neurological diseases is directly linked to neuronal cell damage, neuroinflammation, and brain injury, as well as to its harmful effects on thymic homeostasis and the brain-thymus axis (Ayasoufi et al., 2020). Systemic immunosuppression is mediated by $CD4^+$ and $CD25^+$ regulatory T cells (Tregs), which, in turn, impair the function of cytotoxic T cells. The imbalance in Tregs results in the dysregulation of Th1 and Th2 cytokines in tumors and lymphopenia. The immune responses were suppressed by $CD4^+$ and $CD8^+$ T cells in glioblastomas and in patients with low-grade gliomas. A decline in adaptive immunity and an increase in inflammation result from an imbalance between neutrophils and lymphocytes (Stepanenko et al., 2024).

T-cell elimination in the bone marrow, shrinkage of lymphoid organs, early activation of T-cell signaling, defective calcium mobilization, and blockage of T-cell proliferation and function lead to immunosuppression. In ischemic stroke, peripheral immunosuppression occurs after pneumonia infection, predominantly followed by brain injury, susceptibility to infections, splenic atrophy, and systemic immune dysregulation (Lorrey et al., 2022). The leading cause of death in CNS injury is infection, which induces disruption in the immune system and CNS that leads to immunodeficiency and suppression. The ANS responds immediately to the injuries and systemic infections by producing anti-inflammatory molecules. Both brain and spinal cord injuries result in the secretion of inflammatory molecules, disruption of neural-immune interactions, and downregulation of innate and adaptive immune responses. Phagocytosis by granulocytes was compromised by monocyte deactivation induced by brain immunosuppression. Monocyte inactivation is associated with decreased expression of membrane-bound secretory molecules, impaired antigen presentation, and reduced lymphocyte proliferation (Meisel et al., 2005).

The neuroendocrine signals modulate immune mediators, control inflammation, coordinate immune responses with the fight-or-flight response and stress responses, and feed back to the brain to regulate neurotransmitter activity. The HPA axis secretes glucocorticoids, and the SNS secretes noradrenaline to regulate immune cells (Irwin & Cole, 2011). The immune mediators, neurotransmitters, and neuropeptides activate similar signaling pathways via G protein-coupled receptors. The immune cells also have receptors for signaling molecules, neurotransmitters, and neuropeptides, which activate the molecular machinery. The effects of neurotrophic factors on immune cells and their responses remain incompletely understood (Sternberg, 2006). Neuroinflammation was arrested at the injury site in the CNS by microglia and astrocytes. Immune regulation that compensates for inflammatory reactions in the brain is crucial for reducing damage and dysregulation of immune cells, which can lead to an imbalance and failure to restore brain homeostasis. Interpreting injuries and infections in specific brain regions and identifying the molecular pathways associated with them are crucial for the development of effective immunomodulatory therapies and anti-inflammatory drugs. A substantial body of research is required to elucidate the intricacies of neural-immune interactions, the mechanisms of neural-immune regulation, the roles of inflammatory molecules, and the significance of T cells and their signals in CNS perturbations (Russo & McGavern, 2015).

Acute and chronic intracellular infections, as well as the tumor microenvironment, activate Th1 cells, which secrete the proinflammatory cytokine IFN-γ, thereby recruiting immune cells to the CNS. Th1 cells target glial cells, inducing the release of pro-inflammatory cytokines (TNF-α, IL-1β), nitric oxide, and reactive oxygen species, thereby creating a cytotoxic microenvironment. These proinflammatory cytokines impair neuronal function and oligodendrocyte function, leading to neuronal death and further enhancing peripheral immune invasion by destabilizing the BBB (Angelini et al., 2023; Valiukas et al., 2025). Chronic inflammation triggers Th17 cells, which may initiate CNS tissue damage, drive inflammatory responses, and contribute to neurodegeneration. IL-17 induces endothelial cell dysfunction in the brain, increasing BBB permeability and facilitating the entry of pathogenic T cells from the periphery (Shi et al., 2022). Tregs maintain immune homeostasis and inhibit autoimmunity, thereby reducing the risk of inflammatory diseases. Anti-inflammatory cytokines are produced by Tregs to suppress T-cell and microglial activation and the production of proinflammatory cytokines and costimulatory molecules (Wan, 2010).

The pattern recognition receptors detect damage-associated molecular patterns (DAMPs) or pathogen-associated molecular patterns (PAMPs) in neuroinflammation. Damaged neurons activate NF-κB and upregulate the production of proinflammatory cytokines. Cytotoxicity signals, such as caspase-1 activation, mitochondrial dysfunction, protein aggregation, and extracellular ATP, are detected by the nucleotide-binding domain-like receptor protein 3 (NLRP3) inflammasome. Communication between neurons and glial cells is disrupted by sustained immune cell activation (Hu et al., 2025). The contribution of DAMPs to neuroinflammation arises from their stimulation of glial cells, their induction of BBB injury, and their release of proinflammatory cytokines. Neuroinflammation triggers the disease progression in aging, stroke, infections and trauma by abnormal activation of NLRP3. Chronic inflammatory condition, continued activation of glial cells, and demyelination are observed in Multiple Sclerosis (MS) and autoimmune diseases of the CNS. Neuroinflammation is associated with numerous brain pathologies, including amyloid-β plaque deposition, neurofibrillary tangle formation, hyperphosphorylation of tau proteins in AD, loss of dopaminergic neurons, α-synuclein aggregation, and motor dysfunction in PD (Domínguez Rojo et al., 2024; Zhang et al., 2024). The tumor microenvironment (TME) in the brain induces hypoxic conditions, aberrant angiogenesis, and tissue remodeling, thereby triggering an inflammatory response via disruption of the BBB. Immune cell infiltration exacerbates inflammation by compromising BBB integrity (Alghamri et al., 2021).

1.1 Cellular and molecular signaling pathways

The Rel family transcription factor NF-κB plays an important role in cell survival, immune response and inflammation. Compared with peripheral tissues, NF-κB expression is abundant in the brain, particularly in glutamatergic neurons, the cerebral cortex, and the hippocampus. At the molecular level, NF-κB induces inflammation, which is regulated by various transcription factors and molecules. In neurodegenerative diseases such as AD and PD, NF-κB activation can lead to nitric oxide (NO) synthesis, microglial activation, and the release of ROS and proinflammatory cytokines (Niranjan, 2013; Shih et al., 2015). In AD, NF-κB signaling increases proinflammatory cytokine levels, regulates BACE1 gene expression, and contributes to neurodegeneration. The translocation of NF-κB in dopaminergic neurons recruits genes encoding proinflammatory cytokines, ROS, and dopamine autooxidation in PD. ROS damage neurons, inducing apoptosis, stimulate α-synuclein aggregation in the substantia nigra, and lead to neurodegeneration (Singh & Singh, 2020).

The Janus kinase and signal transducer and activator of transcription (JAK/STAT) pathway is primarily activated by cytokines to drive inflammatory and immune responses, including the initiation of innate and adaptive immunity. This pathway is important in hippocampal synaptic plasticity, synchronises the function of myeloid and lymphoid cells, and plays a dual role in cell proliferation and death. Impairment of the JAK/STAT pathway activates T cells into pathogenic forms and induces neuroinflammation and cell death in AD and PD (Liu et al., 2015). STAT1 regulates immune functions, controls cytokine production, and inhibits apoptosis in immune cells. IFN-mediated STAT1 signaling modulates the balance between Th1 and Th2 cells. Astrocytes activate various intracellular signaling pathways, NF-κB, JAK/STAT and MAPK, in response to extracellular signals such as growth factors, nucleotides, and cytokines. The JAK/STAT3 pathway is activated in disease conditions such as multiple sclerosis (MS), stroke, AD, PD, spinal cord injury, and epilepsy, independent of neuroinflammation (Jain et al., 2022).

The central facilitator of the immune response triggered by DNA is Cyclic guanosine monophosphate-adenosine monophosphate synthase-stimulator of interferon genes (cGAS-STING) signaling pathway. It activates type I interferon signaling in inflammatory conditions that, in turn, leads to neurodegeneration (Paul et al., 2021). Inflammatory conditions and the production of proinflammatory cytokines and chemokines are activated by STING through inhibition of the inhibitor of kappa B kinase (IKK), thereby activating NF-κB. Unusual activation of cGAS-STING drives glial activation, sustained neuroinflammation, motor neuron degeneration, and neuronal damage in neurodegenerative diseases such as AD, HD, and PD (Dhapola et al., 2025). Mitochondrial DNA (mtDNA) is released in the cytosolic region in neurodegenerative diseases due to oxidative stress, and mitochondrial dysfunction activates cGAS, which aggravates neuroinflammation (Min et al., 2025).

2. Immunosuppression in the brain

The tumor microenvironment (TME) and brain cancers cause severe systemic T-cell deficits and dysfunctions at the molecular level, leading to immunosuppression. DNA damage, including telomere shortening due to excess ROS production, induces T-cell senescence in the brain. Thymic involution, a reduction in naïve T-cell populations in the thymus, and decreased T-cell receptor levels were correlated with cancer. The tumor microenvironment alters T-cell function both centrally and peripherally, thereby preventing the anti-tumor response. T-cells are prevented from encountering antigenic determinants by the blood-brain barrier and tumor cells, resulting in T-cell ignorance (Grabowski et al., 2021). The immunosuppression in tumor cells is characterized by the secretion of cytokines by tumor cells, glial cells, and macrophages. IL-6, IL-10, and TGF-β mutually inhibit innate and adaptive immune responses by silencing NK-cell activity, activating T cells, promoting apoptosis, and downregulating major histocompatibility complex class I expression. Tissue hypoxia, resulting from the higher oxygen consumption in tumors, activates the immunosuppressive STAT3 pathway, leading to the synthesis of hypoxia-inducible factor-1 alpha (HIF-1α), the activation of regulatory T cells, and the secretion of vascular endothelial growth factor (VEGF) (Brown et al., 2018). Antigen presentation is inhibited by NK cells as TGF-β suppresses the activation of lymphocytes and NK cells. Cytotoxic T cells have been depleted during tumor growth in the CNS. A neural circuit is formed among the CNS, PNS, and immune cells, relaying information from the brain to tumors and immune cells and conveying information back to the brain. The sensory and vagus nerves collect information from tumors and immune cells and send it back to the brain. The suprachiasmatic nucleus coordinates peripheral tissues and the circadian rhythm of the CNS through the gut-brain and hypothalamic-pituitary-adrenal (HPA) axes. The SNS activates neurons in the central nucleus of the amygdala and the paraventricular nucleus, thereby inducing the secretion of corticotropin-releasing hormone (CRH) in the TME (Pu et al., 2025). Microglia activate pro-inflammatory (M1 phenotype) cytokines or anti-inflammatory cytokines (M2 phenotype) during tissue damage and repair. Regulatory T cells (Tregs) and tumor-associated macrophages are immunosuppressive cells in tumors that affect the immune response (Mathur et al., 2024).

3. Systemic and local immunosuppression in the brain

The immune-modulating therapies failed in the neurological damage due to stroke, tumors, traumatic brain injury, infections and glioblastoma following suppression in the neural immune function (Ayasoufi et al., 2019). The exact mechanism of immunosuppression remains unclear. The primary and secondary lymphoid organs were affected by local immunosuppression induced by neurological disorders (Ritzel et al., 2018). The functions of the immune cells in the periphery are affected by CNS infections in aging through neuronal signaling and the release of soluble signaling molecules. The etiology of immunosuppression at both systemic and local sites remains unknown (Hazeldine et al., 2015).

Recent studies have shown that synaptic connections exist directly between neurons and tumor cells, as well as between paracrine growth factors and excitatory neurons in the brain, which may induce neuronal hyperexcitability. Bidirectional communication occurs between tumors and their associated macrophages, with tumors stimulating cell proliferation and T-cell immune function (Nejo et al., 2025). Deficits in the number and function of T-cells were the foremost observed changes in tumors. Increased ROS production induces DNA damage and telomere shortening, hallmarks of T-cell senescence. The reaction to self-antigens is mediated through negative selection in the thymus, resulting in central tolerance (Theofilopoulos et al., 2017). The suppression of regulatory T cells, followed by their deletion, is a key pathological condition in the development of peripheral tolerance. This peripheral mechanism is hijacked by tumors in the brain, thereby preventing activation of the immune response (Wing & Sakaguchi, 2010). Imperfect activation of the RAS/MAPK pathway and its downstream transcription factors impairs T-cell proliferation and activation, contributing to their dysfunction (Grabowski et al., 2021). The tumor microenvironment inhibits T cell checkpoint signaling in tumor cells and innate immune cells, thereby promoting local immunosuppression (Pinton et al., 2019). Systemic immunosuppression in intracranial malignancies may compromise the naïve T cell population and alter T cell trafficking through adrenergic signaling. A decrease in the $CD4^+$ T helper cell population leads to increased TGF-β expression, resulting in systemic immunosuppression. Damages CD8 T cell cytotoxic activity (Song et al., 2025). The tumors have a higher proportion of microglia and macrophages, as well as myeloid cells. The production of pro-inflammatory cytokines, upregulation of the STAT1 pathway, CD80, and phagocytosis of tumor cells were characteristic features of the M1 phenotype, whereas the M2 phenotype was characterized by the activation of the STAT3 pathway, followed by the production of anti-inflammatory cytokines (Locarno et al., 2019). Glioblastoma induces local and systemic immunosuppression by downregulating MHC class I and II expression. In glioblastoma, immunosuppression is activated through diverse signaling mechanisms, including tumor-associated macrophages, myeloid-derived suppressor cells, and a dysfunctional antitumor immune response. A decrease in T cell function, reduced class II MHC expression, and activation of secondary lymphoid organs initiate systemic immunosuppression in glioblastoma (Narsinh et al., 2024).

3.1 Antigenic invasion

The CNS was considered an immune-privileged site due to the presence of the BBB and tight endothelial junctions. The CNS exhibits a deficient immune response due to the scarcity of the lymphatic system, dendritic cells, and antigen-presenting cells, as well as a lack of class I and II MHC molecules and an insufficiency in T cell initiation (Aloisi, 1999). Disturbance between the immune and nervous systems, resulting from injury/damage and infection, triggers immunosuppression in the brain. Peripheral immune cells, such as T and B cells, dendritic cells, NK cells, and macrophages, guard the CNS by entering the parenchyma and establish a tough line of defense against infectious agents and noxious stimuli. T cells enter the CNS through the choroid plexus and meninges, while dendritic cells are found in the parenchyma and the choroid plexus in the healthy human brain (Ousman & Kubes, 2012). Dendritic cells detect antigens in the CNS and send them to the T cells in the periphery. Expression of Fas ligand in CNS neurons stimulates Fas-mediated death of infiltrating immune cells. In addition to infections, trauma can elicit or suppress immune responses. Injuries to the brain and spinal cord inhibit the synaptic signaling and hinder the immune response (McDonald et al.,

2010). Accumulation of myelin debris enhances the presence of inhibitors associated with myelin for neurite outgrowth. Secondary damage and neuronal degeneration can be mitigated by the secretion of neurotrophic factors, axonal regeneration, and angiogenesis, which help mitigate excitotoxicity (Li et al., 2005). The regulation of immune cells and their functions in the CNS remains unclear. Reports show that the insular cortex projects to the dorsal motor nucleus of the vagus and the rostral ventrolateral medulla of the ANS. Disruption of the BBB allows the entry of T cells, B cells, and macrophages from the periphery, thereby establishing an immunosuppressive environment in the brain. Immune cells, such as NK cells, dendritic cells, and Tregs, are sparsely, densely, or unevenly distributed in the brain, which affects the immune response (Pu et al., 2025). The functions of dendritic cells, monocytes, NK cells, macrophages, T cells, and B cells were inhibited by the $CD4^+$ Tregs (Arifianto et al., 2023). The tumor cytokine environment shifted toward immunosuppression due to Treg proliferation, concomitant with a poor prognosis. The functions of infiltrating T cells were restricted by Tregs, which inhibited IL-1 production and CCL22 and CCL2 secretion in tumors. The activation of T lymphocytes in the early stages was mediated by cytotoxic T-lymphocyte antigen-4 (CTLA-4) (DeCordova et al., 2020). Activation of FoxP3+ regulatory T cells leads to the production of immunosuppressive cytokines, which inhibit T-cell proliferation and induce tissue hypoxia. IL-6, IL-10, TGF-β, and prostaglandin E2 were immunosuppressive cytokines present in the TME, and tumor-promoting cytokines such as IL-1 and basic fibroblast growth factor were also present. T-cell activation and proliferation are blocked, thereby inhibiting IL-2 production. NK cell activity was suppressed by TGF-β-mediated immune suppression (Razavi et al., 2016).

3.2 Chronic stress and immunosuppression

The SNS and HPA axis are the two key pathways that connect stress through the activation of the neuroendocrine system, which in turn triggers the microglia, the resident immune cells of the brain, and releases the stress hormone cortisol, as well as modulates the synthesis of neurotransmitters in the brain. Chronic stress increases cortisol levels in the brain, suppresses immune cell function, and alters cytokine production through the HPA axis (Segerstrom & Miller, 2004). A decline in circulating T cells and NK cells, along with decreased antibody production, weakens immune function, thereby augmenting infections and chronic inflammatory conditions under stress (Cohen et al., 2007). In individuals with chronic stress conditions and insomnia, there was a decrease in lymphocyte proliferation, indicating impaired immune function (Dressle et al., 2022). SNS plays a major role in the release of catecholamines during its activation. Adrenaline and noradrenaline released during stress conditions enhance the functions of NK cells and macrophages, while inhibiting the adaptive immune function by altering the functions of T and B cells. Persistent exposure to catecholamine downregulates the $CD4^+$ and $CD8^+$ T cell receptor expression and leads to a decline in T cell activation and proliferation (Zefferino et al., 2020). Alteration of gene expression is a causative factor in prolonged inflammatory conditions that is concomitant with various health issues like mental disorders, anxiety and depression. An imbalance between pro- and anti-inflammatory cytokines may contribute to immune dysregulation under chronic stress (Illi et al., 2012). SNS activity was regulated by the circadian rhythm, but this rhythm was disrupted by chronic stress. Adaptive immune responses were impaired by cortisol and norepinephrine, thereby disrupting homeostasis and influencing disease progression (Dumbell et al., 2016). Stress increases the number of Treg cells and augments immunoregulation, while cytotoxic T cell and NK cell activity is suppressed, thereby diminishing immune cell activity and increasing vulnerability to infection and tumor development (Balakin et al., 2025).

4. Strategies for suppressing the immune response in the brain

4.1 Immunotherapy

Immunotherapy modulates the host's innate immune response by either enhancing or suppressing the immune response to target cells. Several immunotherapies were under investigation due to the challenges in the BBB. Immunotherapy promotes T-cell activation and enhances their cytotoxicity by targeting the cytotoxic T-lymphocyte-associated protein (CTLA-4) and regulating the immune microenvironment. Tumor-associated antigens, cytotoxic T lymphocytes, checkpoint inhibitors such as PD-1, and the transfer of immune cells were under consideration (Riley et al., 2019). Peptides, aptamers, and antibodies can target tumor-cell receptors and enhance therapeutic efficacy by reprogramming immune cells from pro-tumorigenic to anti-tumorigenic states. Immunosuppressive factors can be neutralized to enhance immune cell infiltration (Hristova-Panusheva et al., 2024). Immune stimulators might be used to activate the immune cells, such as dendritic cells and macrophages, for immunotherapy in neurological complications (Gao et al., 2019). The integration of nanoparticles with immune-specific ligands may enable the precise delivery of immunotherapeutic agents. The nanoparticle-coated drug delivery system, engineered with specific ligands, improves its ability to cross the BBB (Juhairiyah & de Lange, 2021). Nanogel-based immunotherapy can be suggested with various ligands and polymers to target brain tumors and enhance therapeutic efficiency. Nanogels are cross-linked polymers of antigens and biomolecules that, when combined with immune checkpoint inhibitors, enhance the therapeutic efficacy of these agents, making them suitable for systemic delivery in immunotherapy (Myint et al., 2023). Polypeptides, antibodies, and nucleic acids are effective immune agents used in immunotherapy and play a crucial role in regulating both humoral and cell-mediated immune responses (Mesquita et al., 2022). Polymeric substances that are biocompatible and biodegradable can load immune substances with high loading capacity, making them suitable for brain immunotherapy (Mohanty et al., 2020). Polymeric substances act as immune stimulators, activate T cells, and present antigens effectively by targeting specific receptors, thereby increasing cellular uptake in immunotherapy (Yalamandala et al., 2025).

Adoptive T-cell therapies show promise as a therapeutic approach for tumors, in which T cells are isolated from patients, expanded ex vivo, and then transferred back to the patients (Zhang et al., 2022). Chimeric antigen receptor (CAR) T-cell therapy links the antibody's antigen-recognition domain with the T-cell activation domain to express CARs (Choi et al., 2019). CAR-T cells bypass antigen presentation and, by targeting tumor antigens in an MHC-independent manner, identify and kill cancer cells. CAR-T-cell therapy shows a positive response in patients with acute lymphoblastic leukemia and B-cell lymphoma, but is still challenging for solid brain tumors (Bhardwaj et al., 2018). A pilot study was conducted using intrathecal CAR-T-cell infusion into the ventricular system for tumors in the intracranial and spinal cord. The severity and toxicity of tumors were reduced following intracranial infusion. There was a reduction in tumor burden and necrosis in patients who received intracranial administration of IL-13Rα2 and recombinant human IL-2 for GBM, resulting in improved clinical outcomes in 50% of patients (Mende et al., 2021). Immune checkpoint inhibitors maintain tolerance to self-antigens and prevent autoimmunity. Immune checkpoint molecules such as PD-1, PD-L1, and

CTLA-4 were associated with a higher incidence of tumor recovery. PD-1 is initiated by CD274, which is expressed on antigen-presenting cells and is associated with programmed cell death. PD-1 expression was associated with solid gliomas in the brain, and administration of a PD-1 inhibitor increased the immune response in these tumors (Majd et al., 2020). In GBM, the efficiency of immunotherapy was hampered by the immunosuppressive environment. NK cells, without the help of antigen-presenting cells, coordinate crosstalk between T cells and dendritic cells, thereby facilitating the elimination of malignant cells. NK cells influence immunity by activating T cells, mediated by dendritic cells, through the recognition and elimination of cells that lack self-MHC class I molecules (Gunaydin & Bilge, 2018).

4.2 Anti-inflammatory drugs

Anti-inflammatory medications were designed to mitigate pro-inflammatory signaling, repair immune dysfunction, and lessen the harmful effects of inflammation on neuronal functions. These drugs suppressed cyclooxygenase (COX) activity, thereby reducing prostaglandin and inflammatory molecule synthesis (Reichardt et al., 2021). Anti-inflammatory molecules, such as corticosteroids, repress the immune response through glucocorticoid receptor signaling. They are used to reduce swelling in TBI conditions, immunosuppression, metabolic abnormalities, and acute neuroinflammatory conditions (Sampson et al., 2020). Anti-inflammatory medications play a complex role in brain immunotherapy, influencing the control of harmful immune responses and the effectiveness of treatment. They are essential components of therapeutic strategies for brain disorders, particularly brain tumors and neurodegenerative diseases, owing to their dual capacity to reduce neuroinflammation and modulate immune cell activity (Mehta et al., 2019).

Anti-inflammatory drugs, especially corticosteroids and nonsteroidal anti-inflammatory drugs (NSAIDs), act by reducing the production of proinflammatory cytokines and by blocking signals that facilitate the migration of immune cells into the brain. By limiting inflammation, these drugs protect fragile nerve structures from immune-mediated damage, which is especially important during immunotherapy. In treating brain tumors and neurodegenerative diseases, these drugs are often given with immunotherapies to manage side effects like immune-related adverse events (irAEs), brain swelling, and inflammation caused by immune checkpoint blockade. Both experimental and clinical studies demonstrate that anti-inflammatory treatments can mitigate harmful neuroinflammatory responses, maintain blood-brain barrier integrity, and improve neurological outcomes (Pacelli et al., 2015).

However, suppressing immune activity in the brain can also inadvertently reduce the effectiveness of immunotherapies in activating anti-tumor immune responses (Bianchi et al., 2000). This can ultimately weaken treatment effectiveness. For example, corticosteroids like dexamethasone are commonly used to manage cerebral edema. However, they can interfere with the recruitment and activation of cytotoxic T cells. This limits the effectiveness of immunotherapies in targeting cancer cells in conditions like glioblastoma (Xing et al., 2015). Recent findings show that reducing both the dose and duration of immunosuppressive drugs during immunotherapy is crucial for increasing anti-tumor (Kartolo et al., 2021). This highlights the need for careful clinical management and the development of selective agents that maintain beneficial immune responses while limiting harmful inflammation (Tables 3.1 and 3.2).

Corticosteroids, such as dexamethasone, are the primary intervention for treating central nervous system (CNS) inflammation during immunotherapies, particularly for patients receiving immune checkpoint inhibitors (ICIs) or those with edema secondary to brain tumors (Goodman et al., 2023). These medications effectively suppress the inflammatory cascade by inhibiting pro-inflammatory cytokines and suppressing T cell activation. The onset of dexamethasone's mechanism of action provides timely symptom relief in patients and rapidly reverses cerebral edema and, hence, mass effect, which is valuable in the acute neurological setting (Nieblas-Bedolla et al., 2021). Nevertheless, because of their broad immunosuppressive mechanisms, steroids can do more than relieve symptoms; they may also affect critical processes underlying antitumor immunity, such as lymphocyte trafficking and tumor antigen recognition (Ellingson et al., 2017). Clinical trials subject to bias and even animal-based research have consistently demonstrated that the use of steroids, particularly in conjunction with immunotherapy, can dampen the activity of effector immune cells, preventing the potential therapeutic effect of other anti-tumor therapies, including checkpoint blockade, and result in worse survival outcomes in preclinical and clinical patient populations with brain tumors (Goldman et al., 2022).

Given these opposing effects, the timing, dosage, and selection of steroids should be carefully considered to preserve the advantages of immunotherapeutic approaches (Ekdahl et al., 2003). Retrospective studies and clinical trial evidence suggest that steroid administration before and/or during initiation of immunotherapy is associated with lower response rates, shorter progression-free survival, and reduced overall survival in patients with glioblastoma and brain metastases (Somera-Molina et al., 2007). To mitigate the risk of steroid immunosuppression, clinicians are generally encouraged to use the lowest effective steroid dose for the minimum time necessary (typically tapering the dose as symptoms improve). The development of novel therapeutic options and more selective anti-inflammatory agents aims to lessen the dependence on steroid medications and optimize immunotherapeutic strategies in neuro-oncological practice (Lonergan et al., 2002).

Novel strategies targeting neuroinflammation in the brain have begun to focus on selective inhibition of specific inflammatory mediators to treat neurological diseases and cancers with minimal immunosuppression (Jenrow et al., 2013). Such strategies involve developing small-molecule inhibitors that target selective pathways, such as inhibiting pro-inflammatory cytokine production by activated microglial cells and the signaling molecules *P*38α MAPK, STAT3, and iNOS (Miller et al., 2021). In preclinical animal studies, agents such as MW-151, a selective inhibitor of microglial cytokine production, have been shown to reduce neuroinflammation, preserve hippocampal neurogenesis, and improve cognition after brain irradiation (Ribas & Wolchok, 2018). Importantly, these results demonstrate the agent's ability to limit injury while promoting neuronal recovery. Selective agents can, in effect, inhibit the pathological activation of resident immune cells in the brain while allowing innate protective pathways to be engaged, thereby reducing the adverse effects typically observed with systemic immunosuppressive agents (Wang et al., 2020).

4.3 Immunomodulating agents

Immunomodulating agents are a crucial class of drugs that modulate immune responses in the central nervous system. This is particularly relevant for conditions such as neuroinflammation and brain tumors (Liu et al., 2024). These agents either reduce excessive immune activity or improve certain immune functions. By doing so, they maintain a balance between effective treatment and the avoidance of brain damage from therapy (Mariuzza et al., 2024).

Table 3.1 Immunosuppressive agents and their targets.

S.No.	Classical anti-inflammatory and immunosuppressive agents	Targeted inhibitors of immune signaling pathways	Cytokine/chemokine modulation
1	Corticosteroids (Prednisolone, Dexamethasone)	JAK inhibitors (Tofacitinib, Baricitinib)	Anti-TNF-α agents (Infliximab, Adalimumab)
2	Non-steroidal anti-inflammatory drugs (NSAIDs: Aspirin, Ibuprofen)	NF-κB pathway inhibitors	IL-6 inhibitors (Tocilizumab, Sarilumab)
3	Calcineurin inhibitors (Cyclosporine, Tacrolimus)	MAPK pathway inhibitors	IL-1 inhibitors (Anakinra, Canakinumab)
4	Antimetabolites (Methotrexate, Azathioprine)	PI3K/Akt/mTOR inhibitors (Sirolimus)	IL-17 inhibitors (Secukinumab)
5	Alkylating agents (Cyclophosphamide)	SYK inhibitors	Chemokine receptor antagonists (CCR5, CXCR4 inhibitors)
6	Mycophenolate mofetil	BTK inhibitors (ibrutinib)	Interferon modulation (IFN-γ, IFN-γ inhibitors)

One example is interferon-beta (IFN-β), which is used to treat multiple sclerosis. It helps reduce neuroinflammation and modulates cytokine release to manage T-cell activation and movement across the blood-brain barrier. Other promising methods involve using targeted delivery of microRNAs and oligonucleotides to immune cells (Feins et al., 2019). These approaches have been effective in experimental autoimmune encephalomyelitis, a preclinical model for multiple sclerosis (Brahm et al., 2020).

Immune checkpoint inhibitors (ICIs), such as ipilimumab and nivolumab, along with new targets like TIM-3, LAG-3, and TIGIT, have revolutionized brain tumor immunotherapy (Brahm et al., 2020). They aim to restore the body's ability to fight tumors within the unique environment of the central nervous system. These agents work by blocking inhibitory pathways on immune cells. This helps reactivate exhausted T cells and improves their ability to detect and eliminate tumor cells in the brain. However, the effectiveness of ICIs in treating primary and metastatic brain tumors is often limited. The brain has a naturally suppressive environment, and the significant diversity among brain tumor cells allows them to dodge immune detection (Umemura et al., 2023). As a result, response rates are typically low, and maintaining tumor control is difficult, especially in cases such as glioblastoma, where the suppressive microenvironment is most severe (Li et al., 2020).

In addition to immune checkpoint inhibitors (ICIs), certain chemotherapy drugs, such as temozolomide, affect the function and distribution of regulatory and effector T cells. This complicates the balance between immune suppression and activation during treatment (Ranjan et al., 2024). To tackle

Table 3.2 Neurological disorders and immunotherapy.

S.No.	Neurologic condition	Targeted immune pathway	Immunotherapy strategy
1	Multiple sclerosis (MS)	Autoreactive T & B cells	Monoclonal antibodies, immune modulators
2	Alzheimer's disease	Amyloid-β, Tau pathology	Passive & active immunotherapy
3	Parkinson's disease	α-synuclein aggregation	Monoclonal antibodies, vaccines
4	Amyotrophic lateral sclerosis (ALS)	Neuroinflammation, microglial activation	Anti-inflammatory immunotherapy
5	Myasthenia gravis	Autoantibodies (AChR, MuSK)	B-cell depletion, complement inhibition
6	Neuromyelitis Optica (NMOSD)	Aquaporin-4 antibodies	Complement & IL-6 blockade
7	Stroke	Post-ischemic inflammation	Immune modulation, cytokine inhibition
8	Brain tumors (glioblastoma)	Tumor immune evasion	Immune checkpoint inhibitors, CAR-T
9	Epilepsy (autoimmune)	Autoimmune synaptic dysfunction	IVIG, plasmapheresis
10	Peripheral neuropathies (GBS, CIDP)	Autoimmune demyelination	Immunoglobulin therapy

these issues, researchers are exploring combination strategies. They are integrating ICIs with other methods, such as vaccines, adoptive cell therapies, and novel delivery techniques, including focused ultrasound. These aim to enhance local immune activity without inducing systemic immune suppression or additional side effects (Akasaki et al., 2016). Recent systematic reviews and analyses of clinical trials suggest that these multifaceted approaches are most promising for addressing challenges in brain tumor immunotherapy. However, more studies on mechanisms and improved treatment plans are needed to achieve lasting benefits (Antonios et al., 2016).

Immunomodulating agents play a crucial role in the treatment of brain diseases in contemporary medicine, serving as potent regulators of the immune environment within the nervous system. These immunomodulating agents include, but are not limited to, monoclonal antibodies, small-molecule inhibitors, and biologics, which may aim to increase immune responses or suppress immune activity, depending on the stage of disease pathophysiology (Bouffet et al., 2016). In neuro-oncological settings, for example, immune checkpoint inhibitors such as ipilimumab (a CTLA-4 inhibitor) and nivolumab (a PD-1 inhibitor) have emerged as the tools of choice for immunomodulating brain tumors (Crane et al., 2012). Immune checkpoint inhibitors work by blocking inhibitory pathways on T cells, thereby enhancing the immune response to tumors. With increased T-cell activity, however, comes the need to manage potentially neurotoxic or autoimmune reactions; therefore, careful medical intervention and evaluation are paramount (Alghamri et al., 2021).

Beyond checkpoint inhibitors, agents targeting cytokines and chemokines are being actively explored for their ability to disrupt deleterious inflammatory signaling cascades. For instance, drugs that block IL-6, TNF-alpha, or interferon gamma have shown promise in dampening neuroinflammatory processes implicated in both tumor progression and neurodegenerative disorders (Moore et al., 2021). Likewise, selective modulators, such as *P*38α MAPK inhibitors, have been shown to attenuate microglial activation and cytokine release without completely abolishing immune function, thereby maintaining protective responses against infection and repair. These targeted therapies represent a significant advancement over conventional broad-spectrum immunosuppressants, as they can preserve host defense while suppressing pathological immune activation (Sur et al., 2020).

Adoptive cell therapies and therapeutic vaccines are also being refined as immunomodulatory interventions for the brain. Regulatory T cell (Treg)-enhancing drugs, for example, can suppress excessive inflammation without completely silencing effector immune cells, making them valuable in settings such as autoimmune encephalitis and transplant tolerance (Kirit et al., 2025). Engineered T cells, dendritic cell vaccines, and oncolytic viruses are among the cell-based innovations that can target CNS lesions, induce antigen-specific immune responses, and help recalibrate the neuroimmune balance. These modalities are often paired with targeted molecular therapies to enhance specificity and minimize off-target effects, thereby advancing the standard of care for complex and refractory brain conditions (Shetty et al., 2025).

Nanotherapeutic approaches and targeted drug delivery systems are emerging to address the challenge posed by the blood-brain barrier while expanding immunomodulatory capacity. Using nanoparticles, liposomes, or focused ultrasound-assisted delivery, clinicians and researchers can enhance the CNS penetration of immunomodulating agents and maximize local efficacy while minimizing systemic toxicities (Harkins et al., 2024a). This precision in drug delivery increases the likelihood of achieving therapeutic concentrations at the disease site, thereby facilitating safer and more effective treatment protocols. Collectively, the continuous evolution of immunomodulating agents and delivery strategies underscores a shift toward tailored interventions that recalibrate neural immune responses to optimize therapeutic benefit (Zhu et al., 2022).

4.4 Gene and RNA-based therapies

Ever since the Human Genome Project, Gene- and RNA-based therapies for diseases across various systems have been at the forefront of innovation. Such therapeutic approaches have also been investigated for suppressing immune responses in the brain and CNS to maximize therapeutic benefit and reduce neuroinflammatory and off-target effects that may otherwise be detrimental (Harkins et al., 2024). In this context, Adeno-associated virus (AAV) vector-mediated therapeutics have been the pioneers. Here, the route of administration directly affects therapeutic potential, with each route offering distinct advantages. Injecting directly into the parenchyma shows a relatively mild and predominantly local immune response, whereas intraparenchymal administration proves advantageous for patients with anti-AAV immunity to be treated, as they bypass circulating antibodies, as the BBB blocks contact with the antibodies. Such local administration of AAV-based therapeutics results in a mild increase in anti-AAV antibodies, with an almost negligible immune response in the CSF and/or T cell and glial activation. On the other hand, systemic targeting via CSF or IV allows easy penetration of vectors across CNS barriers and the peripheral immune system, increasing the risk of B- and T-cell activation, infiltration, and downstream inflammation (Zhao et al., 2015). Although systemic administration has the disadvantages mentioned above, it is often used in combination with immunosuppressive drugs to mitigate activation of both innate and adaptive immune responses. However, these approaches rarely ever refresh immune memory. Hence, research and innovation in capsid engineering using CNS-tropic AAV variants are increasing (Harkins et al., 2024). Other RNA-based therapeutics, including small interfering RNAs (siRNAs), microRNAs (miRNAs), antisense oligonucleotides (ASOs), and in vitro transcribed mRNA, have also been explored for suppressing immune responses in the brain. RNA-based therapeutics offer the advantage of directly modulating gene regulatory pathways and inflammatory cascades, unlike DNA- or protein-based interventions. ASOs function by promoting the degradation of transcripts of immune importance, inhibiting splicing and translation of immunogenic targets within the nervous system (Zhao et al., 2015). These drugs are often used after undergoing a series of chemical modifications, primarily aimed at reducing the activation of immune receptors such as TLRs and RIG-I and at increasing resistance to nucleases (Wan & Seth, 2016).

Additionally, siRNAs and miRNAs can be utilized via the RNA interference (RNAi) pathway to downregulate immune-response-specific genes. In this context, preclinical data provide evidence for their efficacy in silencing inflammatory cytokines and chemokines, preventing neuroinflammation. Nucleotide modification is a common approach in RNA therapeutics, in which modifications such as the addition of pseudouridine or methylcytidine are preferred to target immune receptors and suppress inflammation in the CNS (Zhao et al., 2015). As carriers, lipid nanoparticles, among others, enable targeted delivery, minimizing off-target toxic effects (Gilleron et al., 2013). Recently, the field has seen an increase in exosome and nanoparticle-mediated gene delivery, offering a safer route to traverse the BBB and target the cells precisely with minimal to no toxicity (Harkins et al., 2024). In conclusion, gene and RNA-based therapeutic approaches, when rationally designed for targeted, local administration via nucleotide modification and the addition of specific groups, along with the administration of immunosuppressive drugs if required, hold promise for this area.

4.5 Stem cell therapies

Inflammation and mitochondrial dysfunction were the important features in the pathophysiology and progression of immunosuppression in neurological diseases (Wyss-Coray, 2016). ROS production increases, and bioenergetics are diminished due to mitochondrial dysfunction, which, in turn, triggers the inflammatory response. Cellular damage results from a deficit in protein homeostasis, which ultimately leads to immunosuppression and inflammation. Exacerbation of microglia in the primed state progresses the brain injury and neurodegenerative diseases (Norden et al., 2015). Stem cells possess high proliferative capacity and hold promise as therapeutic targets for many neurological disorders. Various studies in animal models have reported that stem cells can replace dying neurons in the brain and normalize immune function by modulating inflammatory responses and increasing the secretion of therapeutic molecules (Lindvall et al., 2012). Stem cells in the CNS have immunomodulatory properties and inhibit proinflammatory cytokine production in the brain via mesenchymal stem cells. It also influences anti-inflammatory effects by regulating Treg cells, thereby suppressing the production of pro-inflammatory cytokines, and accelerates brain repair after trauma (Neal et al., 2018). The detrimental effects of aging and disease, as well as the therapeutic potential, were mitigated by stem cell therapy (Nguyen et al., 2018). Therapeutic applications of stem cells include the regeneration of neurotrophic factors, immunomodulation, repair of endogenous molecules, and replacement of neuronal cells. Stem cells can differentiate into neuronal and glial cells, promoting the functions of neurotrophic factors and signaling molecules by integrating with the neural circuits of host cells in adverse neurological conditions (Trounson & DeWitt, 2016). Stem cells secrete growth factors that can promote endogenous neural cell regeneration and survival, augment angiogenesis, and enhance neuroplasticity by modulating the immune response (Li et al., 2022). Mesenchymal stem cells (MSCs) interact with microglia, T and B lymphocytes, and regulate their activity through the secretion of soluble factors that support neural repair and restore function. MSCs and adipose-derived stem cells ADSCs) supports nerve regeneration and remyelination following peripheral nerve injury, resulting in sensory and motor deficits (Darehbagh et al., 2024). Stem cells can be delivered to the injured nerve or transplanted to other biomaterial scaffolds. Early-stage clinical trials reported improved sensory and motor function following stem cell therapy in peripheral nerve injuries (Vijayavenkataraman, 2020). Damaged and dead neurons were replaced by activating neural stem cells (NSCs) and differentiating them into neurons or oligodendrocytes, thereby accelerating nerve function. NSCs secrete neurotrophic factors, including NGF and BDNF, and repair damaged nerve cells. Angiogenesis promotes VEGF secretion, generates new blood vessels that provide sufficient nutrients and oxygen to damaged tissues, repairs damaged nerve cells, and enhances nerve tissue to facilitate self-repair (Lu et al., 2003).

5. Conclusion

The maintenance of immune homeostasis is critically dependent on the brain's regulatory capacity and its bidirectional communication with the immune system. This neuroimmune interface ensures coordinated control of systemic and central immune responses, safeguarding physiological integrity. Aging, however, remains the dominant determinant of immune decline, driving immunosenescence that compromises both peripheral and central immune competence. The resulting attenuation of humoral and cell-mediated immunity contributes to increased susceptibility to infection, neurodegeneration, and chronic inflammatory states.

Immunosuppression can arise under diverse pathological conditions, including antigenic challenge, organ transplantation, neoplastic growth, and chronic stress, each of which perturbs neuroimmune equilibrium. Mechanistically, activation of neuroinflammatory pathways and sympathetic nervous system signaling further amplifies immune dysregulation by releasing proinflammatory cytokines and stress mediators.

Therapeutic advances targeting neuroimmune pathways—ranging from anti-inflammatory and immunomodulatory agents to gene, RNA, and stem cell–based interventions—offer promising routes to counteract age-related immune decline. Of particular interest are corticosteroid and other immunomodulatory therapies that modulate the neuroendocrine axis, restoring balance between neural and immune signaling networks. Future work should prioritize integrative approaches to delineate the molecular mechanisms linking neuroimmune communication with systemic immunocompetence, paving the way for targeted interventions to preserve immune health across the lifespan.

The intricate interplay between the nervous and immune systems underscores the fundamental importance of neuroendocrine signaling in maintaining homeostasis within the central nervous system (CNS). Neuroendocrine pathways modulate immune mediators, regulate inflammatory processes, and coordinate immune activity with physiological stress and adaptive responses. Activation of the hypothalamic–pituitary–adrenal (HPA) axis and the sympathetic nervous system (SNS) results in the release of glucocorticoids and noradrenaline, respectively, which exert profound regulatory effects on immune cell function. These interactions are largely mediated by shared signaling cascades, particularly those involving G-protein-coupled receptors. Moreover, the expression of receptors for neurotransmitters, neuropeptides, and other signaling molecules on immune cells facilitates bidirectional communication between neural and immune components.

Despite growing insight into these mechanisms, the influence of neurotrophic factors on immune cell dynamics remains incompletely understood. Within the CNS, microglia and astrocytes play central roles in constraining neuroinflammation and restoring tissue integrity following injury. Precise immune regulation is therefore essential to prevent excessive inflammation, limit secondary neuronal damage, and preserve neural homeostasis.

A deeper understanding of region-specific neural injuries, infection-driven immune responses, and the molecular pathways linking neural and immune networks will be critical for the rational design of targeted immunomodulatory and anti-inflammatory interventions. Future research should delineate the roles of inflammatory mediators, T-cell subsets, and neuroimmune signaling mechanisms in CNS perturbations to inform the development of effective neuroprotective and restorative therapies.

References

Akasaki, Y., Kikuchi, T., Homma, S., Koido, S., Ohkusa, T., Tasaki, T., et al. (2016). Phase I/II trial of combination of temozolomide chemotherapy and immunotherapy with fusions of dendritic and glioma cells in patients with glioblastoma. *Cancer Immunology Immunotherapy, 65*, 1499–1509. https://doi.org/10.1007/s00262-016-1905-7

Alghamri, M. S., McClellan, B. L., Hartlage, C. S., Haase, S., Faisal, S. M., Thalla, R., Dabaja, A., Banerjee, K., Carney, S. V., Mujeeb, A. A., Olin, M. R., Moon, J. J., Schwendeman, A., Lowenstein, P. R., & Castro, M. G. (2021). Targeting neuroinflammation in brain cancer: Uncovering mechanisms, pharmacological targets, and neuropharmaceutical developments. *Frontiers in Pharmacology, 12*, Article 680021. https://doi.org/10.3389/fphar.2021.680021

Aloisi, F. (1999). Antigen presentation in the central nervous system. In G. Martino, & L. Adorini (Eds.), *From basic immunology to immune-mediated demyelination. Topics in neuroscience*. Milano: Springer. https://doi.org/10.1007/978-88-470-2143-3_10

Angelini, G., Bani, A., Constantin, G., & Rossi, B. (2023). The interplay between T helper cells and brain barriers in the pathogenesis of multiple sclerosis. *Frontiers in Cellular Neuroscience, 17*, Article 1101379. https://doi.org/10.3389/FNCEL.2023.1101379

Antonios, J. P., Soto, H., Everson, R. G., Orpilla, J., Moughon, D., Shin, N., et al. (2016). PD-1 blockade enhances the vaccination-induced immune response in Glioma. *JCI Insight, 1*. https://doi.org/10.1172/jci.insight.87059

Arifianto, M. R., Meizikri, R., Haq, I. B., Susilo, R. I., Wahyuhadi, J., Hermanto, Y., & Faried, A. (2023). Emerging hallmark of gliomas microenvironment in evading immunity: A basic concept. *The Egyptian Journal of Neurology, Psychiatry and Neurosurgery, 59*(1), 1–14. https://doi.org/10.1186/s41983-023-00635-5

Ayasoufi, K., K Pfaller, C., H Khadka, R., Jin, F., Zheng, J., R Schuelke, M., Evgin, L., J Hansen, M., T Himes, B., E Fain, C., P Tritz, Z., N Goddery, E., T Yokanovich, L., R Pease, L., G Vile, R., & J Johnson, A. (2019). Scidot-34. Brain injury signals systemic immunosuppression through thymic involution. *Neuro-Oncology, 21* (Suppl. ment_6), vi278–vi279. https://doi.org/10.1093/neuonc/noz175.1170

Ayasoufi, K., Pfaller, Vile, R. G., & Johnson, A. J. (2020). Brain cancer induces systemic immunosuppression through release of non-steroid soluble mediators. *Brain, 143*(12), 3629–3652. https://doi.org/10.1093/brain/awaa343

Balakin, E., Yurku, K., Ivanov, M., Izotov, A., Nakhod, V., & Pustovoyt, V. (2025). Regulation of stress-induced immunosuppression in the context of neuroendocrine, cytokine, and cellular processes. *Biology, 14*(1), 76. https://doi.org/10.3390/biology14010076

Bao, Y., Chen, Z., Su, Y., Guo, T., Du, H., & Jia, X. (2025). From neuroinflammation to gliomagenesis: Immune drivers of malignant transformation in the CNS. *Frontiers in Immunology, 16*, Article 1682030. https://doi.org/10.3389/fimmu.2025.1682030

Bhardwaj, R., Suzuki, A., Leland, P., et al. (2018). Identification of a novel role of IL-13Rα2 in human glioblastoma multiforme: Interleukin-13 mediates signal transduction through AP-1 pathway. *Journal of Translational Medicine, 16*, 369. https://doi.org/10.1186/s12967-018-1746-6

Bianchi, M., Meng, C., & Ivashkiv, L. B. (2000). Inhibition of IL-2-induced Jak-STAT signaling by glucocorticoids. *Proceedings of the National Academy of Sciences, 97*(17), 9573–9578.

Bouffet, E., Larouche, V., Campbell, B. B., Merico, D., de Borja, R., Aronson, M., et al. (2016). Immune checkpoint inhibition for hypermutant glioblastoma multiforme resulting from germline Biallelic mismatch repair deficiency. *Jco, 34*, 2206–2211. https://doi.org/10.1200/jco.2016.66.6552

Brahm, C. G., van Linde, M. E., Enting, R. H., et al. (2020). The current status of immune checkpoint inhibitors in neuro-oncology: A systematic review. *Cancers (Basel), 12*(3), 586. https://doi.org/10.3390/cancers12030586. Published 2020 Mar 4.

Brown, N. F., Carter, T. J., Ottaviani, D., & Mulholland, P. (2018). Harnessing the immune system in glioblastoma. *British Journal of Cancer, 119*(10), 1171–1181. https://doi.org/10.1038/s41416-018-0258-8

Choi, B. D., Yu, X., Castano, A. P., Bouffard, A. A., Schmidts, A., Larson, R. C., et al. (2019). CAR-T cells secreting BiTEs circumvent antigen escape without detectable toxicity. *Nature Biotechnology, 37*(9), 1049–1058. https://doi.org/10.1038/s41587-019-0192-1

Cohen, S., Janicki-Deverts, D., & Miller, G. E. (2007). Psychological stress and disease. *JAMA, 298*, 1685. https://doi.org/10.1001/jama.298.14.1685

Crane, C. A., Ahn, B. J., Han, S. J., & Parsa, A. T. (2012). Soluble factors secreted by glioblastoma cell lines facilitate recruitment, survival, and expansion of regulatory T cells: Implications for immunotherapy. *Neuro-Oncology, 14*, 584–595. https://doi.org/10.1093/neuonc/nos014

Darehbagh, R. R., Seyedoshohadaei, S. A., Ramezani, R., & Rezaei, N. (2024). Stem cell therapies for neurological disorders: Current progress, challenges, and future perspectives. *European Journal of Medical Research, 29*, 386. https://doi.org/10.1186/s40001-024-01987-1

DeCordova, S., Shastri, A., Tsolaki, A. G., Yasmin, H., Klein, L., Singh, S. K., & Kishore, U. (2020). Molecular heterogeneity and immunosuppressive microenvironment in glioblastoma. *Frontiers in Immunology, 11*, Article 535080. https://doi.org/10.3389/fimmu.2020.01402

Dhapola, R., Paidlewar, M., Kumari, S., Sharma, P., Vellingiri, B., Medhi, B., & HariKrishnaReddy, D. (2025). CGAS-STING and neurodegenerative diseases: A molecular crosstalk and therapeutic perspective. *International Immunopharmacology, 159*, Article 114902. https://doi.org/10.1016/j.intimp.2025.114902

Domínguez Rojo, N., Blanco Benítez, M., Cava, R., Fuentes, J. M., Canales Cortés, S., & González Polo, R. A. (2024). Convergence of neuroinflammation, microbiota, and parkinson's disease: Therapeutic insights and prospects. *International Journal of Molecular Sciences, 25*, Article 11629.

Dressle, R. J., Feige, B., Spiegelhalder, K., Schmucker, C., Benz, F., Mey, N. C., & Riemann, D. (2022). HPA axis activity in patients with chronic insomnia: A systematic review and meta-analysis of case–control studies. *Sleep Medicine Reviews, 62*, Article 101588. https://doi.org/10.1016/j.smrv.2022.101588

Dumbell, R., Matveeva, O., & Oster, H. (2016). Circadian clocks, stress, and immunity. *Frontiers in Endocrinology, 7*, 37. https://doi.org/10.3389/fendo.2016.00037

Ekdahl, C. T., Claasen, J. H., Bonde, S., Kokaia, Z., & Lindvall, O. (2003). Inflammation is detrimental for neurogenesis in adult brain. *PNAS, 100*, 13632–13637. https://doi.org/10.1073/pnas.2234031100

Ellingson, B. M., Chung, C., Pope, W. B., Boxerman, J. L., & Kaufmann, T. J. (2017). Pseudoprogression, radionecrosis, inflammation or true tumor progression? Challenges associated with glioblastoma response assessment in an evolving therapeutic landscape. *Journal of Neuro-Oncology, 134*, 495–504. https://doi.org/10.1007/s11060-017-2375-2

Feins, S., Kong, W., Williams, E. F., Milone, M. C., & Fraietta, J. A. (2019). An introduction to chimeric antigen receptor (CAR) T-cell immunotherapy for human cancer. *American Journal of Hematology, 94*, S3–S9.

Gao, S., Yang, D., Fang, Y., Lin, X., Jin, X., Wang, Q., Wang, X., Ke, L., & Shi, K. (2019). Engineering nanoparticles for targeted remodeling of the tumor microenvironment to improve cancer immunotherapy. *Theranostics, 9*, 126–151.

Gilleron, J., Querbes, W., Zeigerer, A., Borodovsky, A., Marsico, G., Schubert, U., et al. (2013). Image-based analysis of lipid nanoparticle-mediated siRNA delivery, intracellular trafficking and endosomal escape. *Nature Biotechnology, 31*, 638–646.

Goldman, M., Lucke-Wold, B., Martinez-Sosa, M., et al. (2022). Steroid utility, immunotherapy, and brain tumor management: An update on conflicting therapies. *Exploration of Targeted Anti-tumor Therapy, 3*(5), 659–675. https://doi.org/10.37349/etat.2022.00106

Goodman, R. S., Johnson, D. B., & Balko, J. M. (2023). Corticosteroids and cancer immunotherapy. *Clinical Cancer Research, 29*(14), 2580–2587. https://doi.org/10.1158/1078-0432.CCR-22-3181

Grabowski, M. M., Sankey, E. W., Ryan, K. J., et al. (2021). Immune suppression in gliomas. *Journal of Neuro-Oncology, 151*, 3–12. https://doi.org/10.1007/s11060-020-03483-y

Gunaydin, C., & Bilge, S. S. (2018). Effects of nonsteroidal anti-inflammatory drugs at the molecular level. *Eurasian Journal of Medicine, 50*, 116–121.

Hanisch, U. K., & Kettenmann, H. (2007). Microglia: Active sensor and versatile effector cells in the normal and pathologic brain. *Nature Neuroscience, 10*(11), 1387–1394. https://doi.org/10.1038/nn1997

Harkins, A. L., Ambegaokar, P. P., & Keeler, A. M. (2024a). Immune responses to central nervous system directed adeno-associated virus gene therapy: Does direct CNS delivery make a difference? *Neurotherapeutics: The Journal of the American Society for Experimental NeuroTherapeutics, 21*(4), Article e00435.

Hazeldine, J., Lord, J. M., & Belli, A. (2015). Traumatic brain injury and peripheral immune suppression: Primer and prospectus. *Frontiers in Neurology, 6*, Article 165019. https://doi.org/10.3389/fneur.2015.00235

Hristova-Panusheva, K., Xenodochidis, C., Georgieva, M., & Krasteva, N. (2024). Nanoparticle-mediated drug delivery systems for precision targeting in oncology. *Pharmaceuticals, 17*, 677.

Hu, X., Qi, D., Li, S., Ye, S., Chen, Y., Cao, W., et al. (2025). Development and validation of an interpretable machine learning model for prediction of the risk of clinically ineffective reperfusion in patients following thrombectomy for ischemic stroke. *Therapeutics and Clinical Risk Management, 21*, 621–631. https://doi.org/10.2147/tcrm.S520362

Illi, J., Miaskowski, C., Cooper, B., Levine, J. D., Dunn, L., West, C., Dodd, M., Dhruva, A., Paul, S. M., Baggott, C., et al. (2012). Association between Pro- and anti-inflammatory cytokine genes and a symptom cluster of pain, fatigue, sleep disturbance, and depression. *Cytokine, 58*, 437–447. https://doi.org/10.1016/j.cyto.2012.02.015

Irwin, M., & Cole, S. (2011). Reciprocal regulation of the neural and innate immune systems. *Nature Reviews Immunology, 11*, 625–632. https://doi.org/10.1038/nri3042

Jain, M., Singh, M. K., Shyam, H., Mishra, A., Kumar, S., Kumar, A., & Kushwaha, J. (2022). Role of JAK/STAT in neuroinflammation and its association with neurological disorders. *Annals of Neurosciences, 28*(3–4), 191. https://doi.org/10.1177/09727531211070532

Jassam, Y. N., Izzy, S., Whalen, M., McGavern, D. B., & El Khoury, J. (2017). Neuroimmunology of traumatic brain injury: Time for a paradigm shift. *Neuron, 95*, 1246–1265.

Jenrow, K. A., Brown, S. L., Lapanowski, K., Naei, H., Kolozsvary, A., & Kim, J. H. (2013). Selective inhibition of microglia-mediated neuroinflammation mitigates radiation-induced cognitive impairment. *Radiation Research, 179*(5), 549–556. https://doi.org/10.1667/RR3026.1. Epub 2013 Apr 5. PMID: 23560629; PMCID: PMC3673739.

Juhairiyah, F., & de Lange, E. C. M. (2021). Understanding drug delivery to the brain using liposome-based strategies: Studies that provide mechanistic insights are essential. *AAPS Journal, 23*, 114.

Kartolo, A., Deluce, J., Holstead, R., Hopman, W., Lenehan, J., & Baetz, T. (2021). Impact of baseline corticosteroids on immunotherapy efficacy in patients with advanced melanoma. *Journal of Immunotherapy, 44*(4), 167–174.

Kirit, E., Gokce, C., Altun, B., & Yilmazer, A. (2025). Nanotherapeutic strategies for overcoming the blood–brain barrier: Applications in disease modeling and drug delivery. *ACS Omega, 10*(30), Article 32606. https://doi.org/10.1021/acsomega.5c02206

Ladomersky, E., Zhai, L., Lauing, K. L., Zhang, B., & Wainwright, D. A. (2020). Advanced age increases immunosuppression in the brain and decreases immunotherapeutic efficacy in subjects with glioblastoma. *Clinical Cancer Research, 26*(19), 5232–5245. https://doi.org/10.1158/1078-0432.CCR-19-3874

Li, M., Jiang, Y., Hou, Q., Zhao, Y., Zhong, L., & Fu, X. (2022). Potential pre-activation strategies for improving therapeutic efficacy of mesenchymal stem cells: Current status and future prospects. *Stem Cell Research & Therapy, 13*(1), 146. https://doi.org/10.1186/s13287-022-02822

Li, C., Jiang, P., Wei, S., Xu, X., & Wang, J. (2020). Regulatory T cells in tumor microenvironment: New mechanisms, potential therapeutic strategies and future prospects. *Molecular Cancer, 19*, 116.

Li, W. W., Setzu, A., Zhao, C., & Franklin, R. J. (2005). Minocycline-mediated inhibition of microglia activation impairs oligodendrocyte progenitor cell responses and remyelination in a non-immune model of demyelination. *Journal of Neuroimmunology, 158*, 58–66.

Lindvall, O., Barker, R. A., Brustle, O., Isacson, O., & Svendsen, C. N. (2012). Clinical translation of stem cells in neurodegenerative disorders. *Cell Stem Cell, 10*, 151–155. https://doi.org/10.1016/j.stem.2012.01.009

Liu, Y., Gibson, S. A., Benveniste, E. N., et al. (2015). Opportunities for bench-to-bedside translation: Therapeutic intervention targeting the JAK/STAT pathway in neuroinflammatory diseases. *Critical Reviews in Immunology, 35*(6), 505–527.

Liu, Y., Zhou, F., Ali, H., et al. (2024). Immunotherapy for glioblastoma: Current state, challenges, and future perspectives. *Cellular and Molecular Immunology, 21*, 1354–1375. https://doi.org/10.1038/s41423-024-01226-x

Locarno, C. V., Simonelli, M., Carenza, C., Capucetti, A., Stanzani, E., Lorenzi, E., Persico, P., Della Bella, S., Passoni, L., Mavilio, D., Bonecchi, R., Locati, M., & Savino, B. (2019). Role of myeloid cells in the immunosuppressive microenvironment in gliomas. *Immunobiology, 225*(1), Article 151853. https://doi.org/10.1016/j.imbio.2019.10.002

Lonergan, P. E., Martin, D. S. D., Horrobin, D. F., & Lynch, M. A. (2002). Neuroprotective effect of eicosapentaenoic acid in hippocampus of rats exposed to γ-irradiation. *Journal of Biological Chemistry, 277*, 20804–20811. https://doi.org/10.1074/jbc.M202387200

Lorrey, S. J., Waibl Polania, J., Wachsmuth, L. P., Tritz, Z. P., Edwards, R., Wolf, D. M., Johnson, A. J., Fecci, P. E., & Ayasoufi, K. (2022). Systemic immune derangements are shared across various CNS pathologies and reflect novel mechanisms of immune privilege. *Neuro-Oncology Advances, 5*(1). https://doi.org/10.1093/noajnl/vdad035

Lu, P., Jones, L. L., Snyder, E. Y., & Tuszynski, M. H. (2003). Neural stem cells constitutively secrete neurotrophic factors and promote extensive host axonal growth after spinal cord injury. *Experimental Neurology, 181*(2), 115–129. https://doi.org/10.1016/s0014-4886(03)00037

Majd, N., Dasgupta, P., & de Groot, J. (2020). Immunotherapy for neuro-oncology. In A. Naing, & J. Hajjar (Eds.), *Immunotherapy. Advances in experimental medicine and biology* (Vol 1244). Cham: Springer. https://doi.org/10.1007/978-3-030-41008-7_8

Mariuzza, R. A., Shahid, S., & Karade, S. S. (2024). The immune checkpoint receptor LAG3: Structure, function, and target for cancer immunotherapy. *Journal of Biological Chemistry, 300*, Article 107241.

Mathur, R., Wang, Q., Schupp, P. G., Nikolic, A., Hilz, S., Hong, C., Grishanina, N. R., Kwok, D., Stevers, N. O., Jin, Q., Youngblood, M. W., Stasiak, L. A., Hou, Y., Wang, J., Yamaguchi, T. N., Lafontaine, M., Shai, A.,

Smirnov, I. V., Solomon, D. A., … Costello, J. F. (2024). Glioblastoma evolution and heterogeneity from a 3D whole-tumor perspective. *Cell, 187*(2), 446–463.e16. https://doi.org/10.1016/j.cell.2023.12.013. PMID: 38242087; PMCID: PMC10832360.

McDonald, B., et al. (2010). Intravascular danger signals guide neutrophils to sites of Sterile inflammation. *Science, 330*, 362–366.

Mehta, A., Mahale, R., Buddaraju, K., Javali, M., Acharya, P., & Srinivasa, R. (2019). Efficacy of neuroprotective drugs in acute ischemic stroke: Is it helpful? *Journal of Neurosciences in Rural Practice, 10*, 576–581. https://doi.org/10.1055/s-0039-1700790

Meisel, C., Schwab, J., Prass, K., et al. (2005). Central nervous system injury-induced immune deficiency syndrome. *Nature Reviews Neuroscience, 6*, 775–786. https://doi.org/10.1038/nrn1765

Mende, A. L., Schulte, J. D., Okada, H., & Clarke, J. L. (2021). Current advances in immunotherapy for glioblastoma. *Current Oncology Reports, 23*(2), 21. https://doi.org/10.1007/s11912-020-01007-5

Mesquita, B. S., Fens, M. H. A. M., Di Maggio, A., Bosman, E. D. C., Hennink, W. E., Heger, M., & Oliveira, S. (2022). The impact of nanobody density on the targeting efficiency of pegylated liposomes. *International Journal of Molecular Sciences, 23*, Article 14974.

Miller, K. D., Ostrom, Q. T., Kruchko, C., Patil, N., Tihan, T., Cioffi, G., et al. (2021). Brain and other central nervous system tumor statistics, 2021. *CA: A Cancer Journal for Clinicians, 71*, 381–406.

Min, Y., Lee, Y. S., Lee, J., Keum, D. Y., Gwag, J. Y., Jeon, S. M., Jo, H., & Kang, S. U. (2025). The cGAS–STING pathway in dementia: An emerging mechanism of neuroinflammation. *Brain Sciences, 15*(11). https://doi.org/10.3390/brainsci15111241

Mohanty, A., Uthaman, S., & Park, I. K. (2020). Utilization of polymer-lipid hybrid nanoparticles for targeted anti-cancer therapy. *Molecules, 25*, 4377.

Moore, E. M., Maestas, D. R., Comeau, H. Y., & Elisseeff, J. H. (2021). The immune system and its contribution to variability in regenerative medicine. *Tissue Engineering, Part B: Reviews, 27*, 39–47.

Myint, S. S., Laomeephol, C., Thamnium, S., Chamni, S., & Luckanagul, J. A. (2023). Hyaluronic acid nanogels: A promising platform for therapeutic and theranostic applications. *Pharmaceutics, 15*, 2671.

Narsinh, K. H., Perez, E., Haddad, A. F., et al. (2024). Strategies to improve drug delivery across the blood–brain barrier for glioblastoma. *Current Neurology and Neuroscience Reports, 24*, 123–139. https://doi.org/10.1007/s11910-024-01338-x

Neal, E. G., Acosta, S. A., Kaneko, Y., Ji, X., & Borlongan, C. V. (2018). Regulatory T-cells within bone marrow-derived stem cells actively confer immunomodulatory and neuroprotective effects against stroke. *Journal of Cerebral Blood Flow & Metabolism, 271678X18766172.*

Nejo, T., Krishna, S., Yamamichi, A., Lakshmanachetty, S., Jimenez, C., Lee, K. Y., Baker, D. L., Young, J. S., Chen, T., Phyu, S. S., Phung, L., Gallus, M., Maldonado, G. C., Okada, K., Ogino, H., Watchmaker, P. B., Diebold, D., Choudhury, A., Daniel, A. G., … Okada, H. (2025). Glioma-neuronal circuit remodeling induces regional immunosuppression. *Nature Communications, 16*(1), 1–19. https://doi.org/10.1038/s41467-025-60074-z

Nguyen, H., Zarriello, S., Coats, A., Nelson, C., Kingsbury, C., Gorsky, A., Rajani, M., Neal, E. G., & Borlongan, C. V. (2018). Stem cell therapy for neurological disorders: A focus on aging. *Neurobiology of Disease, 126*, 85. https://doi.org/10.1016/j.nbd.2018.09.011

Nieblas-Bedolla, E., Nayyar, N., Singh, M., Sullivan, R. J., & Brastianos, P. K. (2021). Emerging immunotherapies in the treatment of brain metastases. *The Oncologist, 26*, 231–241. https://doi.org/10.1002/onco.13575

Niranjan, R. (2013). Molecular basis of etiological implications in Alzheimer's disease: Focus on neuroinflammation. *Molecular Neurobiology, 48*, 412–428. https://doi.org/10.1007/s12035-013-8428-4

Norden, D. M., Muccigrosso, M. M., & Godbout, J. P. (2015). Microglial priming and enhanced reactivity to secondary insult in aging, and traumatic CNS injury, and neurodegenerative disease. *Neuropharmacology, 96*, 29–41. https://doi.org/10.1016/j.neuropharm.2014.10.028

Ousman, S., & Kubes, P. (2012). Immune surveillance in the central nervous system. *Nature Neuroscience, 15*, 1096–1101. https://doi.org/10.1038/nn.3161

Pacelli, C., Giguere, N., Bourque, M. J., Levesque, M., Slack, R. S., & Trudeau, L. E. (2015). Elevated mitochondrial bioenergetics and axonal arborization size are key contributors to the vulnerability of dopamine neurons. *Current Biology, 25*, 2349–2360. https://doi.org/10.1016/j.cub.2015.07.050

Paul, B. D., Snyder, S. H., & Bohr, V. A. (2021). Signaling by cGAS–STING in neurodegeneration, neuroinflammation, and aging. *Trends in Neurosciences, 44*(2), 83–96. https://doi.org/10.1016/j.tins.2020.10.008

Pinton, L., Masetto, E., Vettore, M., Solito, S., Magri, S., D'Andolfi, M., et al. (2019). The immune suppressive microenvironment of human gliomas depends on the accumulation of bone marrow-derived macrophages in the center of the lesion. *Journal for ImmunoTherapy of Cancer, 7*, 58. https://doi.org/10.1186/s40425-019-0536-x

Pu, T., Sun, J., Ren, G., & Li, H. (2025). Neuro-immune crosstalk in cancer: Mechanisms and therapeutic implications. *Signal Transduction and Targeted Therapy, 10*(1), 1–33. https://doi.org/10.1038/s41392-025-02241-8

Plata-Salaman, R. C. (1998). Brain injury and immunosuppression. *Nature Medicine, 4*(7), 768–769. https://doi.org/10.1038/nm0798-768

Ranjan, T., Podder, V., Margolin, K., Velcheti, V., Maharaj, A., & Ahluwalia, M. S. (2024). Immune checkpoint inhibitors in the management of brain metastases from non-small cell lung cancer: A comprehensive review of current trials, guidelines and future directions. *Cancers (Basel), 16*(19), 3388. https://doi.org/10.3390/cancers16193388. Published 2024 Oct 3.

Razavi, M., Lee, K. E., Jin, B. E., Aujla, P. S., Gholamin, S., & Li, G. (2016). Immune evasion strategies of glioblastoma. *Frontiers in Surgery, 3*, 11. https://doi.org/10.3389/fsurg.2016.00011

Reichardt, S. D., Amouret, A., Muzzi, C., Vettorazzi, S., Tuckermann, J. P., Lühder, F., & Reichardt, H. M. (2021). The role of glucocorticoids in inflammatory diseases. *Cells, 10*, 2921.

Ribas, A., & Wolchok, J. D. (2018). Cancer immunotherapy using checkpoint blockade. *Science., 359*, 1350–1355.

Riley, R. S., June, C. H., Langer, R., & Mitchell, M. J. (2019). Delivery technologies for cancer immunotherapy. *Nature Reviews Drug Discovery, 18*, 175–196.

Ritzel, R. M., Doran, S. J., Barrett, J. P., Henry, R. J., Ma, E. L., Faden, A. I., & Loane, D. J. (July 1, 2018). Chronic alterations in systemic immune function after traumatic brain injury. *Journal of Neurotrauma, 35*(13), 1419–1436. https://doi.org/10.1089/neu.2017.5399. Epub 2018 May 3. PMID: 29421977; PMCID: PMC5998829.

Rodgers, K. R., Lin, Y., Langan, T. J., Iwakura, Y., & Chou, R. C. (2020). Innate immune functions of astrocytes are dependent upon tumor necrosis factor-alpha. *Scientific Reports, 10*, 7047.

Russo, M., & McGavern, D. B. (2015). Immune surveillance of the CNS following infection and injury. *Trends in Immunology, 36*(10), 637. https://doi.org/10.1016/j.it.2015.08.002

Sampson, J. H., Gunn, M. D., Fecci, P. E., & Ashley, D. M. (2020). Brain immunology and immunotherapy in brain tumours. *Nature Reviews Cancer, 20*(1), 12–25. https://doi.org/10.1038/s41568-019-0224-7

Segerstrom, S. C., & Miller, G. E. (2004). Psychological stress and the human immune system: A meta-analytic study of 30 years of inquiry. *Psychological Bulletin, 130*, 601–630. https://doi.org/10.1037/0033-2909.130.4.601

Shetty, C., Tamatta, R., Dhas, N., & Singh, A. K. (2025). Evolving therapeutic strategies in glioblastoma: Traditional approaches and novel interventions. *3 Biotech, 15*(9), 318. https://doi.org/10.1007/s13205-025-04493-1

Shi, Y., Wei, B., Li, L., et al. (2022). Th17 cells and inflammation in neurological disorders: Possible mechanisms of action. *Frontiers in Immunology, 13*, Article 932152. https://doi.org/10.3389/FIMMU.2022.932152

Shih, R. H., Wang, C. Y., & Yang, C. M. (2015). NF-kappaB signaling pathways in neurological inflammation: A mini review. *Frontiers in Molecular Neuroscience, 8*, 77. https://doi.org/10.3389/fnmol.2015.00077

Singh, S., & Singh, T. G. (2020). Role of nuclear factor kappa B (NF-KB) signalling in neurodegenerative diseases: An mechanistic approach. *Current Neuropharmacology, 18*(10), 918. https://doi.org/10.2174/1570159X18666200207120949

Smith, T. W., Girolami, U. D., & Hickey, W. F. (1992). Neuropathology of immunosuppression. *Brain Pathology, 2*(3), 183–194. https://doi.org/10.1111/j.1750-3639.1992.tb00691.x

Somera-Molina, K. C., Robin, B., Somera, C. A., Anderson, C., Stine, C., Koh, S., et al. (2007). Glial activation links early-life seizures and long-term neurologic dysfunction: Evidence using a small molecule inhibitor of proinflammatory cytokine upregulation. *Epilepsia, 48*, 1785–1800. https://doi.org/10.1111/j.1528-1167.2007.01135.x

Song, K., Lim, M., & Monje, M. (2025). Complex neural-immune interactions shape glioma immunotherapy. *Immunity, 58*(5), 1140–1160. https://doi.org/10.1016/j.immuni.2025.04.017

Stepanenko, A. A., Sosnovtseva, A. O.,O. V., Pavlov, K. A., & Chekhonin, V. P. (2024). Systemic and local immunosuppression in glioblastoma and its prognostic significance. *Frontiers in Immunology, 15*, Article 1326753. https://doi.org/10.3389/fimmu.2024.1326753

Sternberg, E. (2006). Neural regulation of innate immunity: A coordinated nonspecific host response to pathogens. *Nature Reviews Immunology, 6*, 318–328. https://doi.org/10.1038/nri1810

Sur, D., Havasi, A., Cainap, C., Samasca, G., Burz, C., Balacescu, O., Lupan, I., Deleanu, D., & Irimie, A. (2020). Chimeric antigen receptor T-cell therapy for colorectal cancer. *Journal of Clinical Medicine, 9*, 182. https://doi.org/10.3390/jcm9010182

Theofilopoulos, A. N., Kono, D. H., & Baccala, R. (2017). The multiple pathways to autoimmunity. *Nature Immunology, 18*, 716–724.

Trounson, A., & DeWitt, N. D. (2016). Pluripotent stem cells progressing to the clinic. *Nature Reviews Molecular Cell Biology, 17*(3), 194–200. https://doi.org/10.1038/nrm.2016.10

Umemura, Y., Orringer, D., Junck, L., Varela, M. L., West, M. E. J., Faisal, S. M., et al. (2023). Combined cytotoxic and immune-stimulatory gene therapy for primary adult high-grade glioma: A phase 1, first-in-human trial. *The Lancet Oncology, 24*, 1042–1052.

Valiukas, Z., Tangalakis, K., Apostolopoulos, V., & Feehan, J. (2025). Microglial activation states and their implications for Alzheimer's disease. *The Journal of Prevention of Alzheimers' Disease, 12*, Article 100013. https://doi.org/10.1016/j.tjpad.2024.100013

Vijayavenkataraman, S. (2020). Nerve guide conduits for peripheral nerve injury repair: A review on design, materials and fabrication methods. *Acta Biomaterialia, 1*(106), 54–69. https://doi.org/10.1016/j.actbio.2020.02.003

Wan, Y. Y. (2010). Regulatory t cells: Immune suppression and beyond. *Cellular and Molecular Immunology, 7*, 204. https://doi.org/10.1038/CMI.2010.20

Wan, W. B., & Seth, P. P. (2016). The medicinal chemistry of therapeutic oligonucleotides. *Journal of Medicinal Chemistry, 59*(21), 9645–9667.

Wang, J., Shen, F., Yao, Y., Wang, L. L., Zhu, Y., & Hu, J. (2020). Adoptive cell therapy: A novel and potential immunotherapy for glioblastoma. *Frontiers in Oncology, 10*, 59.

Wing, K., & Sakaguchi, S. (2010). Regulatory T cells exert checks and balances on self tolerance and autoimmunity. *Nature Immunology, 11*, 7–13.

Wyss-Coray, T. (2016). Ageing, neurodegeneration and brain rejuvenation. *Nature, 539*, 180–186. https://doi.org/10.1038/nature20411

Xing, K., Gu, B., Zhang, P., & Wu, X. (2015). Dexamethasone enhances programmed cell death 1 (PD-1) expression during T cell activation: An insight into the optimum application of glucocorticoids in anti-cancer therapy. *BMC Immunology, 16*(1), 39.

Yalamandala, B. N., Huynh, T. M. H., Lien, H. W., et al. (2025). Advancing brain immunotherapy through functional nanomaterials. *Drug Delivery and Translational Research*. https://doi.org/10.1007/s13346-024-01778-5

Zefferino, R., Di Gioia, S., & Conese, M. (2020). Molecular links between endocrine, nervous and immune system during chronic stress. *Brain and Behavior, 11*, Article e01960. https://doi.org/10.1002/brb3.1960

Zhang, J., Zhang, Y., Wang, J., Xia, Y., Zhang, J., & Chen, L. (2024). Recent advances in Alzheimer's disease: Mechanisms, clinical trials and new drug development strategies. *Signal Transduction and Targeted Therapy, 9*, 211.

Zhang, X., Zhao, L., Zhang, H., Zhang, Y., Ju, H., Wang, X., Ren, H., Zhu, X., & Dong, Y. (2022). The immunosuppressive microenvironment and immunotherapy in human glioblastoma. *Frontiers in Immunology, 13*, Article 1003651. https://doi.org/10.3389/fimmu.2022.1003651

Zhao, Z., Nelson, A. R., Betsholtz, C., & Zlokovic, B. V. (2015). Establishment and dysfunction of the blood-brain barrier. *Cell, 163*(5), 1064–1078. https://doi.org/10.1016/j.cell.2015.10.067

Zhu, Y., Zhu, L., Wang, X., & Jin, H. (2022). RNA-Based therapeutics: An overview and prospectus. *Cell Death & Disease, 13*(7), 644.

Zou, Z., Li, L., Li, Q., Zhao, P., Zhang, K., Liu, C., Cai, D., Maegele, M., Gu, Z., & Huang, Q. (2022). The role of S100B/RAGE-enhanced ADAM17 activation in endothelial glycocalyx shedding after traumatic brain injury. *Journal of Neuroinflammation, 19*, 46.

CHAPTER

Modulating brain immunity with recombinant proteins

4

Spoorthy Pathikonda[1] **and Clement Arava**[2]
[1]*City University of Hong Kong, Department of Chemistry, Hong Kong, China;* [2]*Université de Rouen Normandie, Laboratoire Sciences et Méthodes Séparatives, Rouen, France*

1. Introduction

The brain, once conceptualized as an immune-privileged organ, is now recognized as a dynamic interface between neural and immune systems (Müller et al.). Far from being isolated, the central nervous system (CNS) maintains continuous bidirectional communication with peripheral immunity through structural gateways, such as the meninges, choroid plexus, and recently characterized meningeal lymphatic vessels (Zhang, Niu et al., 2025). These systems orchestrate neuroprotective responses but can also propagate pathological inflammation when homeostatic equilibrium fails (Müller et al., 2025a).

Neuroimmune dysfunction lies at the core of numerous neurological disorders (Eva et al., 2023). In Alzheimer's disease (AD), microglial overactivation leads to excessive release of pro-inflammatory mediators such as IL-1β, IL-6, and TNF-α, which accelerate amyloidogenesis and tau hyperphosphorylation (Miao et al., 2023). Similarly, Parkinson's disease and multiple sclerosis feature aberrant T cell infiltration, dysregulated innate immunity, and impaired neurorepair (Garretti et al., 2019). The recognition of these mechanisms has catalyzed efforts to develop targeted immunomodulatory approaches that can recalibrate these systems without suppressing essential immune surveillance (Strzelec et al., 2023).

Among these emerging strategies, recombinant protein therapeutics have shown striking promise. Initially designed for systemic inflammation and oncology applications, these engineered molecules now represent a frontier for neuroimmunotherapy (Kintzing et al., 2016). They are capable of restoring immune balance through precisely regulated mechanisms, such as blocking pro-inflammatory receptor activation, enhancing antiinflammatory cytokine activity, or promoting neurotrophic signaling (Markovics et al., 2021). Key examples include recombinant plasma gelsolin, which scavenges actin and inflammatory mediators to prevent neuronal injury; recombinant FOXN1 protein, which reconstitutes thymic function to rejuvenate immune regulation in aged brains; and chimeric fusion proteins engineered to cross the Blood–Brain Barrier (BBB) and deliver targeted payloads to neurons or glia (Zhang et al., 2011).

The past decade has seen a marked expansion in our understanding of how recombinant proteins can modulate brain immunity at molecular and systems levels (Chen et al., 2025). Preclinical studies

Immunotherapies for Neurological Disorders. https://doi.org/10.1016/B978-0-443-44631-3.00009-3

have demonstrated their ability to reduce microglial activation, limit leukocyte infiltration, and enhance neural survival following trauma or neurodegeneration (Zhao et al., 2025). Clinical explorations, meanwhile, underscore the potential for recombinant cytokines such as GM-CSF and IL-2 derivatives to restore cognitive and motor functions in neurodegenerative disease models (Ogunmokun et al., 2021). These effects are mediated through immune rebalancing, tilting the system from cytotoxic T helper-17 and M1 macrophage dominance toward regulatory T cell and M2 microglial phenotypes (Peng et al., 2023).

From a mechanistic viewpoint, recombinant proteins exert their influence across key signaling cascades, including the PI3K/Akt/NF-κB, JAK/STAT, and AMPK/mTOR pathways (Charles & Prince, 2024; Wen et al., 2022). These pathways govern neuronal plasticity, microglial polarization, oxidative stress, and transport across the BBB (Müller & Di Benedetto, 2025). Modern advances in protein engineering now make it possible to tailor molecular interactions within these cascades to achieve spatially targeted immunomodulation (Zhang, Wang, et al., 2025). This fine control enables enhanced efficacy with minimal systemic toxicity.

Moreover, technological progress, such as the integration of nanocarriers, PEGylation, and encapsulated cellular delivery platforms, has significantly improved the pharmacokinetic profiles of recombinant proteins (Zeb et al., 2020). These strategies extend their half-life, improve bioavailability, and enable sustained local release directly in affected brain regions (Karnwal et al., 2024). Together, these innovations make recombinant protein immunotherapy a viable modality for diseases previously resistant to pharmacological intervention.

In summary, recombinant proteins mark a paradigm shift in neuroimmunology, transforming therapeutic design from symptom management to immune recalibration and tissue repair. This chapter aims to dissect the scientific foundations, molecular mechanisms, and translational opportunities of recombinant protein-based modulation of brain immunity. It also discusses engineering strategies to optimize delivery, safety, and efficacy, paving the way toward next-generation immunotherapies for complex neurological disorders.

2. Overview of brain immunity

The central nervous system (CNS) is no longer perceived as a passive or immune-isolated domain; it represents an active immunological interface where neural, glial, and peripheral immune elements converge to maintain homeostasis (Li et al., 2025). The CNS immune landscape integrates resident glial networks, peripheral immune infiltration pathways, and the barrier systems that regulate molecular communication between the brain and the systemic circulation (Norris & Kipnis, 2019). This orchestration allows for constant surveillance and finely tuned responses to tissue stress, pathogens, and degenerative stimuli (Schroeder et al., 2024).

2.1 Microglia: The innate immune core

Microglia serve as the primary innate immune sentinels in the CNS (Qin et al., 2023). Under homeostatic conditions, they monitor the local environment with elaborate processes, maintaining synaptic pruning and neuroplasticity (Turrigiano, 2012). Upon activation, microglia can polarize into functionally distinct phenotypes: the proinflammatory M1 type, which releases cytokines such as

IL-1β, TNF-α, and IL-12; and the antiinflammatory M2 type, which secretes IL-10, TGF-β, and neurotrophic factors that promote repair (Guo et al., 2022). Dysregulated microglial activation is a central feature of chronic neuroinflammation, leading to synaptic dysfunction, demyelination, and neuronal death (Qin et al., 2023). Recombinant protein therapies, such as IL-1 receptor antagonists or engineered TGF-β analogs, aim to shift microglial polarization toward regeneration while mitigating inflammatory cytotoxicity (Ning et al., 2024).

2.2 Astrocytes and oligodendrocytes as immunomodulators

Astrocytes, traditionally considered metabolic and structural supporters, have critical immunomodulatory functions (Naveed et al., 2025). They express pattern recognition receptors (PRRs) including Toll-like receptors (TLRs), enabling them to detect pathogen-associated and damage-associated molecular patterns (PAMPs and DAMPs) (Land, 2015). Activation of astrocytic NF-κB and STAT3 pathways leads to cytokine and chemokine release that influences microglial recruitment and T cell infiltration (Palmer et al., 2026). Conversely, astrocytic secretion of IL-33 and apoE can aid synapse stabilization and repair, suggesting that recombinant mimicry of these signals represents a novel therapeutic direction (Wang et al., 2021). Oligodendrocytes, while primarily myelinating cells, also interact with immune mediators; recombinant neuregulin and BDNF analogs can protect oligodendrocyte progenitor cells against inflammatory insults, preserving conduction and network integrity (Wellman et al., 2018).

2.3 Blood–brain barrier (BBB) and neurovascular unit

The BBB forms a selective permeability interface controlling the passage of immune cells and molecules into the nervous tissue (Wu et al., 2023). It comprises endothelial cells, pericytes, astrocytic end-feet, and a basal lamina that together maintain CNS homeostasis (Daneman & Prat, 2015). In disease, inflammatory cytokines such as TNF-α and IL-6 disrupt endothelial tight junctions (e.g., claudins and occludins), allowing leukocyte infiltration (Wang, Guan, et al., 2025). Recombinant protein therapies can stabilize BBB integrity through several mechanisms, for example, recombinant VEGF derivatives and angiopoietin-1 mimetics enhance endothelial survival, while engineered TNF antagonists decrease paracellular leakage (Shen et al., 2011). Furthermore, recombinant cytokine-growth factor hybrids are being explored for targeted delivery across the BBB, employing receptor-mediated transcytosis mechanisms.

2.4 Peripheral-CNS immune crosstalk

Recent discoveries reveal that the CNS communicates dynamically with peripheral immunity through the meninges, choroid plexus, and cervical lymphatics (Zhang, Niu et al., 2025). Activated monocytes, T cells, and B cells can transmigrate via these interfaces under inflammatory conditions, shaping CNS immune tone (Man et al., 2007). In healthy states, low-level surveillance by these cells supports antigen presentation and cytokine equilibrium (Ousman & Kubes, 2012). Aberrant trafficking, however, fuels chronic disease. Recombinant proteins that regulate chemokine receptor expression, such as modified CXCL12 or CCL2 inhibitors, are under investigation to selectively block pathogenic immune entry while preserving physiological immune exchange (Cambier et al., 2023).

2.5 Cytokine networks and signaling convergence

At the molecular level, neuroimmune signaling depends on a network of cytokines and their receptor systems (Dantzer, 2018). Proinflammatory mediators, IL-1β, IL-12, and IFN-γ activate cascades through NF-κB and MAPK, promoting glial proliferation and oxidative stress (Conti et al., 2010). Antiinflammatory cytokines, IL-4, IL-10, and TGF-β, activate the JAK/STAT and PI3K/Akt axes, encouraging repair and resolution (Deng et al., 2024). Recombinant cytokine therapy leverages these dynamics by introducing synthetically balanced cytokine ratios or receptor agonists that restore this equilibrium (Donnelly et al., 2009). Importantly, the capacity of recombinant proteins to selectively activate intracellular signaling nodes offers precision beyond traditional antiinflammatory drugs (Hegde et al., 2025).

2.6 Meningeal and lymphatic interfaces

The rediscovery of cerebral lymphatic vessels has revolutionized the understanding of neuroimmune homeostasis. These channels drain cerebrospinal fluid, soluble antigens, and immune cells to cervical lymph nodes (Zhang, Niu et al., 2025). Alterations in glymphatic flow or lymphatic structure contribute to protein aggregation and immune dysregulation in neurodegenerative diseases (Gao et al., 2023). Recombinant proteins that enhance lymphatic endothelial function, such as engineered VEGF-C variants, can improve immune clearance and reduce amyloid deposition, representing a potential adjunct to immunotherapeutic interventions (Guo et al.).

2.7 Integrative perspective

Collectively, the brain's immune system is a tightly coordinated biological network in constant negotiation between protection and pathology (Müller et al., 2025b). Recombinant proteins provide a molecular toolkit to reprogram this balance by suppressing maladaptive inflammatory cascades, enhancing regenerative pathways, and stabilizing vascular interfaces (Leiba et al., 2023). Understanding this ecosystem is fundamental to designing therapies that safely exploit immune plasticity for brain repair (Gazerani, 2025). As the subsequent sections will discuss, recombinant proteins have emerged not merely as modulators, but as precision architects of the neuroimmune environment.

3. Recombinant proteins as therapeutic modulators

Recombinant protein technologies have transformed modern immunotherapy, offering tools capable of reshaping the mechanistic and cellular landscape of neuroinflammation (Thombre et al.). In neurological disease contexts, recombinant proteins serve as precision-engineered biologicals designed to correct disrupted signaling, mitigate immune-driven cytotoxicity, and promote repair within the central nervous system (CNS). Their versatility spans recombinant cytokines, growth factors, and hybrid fusion constructs that can modulate immune networks across molecular and cellular scales (Khodve et al., 2025).

3.1 Mechanistic basis for recombinant protein immunotherapy

Neuroimmune dysfunction in the brain is characterized by chronic activation of microglia and astrocytes, accumulation of pro-inflammatory cytokines, and disruption of barrier and synaptic integrity (Adamu et al., 2024). Recombinant proteins can intervene at multiple junctures:

- **Receptor-level modulation:** Recombinant antagonists (e.g., IL-1Ra, TNF receptor–Fc fusion proteins) prevent excessive cytokine receptor signaling, dampening chronic inflammation (Wang, Luo, et al., 2025).
- **Signal transduction corrections:** Recombinant proteins such as TGF-β1 analogs activate regulatory pathways that restrain NF-κB-mediated inflammation while promoting neuronal survival (Qian et al., 2008).
- **Tissue repair augmentation:** Recombinant trophic factors restore synaptic connectivity and remyelination by supporting neuronal progenitor differentiation (Fischer et al., 2020).

Through these actions, recombinant proteins enable the reprogramming of immune dynamics in the brain, from hyperinflammatory to reparative states, without completely suppressing host defense.

3.2 Recombinant cytokine-based modulators

Cytokines stand at the forefront of neuroimmune signaling, making them ideal templates for recombinant therapeutic design (Donnelly et al., 2009). Recent advances leverage structural biology and site-directed mutagenesis to preserve beneficial cytokine activity while minimizing systemic toxicity (Aung et al., 2023).

3.2.1 Interleukin family

Recombinant IL-1 Receptor Antagonist (IL-1Ra): By blocking IL-1β binding to IL-1R1, IL-1Ra prevents propagation of glial activation and nociceptive sensitization (Mailhot et al., 2020). In animal models, IL-1Ra delivery attenuates NLRP3 inflammasome activation, reducing IL-6 secretion and neuronal hyperexcitability (Meng et al., 2014).

Recombinant IL-10 and IL-4: These cytokines enhance the antiinflammatory M2 microglial phenotype while stimulating neuronal autophagy and synaptic pruning repair. Engineered IL-10 fusion proteins designed for BBB transport show extended half-life and localized CNS action (Cherry et al., 2014).

IL-2 Derivatives: Low-dose recombinant IL-2 selectively expands regulatory T cells (Tregs). This mechanism reestablishes neuroimmune equilibrium in models of multiple sclerosis and Parkinson's disease, mitigating inflammatory demyelination (Markovic et al.).

3.2.2 Colony-stimulating factors

Granulocyte-Macrophage Colony-Stimulating Factor (GM-CSF/Sargramostim): Recombinant GM-CSF enhances dendritic and microglial repair capacity, suppresses neurotoxic inflammation, and promotes neurogenesis in Alzheimer's disease models. Clinical trials indicate improved cognitive functions via Treg expansion and microglial reprogramming (Kiyota et al., 2018).

3.2.3 Transforming growth factor family

Recombinant TGF-β1: Exhibits dual roles, neuronal excitability modulation and glial cell suppression. Its canonical pathway upregulates Smad2/3 transcription, reducing pro-inflammatory cytokine release and oxidative stress within the spinal cord and cortex (Meyers & Kessler, 2017).

3.3 Recombinant growth factors and structural proteins

Recombinant growth factors contribute to both immune regulation and structural regeneration. Their signaling actions integrate tightly with immunomodulatory cascades (Butenko et al., 2023).

Recombinant Brain-Derived Neurotrophic Factor (BDNF): Supports neuronal survival, plasticity, and synaptogenesis. It suppresses microglial reactivity through TrkB-mediated PI3K/Akt activation and inhibition of NF-κB (Toader et al., 2025).

Recombinant Plasma Gelsolin (rhu-pGSN): Acts as an extracellular scavenger of F-actin and inflammatory microparticles, reducing oxidative stress and promoting recovery following CNS injury (Bhat et al., 2024). In stroke models, rhu-pGSN dampens IL-6 and TNF-α release while restoring vascular homeostasis (Zhi et al., 2024).

3.4 Chimeric and fusion proteins

Fusion and chimeric proteins represent the most sophisticated generation of recombinant constructs, capable of integrating immunomodulatory efficacy with target specificity and BBB penetrance (Baldo, 2015).

3.4.1 Cytokine fusion constructs

Recombinant fusion molecules such as IL-2–anti-CD25 chimeras concentrate immunoregulatory action on Tregs while avoiding systemic expansion of effector T cells (Ward et al., 2018). Similarly, IL-10–albumin fusions prolong circulating half-life and enhance CNS bioavailability (Linciano et al., 2024).

3.4.2 BBB-penetrant chimeras

Crossing the BBB remains a central challenge. Chimeric proteins combining therapeutic domains (e.g., IL-1Ra, TNFR-Fc) with transferrin or insulin receptor–binding peptides facilitate transcytotic entry into brain tissue. Once inside, they sustain local cytokine suppression without causing immunodeficiency (De et al., 2025).

3.4.3 Recombinant antibody-fusion proteins

Neuroprotective antibodies coupled with cytokine or enzymatic domains can neutralize pathogenic aggregates while providing immunoregulatory benefits (Niazi et al., 2024). Examples include anti-Aβ-GM-CSF hybrids that boost amyloid clearance while mitigating microglial toxicity (Valiukas et al., 2025).

3.5 Mechanism–effect relationships

The following Table 4.1 summarizes representative recombinant proteins, their molecular mechanisms, and corresponding neuroimmune effects.

The table summarizes representative recombinant proteins, their principal molecular mechanisms, signaling targets, and neuroimmune outcomes relevant to therapeutic interventions in neurological disorders. IL-1Ra and IL-10 fusion proteins act via NF-κB inhibition to attenuate inflammation; GM-CSF operates through JAK/STAT-mediated immune rebalancing; rhu-pGSN activates PI3K/Akt to stabilize the BBB; and chimeric IL-1Ra–Transferrin constructs enable receptor-mediated transcytosis for targeted cytokine neutralization.

Table 4.1 Key recombinant proteins and their primary mechanisms of action in neuroimmune modulation.

Recombinant protein	Primary mechanism	Target pathway	Neuroimmune effect	Therapeutic context
IL-1Ra	IL-1R1 blockade	NF-κB inhibition	Reduced microglial activation; decreased cytokine production	Neuroinflammation, neuropathic pain (Dinarello, 2011; Gui et al., 2016)
GM-CSF (Sargramostim)	Treg and microglial modulation	JAK/STAT	Immune rebalancing; neurogenesis	Alzheimer's, Parkinson's (Boyd et al., 2010; Potter et al., 2021; Sanchez-Ramos et al., 2009)
rhu-pGSN	Actin scavenging, microparticle clearance	PI3K/Akt	BBB stabilization; antioxidative effects	Stroke, TBI (Guo et al., 2011; Le et al., 2011)
IL-10 fusion protein	Cytokine-mediated immune suppression	NF-κB inhibition	Antiinflammatory reprogramming	Multiple sclerosis (Kwilasz et al., 2015; Moore et al., 2001)
Chimeric IL-1Ra–Transferrin	BBB transport and cytokine inhibition	Receptor-mediated transcytosis	Targeted cytokine neutralization	CNS inflammatory diseases (Pardridge, 2012; Yu et al., 2014)

3.6 Integrative summary

The modular versatility of recombinant proteins makes them uniquely suited for reprogramming maladaptive immune responses in the brain (Lin & Liu, 2016). Through combinations of cytokine mimicry, trophic factor replenishment, and molecular fusion design, these therapeutics bridge neuroimmunology and bioengineering (Milo & Panitch, 2011). Unlike conventional small-molecule drugs, recombinant proteins display high biochemical specificity, limited off-target toxicity, and customizable pharmacokinetics (Kumar et al., 2024). As subsequent sections will explore, achieving sustained therapeutic benefit requires parallel innovation in delivery systems and mechanistic understanding of neuroimmune feedback circuits (Wang, Xing, et al., 2025).

4. Molecular mechanisms and signaling pathways

Understanding the molecular signaling pathways modulated by recombinant proteins is essential for elucidating how neuroimmune balance is restored in neurological disorders (Yuasa-Kawada et al., 2025). Recombinant therapeutic proteins influence multiple interconnected intracellular cascades that govern inflammatory responses, cellular survival, and regenerative processes within the central nervous system (CNS) (Zavvarian et al., 2024).

4.1 PI3K/Akt/NF-κB pathway

The phosphoinositide 3-kinase (PI3K)/Akt pathway is a critical regulator of cell survival and inflammation (Fig. 4.1) (Acosta-Martinez & Cabail, 2022). Activation of PI3K leads to phosphorylation of Akt, which subsequently inhibits the nuclear translocation of nuclear factor kappa B (NF-κB), a transcription factor central to the expression of pro-inflammatory cytokines such as TNF-α, IL-1β, and IL-6 (Acosta-Martinez & Cabail, 2022). Recombinant proteins like plasma gelsolin (rhu-pGSN) and brain-derived neurotrophic factor (BDNF) exert neuroprotective effects by enhancing PI3K/Akt signaling, thereby suppressing NF-κB-mediated neuroinflammation and oxidative stress (Bhat et al., 2024).

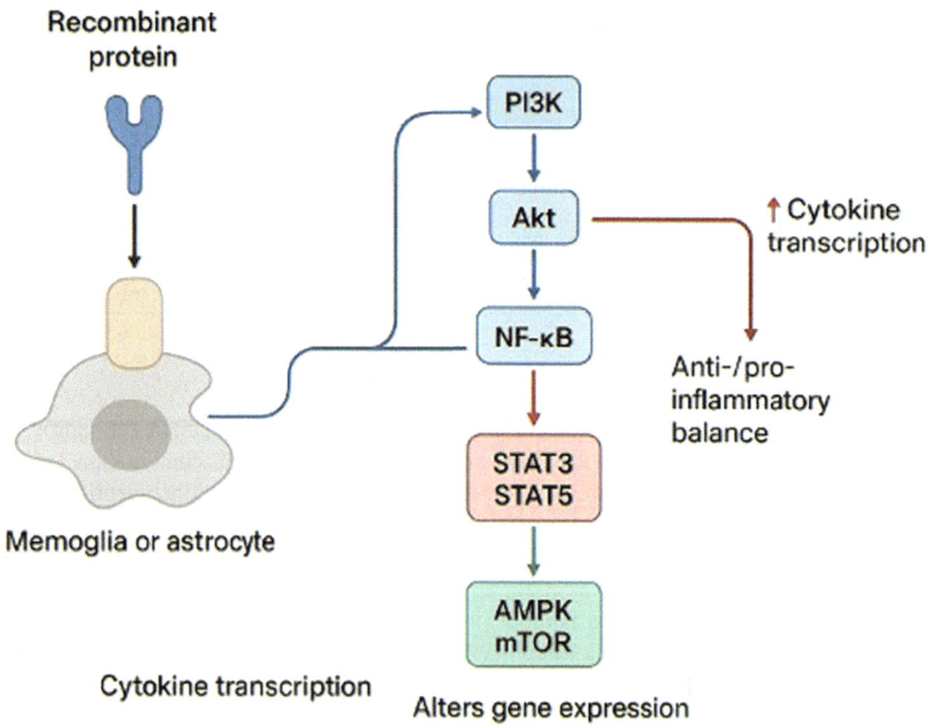

FIGURE 4.1 Recombinant protein interaction with cell surface receptors and downstream pathways.
The schematic illustrates how a recombinant protein binds to a membrane receptor on a microglial or astrocytic cell, initiating activation of the PI3K–Akt–NF-κB axis, the STAT3/STAT5 branch, and the AMPK–mTOR pathway. These cascades converge to regulate cytokine transcription, shift the anti/proinflammatory balance, and alter gene expression profiles that collectively influence neuroimmune homeostasis.

4.2 JAK/STAT signaling

The Janus kinase (JAK)/signal transducer and activator of transcription (STAT) pathway orchestrates responses to cytokines and growth factors (Harrison, 2012). Recombinant cytokines, such as GM-CSF and IL-10 derivatives, modulate this pathway to promote antiinflammatory phenotypes in microglia and T cells (Akhmetzyanova et al., 2019). Activation of STAT3, in particular, induces expression of suppressors of cytokine signaling (SOCS) proteins that negatively regulate inflammatory mediators (Tinè et al., 2024). This pathway is pivotal in expanding regulatory T cell populations that facilitate immunotolerance and neuroprotection (Fu et al., 2025).

4.3 AMPK/mTOR axis

The AMP-activated protein kinase (AMPK)/mechanistic target of rapamycin (mTOR) axis integrates cellular energy status with growth and inflammatory responses (Fig. 4.2) (Panwar et al., 2023).

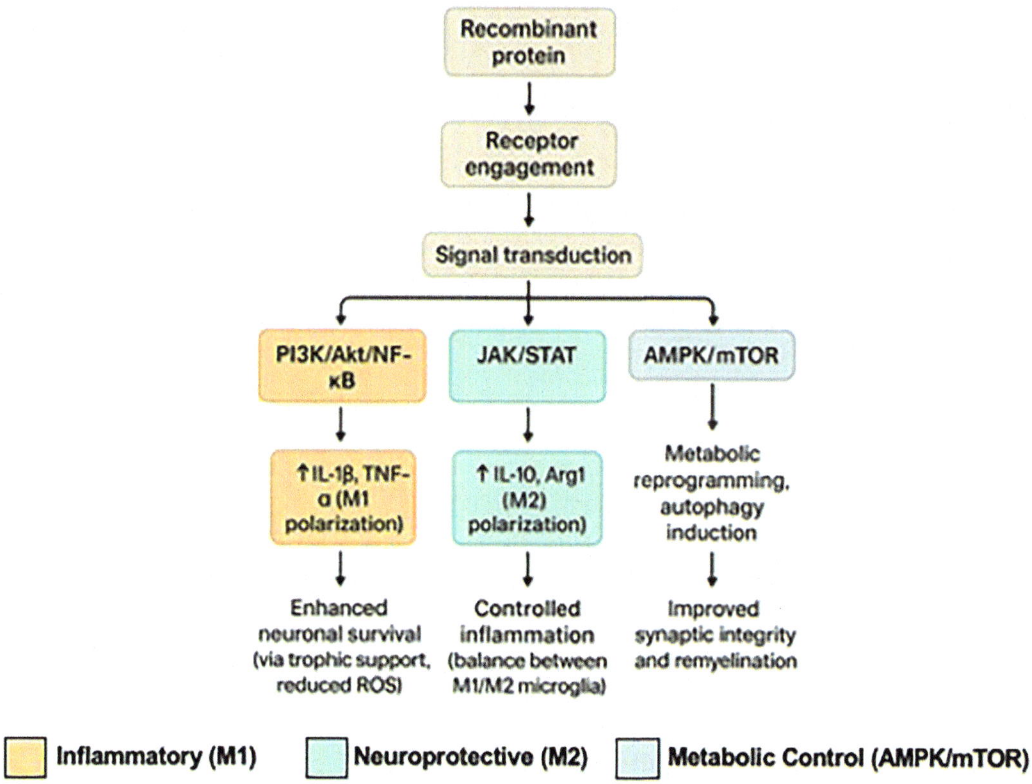

FIGURE 4.2 Flowchart of downstream effects on cytokine production, microglial polarization, and neuronal survival.

Receptor engagement by recombinant proteins activates PI3K/Akt/NF-κB, JAK/STAT, and AMPK/mTOR cascades, which coordinate cytokine expression, microglial polarization (M1 vs. M2), metabolic adaptation, and neuronal survival. Color coding indicates inflammatory (*orange*), neuroprotective (*blue*), and metabolic (*gray*) functional pathways.

Recombinant proteins such as CTRP9 modulate AMPK activation, leading to inhibition of mTOR signaling and downstream NF-κB activation, reducing production of inflammatory cytokines and cerebral edema after injury (Zhao et al., 2018). This pathway also enhances autophagy, promoting clearance of damaged organelles and aggregated proteins implicated in neurodegeneration (Jaeger & Wyss-Coray, 2009).

4.4 Immune checkpoint modulation (PD-1/PD-L1)

Immune checkpoints serve as brakes on excessive immune activation. Recombinant fusion proteins targeting the PD-1/PD-L1 axis within the CNS offer a mechanism to restrain autoreactive T cells and mitigate chronic neuroinflammation (Sherafat et al., 2025). As illustrated in Fig. 4.3, these engineered

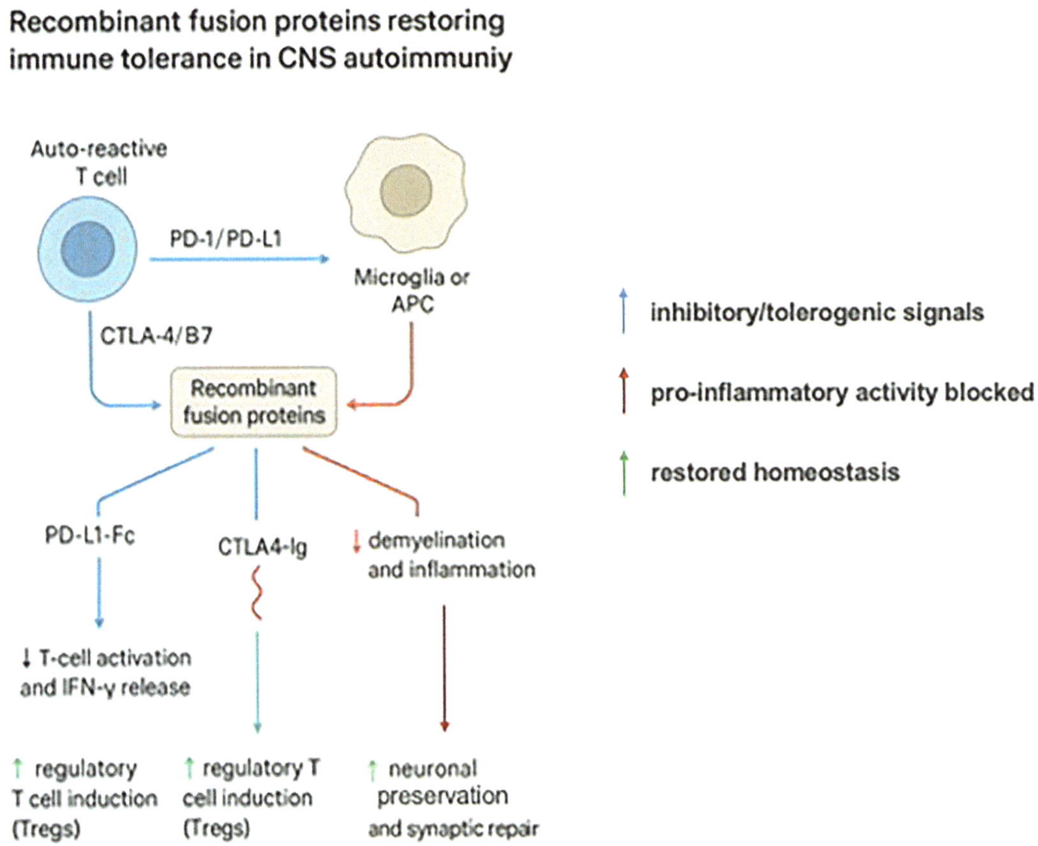

FIGURE 4.3 Schematic of immune checkpoint pathways modulated by recombinant fusion proteins in CNS autoimmunity.

Recombinant fusion proteins targeting PD-1/PD-L1 and CTLA-4 pathways enhance inhibitory signaling between autoreactive T cells and microglia/APCs, suppressing pro-inflammatory cytokine release and demyelinating inflammation while promoting regulatory T-cell induction and neuronal preservation, thereby restoring immune homeostasis.

constructs enhance inhibitory signaling between immune cells, promoting regulatory T-cell responses while suppressing pro-inflammatory cytokine activity (Kim et al., 2025). These recombinant immune checkpoint modulators re-establish microglial homeostasis and prevent demyelination in multiple sclerosis models (Manenti et al., 2022).

4.5 Crosstalk and integration

These pathways function not in isolation but exhibit extensive crosstalk. For example, Akt can phosphorylate and inhibit components upstream of NF-κB, while SOCS proteins link JAK/STAT signaling to mitigate PI3K/Akt activity. This regulatory network ensures feedback control of neuro-inflammatory processes, which recombinant proteins leverage to bias immune responses toward repair and regeneration rather than cytotoxicity (Hu et al., 2021).

5. Delivery systems and pharmacological challenges

Effective delivery of recombinant proteins to the central nervous system (CNS) is a fundamental challenge due to the restrictive nature of the blood–brain barrier (BBB) (Vargas et al., 2025). The BBB, composed of tightly joined endothelial cells, pericytes, and astrocyte end-feet, strictly regulates molecular trafficking, limiting the passage of large biologics such as recombinant proteins. To realize their neuroimmune modulatory potential, recombinant proteins must be engineered to traverse or bypass this barrier while retaining biological activity and minimizing systemic side effects (Chow & Gu, 2015).

5.1 Blood–brain barrier penetration strategies

The primary method to enhance CNS delivery involves receptor-mediated transcytosis (RMT) (Haqqani et al., 2024). This approach exploits endogenous BBB transporters such as the transferrin receptor (TfR) and insulin receptor (IR), which naturally ferry peptides and proteins into the brain (Pardridge, 2020). Recombinant proteins can be fused with monoclonal antibodies (MAbs) or peptides targeting these receptors, acting as "molecular Trojan horses" that shuttle therapeutic payloads across the BBB (Stanimirovic et al., 2018).

- **Transferrin receptor-mediated transport:** Fusion of therapeutic proteins with anti-TfR MAbs enhances receptor binding and subsequent endocytosis into brain endothelial cells, facilitating transcytosis into brain parenchyma. This strategy achieves brain uptake comparable to small molecules (~2–3% of the injected dose), a significant advancement for large biologics (Vega et al., 2025).
- **Insulin receptor targeting:** Human insulin receptor monoclonal antibodies (HIRMAbs) also serve as Trojan horses, promoting transport across the BBB, particularly in primate models. These chimeric proteins preserve endogenous receptor functionality while delivering fused recombinant therapeutics (Coloma et al., 2000).

5.2 Alternative delivery approaches

- **Intracerebroventricular or Intrathecal Administration:** Direct injection into cerebrospinal fluid (CSF) bypasses the BBB but suffers from limited parenchymal penetration due to rapid CSF clearance. This method is often reserved for acute interventions or preclinical studies (Schreiner et al., 2025).
- **Nanoparticle and Liposomal Encapsulation:** Recombinant proteins can be packaged in biodegradable nanoparticles or liposomes functionalized with BBB-targeting ligands. This encapsulation protects them from degradation and enhances receptor-mediated uptake (Muolokwu et al., 2024).
- **Peptide-mediated Delivery:** Short peptides derived from BBB transporters or viral vectors can be coupled to recombinant proteins, facilitating receptor-independent or less receptor-restricted transcytosis (Bickel et al., 2001).

5.3 Pharmacokinetic considerations and protein stability

The fusion of recombinant proteins with Fc regions of immunoglobulins or albumin-binding domains can prolong systemic half-life by engaging neonatal Fc receptors, reducing renal clearance, and improving bioavailability (Rath et al., 2015). However, this may alter tissue distribution and necessitates carefully balanced dosing regimens to limit peripheral side effects.

Moreover, recombinant proteins must retain conformational integrity post-fusion and transport, requiring advanced protein engineering to mitigate aggregation, proteolysis, or loss of affinity (Rahban et al.).

5.4 Encapsulated cell implants and sustained release systems

Sustained local delivery of recombinant proteins within the CNS is achievable using encapsulated cell technologies, whereby genetically engineered cells produce proteins continuously within biocompatible implants implanted in or near target brain areas (Lathuilière et al., 2015). This method circumvents systemic clearance and repeat injections, offering stable therapeutic concentrations while minimizing immunogenicity (Lathuilière et al., 2015).

6. Preclinical and clinical evidence

Recombinant proteins have demonstrated significant therapeutic potential in modulating neuroimmune responses both in preclinical models and initial clinical trials targeting neurological disorders Table 4.2. These studies highlight their capacity to mitigate neuroinflammation, promote tissue repair, and improve functional outcomes (Wang, Xing, et al., 2025).

The table outlines selected recombinant protein therapeutics evaluated across major neurological disease models and early clinical trials. GM-CSF and IL-2 promote immune rebalancing and neuroprotection; IL-10 fusion proteins suppress autoimmune demyelination; recombinant plasma gelsolin reduces neuroinflammation and edema; and mRNA-encoded recombinant proteins demonstrate efficient in vivo expression and symptomatic improvement.

Table 4.2 Summary of key preclinical and clinical studies on recombinant proteins in neurological disorders.

Disorder	Recombinant protein	Model/Trial type	Key findings	Status
Alzheimer's disease	GM-CSF (Sargramostim)	Mouse models; phase II	Reduced amyloid, cognitive improvement	Clinical trials (Butterfield & Boyd-Kimball, 2004; Schneider, 2015)
Multiple sclerosis	IL-10 fusion proteins	EAE models; early trials	Suppressed autoimmune demyelination	Preclinical (Imitola et al., 2005; Mari et al., 2015)
Parkinson's disease	GM-CSF, low-dose IL-2	Rodent models; trials	Treg expansion, neuroprotection	Preclinical/Trials (Kosloski et al., 2013; Rosenzwajg et al., 2015)
Stroke/TBI	Recombinant plasma gelsolin	Animal models	Reduced inflammation, edema	Preclinical (Beis et al., 2004; Fuster-Matanzo et al., 2013)
Inherited metabolic	mRNA-encoded recombinant proteins	Animal models; phase I	Efficient protein expression, symptom alleviation	Preclinical/Trials (Sahin et al., 2014; Yin et al., 2014)

6.1 Preclinical studies

Animal models of neurological diseases such as Alzheimer's disease (AD), Parkinson's disease (PD), multiple sclerosis (MS), intracerebral hemorrhage (ICH), and traumatic brain injury (TBI) have been extensively used to study recombinant protein therapies (Dawson et al., 2018).

- **Alzheimer's Disease:** Recombinant Granulocyte-Macrophage Colony-Stimulating Factor (GM-CSF) has been shown to reprogram microglia toward a neuroprotective phenotype, decrease amyloid plaque burden, and enhance cognitive function in AD mouse models (Kiyota et al., 2018). Recombinant plasma gelsolin administration in ischemic stroke models reduces infarct size and inflammation by scavenging extracellular actin and inflammatory microparticles (Piktel et al., 2018). Patient-derived induced pluripotent stem cell (iPSC) models and 3D brain organoids expressing AD pathology have further enabled drug screening of recombinant protein candidates that target amyloid aggregation and tau phosphorylation (Ji et al., 2025).
- **Parkinson's Disease:** Recombinant GM-CSF and IL-2 derivatives have shown promise in expanding regulatory T cell populations, reducing microglial activation, and preserving dopaminergic neurons in preclinical PD models (Markovic et al.). Recombinant neurotrophic factors such as BDNF analogs promote neuronal survival and functional recovery (Bathina & Das, 2015).
- **Multiple Sclerosis:** Recombinant IL-10 fusion proteins and PD-1/PD-L1 immune checkpoint modulators effectively suppress autoreactive T cell responses and demyelination in experimental autoimmune encephalomyelitis models (Mi et al., 2021). Chimeric fusion proteins designed for BBB penetration provide targeted immunomodulation with minimized systemic immunosuppression (Gampa et al., 2026).

- **Intracerebral Hemorrhage and Traumatic Brain Injury:** Recombinant CTRP9 reduces neuroinflammation and brain edema via AMPK/NF-κB pathway inhibition, improving neurological outcomes in hemorrhagic stroke models (Zhao et al., 2018). Recombinant plasma gelsolin has shown similar neuroprotective effects post-TBI (Zhang et al., 2011).

6.2 Clinical trials and translational advances

Several recombinant proteins have progressed into clinical trials for neurological disorders with encouraging safety and efficacy profiles.

- **GM-CSF (Sargramostim):** Phase II trials in AD patients demonstrated improved cognitive scores and increased numbers of regulatory T cells, with acceptable tolerability (University of Colorado, 2025). These findings support its potential for modulating neuroinflammation in human subjects.
- **Recombinant IL-2:** Low-dose IL-2 therapy trials in multiple sclerosis and PD aim to expand Treg populations to rebalance immune homeostasis, with ongoing investigations of dosing and long-term safety (Matsuoka et al., 2013).
- **Recombinant plasma gelsolin:** Clinical trials are underway exploring its role in ischemic stroke and neuroinflammatory disorders due to its multifunctional antiinflammatory effects (Bhat et al., 2024).
- **mRNA-Encoded Recombinant Proteins:** Novel mRNA therapeutics encoding recombinant proteins are emerging, with preclinical models showing robust protein expression and functional recovery (Shi et al., 2024). Early-phase clinical trials for inherited metabolic and neurodegenerative diseases underscore the translational promise of mRNA-based recombinant protein delivery (Castro-Alpízar et al., 2026).

6.3 Challenges and considerations in clinical translation

While progress is promising, challenges include ensuring effective CNS delivery, minimizing immunogenicity, and validating biomarkers of therapeutic response. Patient stratification and combinatorial approaches with small molecules or gene therapy may enhance outcomes (Puhl et al., 2019).

7. Limitations and safety considerations

While recombinant proteins hold extraordinary promise for modulating brain immunity, myriad safety and translational challenges remain to be addressed before widespread clinical adoption (Rohner et al., 2022).

7.1 Blood-brain barrier bioavailability and dosing concerns

A critical challenge is achieving sufficient brain bioavailability. The blood-brain barrier (BBB) limits entry of large biologics, necessitating high systemic doses that can increase off-target toxicity (Jiao et al., 2024). Even with receptor-mediated transcytosis using transferrin or insulin receptor fusion strategies, typically less than 2%–3% of administered recombinant protein reaches the CNS (Xiao & Gan, 2013). This low CNS penetration necessitates careful dose optimization to balance efficacy and systemic adverse events.

7.2 Immunogenicity and off-target immune activation

Recombinant proteins, especially fusion proteins, risk eliciting immune responses including neutralizing antibodies, hypersensitivity, or systemic immune activation (Dingman & Balu-Iyer, 2019). Such immune reactions can reduce therapeutic effect or cause adverse events (Dingman & Balu-Iyer, 2019). Protein engineering aiming to humanize sequences and remove immunogenic epitopes partially overcomes this issue but may not fully eliminate risks.

7.3 Safety profile in clinical trials

Some recombinant protein therapies targeting neurological diseases, such as monoclonal antibodies against amyloid-beta (aducanumab, lecanemab, and donanemab), have demonstrated limited clinical efficacy and concerning adverse effects including amyloid-related imaging abnormalities (ARIA), brain edema, and microhemorrhages (Nitrini & Studart-Neto, 2025). The FDA recall of aducanumab underlines the need for rigorous assessment of risk-benefit ratios (Nitrini & Studart-Neto, 2025).

7.4 Long-term neurological and cognitive effects

Chronic modulation of innate immunity poses risks of altering neuroplasticity or immune surveillance, potentially exacerbating neurodegeneration or promoting gliosis (Shastri et al., 2013). Longitudinal studies are necessary to evaluate the effects of sustained recombinant protein exposure on cognitive functions and brain homeostasis (Coelho-Júnior et al., 2021).

7.5 Regulatory and ethical considerations

The complex biology of the CNS combined with patient vulnerability necessitates strict ethical standards in trial design (Waykar & Kulkarni, 2025). Ensuring informed consent includes disclosure of known uncertainties related to recombinant protein immunotherapies is mandatory.

8. Emerging directions

The field of recombinant protein therapeutics for brain immunity is rapidly evolving, driven by advances in molecular engineering, delivery strategies, and synthetic biology (Hersh et al., 2016). Several promising avenues are poised to transform current approaches and overcome existing limitations related to blood-brain barrier (BBB) penetration, specificity, and durability of therapeutic effects (Hersh et al., 2016).

8.1 mRNA-based recombinant protein therapeutics

Messenger RNA (mRNA) technology enables in situ synthesis of recombinant proteins directly within target CNS cells (Wadhwa et al., 2020). This approach bypasses the challenges of systemic protein delivery and rapid degradation (Wadhwa et al., 2020). Recent advances have demonstrated robust expression of therapeutic proteins following delivery of synthetic mRNA encapsulated in lipid nanoparticles, achieving long-lasting effects in preclinical neurodegenerative disease models

(Moosavi et al., 2025). Ongoing trials are exploring mRNA platforms for producing antiinflammatory cytokines and growth factors on demand within the brain, which could revolutionize dosing frequency and patient compliance (Huang et al.).

8.2 Gene therapy and viral vector delivery

Recombinant proteins can be expressed via viral vectors such as adeno-associated virus (AAV) or lentivirus, providing long-term, localized expression in neural tissues. This approach is particularly attractive for chronic neurodegenerative disorders requiring sustained immunomodulation (Słyk et al., 2024). Direct intracerebral or intrathecal administration of these vectors enables high concentrations in affected regions, while advancements in vector tropism and promoter design improve cell specificity and safety (Schreiner et al., 2025).

8.3 Synthetic biology and protein engineering

Synthetic biology techniques facilitate the design of chimeric proteins with multi-functionality, combining BBB-targeting domains, receptor-binding elements, and catalytic or signaling units into compact constructs (Yan et al., 2023). Engineering protease-cleavable linkers allows release of active therapeutic moieties once inside the CNS, minimizing systemic exposure (Dal Corso et al., 2017). Directed evolution and computational modeling are further optimizing stability, immunogenicity, and pharmacokinetics of recombinant proteins.

8.4 Nanotechnology and novel carriers

Hybrid delivery platforms combining recombinant proteins with nanocarriers (lipid nanoparticles, exosomes, polymeric particles) offer targeted, sustained release with enhanced BBB transcytosis. Surface functionalization with antibodies or peptides further improves cell-specific uptake and intracellular trafficking, reducing off-target effects (Sanadgol et al., 2025).

8.5 Combination immunotherapy

Combining recombinant protein therapy with other modalities, such as immune checkpoint inhibitors, small-molecule modulators, or neuromodulation techniques (e.g., focused ultrasound) may synergize to recalibrate brain immunity more effectively. This integrated approach holds promise for refractory neurological conditions marked by complex immune dysregulation (Nourizadeh et al., 2025).

8.6 Systems biology and AI-driven design

The integration of multi-omics data, computational modeling, and artificial intelligence accelerates discovery of novel recombinant protein targets and optimizes therapeutic designs by predicting efficacy, safety, and delivery outcomes. This paradigm allows the iterative refinement of protein therapeutics tailored to patient-specific neuroimmune profiles (Ivanisevic & Sewduth, 2023).

9. Conclusion and future outlook

Recombinant protein therapeutics have ushered in a new era in the modulation of brain immunity, offering unprecedented opportunities to recalibrate neuroinflammatory processes pivotal in neurological disorders (Khanal et al., 2025). Through precise targeting of key immune signaling cascades, stabilization of the blood-brain barrier, and enhancement of regenerative pathways, these biologics have demonstrated capacity not only to attenuate pathological inflammation but also to promote neural repair and functional recovery (Lemarchant et al., 2025). The integration of molecular engineering, innovative delivery technologies, and expanding mechanistic insights has facilitated recombinant proteins in overcoming traditional challenges of CNS drug delivery and specificity (Lu et al., 2014).

Preclinical and early clinical evidence underscores the therapeutic promise of diverse recombinant proteins, from cytokine analogs and trophic factors to fusion constructs capable of traversing the blood-brain barrier (Yi et al., 2014). Emerging modalities such as mRNA-based recombinant protein synthesis and gene therapy vectors further extend the versatility and durability of these interventions (Vavilis et al., 2023). Despite persistent challenges related to immunogenicity, delivery efficiency, and long-term safety, ongoing advances in synthetic biology and systems medicine continue to drive this field toward clinical translation (Makkar, 2025).

Looking forward, the convergence of recombinant protein engineering with artificial intelligence-guided design and combinatory immunotherapeutic strategies positions these agents at the forefront of personalized neurological care. Realizing their full potential will require rigorous multidisciplinary collaboration, sustained investment in translational research, and thoughtfully designed clinical trials. Ultimately, recombinant protein-based immunotherapies hold transformative promise for unlocking the brain's defenses and mitigating the burden of neurological diseases.

References

Acosta-Martinez, M., & Cabail, M. Z. (2022). The PI3K/Akt pathway in meta-inflammation. *International Journal of Molecular Sciences, 23*(23), Article 15330. https://doi.org/10.3390/ijms232315330

Adamu, A., Li, S., Gao, F., & Xue, G. (2024). The role of neuroinflammation in neurodegenerative diseases: Current understanding and future therapeutic targets. *Frontiers in Aging Neuroscience, 16*, Article 1347987. https://doi.org/10.3389/fnagi.2024.1347987

Akhmetzyanova, E., Kletenkov, K., Mukhamedshina, Y., & Rizvanov, A. (2019). Different approaches to modulation of microglia phenotypes after spinal cord injury. *Frontiers in Systems Neuroscience, 13*, 37. https://doi.org/10.3389/fnsys.2019.00037

Aung, T., Grubbe, W. S., Nusbaum, R. J., & Mendoza, J. L. (2023). Recent and future perspectives on engineering interferons and other cytokines as therapeutics. *Trends in Biochemical Sciences, 48*(3), 259–273. https://doi.org/10.1016/j.tibs.2022.09.005

Baldo, B. A. (2015). Chimeric fusion proteins used for therapy: Indications, mechanisms, and safety. *Drug Safety, 38*(5), 455–479. https://doi.org/10.1007/s40264-015-0285-9

Bathina, S., & Das, U. N. (2015). Brain-derived neurotrophic factor and its clinical implications. *Archives of Medical Science, 11*(6), 1164–1178. https://doi.org/10.5114/aoms.2015.56342

Beis, J. M., Keller, C., Morin, N., et al. (2004). Right spatial neglect after left hemisphere stroke: Qualitative and quantitative study. *Neurology, 63*(9), 1600–1605. https://doi.org/10.1212/01.wnl.0000142967.60579.32

Bhat, A. R., Arya, A. K., Bhopale, V. M., Imtiyaz, Z., & Thom, S. R. (2024). Recombinant human plasma gelsolin suppresses persistent neuroinflammation and restores hippocampal neurogenesis in murine model of decompression sickness. *Journal of Neurophysiology, 132*(6), 1877–1886. https://doi.org/10.1152/jn.00332.2024

Bickel, U., Yoshikawa, T., & Pardridge, W. M. (2001). Delivery of peptides and proteins through the blood–brain barrier. *Advanced Drug Delivery Reviews, 46*(1), 247–279. https://doi.org/10.1016/S0169-409X(00)00139-3

Boyd, T. D., Bennett, S. P., Mori, T., et al. (2010). GM-CSF upregulated in rheumatoid arthritis reverses cognitive impairment and amyloidosis in alzheimer mice. *Journal of Alzheimer's Disease JAD, 21*(2), 507–518. https://doi.org/10.3233/JAD-2010-091471

Butenko, S., Miwa, H., Liu, Y., Plikus, M. V., Scumpia, P. O., & Liu, W. F. (2023). Engineering immunomodulatory biomaterials to drive skin wounds toward regenerative healing. *Cold Spring Harbor Perspectives in Biology, 15*(5), Article a041242. https://doi.org/10.1101/cshperspect.a041242

Butterfield, D. A., & Boyd-Kimball, D. (2004). Amyloid beta-peptide(1-42) contributes to the oxidative stress and neurodegeneration found in alzheimer disease brain. *Brain Pathology, 14*(4), 426–432. https://doi.org/10.1111/j.1750-3639.2004.tb00087.x

Cambier, S., Gouwy, M., & Proost, P. (2023). The chemokines CXCL8 and CXCL12: Molecular and functional properties, role in disease and efforts towards pharmacological intervention. *Cellular & Molecular Immunology, 20*(3), 217–251. https://doi.org/10.1038/s41423-023-00974-6

Castro-Alpízar, J. A., Lenderink, M. J., Nieuwenhuis, E. E. S., Kooijmans, S. A. A., & Fuchs, S. A. (2026). Navigating molecular therapies: The emerging role of mRNA in treating inherited metabolic diseases. *Molecular Genetics and Metabolism, 147*(1), Article 109698. https://doi.org/10.1016/j.ymgme.2025.109698

Charles, D. A., & Prince, S. E. (2024). Deciphering the molecular mechanism of NLRP3 in BPA-mediated toxicity: Implications for targeted therapies. *Heliyon, 10*(7), Article e28917. https://doi.org/10.1016/j.heliyon.2024.e28917

Chen, J., Wang, C., Chen, S., et al. (2025). Trained immunity modulators: A new frontier in immunoregulation and disease intervention. *Journal of Advanced Research, 18*. https://doi.org/10.1016/j.jare.2025.09.029

Cherry, J. D., Olschowka, J. A., & O'Banion, M. K. (2014). Neuroinflammation and M2 microglia: The good, the bad, and the inflamed. *Journal of Neuroinflammation, 11*, 98. https://doi.org/10.1186/1742-2094-11-98

Chow, B. W., & Gu, C. (2015). The molecular constituents of the blood-brain barrier. *Trends in Neurosciences, 38*(10), 598–608. https://doi.org/10.1016/j.tins.2015.08.003

Coelho-Júnior, H. J., Calvani, R., Landi, F., Picca, A., & Marzetti, E. (2021). Protein intake and cognitive function in older adults: A systematic review and meta-analysis. *Nutrition and Metabolic Insights, 14*. https://doi.org/10.1177/11786388211022373, 11786388211022373.

Coloma, M. J., Lee, H. J., Kurihara, A., et al. (2000). Transport across the primate blood-brain barrier of a genetically engineered chimeric monoclonal antibody to the human insulin receptor. *Pharmaceutical Research, 17*(3), 266–274. https://doi.org/10.1023/a:1007592720793

Conti, A., Gulì, C., La Torre, D., Tomasello, C., Angileri, F. F., & Aguennouz, M. (2010). Role of inflammation and oxidative stress mediators in gliomas. *Cancers, 2*(2), 693–712. https://doi.org/10.3390/cancers2020693

Dal Corso, A., Cazzamalli, S., Gébleux, R., Mattarella, M., & Neri, D. (2017). Protease-cleavable linkers modulate the anticancer activity of non-internalizing antibody-drug conjugates. *Bioconjugate Chemistry, 28*(7), 1826–1833. https://doi.org/10.1021/acs.bioconjchem.7b00304

Daneman, R., & Prat, A. (2015). The blood–brain barrier. *Cold Spring Harbor Perspectives in Biology, 7*(1), Article a020412. https://doi.org/10.1101/cshperspect.a020412

Dantzer, R. (2018). Neuroimmune interactions: From the brain to the immune system and vice versa. *Physiological Reviews, 98*(1), 477–504. https://doi.org/10.1152/physrev.00039.2016

Dawson, T. M., Golde, T. E., & Tourenne, C. L. (2018). Animal models of neurodegenerative diseases. *Nature Neuroscience, 21*(10), 1370–1379. https://doi.org/10.1038/s41593-018-0236-8

De, R., Shi, S., & Kim, K. T. (2025). Crossing the blood-brain barrier with molecularly imprinted polymeric nanocarriers: An emerging frontier in brain disease therapy. *Advanced Science, 29*, Article e17004. https://doi.org/10.1002/advs.202517004

Deng, Z., Fan, T., Xiao, C., et al. (2024). TGF-β signaling in health, disease and therapeutics. *Signal Transduction and Targeted Therapy, 9*, 61. https://doi.org/10.1038/s41392-024-01764-w

Dinarello, C. A. (2011). Interleukin-1 in the pathogenesis and treatment of inflammatory diseases. *Blood, 117*(14), 3720–3732. https://doi.org/10.1182/blood-2010-07-273417

Dingman, R., & Balu-Iyer, S. V. (2019). Immunogenicity of protein pharmaceuticals. *Journal of Pharmaceutical Science, 108*(5), 1637–1654. https://doi.org/10.1016/j.xphs.2018.12.014

Donnelly, R. P., Young, H. A., & Rosenberg, A. S. (2009). An overview of cytokines and cytokine antagonists as therapeutic agents. *Annals of the New York Academy of Sciences, 1182*, 1–13. https://doi.org/10.1111/j.1749-6632.2009.05382.x

Eva, L., Ples, H., Covache-Busuioc, R. A., et al. (2023). A comprehensive review on neuroimmunology: Insights from multiple sclerosis to future therapeutic developments. *Biomedicines, 11*(9), 2489. https://doi.org/10.3390/biomedicines11092489

Fischer, I., Dulin, J. N., & Lane, M. A. (2020). Transplanting neural progenitor cells to restore connectivity after spinal cord injury. *Nature Reviews Neuroscience, 21*(7), 366–383. https://doi.org/10.1038/s41583-020-0314-2

Fu, Y., Wang, B., Alu, A., et al. (2025). Immunosenescence: Signaling pathways, diseases and therapeutic targets. *Signal Transduction and Targeted Therapy, 10*, 250. https://doi.org/10.1038/s41392-025-02371-z

Fuster-Matanzo, A., Llorens-Martín, M., Hernández, F., & Avila, J. (2013). Role of neuroinflammation in adult neurogenesis and alzheimer disease: Therapeutic approaches. *Mediators of Inflammation, 2013*, Article 260925. https://doi.org/10.1155/2013/260925

Gampa, G., Vadlakonda, R., Stefanich, E., Kamath, A. V., Sadekar, S., & Shivva, V. (2026). Bridging the blood-brain barrier: Strategies to improve delivery of biologics to tumors in the brain. *Fluids and Barriers of the CNS, 23*, 25. https://doi.org/10.1186/s12987-026-00760-2

Gao, Y., Liu, K., & Zhu, J. (2023). Glymphatic system: An emerging therapeutic approach for neurological disorders. *Frontiers in Molecular Neuroscience, 16*, Article 1138769. https://doi.org/10.3389/fnmol.2023.1138769

Garretti, F., Agalliu, D., Lindestam Arlehamn, C. S., Sette, A., & Sulzer, D. (2019). Autoimmunity in parkinson's disease: The role of α-Synuclein-Specific T cells. *Frontiers in Immunology, 10*, 303. https://doi.org/10.3389/fimmu.2019.00303

Gazerani, P. (2025). The neuroplastic brain: Current breakthroughs and emerging frontiers. *Brain Research, 1858*, Article 149643. https://doi.org/10.1016/j.brainres.2025.149643

Gui, W. S., Wei, X., Mai, C. L., et al. (2016). Interleukin-1β overproduction is a common cause for neuropathic pain, memory deficit, and depression following peripheral nerve injury in rodents. *Molecular Pain, 12*, Article 1744806916646784. https://doi.org/10.1177/1744806916646784

Guo, X. C., Luo, B. Y., Li, X. F., Yang, D. G., Zheng, X. N., & Zhang, K. (2011). Plasma gelsolin levels and 1-year mortality after first-ever ischemic stroke. *Journal of Critical Care, 26*(6), 608–612. https://doi.org/10.1016/j.jcrc.2011.02.007

Guo, S., Wang, H., & Yin, Y. (2022). Microglia polarization from M1 to M2 in neurodegenerative diseases. *Frontiers in Aging Neuroscience, 14*, Article 815347. https://doi.org/10.3389/fnagi.2022.815347

Guo X, Zhang G, Peng Q, Huang L, Zhang Z, & Zhang Z. Emerging roles of meningeal lymphatic vessels in alzheimer's disease, Journal of Alzheimer's Disease. 94(Suppl. 1):S355–S366.

Haqqani, A. S., Bélanger, K., & Stanimirovic, D. B. (2024). Receptor-mediated transcytosis for brain delivery of therapeutics: Receptor classes and criteria. *Frontiers in Drug Delivery, 4*, Article 1360302. https://doi.org/10.3389/fddev.2024.1360302

Harrison, D. A. (2012). The Jak/STAT pathway. *Cold Spring Harbor Perspectives in Biology, 4*(3), Article a011205. https://doi.org/10.1101/cshperspect.a011205

Hegde, M., Mishra, A., Banerjee, R., et al. (2025). Bioresponsive engineered nanoparticles for immunomodulation. *BMC Medicine, 23*, 595. https://doi.org/10.1186/s12916-025-04305-6

Hersh, D. S., Wadajkar, A. S., Roberts, N. B., et al. (2016). Evolving drug delivery strategies to overcome the blood brain barrier. *Current Pharmaceutical Design, 22*(9), 1177–1193. https://doi.org/10.2174/1381612822666151221150733

Hu, X., li, J., Fu, M., Zhao, X., & Wang, W. (2021). The JAK/STAT signaling pathway: From bench to clinic. *Signal Transduction and Targeted Therapy, 6*, 402. https://doi.org/10.1038/s41392-021-00791-1

Huang X, Ma Y, Ma G, & Xia Y. Unlocking the therapeutic applicability of LNP-mRNA: Chemistry, formulation, and clinical strategies. Research: Ideas for Today's Investors 7:0370..

Imitola, J., Chitnis, T., & Khoury, S. J. (2005). Cytokines in multiple sclerosis: From bench to bedside. *Pharmacology & Therapeutics, 106*(2), 163–177. https://doi.org/10.1016/j.pharmthera.2004.11.007

Ivanisevic, T., & Sewduth, R. N. (2023). Multi-omics integration for the design of novel therapies and the identification of novel biomarkers. *Proteomes, 11*(4), 34. https://doi.org/10.3390/proteomes11040034

Jaeger, P. A., & Wyss-Coray, T. (2009). All-you-can-eat: Autophagy in neurodegeneration and neuroprotection. *Molecular Neurodegeneration, 4*, 16. https://doi.org/10.1186/1750-1326-4-16

Ji, Y., Chen, X., Wang, Z., et al. (2025). Alzheimer's disease patient brain extracts induce multiple pathologies in novel vascularized neuroimmune organoids for disease modeling and drug discovery. *Molecular Psychiatry, 30*(10), 4558–4575. https://doi.org/10.1038/s41380-025-03041-w

Jiao, Y., Yang, L., Wang, R., et al. (2024). Drug delivery across the blood–brain barrier: A new strategy for the treatment of neurological diseases. *Pharmaceutics, 16*(12), 1611. https://doi.org/10.3390/pharmaceutics16121611

Karnwal, A., Sharma, V., Kumar, G., Jassim, A. Y., Dohroo, A., & Sivanesan, I. (2024). Transforming medicine with nanobiotechnology: Nanocarriers and their biomedical applications. *Pharmaceutics, 16*(9), 1114. https://doi.org/10.3390/pharmaceutics16091114

Khanal, P., Chikhale, R., & Machhi, J. (2025). Editorial: Targeting neuroinflammation for novel therapeutics in neurodegenerative diseases. *Frontiers in Pharmacology, 16*, Article 1602495. https://doi.org/10.3389/fphar.2025.1602495

Khodve, G., Banerjee, S., Kumari, M., Ravichandiran, V., Banerjee, S., & Roy, S. (2025). Exploration of biomaterial and stem cell-based strategies for promoting neuronal regeneration and creating engineered 3D in-vitro disease models. *Journal of Translational Medicine, 23*, 1197. https://doi.org/10.1186/s12967-025-07266-9

Kim, S., Heo, S. H., Baek, H., & Hwang, S. S. (2025). Cytokine engineering in CAR-T cell therapy: Next-generation strategies. *Immune Network, 25*(6), Article e43. https://doi.org/10.4110/in.2025.25.e43

Kintzing, J. R., Filsinger Interrante, M. V., & Cochran, J. R. (2016). Emerging strategies for developing next-generation protein therapeutics for cancer treatment. *Trends in Pharmacological Sciences, 37*(12), 993–1008. https://doi.org/10.1016/j.tips.2016.10.005

Kiyota, T., Machhi, J., Lu, Y., et al. (2018). Granulocyte-macrophage colony-stimulating factor neuroprotective activities in Alzheimer's disease mice. *Journal of Neuroimmunology, 319*, 80–92. https://doi.org/10.1016/j.jneuroim.2018.03.009

Kosloski, L. M., Kosmacek, E. A., Olson, K. E., Mosley, R. L., & Gendelman, H. E. (2013). GM-CSF induces neuroprotective and anti-inflammatory responses in 1-methyl-4-phenyl-1,2,3,6-tetrahydropyridine intoxicated mice. *Journal of Neuroimmunology, 265*(1–2), 1–10. https://doi.org/10.1016/j.jneuroim.2013.10.009

Kumar, V., Barwal, A., Sharma, N., Mir, D. S., Kumar, P., & Kumar, V. (2024). Therapeutic proteins: Developments, progress, challenges, and future perspectives. *3 Biotech, 14*(4), 112. https://doi.org/10.1007/s13205-024-03958-z

Kwilasz, A. J., Grace, P. M., Serbedzija, P., Maier, S. F., & Watkins, L. R. (2015). The therapeutic potential of interleukin-10 in neuroimmune diseases. *Neuropharmacology, 96*(Pt A), 55–69. https://doi.org/10.1016/j.neuropharm.2014.10.020

Land, W. G. (2015). The role of damage-associated molecular patterns in human diseases. *Sultan Qaboos University Medical Journal, 15*(1), e9–e21.
Lathuilière, A., Mach, N., & Schneider, B. L. (2015). Encapsulated cellular implants for recombinant protein delivery and therapeutic modulation of the immune system. *International Journal of Molecular Sciences, 16* (5), 10578–10600. https://doi.org/10.3390/ijms160510578
Le, H. T., Hirko, A. C., Thinschmidt, J. S., et al. (2011). The protective effects of plasma gelsolin on stroke outcome in rats. *Experimental & Translational Stroke Medicine, 3*(1), 13. https://doi.org/10.1186/2040-7378-3-13
Leiba, J., Özbilgiç, R., Hernández, L., et al. (2023). Molecular actors of inflammation and their signaling pathways: Mechanistic insights from zebrafish. *Biology, 12*(2), 153. https://doi.org/10.3390/biology12020153
Lemarchant, S., Engelhardt, B., Cicchetti, F., et al. (2025). Restoring brain barriers: An innovative approach for treating neurological disorders. *Fluids and Barriers of the CNS, 22*, 72. https://doi.org/10.1186/s12987-025-00688-z
Li, T., Qiu, T., Jiang, F., Cai, H., & Le, W. (2025). Microglia in the crosstalk between peripheral and central nervous systems in Parkinson's disease. *Translational Neurodegeneration, 14*, 66. https://doi.org/10.1186/s40035-025-00531-3
Lin, C yu, & Liu, J. C. (2016). Modular protein domains: An engineering approach towards functional biomaterials. *Current Opinion in Biotechnology, 40*, 56–63. https://doi.org/10.1016/j.copbio.2016.02.011
Linciano, S., Vigolo, E., Rosato, A., Kumada, Y., & Angelini, A. (2024). Albumin-based strategies to effectively prolong the circulation half-life of small immunomodulatory payloads in cancer therapy. *Current Opinion in Biotechnology, 90*, Article 103218. https://doi.org/10.1016/j.copbio.2024.103218
Lu, C. T., Zhao, Y. Z., Wong, H. L., Cai, J., Peng, L., & Tian, X. Q. (2014). Current approaches to enhance CNS delivery of drugs across the brain barriers. *International Journal of Nanomedicine, 9*, 2241–2257. https://doi.org/10.2147/IJN.S61288
Mailhot, B., Christin, M., Tessandier, N., et al. (2020). Neuronal interleukin-1 receptors mediate pain in chronic inflammatory diseases. *Journal of Experimental Medicine, 217*(9), Article e20191430. https://doi.org/10.1084/jem.20191430
Makkar, S. K. (2025). Advances in RNA-based therapeutics: Current breakthroughs, clinical translation, and future perspectives. *Frontiers in Genetics, 16*, Article 1675209. https://doi.org/10.3389/fgene.2025.1675209
Man, S., Ubogu, E. E., & Ransohoff, R. M. (2007). Inflammatory cell migration into the central nervous system: A few new twists on an old tale. *Brain Pathology, 17*(2), 243–250. https://doi.org/10.1111/j.1750-3639.2007.00067.x
Manenti, S., Orrico, M., Masciocchi, S., Mandelli, A., Finardi, A., & Furlan, R. (2022). PD-1/PD-L axis in neuroinflammation: New insights. *Frontiers in Neurology, 13*, Article 877936. https://doi.org/10.3389/fneur.2022.877936
Mari, E. R., Moore, J. N., Zhang, G. X., & Rostami, A. (2015). Mechanisms of immunological tolerance in central nervous system inflammatory demyelination. *Clinical & Experimental Neuroimmunology, 6*(3), 264–274. https://doi.org/10.1111/cen3.12196
Markovic M, Yeapuri P, & Namminga K.L, et al. Interleukin-2 expands neuroprotective regulatory T cells in Parkinson's disease, NeuroImmune Pharmacology and Therapeutics 1(1):43–50.
Markovics, A., Rosenthal, K. S., Mikecz, K., Carambula, R. E., Ciemielewski, J. C., & Zimmerman, D. H. (2021). Restoring the balance between pro-inflammatory and anti-inflammatory cytokines in the treatment of rheumatoid arthritis: New insights from animal models. *Biomedicines, 10*(1), 44. https://doi.org/10.3390/biomedicines10010044
Matsuoka, K ichi, Koreth, J., Kim, H. T., et al. (2013). Low-dose interleukin-2 therapy restores regulatory T cell homeostasis in patients with chronic graft-versus-host disease. *Science Translational Medicine, 5*(179), Article 179ra43. https://doi.org/10.1126/scitranslmed.3005265

Meng, X. F., Tan, L., Tan, M. S., et al. (2014). Inhibition of the NLRP3 inflammasome provides neuroprotection in rats following amygdala kindling-induced status epilepticus. *Journal of Neuroinflammation, 11*, 212. https://doi.org/10.1186/s12974-014-0212-5

Meyers, E. A., & Kessler, J. A. (2017). TGF-β family signaling in neural and neuronal differentiation, development, and function. *Cold Spring Harbor Perspectives in Biology, 9*(8), Article a022244. https://doi.org/10.1101/cshperspect.a022244

Mi, Y., Han, J., Zhu, J., & Jin, T. (2021). Role of the PD-1/PD-L1 signaling in multiple sclerosis and experimental autoimmune encephalomyelitis: Recent insights and future directions. *Molecular Neurobiology, 58*(12), 6249–6271. https://doi.org/10.1007/s12035-021-02495-7

Miao, J., Ma, H., Yang, Y., et al. (2023). Microglia in Alzheimer's disease: Pathogenesis, mechanisms, and therapeutic potentials. *Frontiers in Aging Neuroscience, 15*. https://doi.org/10.3389/fnagi.2023.1201982

Milo, R., & Panitch, H. (2011). Combination therapy in multiple sclerosis. *Journal of Neuroimmunology, 231* (1–2), 23–31. https://doi.org/10.1016/j.jneuroim.2010.10.021

Moore, K. W., de Waal Malefyt, R., Coffman, R. L., & O'Garra, A. (2001). Interleukin-10 and the interleukin-10 receptor. *Annual Review of Immunology, 19*, 683–765. https://doi.org/10.1146/annurev.immunol.19.1.683

Moosavi, S. G., Rahiman, N., Jaafari, M. R., & Arabi, L. (2025). Lipid nanoparticle (LNP) mediated mRNA delivery in neurodegenerative diseases. *Journal of Controlled Release: Official Journal of the Controlled Release Society, 381*, Article 113641. https://doi.org/10.1016/j.jconrel.2025.113641

Müller, L., & Di Benedetto, S. (2025). Bridging the brain and gut: Neuroimmune mechanisms of neuroinflammation and therapeutic insights. *Frontiers in Cellular Neuroscience, 19*, Article 1590002. https://doi.org/10.3389/fncel.2025.1590002

Müller L, Di Benedetto S, & Müller V. Neuroimmune dynamics and brain aging: Mechanisms and consequences, Frontiers in Aging Neuroscience. 17:1715045.

Müller, L., Di Benedetto, S., & Müller, V. (2025a). From homeostasis to neuroinflammation: Insights into cellular and molecular interactions and network dynamics. *Cells, 14*(1), 54. https://doi.org/10.3390/cells14010054

Müller, L., Di Benedetto, S., & Müller, V. (2025b). The dual nature of neuroinflammation in networked brain. *Frontiers in Immunology, 16*, Article 1659947. https://doi.org/10.3389/fimmu.2025.1659947

Muolokwu, C. E., Chaulagain, B., Gothwal, A., et al. (2024). Functionalized nanoparticles to deliver nucleic acids to the brain for the treatment of Alzheimer's disease. *Frontiers in Pharmacology, 15*, Article 1405423. https://doi.org/10.3389/fphar.2024.1405423

Naveed, M., Smedlund, K., Zhou, Q. G., Cai, W., & Hill, J. W. (2025). Astrocyte involvement in metabolic regulation and disease. *Trends in Endocrinology and Metabolism: TEM, 36*(3), 219–234. https://doi.org/10.1016/j.tem.2024.08.001

Niazi, S. K., Mariam, Z., & Magoola, M. (2024). Engineered antibodies to improve efficacy against neurodegenerative disorders. *International Journal of Molecular Sciences, 25*(12), 6683. https://doi.org/10.3390/ijms25126683

Ning, W., Lv, S., Wang, Q., & Xu, Y. (2024). The pivotal role of microglia in injury and the prognosis of subarachnoid hemorrhage. *Neural Regeneration Research, 20*(7), 1829–1848. https://doi.org/10.4103/NRR.NRR-D-24-00241

Nitrini, R., & Studart-Neto, A. (2025). Monoclonal antibodies against beta-amyloid protein (lecanemab and donanemab) should not be used in the treatment of Alzheimer's disease. *Arquivos de Neuro-Psiquiatria, 83*(5), Article s00451808082. https://doi.org/10.1055/s-0045-1808082

Norris, G. T., & Kipnis, J. (2019). Immune cells and CNS physiology: Microglia and beyond. *Journal of Experimental Medicine, 216*(1), 60–70. https://doi.org/10.1084/jem.20180199

Nourizadeh, M., Mounesyar, S. M., Movahhed, M. S., et al. (2025). Current strategies and novel immunotherapeutic approaches for overcoming immune resistance in glioblastoma. *Discover Oncology, 16*, 1952. https://doi.org/10.1007/s12672-025-03807-2

Ogunmokun, G., Dewanjee, S., Chakraborty, P., et al. (2021). The potential role of cytokines and growth factors in the pathogenesis of alzheimer's disease. *Cells, 10*(10), 2790. https://doi.org/10.3390/cells10102790

Ousman, S. S., & Kubes, P. (2012). Immune surveillance in the central nervous system. *Nature Neuroscience, 15* (8), 1096–1101. https://doi.org/10.1038/nn.3161

Palmer, A. L., Wang, R., Zonta, Y. R., Bailey, Z. D. J., Kuipers, H. F., & Ousman, S. S. (2026). Cytokine and chemokine production by astrocytes is influenced by cystatin C. *Journal of Neuroimmunology, 410*, Article 578801. https://doi.org/10.1016/j.jneuroim.2025.578801

Panwar, V., Singh, A., Bhatt, M., et al. (2023). Multifaceted role of mTOR (mammalian target of rapamycin) signaling pathway in human health and disease. *Signal Transduction and Targeted Therapy, 8*, 375. https://doi.org/10.1038/s41392-023-01608-z

Pardridge, W. M. (2012). Drug transport across the blood-brain barrier. *Journal of Cerebral Blood Flow and Metabolism: Official Journal of the International Society of Cerebral Blood Flow and Metabolism,, 32*(11), 1959–1972. https://doi.org/10.1038/jcbfm.2012.126

Pardridge, W. M. (2020). Blood-brain barrier and delivery of protein and gene therapeutics to brain. *Frontiers in Aging Neuroscience, 11*, 373. https://doi.org/10.3389/fnagi.2019.00373

Peng, Y., Zhou, M., Yang, H., et al. (2023). Regulatory mechanism of M1/M2 macrophage polarization in the development of autoimmune diseases. *Mediators of Inflammation, 2023.* https://doi.org/10.1155/2023/8821610

Piktel, E., Levental, I., Durnaś, B., Janmey, P. A., & Bucki, R. (2018). Plasma gelsolin: Indicator of inflammation and its potential as a diagnostic tool and therapeutic target. *International Journal of Molecular Sciences, 19* (9), 2516. https://doi.org/10.3390/ijms19092516

Potter, H., Woodcock, J. H., Boyd, T. D., et al. (2021). Safety and efficacy of sargramostim (GM-CSF) in the treatment of Alzheimer's disease. *Alzheimer's & Dementia: Translational Research & Clinical Interventions, 7*(1), Article e12158. https://doi.org/10.1002/trc2.12158

Puhl, D. L., D'Amato, A. R., & Gilbert, R. J. (2019). Challenges of gene delivery to the central nervous system and the growing use of biomaterial vectors. *Brain Research Bulletin, 150*, 216–230. https://doi.org/10.1016/j.brainresbull.2019.05.024

Qian, L., Wei, S. J., Zhang, D., et al. (2008). Potent anti-inflammatory and neuroprotective effects of TGFβ1 are mediated through the inhibition of ERK and p47phox-Ser345 phosphorylation and translocation in microglia. *The Journal of Immunology: Official Journal of the American Association of Immunologists, 181*(1), 660–668. https://doi.org/10.4049/jimmunol.181.1.660

Qin, J., Ma, Z., Chen, X., & Shu, S. (2023). Microglia activation in central nervous system disorders: A review of recent mechanistic investigations and development efforts. *Frontiers in Neurology, 14*, Article 1103416. https://doi.org/10.3389/fneur.2023.1103416

Rahban M, Ahmad F, Piatyszek M.A, Haertlé T, Saso L, & Saboury A.A. Stabilization challenges and aggregation in protein-based therapeutics in the pharmaceutical industry, RSC Advances. 13(51):35947-35963.

Rath, T., Baker, K., Dumont, J. A., et al. (2015). Fc-fusion proteins and FcRn: Structural insights for longer-lasting and more effective therapeutics. *Critical Reviews in Biotechnology, 35*(2), 235–254. https://doi.org/10.3109/07388551.2013.834293

Rohner, E., Yang, R., Foo, K. S., Goedel, A., & Chien, K. R. (2022). Unlocking the promise of mRNA therapeutics. *Nature Biotechnology, 40*(11), 1586–1600. https://doi.org/10.1038/s41587-022-01491-z

Rosenzwajg, M., Churlaud, G., Mallone, R., et al. (2015). Low-dose interleukin-2 fosters a dose-dependent regulatory T cell tuned milieu in T1D patients. *Journal of Autoimmunity, 58*, 48–58. https://doi.org/10.1016/j.jaut.2015.01.001

Sahin, U., Karikó, K., & Türeci, Ö. (2014). mRNA-based therapeutics–developing a new class of drugs. *Nature Reviews Drug Discovery, 13*(10), 759–780. https://doi.org/10.1038/nrd4278

Sanadgol, N., Abedi, M., Hashemzaei, M., et al. (2025). Exosomes as nanocarriers for brain-targeted delivery of therapeutic nucleic acids: Advances and challenges. *Journal of Nanobiotechnology, 23*, 453. https://doi.org/10.1186/s12951-025-03528-2

Sanchez-Ramos, J., Song, S., Sava, V., et al. (2009). Granulocyte colony stimulating factor decreases brain amyloid burden and reverses cognitive impairment in Alzheimer's mice. *Neuroscience, 163*(1), 55–72. https://doi.org/10.1016/j.neuroscience.2009.05.071

Schneider, L. S. (2015). Introducing Alzheimer's & dementia: Translational research & clinical interventions, an open access journal of the Alzheimer's association. *Alzheimer's & Dementia : Translational Research & Clinical Interventions, 1*(1), 91–93. https://doi.org/10.1016/j.trci.2015.06.002

Schreiner, T. G., Menéndez-González, M., Schreiner, O. D., & Ciobanu, R. C. (2025). Intrathecal therapies for neurodegenerative diseases: A review of current approaches and the urgent need for advanced delivery systems. *Biomedicines, 13*(9), 2167. https://doi.org/10.3390/biomedicines13092167

Schroeder, H. T., De Lemos Muller, C. H., Heck, T. G., Krause, M., & Homem de Bittencourt, P. I. (2024). Heat shock response during the resolution of inflammation and its progressive suppression in chronic-degenerative inflammatory diseases. *Cell Stress & Chaperones, 29*(1), 116–142. https://doi.org/10.1016/j.cstres.2024.01.002

Shastri, A., Bonifati, D. M., & Kishore, U. (2013). Innate immunity and neuroinflammation. *Mediators of Inflammation, 2013*, Article 342931. https://doi.org/10.1155/2013/342931

Shen, F., Walker, E. J., Jiang, L., et al. (2011). Coexpression of angiopoietin-1 with VEGF increases the structural integrity of the blood–brain barrier and reduces atrophy volume. *Journal of Cerebral Blood Flow & Metabolism, 31*(12), 2343–2351. https://doi.org/10.1038/jcbfm.2011.97

Sherafat, N. S., Keshavarz, A., Mardi, A., et al. (2025). Rationale of using immune checkpoint inhibitors (ICIs) and anti-angiogenic agents in cancer treatment from a molecular perspective. *Clinical and Experimental Medicine, 25*(1), 238. https://doi.org/10.1007/s10238-025-01751-7

Shi, Y., Shi, M., Wang, Y., & You, J. (2024). Progress and prospects of mRNA-based drugs in pre-clinical and clinical applications. *Signal Transduction and Targeted Therapy, 9*(1), 322. https://doi.org/10.1038/s41392-024-02002-z

Słyk, Ż., Stachowiak, N., & Małecki, M. (2024). Recombinant adeno-associated virus vectors for gene therapy of the central nervous system: Delivery routes and clinical aspects. *Biomedicines, 12*(7), 1523. https://doi.org/10.3390/biomedicines12071523

Stanimirovic, D. B., Sandhu, J. K., & Costain, W. J. (2018). Emerging technologies for delivery of biotherapeutics and gene therapy across the blood–brain barrier. *BioDrugs, 32*(6), 547–559. https://doi.org/10.1007/s40259-018-0309-y

Strzelec, M., Detka, J., Mieszczak, P., Sobocińska, M. K., & Majka, M. (2023). Immunomodulation—A general review of the current state-of-the-art and new therapeutic strategies for targeting the immune system. *Frontiers in Immunology, 14*. https://doi.org/10.3389/fimmu.2023.1127704

Thombre K..R, Gupta K.R, Masne T.P, & Umekar M.J. Recombinant proteins: Evolution to their therapeutic potential. https://www.eurekaselect.com/article/149830.

Tinè, M., Balestro, E., Carpi, S., et al. (2024). Suppressor of cytokine signaling-3 expression and its regulation in relation to inflammation in chronic obstructive pulmonary disease. *Frontiers in Immunology, 15*, Article 1320077. https://doi.org/10.3389/fimmu.2024.1320077

Toader, C., Serban, M., Munteanu, O., et al. (2025). From synaptic plasticity to neurodegeneration: BDNF as a transformative target in medicine. *International Journal of Molecular Sciences, 26*(9), 4271. https://doi.org/10.3390/ijms26094271

Turrigiano, G. (2012). Homeostatic synaptic plasticity: Local and global mechanisms for stabilizing neuronal function. *Cold Spring Harbor perspectives in biology, 4*(1), Article a005736. https://doi.org/10.1101/cshperspect.a005736

University of Colorado. (2025). *Phase II trial to evaluate safety and efficacy of GM-CSF/Sargramostim in Alzheimer's disease (SESAD).* https://clinicaltrials.gov/study/NCT04902703.

Valiukas, Z., Tangalakis, K., Apostolopoulos, V., & Feehan, J. (2025). Microglial activation states and their implications for Alzheimer's disease. *The Journal of Prevention of Alzheimer's Disease, 12*(1), Article 100013. https://doi.org/10.1016/j.tjpad.2024.100013

Vargas, R., Martinez-Martinez, N., Lizano-Barrantes, C., et al. (2025). Advancing through the blood-brain barrier: Mechanisms, challenges and drug delivery strategies. *ADMET & DMPK, 13*(5), 2988. https://doi.org/10.5599/admet.2988

Vavilis, T., Stamoula, E., Ainatzoglou, A., et al. (2023). mRNA in the context of protein replacement therapy. *Pharmaceutics, 15*(1), 166. https://doi.org/10.3390/pharmaceutics15010166

Vega, M. R., Hansen, H. H., Jensen, C. S., et al. (2025). Transferrin receptor-binding blood-brain barrier shuttle enhances brain delivery and plaque-clearing efficacy of a therapeutic anti-Aβ antibody. *Fluids and Barriers of the CNS, 22*, 121. https://doi.org/10.1186/s12987-025-00737-7

Wadhwa, A., Aljabbari, A., Lokras, A., Foged, C., & Thakur, A. (2020). Opportunities and challenges in the delivery of mRNA-Based vaccines. *Pharmaceutics, 12*(2), 102. https://doi.org/10.3390/pharmaceutics12020102

Wang, Y., Fu, W. Y., Cheung, K., et al. (2021). Astrocyte-secreted IL-33 mediates homeostatic synaptic plasticity in the adult hippocampus. *Proceedings of the National Academy of Sciences of the United States of America, 118*(1), Article e2020810118. https://doi.org/10.1073/pnas.2020810118

Wang, Y., Guan, Q. N., Zhang, Z. J., & Zhang, Y. M. (2025). Interaction between endothelial injury and immune response in septic shock: From basic research to clinical applications. *Frontiers in Physiology, 16*, Article 1627008. https://doi.org/10.3389/fphys.2025.1627008

Wang, K., Luo, H., Liu, L., Gao, H., Song, Y., & Li, D. (2025). Blockade of IL-1 family cytokines in the treatment of rheumatoid arthritis. *Frontiers in Pharmacology, 16*, Article 1577628. https://doi.org/10.3389/fphar.2025.1577628

Wang, J., Xing, L., Song, Y., et al. (2025). FGFs/FGFRs and neuroinflammatory diseases: Mechanism, drug therapies and delivery systems. *Journal of Advanced Research, 78*, 733–756. https://doi.org/10.1016/j.jare.2025.06.024

Ward, N. C., Yu, A., Moro, A., et al. (2018). IL-2/CD25: A long-acting fusion protein that promotes immune tolerance by selectively targeting the IL-2R on regulatory T cells. *The Journal of Immunology: Official Journal of the American Association of Immunologists, 201*(9), 2579–2592. https://doi.org/10.4049/jimmunol.1800907

Waykar, R., & Kulkarni, Y. A. (2025). Informed consent: Navigating the bioethical complexities of clinical research. *Bioinformation, 21*(9), 2950–2955. https://doi.org/10.6026/973206300212950

Wellman, S. M., Cambi, F., & Kozai, T. D. (2018). The role of oligodendrocytes and their progenitors on neural interface technology: A novel perspective on tissue regeneration and repair. *Biomaterials, 183*, 200–217. https://doi.org/10.1016/j.biomaterials.2018.08.046

Wen, X., Zhang, B., Wu, B., et al. (2022). Signaling pathways in obesity: Mechanisms and therapeutic interventions. *Signal Transduction and Targeted Therapy, 7*, 298. https://doi.org/10.1038/s41392-022-01149-x

Wu, D., Chen, Q., Chen, X., Han, F., Chen, Z., & Wang, Y. (2023). The blood–brain barrier: Structure, regulation and drug delivery. *Signal Transduction and Targeted Therapy, 8*(1), 217. https://doi.org/10.1038/s41392-023-01481-w

Xiao, G., & Gan, L. S. (2013). Receptor-mediated endocytosis and brain delivery of therapeutic biologics. *International Journal of Cell Biology, 2013*, Article 703545. https://doi.org/10.1155/2013/703545

Yan, X., Liu, X., Zhao, C., & Chen, G. Q. (2023). Applications of synthetic biology in medical and pharmaceutical fields. *Signal Transduction and Targeted Therapy, 8*, 199. https://doi.org/10.1038/s41392-023-01440-5

Yi, X., Manickam, D. S., Brynskikh, A., & Kabanov, A. V. (2014). Agile delivery of protein therapeutics to CNS. *Journal of Controlled Release: Official Journal of the Controlled Release Society, 0*, 637–663. https://doi.org/10.1016/j.jconrel.2014.06.017

Yin, H., Kanasty, R. L., Eltoukhy, A. A., Vegas, A. J., Dorkin, J. R., & Anderson, D. G. (2014). Non-viral vectors for gene-based therapy. *Nature Reviews Genetics, 15*(8), 541–555. https://doi.org/10.1038/nrg3763

Yu, Y. J., Atwal, J. K., Zhang, Y., et al. (2014). Therapeutic bispecific antibodies cross the blood-brain barrier in nonhuman primates. *Science Translational Medicine, 6*(261), Article 261ra154. https://doi.org/10.1126/scitranslmed.3009835

Yuasa-Kawada, J., Kinoshita-Kawada, M., Hiramoto, M., et al. (2025). Neuronal guidance signaling in neurodegenerative diseases: Key regulators that function at neuron-glia and neuroimmune interfaces. *Neural Regeneration Research, 21*(2), 612–635. https://doi.org/10.4103/NRR.NRR-D-24-01330

Zavvarian, M. M., Modi, A. D., Sadat, S., Hong, J., & Fehlings, M. G. (2024). Translational relevance of secondary intracellular signaling cascades following traumatic spinal cord injury. *International Journal of Molecular Sciences, 25*(11), 5708. https://doi.org/10.3390/ijms25115708

Zeb, A., Rana, I., Choi, H. I., et al. (2020). Potential and applications of nanocarriers for efficient delivery of biopharmaceuticals. *Pharmaceutics, 12*(12), 1184. https://doi.org/10.3390/pharmaceutics12121184

Zhang, Q. H., Chen, Q., Kang, J. R., et al. (2011). Treatment with gelsolin reduces brain inflammation and apoptotic signaling in mice following thermal injury. *Journal of Neuroinflammation, 8*, 118. https://doi.org/10.1186/1742-2094-8-118

Zhang, Q., Niu, Y., Li, Y., et al. (2025c). Meningeal lymphatic drainage: Novel insights into central nervous system disease. *Signal Transduction and Targeted Therapy, 10*(1), 142. https://doi.org/10.1038/s41392-025-02177-z

Zhang, H., Wang, J., Wei, J., Fu, X., Ma, J., & Chen, J. (2025b). Molecular engineering of recombinant protein hydrogels: Programmable design and biomedical applications. *Gels, 11*(8), 579. https://doi.org/10.3390/gels11080579

Zhao, L., Chen, S., Sherchan, P., et al. (2018). Recombinant CTRP9 administration attenuates neuroinflammation via activating adiponectin receptor 1 after intracerebral hemorrhage in mice. *Journal of Neuroinflammation, 15*(1), 215. https://doi.org/10.1186/s12974-018-1256-8

Zhao, J. Y., Zhou, Y., Zhou, C. W., et al. (2025). Revisiting the critical roles of reactive microglia in traumatic brain injury. *International Journal of Surgery, 111*(6), 3942–3978. https://doi.org/10.1097/JS9.0000000000002420

Zhi, J., Zhao, K. X., Liu, J. H., et al. (2024). The therapeutic potential of gelsolin in attenuating cytokine storm, ARDS, and ALI in severe COVID-19. *Frontiers in Pharmacology, 15*, Article 1447403. https://doi.org/10.3389/fphar.2024.1447403

CHAPTER

5 Peptides and their ligands: A new frontier in immunomodulation

Vineet Arora[1] **and Pardeep Kumar Singh**[2]

[1]*Department of Behavioral Health, Children's Hospital of Philadelphia, Philadelphia, PA, United States;* [2]*Department of Neuroimaging and Interventional Radiology, National Institute of Mental Health and Neurosciences, Bangalore, Karnataka, India*

1. Introduction

The exploration of peptides as promising therapeutics for neurological disorders has gained substantial momentum in recent years, driven by the urgent need for novel treatments capable of addressing the complex pathophysiology of these diseases (Silva-Reis et al., 2023). Neurological disorders, encompassing neurodegenerative conditions such as Alzheimer's disease, Parkinson's disease, and autoimmune diseases like multiple sclerosis, impose considerable burdens on patients and healthcare systems globally (Ding et al., 2022; Kumar et al., 2024). Traditional therapeutic approaches often provide symptomatic relief rather than disease modification and are frequently limited by poor specificity and significant systemic toxicity ((Gokhale & Satyanarayanajois, 2014). In this context, peptides emerge as a highly attractive class of molecules due to their inherent biological functions, which include hormone regulation, neurotransmission, and immune system modulation (Li, 2012).

The importance of targeted immunomodulation with high specificity and low toxicity for neurological disorders cannot be overstated, as these diseases often involve dysregulated immune responses that contribute to neuroinflammation and neurodegeneration (Hu et al., 2018). Peptides offer the ability to engage specific cell surface receptors, enabling precise modulation of immune pathways without the broad immunosuppressive effects associated with many conventional therapies. This selectivity can reduce systemic toxicity, which is particularly critical for chronic neurological conditions requiring long-term treatment (Gokhale & Satyanarayanajois, 2014). Furthermore, peptides' versatile structural properties allow for tailored design to enhance their stability, bioavailability, and ability to cross the blood-brain barrier, addressing one of the primary challenges in CNS therapeutics (Zhang & Eiden, 2019).

The scope and objectives of this chapter include providing a comprehensive overview of the biological roles of peptides in the nervous system, highlighting their therapeutic potential in modulating immune responses in neurological disorders, and discussing current advances and challenges in peptide-based drug development for CNS diseases (Kaspar & Reichert, 2013). The chapter also aims to elucidate innovative delivery approaches, such as chemical modification and nanoparticle encapsulation, which overcome the inherent limitations of peptides, like rapid degradation and poor brain

Immunotherapies for Neurological Disorders. https://doi.org/10.1016/B978-0-443-44631-3.00012-3

penetration (Disha, 2025). Moreover, it seeks to integrate findings from preclinical studies and clinical trials to assess the translational potential of peptide therapeutics in diseases such as multiple sclerosis, Parkinson's disease, and Alzheimer's disease (Metaxakis et al., 2020). Through this analysis, the chapter underscores the transformative promise of peptides as highly specific, low-toxicity immunomodulators in the future landscape of neurological disease treatment (Russo et al., 2016).

2. Importance of targeted immunomodulation in neurological disorders

Targeted immunomodulation is crucial in neurological conditions marked by dysregulated immune responses, neuroinflammation, and neurodegeneration. The immune system plays a significant role in neurodegenerative diseases; in conditions like multiple sclerosis, it is the primary driver, while in diseases such as Alzheimer's disease, amyotrophic lateral sclerosis, and Parkinson's disease, it has an amplifying role. Immunotherapeutic approaches that target both the adaptive and innate immune systems are being investigated for almost all neurological diseases, often with common targets and strategies across different conditions. Microglia, the primary immune cells in the brain, are key contributors to disease pathogenesis and are consequently frequent therapeutic targets (Strzelec et al., 2023). Other therapeutic strategies focus on components of the peripheral immune system, such as regulatory T cells and monocytes, which exert their effects within the central nervous system (CNS) (Weiner, 2025). Additionally, the microbiome is gaining recognition as an emerging therapeutic target that indirectly modulates the immune system (Ma et al., 2024). Understanding the immune mechanisms involved in neurodegenerative diseases is vital for developing immunomodulatory therapies, as these mechanisms often involve peripheral immune cells like T cells and monocytes, as well as CNS-resident cells such as microglia (Cohen et al., 2024). Immunomodulatory therapies aim to alter or modify the immune response, and the specific choice of immunosuppressive therapy is tailored to the type and severity of the neurological disorder (Firdaus & Li, 2024).

2.1 Immune system's contribution to neuroinflammation and neurodegeneration

Immune dysregulation is a central feature linking neuroinflammation to neurodegeneration (DeMaio et al., 2022). Neuroinflammation, the CNS's immune response to injury, infection, or disease, can be acutely protective, clearing pathogens and facilitating tissue repair (Carmelina Gemma, no date). Yet, when chronic or dysregulated, this inflammatory process significantly contributes to neuronal damage, synaptic dysfunction, and cognitive decline (Kim & Lee, 2025). This persistent inflammation, driven by activated glial cells such as microglia and astrocytes, leads to the release of pro-inflammatory cytokines and chemokines, and the infiltration of peripheral leukocytes into the CNS (Fornari Laurindo et al., 2024). In neurodegenerative diseases, protein misfolding and accumulation, such as amyloid plaques and tau tangles in Alzheimer's disease, or α-synuclein aggregates in Parkinson's disease, can trigger and sustain these innate inflammatory responses (Carriba & Comella, 2015). Furthermore, systemic inflammation, potentially exacerbated by immune aging, has been associated with neurodegenerative biomarkers and cognitive dysfunction, suggesting that interventions to reduce systemic inflammation could mitigate neurodegeneration (Klopak & Crimmins, 2023). The intricate balance between beneficial and detrimental inflammatory effects dictates the outcome of neurodegenerative processes, making a precise understanding of immune dysregulation critical for therapeutic intervention.

2.2 Key immune cells: Microglia, T cells, and monocytes

The intricate interplay of specific immune cells is paramount in neurological disorders. Microglia, the CNS's resident macrophages, are central to both maintaining brain homeostasis and mediating neuroinflammatory processes. In healthy brains, microglia constantly survey their microenvironment, clearing damaged cells and pathogens. However, under pathological conditions, microglia become activated, secreting pro-inflammatory mediators that can lead to neuronal dysfunction and neurodegeneration (Nimmerjahn et al., 2005). Their role is complex and dual, sometimes offering neuroprotection and repair, while at other times exacerbating damage in diseases like Alzheimer's and Parkinson's. For instance, over-expressed Interleukin-1 (IL-1) from microglia in Alzheimer's brains can lead to extreme tau phosphorylation, associated with tangle development (Kaushik & Basu, 2013).

T cells, components of the adaptive immune system, also play critical and often paradoxical roles in CNS disorders. While traditionally associated with autoimmune conditions like multiple sclerosis, T cells are increasingly recognized for their involvement in neurodegenerative diseases such as Alzheimer's, Parkinson's, and ALS. T cell dysregulation can lead to detrimental autoimmune responses, but beneficial roles, including tissue protection, neuroregeneration, and immunomodulation, have also been uncovered (DeMaio et al., 2022). Different T cell subsets, such as regulatory T cells (Tregs), can dampen inflammatory responses, and their reduced ability to do so in neurodegenerative disorders can perpetuate a pro-inflammatory environment.

Monocytes, originating from the bone marrow, represent another crucial immune cell population that can infiltrate the brain and contribute to neuroinflammation. These cells act as a first line of defense during inflammation, playing roles in both the pathogenesis and progression of neurological diseases (Savinetti et al., 2021). Monocytes have been implicated in various conditions, including Parkinson's disease and Alzheimer's disease, where their dysregulation is observed in the brain or periphery. Distinguishing the precise functions of monocytes from resident microglia has historically been challenging, but advanced single-cell technologies are improving this understanding. Their ability to infiltrate the CNS and adopt microglia-like phenotypes further highlights their complex role in neuroinflammation (Grabon et al., 2025).

2.3 Therapeutic strategies: Targeting adaptive and innate immune systems

Given the critical involvement of both innate and adaptive immune systems in neurological disorders, therapeutic strategies increasingly focus on targeted immunomodulation. Traditional immunosuppressive treatments, while effective in some cases, often lack disease specificity and can have undesirable side effects, including an increased risk of infections (Nath & Berger, 2012). Newer approaches aim to selectively modify immune responses to benefit the host (Ulevitch, 2004).

Targeting the innate immune system involves modulating proteins like Toll-like receptors (TLRs), NOD-like receptor family pyrin domain containing protein 3 (NLRP3) inflammasome, and myeloid differentiation primary-response protein 88 (MyD88) family members, which play important roles in recognizing pathogens and initiating immune responses. For instance, certain antidepressants can modulate the NLRP3-mediated inflammatory pathway, reducing proinflammatory cytokines (Strzelec et al., 2023). CSF1R antagonists are being explored to deplete or reset microglia as a therapeutic strategy for various neurological disorders, although recent research suggests CSF1R inhibition may also affect T-helper cell differentiation (Barca et al., 2021).

For the adaptive immune system, strategies include inhibiting or potentiating T cell and B cell responses, as well as modulating antibody production and memory (Schäfer et al., 2017). Monoclonal antibodies (mAbs) represent a significant advance, offering highly selective binding capacity against specific immune targets, such as proinflammatory cytokines or surface receptors on immune cells. IFN-β, for example, is used in multiple sclerosis therapy to mitigate inflammatory processes and inhibit T-cell activation and migration across the blood-brain barrier. Genomic editing tools like CRISPR-Cas9 are also emerging as promising, enabling the inactivation or replacement of specific genes, with applications in modifying T cells to combat diseases and understanding autoimmune pathogenesis. RNA interference (RNAi) is another novel approach, utilizing microRNAs (miRNAs) and small interfering RNAs (siRNAs) to inhibit gene expression, with potential for treating inflammatory and autoimmune diseases once delivery challenges are overcome. Mesenchymal stem cells (MSCs) are also being explored due to their immunomodulatory features and ability to suppress T cell proliferation and promote regulatory T cell expansion, showing promise in neurodegenerative diseases and CNS injuries (Strzelec et al., 2023).

2.4 Emerging role of the microbiome

The human microbiome, particularly the gut microbiota, is gaining recognition as a significant modulator of neurological health and disease through the complex gut-brain axis (GBA) (Ijaz et al., 2024, pp. 273–301). Gut dysbiosis—an imbalance in microbial communities—is associated with altered intestinal and blood-brain barrier permeability, activated inflammatory responses, and changes in microbial metabolites, all of which can contribute to the development and progression of neurological disorders like Alzheimer's, Parkinson's, MS, epilepsy, and autism spectrum disorder (Qin et al., 2020).

The gut microbiota influences neuroinflammation and neurodegeneration through various mechanisms, including modulating immune responses, producing neuroactive compounds, and influencing brain development (Qin et al., 2020). For instance, gut microbiota changes can exacerbate neurodegeneration in Alzheimer's disease via pro-inflammatory microorganisms. The potential for microbiota-based therapies, such as probiotics or fecal microbiome transplantation, to normalize gut microbiota and counteract neurological impairment is a burgeoning area of research (Liu et al., 2022). Furthermore, gut microbial extracellular vesicles (EVs) are emerging as pivotal communicators in the gut-brain axis, capable of crossing the blood-brain barrier and exerting regulatory functions on brain cells, suggesting their therapeutic potential in treating neurological disorders (Sun et al., 2023).

2.5 Tailoring immunosuppressive therapies

Tailoring immunosuppressive therapies involves developing personalized treatment regimens that consider the specific immunological dysfunction of a patient, the disease's mechanisms, and the risk-benefit ratio of therapeutic agents (Nath & Berger, 2012). The increasing understanding of immune-mediated neurological conditions and the development of novel immunomodulatory agents necessitate a practical and individualized approach to patient management. For example, early administration of immunosuppressive therapy has been shown to benefit patients in observational studies (Ashraf et al., 2022).

This personalized approach is crucial for optimizing treatment outcomes and minimizing adverse effects, especially given the neurotoxic potential of some immunosuppressive drugs. Tailored therapies consider specific components of the immune system, such as adhesion molecules or surface receptors on particular cell classes, to achieve more precise immunomodulation. For instance, therapies like natalizumab, an $\alpha4\beta1$ integrin inhibitor effective in multiple sclerosis, illustrate the benefits of targeted perturbation while also highlighting the need to understand unique opportunistic infection risks associated with such specific disruptions (Nath & Berger, 2012). The continuous study of new treatment targets and the integration of novel biotechnological and pharmacological techniques are leading to more efficient and safer personalized treatments for neurological diseases of immunological origin (Strzelec et al., 2023). However, challenges remain in translating these findings into clinically viable and broadly applicable therapies, necessitating further research, particularly in randomized clinical trials (Fornari Laurindo et al., 2024).

3. Biological roles of peptides in the nervous system

Peptides play essential roles in the nervous system, acting as neurotransmitters, neuromodulators, hormones, and immunoregulatory agents across the central and peripheral nervous systems. Their actions are primarily mediated through G protein-coupled receptors (GPCRs), a large family of over 800 membrane receptors that respond to diverse extracellular signals, including more than 100 identified neuropeptides. Peptide-binding GPCRs regulate numerous physiological processes, making them key targets for therapies against diseases such as diabetes, cancer, and neurodegeneration, as well as for veterinary and agricultural applications (Azam et al., 2020). Dysfunction of peptide-GPCR signaling is implicated in neurodegenerative and psychiatric disorders, while specific neuropeptides—including POMC-derived peptides, neuropeptide Y, vasoactive intestinal peptide, somatostatin, calcitonin gene-related peptide, and cortistatin—modulate inflammation and pain via GPCRs (Birgül Iyison et al., 2025). Neuropeptides frequently co-exist and co-release with classical neurotransmitters, a phenomenon known as cotransmission, which allows complex regulation of synaptic activity. Examples include cholecystokinin with dopamine, galanin with acetylcholine, substance P and thyrotropin-releasing hormone with serotonin, CRH and substance P with acetylcholine, oxytocin with cholecystokinin, and neuropeptide Y with somatostatin. These co-released peptides can synergistically or antagonistically influence neurotransmitter synthesis, release, reuptake, and receptor activity, with their expression tightly regulated by physiological, chemical, and pathological cues (Crawley, 1990). Advances in GPCR structural biology have illuminated the molecular mechanisms of peptide recognition, facilitating the development of peptide-based therapeutics with improved efficacy.

3.1 Peptides as neurotransmitters and neuromodulators

Neuropeptides are a large and varied class of signaling molecules in the brain, capable of acting directly as neurotransmitters or as modulators of ongoing synaptic activity. They modulate various biological effects, including membrane excitability, synaptic transmission, synaptogenesis, gene expression, and glial cell architecture and function (Casello et al., 2022). Many neuropeptides coexist with classical neurotransmitters, such as acetylcholine and catecholamines, in the same neurons, suggesting intricate interactions. This concept of cotransmission, where peptides intervene in transmission processes, opens new avenues for neurological and psychiatric research. For example, the trace amines in the mammalian central nervous system, including 2-phenylethylamine and tyramine, are hypothesized to function as endogenous neuromodulators of classical monoamine neurotransmitters, altering neuronal sensitivity to monoamines without changing neuronal excitability in their absence (Berry, 2004). Over 25 biologically active peptides have been identified in the CNS, regulating complex cerebral functions like sleep, ingestive and motor behavior, pain, cognition, emotions, and mood. Peptides in the mammalian cochlea, such as enkephalins, dynorphins, and calcitonin gene-related peptide, also serve as efferent neurotransmitters and neuromodulators (Eybalin, 1993). In certain neurological disorders, such as depression and senile dementia, altered levels of neuropeptides like CCK, CRF, NPY, somatostatin, and substance P have been observed in cerebrospinal fluid and cortical extracts, indicating their involvement in pathological states (Tuominen & Leppäluoto, 1987).

3.2 Hormonal regulation and signaling

Peptides in the nervous system also function as neurohormones, playing a critical role in hormonal regulation and signaling (Li, 2012). They are widely distributed throughout the nervous system, gastrointestinal tract, and pancreas of both vertebrate and invertebrate animals, acting as intercellular messengers (Brown & Fisher, 1984). Neuropeptides and peptide hormones are abundant cell-to-cell signaling molecules in both the central nervous system and the endocrine system (Abid et al., 2021). They regulate physiological functions, including energy homeostasis and feeding, through hypothalamic circuits that integrate peripheral signals. Hormonal peptides, such as GLP-1 and melanocortins, modulate synaptic function and behavior, mediating neuroendocrine control and homeostasis via complex intracellular signaling pathways. The concept of a central peptidergic nervous system, distinct but interrelated with other neurotransmitter systems, has emerged, suggesting that products of neurosecretory neurons originally served both neurohormonal and neurotransmitter functions (Krieger, 1979). This system is phylogenetically ancient and involves a distinctive class of neurosecretory neurons. The insulin-like signaling pathway, for example, controls aging, metabolism, and development in Caenorhabditis elegans, with neuronal signaling alone being sufficient to regulate lifespan (Wolkow et al., 2000). Hypothalamic peptides like thyrotropin-releasing factor (TRF), somatostatin, and bombesin-like peptide are present in the brain and are involved in CNS control of visceral functions, including thermoregulation, adrenal epinephrine secretion, gastric acid secretion, heart rate, and blood pressure. Neuropeptide Y, a pleiotropic factor expressed in several areas of the nervous system, is also involved in various regulatory processes. See Fig. 5.1.

3.3 Immune system modulation

Peptides are crucial modulators of the immune system within the nervous system, influencing immune responses and promoting neuroprotection. They act as immunoregulatory agents, interacting with immune cells like lymphocytes and microglia. The peripheral nervous system is connected to lymphoid organs through sensory nerves that release neuropeptides, such as calcitonin gene-related peptide (CGRP), which can influence immune responses (Holzmann, 2013). CGRP inhibits the effector functions of various immune cells and dampens inflammation by amplifying IL-10 production and inducing the transcriptional repressor inducible cAMP early repressor (ICER). Local and systemic levels of CGRP rapidly increase during inflammatory responses, highlighting its role as a potent peptidergic anti-inflammatory pathway (Waschek, 2013). Another example is vasoactive intestinal peptide (VIP), which, along with pituitary adenylyl cyclase-activating peptide (PACAP), exerts

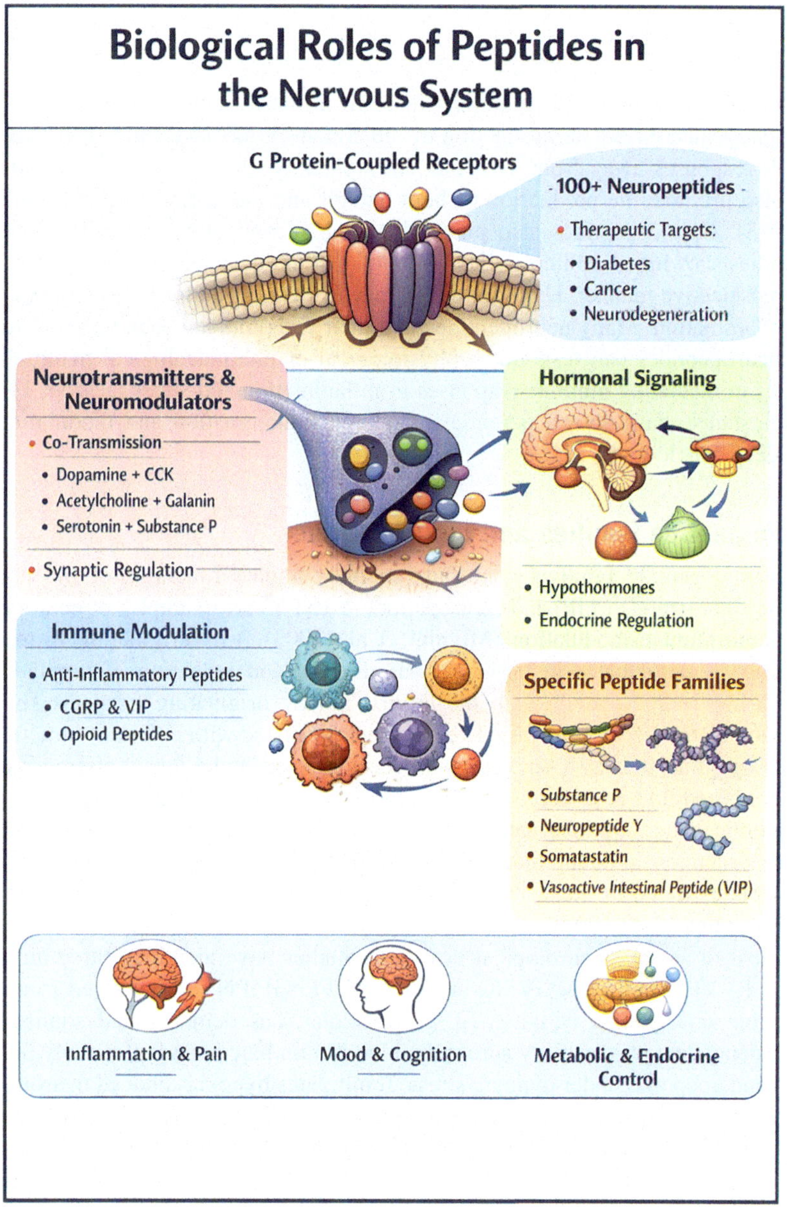

FIGURE 5.1 Biological roles of peptides in the nervous system.

Schematic overview illustrating the multifaceted functions of peptides across the central and peripheral nervous systems. Neuropeptides act as neurotransmitters, neuromodulators, neurohormones, and immunoregulatory agents, primarily signaling through peptide-binding G protein–coupled receptors (GPCRs). These pathways regulate synaptic transmission and cotransmission with classical neurotransmitters, neuronal excitability, hormonal homeostasis via neuroendocrine circuits, and immune responses through interactions with microglia and peripheral immune cells. Representative peptide families, including neuropeptide Y, vasoactive intestinal peptide, substance P, somatostatin, and calcitonin gene-related peptide, are highlighted to emphasize their roles in inflammation, pain modulation, cognition, metabolism, and neuroprotection. Advances in GPCR structural biology have further enabled the rational design of peptide-based therapeutics targeting neurological, neuropsychiatric, and neurodegenerative disorders.

powerful in vivo immunomodulatory actions that are primarily anti-inflammatory. These peptides inhibit macrophage and microglia production of inflammatory mediators like TNF-α and IFN-γ, and polarize T-cell responses away from Th1 and Th17 phenotypes toward a Th2 phenotype. VIP and PACAP can also promote the production of both natural and inducible subsets of regulatory T-cells (Waschek, 2013). Opioid peptides also play a key role in regulating some immune system functions, with studies showing morphine's effect on human granulocyte aggregation and ATP release in a naloxone stereoselective manner. Dynorphin 1–9 may act as a mediator between the central nervous system and inflammation. Many neuropeptides and their receptors are found within immune tissues, and immunoneuropeptides can respond to physiological or pharmacological manipulation, playing important roles in mediating immune responses to inflammation and stress (Jessop, 1998). Bioactive peptides, for instance, have shown potential in treating inflammation and modulating immune responses (Kuldeep Singh et al., 2025).

3.4 Specific peptide families and their functions

Numerous specific peptide families contribute to the complex functions of the nervous system. Vasoactive intestinal peptide (VIP) and Neuropeptide Y (NPY) are examples of neuropeptides widely involved in neuroimmune modulation (Mignini et al., 2003). VIP, originating from intralaryngeal ganglionic neurons, participates in laryngeal vasodilation and reduction of laryngeal seromucous secretion. NPY nerve fibers are few in the larynx, mostly originating from the superior cervical ganglion, and are distributed around blood vessels and associated with excretory structures. Substance P, another neuropeptide, acts as a sensory neurotransmitter in the laryngeal afferent system and regulates laryngeal blood flow and secretion. Calcitonin gene-related peptide (CGRP) is associated with sensory, autonomic, and motor innervation of the larynx. Enkephalin nerve fibers are primarily located near excretory structures, although their precise physiological significance is still being investigated. Other neuropeptides found in the larynx include peptides histidine isoleucine, histidine methionine, and helospectin (Hisa et al., 1999).

In the context of specific neurological disorders, studies have identified three bioactive peptides (YPFPGPIPN, PVVPPFLQPEVMGVSK, and T3-LVYPFPGPIPN (T3)) derived from yak milk residue that exhibit anti-hypoxic activity. T3, in particular, has demonstrated significant time- and concentration-dependent permeability across the blood-brain barrier and effectively inhibits neuronal inflammation and apoptosis under hypoxic stress. It mitigates hypoxia-induced neuroinflammation by regulating L-glutamine metabolism through the RAS/TNF-α/MAPK signaling pathway (Yang et al., 2025). Peptide agonists and antagonists are also being investigated for their potential application in neurological disorders, including neurodegenerative diseases. These peptides can serve as receptor antagonists, inhibitors of protein-protein interactions, and many are either commercial drugs or in clinical trials. Their versatile structural properties allow for tailored design to enhance stability, bioavailability, and blood-brain barrier penetration, addressing key challenges in CNS therapeutics. Despite challenges in bioavailability and metabolic stability, new synthetic strategies and alternative administration routes are being developed to expand the number of peptide-based drugs in preclinical phases (Anna Russo et al., 2015). Neuropeptides such as dynorphin, enkephalin, corticotropin-releasing factor, cholecystokinin, somatostatin, neuropeptide Y, and vasoactive intestinal peptide are expressed in the prefrontal cortex and are being studied for their implications in prefrontal cortical circuit function and as potential therapeutic targets for neuropsychiatric disorders (Casello et al., 2022).

4. Therapeutic potential of peptides in modulating immune responses in neurological disorders

Peptides hold significant therapeutic potential in modulating immune responses in neurological disorders through various mechanisms, including receptor engagement, pathway modulation, reduction of neuroinflammation, promotion of neuroprotection, and enhancement of neuroregeneration (Souza-Moreira et al., 2011; Waschek, 2013). This section delves into these key areas, highlighting how peptides can offer a more targeted and effective approach to treating complex neurological conditions.

4.1 Mechanisms of action: Receptor engagement and pathway modulation

Peptides can modulate immune responses by engaging specific receptors and influencing crucial signaling pathways (Badawi & Siahaan, 2012). For instance, certain neuropeptides produced during inflammation act as endogenous anti-inflammatory agents by regulating the balance between pro-inflammatory and anti-inflammatory factors and by inducing regulatory T cells. Vasoactive intestinal peptide (VIP) serves as an example of an immunomodulatory neuropeptide, with similar characteristics found in adrenomedullin, urocortin, cortistatin, and ghrelin (Souza-Moreira et al., 2011). The neuroimmunomodulatory peptide α-melanocyte-stimulating hormone (α-MSH) has been shown to modulate peripheral inflammation by inhibiting the production of proinflammatory agents like TNF-α through action on melanocortin receptors in host cells. Within the brain, α-MSH also directly modulates local inflammation, reducing TNF-α and nitric oxide production in microglial cells and human astrocytes (Lipton et al., 1998). Peptides can also act as agonists, activating specific receptors to initiate desired cellular responses, or as antagonists, blocking certain cellular processes. They are also valuable specific modulators of protein-mediated signaling, serving as inhibitors of protein-protein interactions (Badawi & Siahaan, 2012). Some peptides modulate the immune response and interact with specific receptors like P2X7, which is a potential therapeutic target (De Souza Oliveira Carneiro et al., 2025).

4.2 Reducing neuroinflammation

Neuroinflammation is a complex inflammatory process in the central nervous system where microglia play a critical role, contributing to the development and progression of various neurological disorders (García-Domínguez, 2025). Peptides are increasingly recognized for their ability to reduce neuroinflammation, offering a promising therapeutic strategy (Mengr et al., 2025). For example, the peptide GPETAFLR, isolated from Lupinus angustifolius L. protein hydrolysates, effectively inhibits LPS-induced upregulation of pro-inflammatory and M1 marker genes in BV-2 microglial cells. It also increases the expression of M2 marker genes and counteracts high-fat diet-induced downregulation of IL-10 and upregulation of pro-inflammatory markers in the mouse brain. This suggests that GPETAFLR can help maintain CNS homeostasis by inhibiting neuroinflammation (Lemus-Conejo et al., 2022).

Neuropeptides, such as proopiomelanocortin (POMC) gene-derived peptides, neuropeptide Y (NPY), vasoactive intestinal peptide (VIP), somatostatin (SST), calcitonin gene-related peptide (CGRP), and cortistatin (CST), can affect inflammatory responses and pain sensitivity by modulating glial cell activity (Carniglia et al., 2017). VIP and pituitary adenylyl cyclase-activating peptide (PACAP), which are upregulated in neurons and immune cells after injury or inflammation, exert powerful in vivo immunomodulatory actions that are primarily anti-inflammatory. These peptides inhibit macrophage and microglia production of inflammatory mediators such as TNF-α and IFN-γ, and shift T-cell responses away from Th1 and Th17 phenotypes toward a Th2 phenotype. Furthermore, they can promote the production of both natural and inducible subsets of regulatory T-cells (Waschek, 2013). The peptide analogue of thymulin (PAT) has also demonstrated potent anti-inflammatory effects in both peripheral tissues and the brain, partly through the activation of cholinergic mechanisms. Short peptides can also exert neuroprotective effects on cerebral ischemia-reperfusion injury by reducing inflammation via the miR-6328/IKKβ/NF-κB axis (Li et al., 2023). Copper-binding peptides have been shown to attenuate microglia inflammation by suppressing the NF-kB pathway (Caetano-Silva et al., 2021). Overall, these studies highlight the potential of peptides to mitigate neuroinflammation, a common underlying mechanism in many neurological conditions (Mengr et al., 2025).

4.3 Promoting neuroprotection

Neurodegeneration, characterized by the progressive loss of neuronal populations, is a hallmark of many neurological disorders. Peptides offer significant promise in promoting neuroprotection by targeting various mechanisms involved in these diseases (Shashi & Rajnish, 2014). Brain-gut peptides, including glucagon-like peptide 1, pituitary adenylate cyclase activating polypeptide, nesfatin-1, and ghrelin, have demonstrated neuroprotective effects in both in vivo and in vitro studies, making them promising treatments for conditions like Parkinson's disease (PD) (Dong et al., 2019). Neurotrophins, neurotrophic factors (such as NGF, BDNF, and GDNF), neuropeptides, mitochondrial-targeted antioxidants/peptides like MitoQ, and β-sheet breaker peptides are all being investigated for their utility in addressing neurodegenerative disorders (Shashi & Rajnish, 2014). The neuroprotective effects of glucagon-like peptide 1 (GLP-1), a peptide hormone and growth factor, have been observed in preclinical studies (Reich & Hölscher, 2022). Neuropeptides such as prolactin-releasing peptide (palm11-PrRP31) and ghrelin have shown neuroprotective properties by reducing Aβ plaque load and microgliosis in Alzheimer's disease mouse models (Mengr et al., 2025). Adropin, another neuropeptide, has been shown to reverse cognitive dysfunction associated with aging in mice. NPY has also been suggested to attenuate the toxic effects of Aβ accumulation and has a neuroprotective role in neural networks, being implicated in several neurological disorders including PD, Huntington's disease, Machado-Joseph disease, and ALS (Yeo et al., 2022). Furthermore, peptides are used to inhibit mitochondrial permeability transition (MPT), a key process in neurodegenerative diseases, with examples such as Ba–V from snake venom (Asmita Yadav et al., 2021).

4.4 Enhancing neuroregeneration

Neuroregeneration, the process of repairing and regenerating nervous tissue, is crucial for functional recovery after neurological injuries and diseases (Tsai et al., 2025). Peptides are being explored for their ability to enhance neuroregeneration, particularly in the central nervous system, which has limited intrinsic repair capabilities (Xiao-Yan Song et al., 2024). The TnP peptide, a synthetic peptide family, has shown a disease-suppressive function in experimental autoimmune encephalomyelitis (EAE), an animal model for multiple sclerosis (MS). TnP ameliorated disease severity, suppressed the accumulation of pro-inflammatory T helper lymphocytes and activated microglia/macrophage populations in the CNS, and promoted remyelination. Compared to existing therapies, TnP was more effective in the long-term control of neuronal degeneration and in reversing leukocyte infiltration into the spinal cord, while also inducing a higher percentage of regulatory cells. This specialized profile for inducing immune tolerance and neuronal regeneration suggests significant therapeutic potential for MS and other autoimmune diseases (Lima et al., 2022).

Synthetic peptides offer a promising approach for neural repair, functioning as soluble drugs or as extracellular matrix (ECM) mimics for cell adhesion through their self-assembly properties. Functionalized self-assembling nanopeptide hydrogels, such as RADA16-SVVYGLR, can facilitate angiogenesis and neurogenesis at brain injury sites. These hydrogels can support endothelial cells in forming tube-like structures and neural stem cells in survival and proliferation, leading to enhanced functional recovery in injured brain models (Wang et al., 2017). Some peptides, like those with the general formula A-B-L-Phe (or L-Ala)-D-Lys-L-Phe-Z-OH, have been identified for their ability to promote axonal regeneration. Peptoids, which are peptidomimetics, also show potential for neurotherapeutic applications, including modulating cell signaling pathways involved in axonal function and promoting anti-inflammatory actions, which can indirectly support regeneration (Tsai et al., 2025). See Fig. 5.2.

5. Current advances and challenges in peptide-based drug development for CNS diseases

The development of peptide-based drugs for central nervous system (CNS) diseases is a rapidly evolving field that holds immense promise for addressing a wide range of neurological disorders, from neurodegenerative conditions like Alzheimer's and Parkinson's to mental health disorders and stroke. Peptides, with their high specificity, potent biological activity, and favorable safety profiles, offer distinct advantages over traditional small-molecule drugs. However, translating these advantages into effective CNS therapies is fraught with challenges, primarily due to their inherent susceptibility to enzymatic degradation, limited bioavailability, and the formidable barrier presented by the blood-brain barrier (BBB).

This section will delve into the cutting-edge advancements in peptide design and synthesis that are revolutionizing the landscape of peptide therapeutics. We will then critically examine the persistent challenges, focusing on issues of stability, bioavailability, and the complex mechanisms of the blood-brain barrier that impede drug delivery to the CNS. Finally, we will explore innovative strategies being developed to overcome these hurdles, paving the way for a new generation of highly effective peptide-based treatments for CNS diseases.

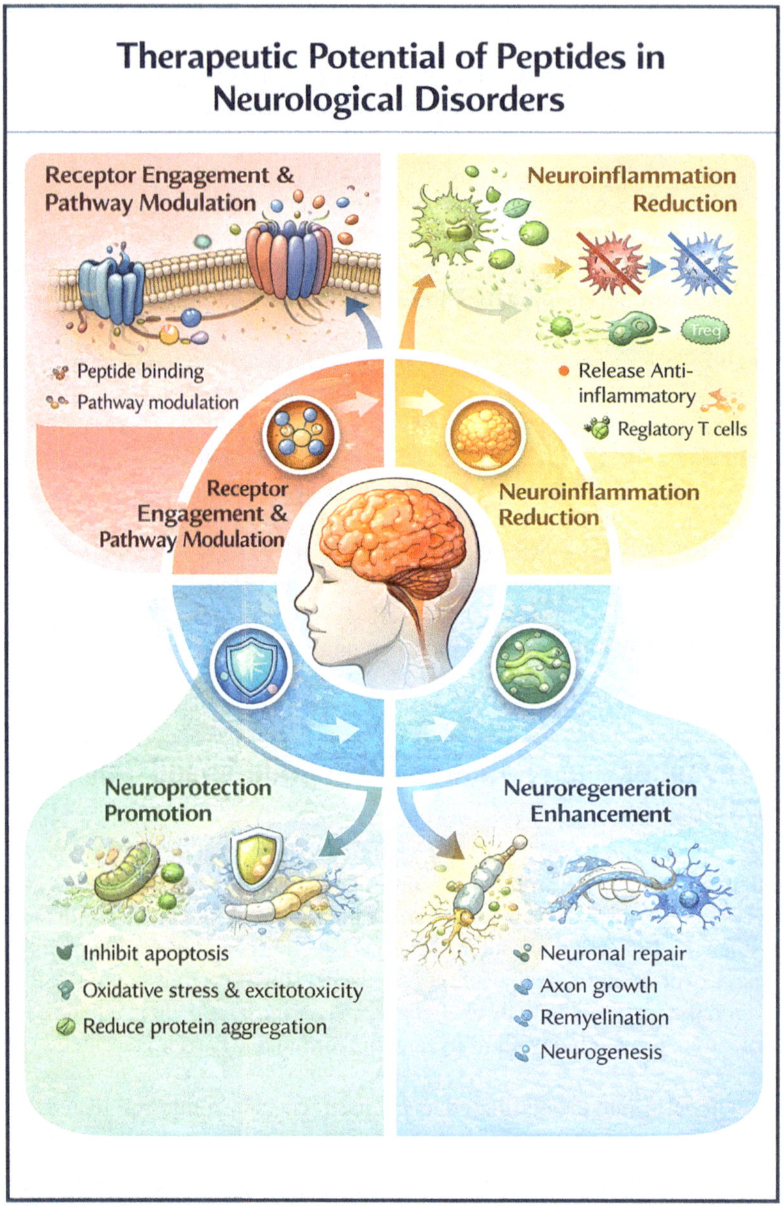

FIGURE 5.2 Therapeutic mechanisms of peptides in modulating immune responses in neurological disorders. Graphical summary illustrating how peptides exert therapeutic effects in the nervous system through four interconnected mechanisms. Peptides engage specific cell-surface receptors to modulate intracellular signaling pathways, suppress neuroinflammation by inhibiting microglial activation and promoting regulatory immune responses, enhance neuroprotection by reducing apoptosis, oxidative stress, and protein aggregation, and support neuroregeneration by promoting axonal growth, remyelination, and neurogenesis. Together, these mechanisms highlight the multifaceted potential of peptide-based interventions for immune-mediated and neurodegenerative disorders.

5.1 Advances in peptide design and synthesis

Recent years have seen substantial developments in biotechnological, pharmacological, and medical techniques that can be used to functionally modulate immune system components (Strzelec et al., 2023). Peptides possess unique advantages, including ease of synthesis, rapid optimization, reduced immune responses, lower toxic side effects, and swift clearance. Significant progress has been made in this area, with numerous peptide drugs on the market and many more undergoing clinical and preclinical studies. These drugs primarily target G protein-coupled receptors (GPCRs) and are often short, synthetic, and long-acting peptides. The field of peptide drug discovery is continuously evolving, with novel wet-lab and computational multi-omic methods contributing to the identification of new therapeutic agents (Vrbnjak & Sewduth, 2024). Further advances include the development of various peptide-based hydrogels for nerve regeneration, such as dipeptide, tripeptide, and oligopeptide hydrogels. Current knowledge about peptides as drugs is significant, with potential applications across various medical practices, including synthesis, biological activities, design strategies, screening methods, and optimization for stability and bioavailability (Xie et al., 2024).

5.2 Challenges: Stability, bioavailability, and blood-brain barrier penetration

Despite their therapeutic potential, peptides face considerable challenges, particularly in their application as central nervous system (CNS) drugs. One major hurdle is their poor metabolic stability and limited bioavailability, which is partly due to their inability to easily cross biological membrane barriers such as the intestinal and blood-brain barriers (BBB) (McGowan et al., 2015). Low oral bioavailability of peptides is often attributed to low absorption and high first-pass metabolism. The instability of therapeutic peptides in vivo further restricts their widespread use (Adessi & Soto, 2002).

The blood-brain barrier (BBB) poses the most significant obstacle for delivering therapeutics to the brain for CNS diseases (Lalatsa et al., 2014). It restricts the entry of over 98% of small-molecule drugs and nearly 100% of large-molecule drugs, including proteins, antibodies, and gene therapy drugs, preventing them from reaching therapeutic concentrations in the brain. This barrier is a specialized, protective structure essential for maintaining proper brain function and nutrient transport. The BBB is composed of cerebral capillary endothelial cells, tight junctions, basement membranes, and pericytes, which together maintain the stability of the CNS internal environment and prevent harmful substances from entering the brain (See Fig. 5.3). The compact nature of the BBB significantly limits the paracellular transport of molecules (Lalatsa et al., 2014).

In addition to the inherent challenges of the BBB, patients with neurodegenerative diseases (NDDs) often experience BBB dysfunction, including disrupted tight junctions and intensified inflammatory responses, which further impede drug delivery. This dysfunction in conditions like Alzheimer's disease can lead to the accumulation of neurotoxic proteins such as beta-amyloid peptide (Aβ) and Tau protein in the cerebral blood vessels and brain parenchyma. Similarly, in Parkinson's disease, abnormal aggregated proteins like α-synuclein cannot be effectively cleared due to impaired BBB function, leading to their deposition and toxic effects on nerve cells (Di, 2015). Moreover, the BBB can be damaged by various factors, altering its permeability and complicating drug delivery control, while abnormal immune responses reduce its effectiveness in treating NDDs (Lalatsa et al., 2014).

For peptide drugs, specific issues include rapid degradation and poor brain penetration. Traditional drug delivery methods, such as systemic administration, often require high doses to achieve effective brain concentrations, leading to increased toxic side effects and limiting clinical application. This

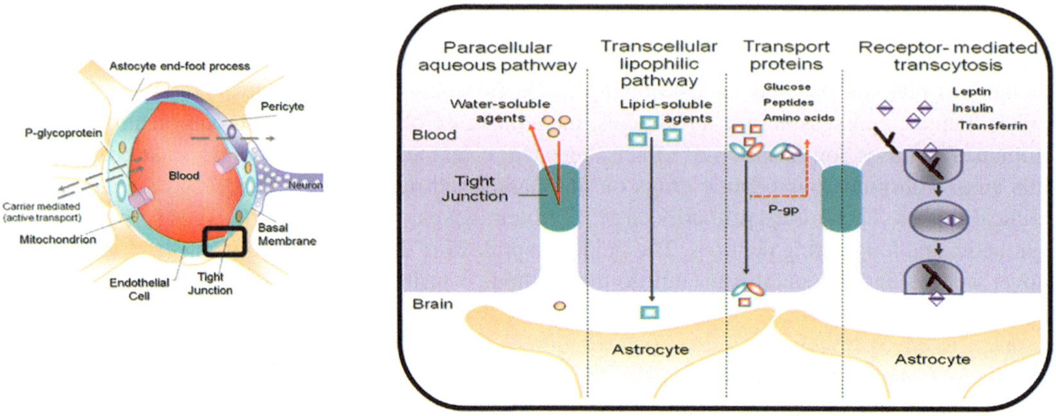

FIGURE 5.3 Structure and transport mechanisms of the blood-brain barrier.

Diagram of the blood-brain barrier illustrating its cellular components—endothelial cells with tight junctions, pericytes, basement membrane, and astrocyte end-feet—and the four main transport pathways: Paracellular aqueous pathway allowing limited passage of water-soluble agents, transcellular lipophilic pathway for lipid-soluble agents, transport proteins facilitating glucose, peptides, and amino acids transport, and receptor-mediated transcytosis enabling uptake of leptin, insulin, and transferrin. The P-glycoprotein efflux pump is shown removing some substances from endothelial cells.

Lalatsa, A., Schatzlein, A. G. & Uchegbu, I. F. (2014). Mol. Pharmaceutics, 11(4), 1081–1093. https://doi.org/10.1021/mp400680d.

problem is compounded by the fact that many peptides also have a short duration of action and require parenteral administration (Adessi & Soto, 2002).

5.3 Strategies to overcome challenges

To address the stability, bioavailability, and BBB penetration issues of peptide-based drugs for CNS diseases, various innovative strategies are being explored (Zhang et al., 2025). These approaches aim to improve drug stability, enhance absorption, and facilitate transport across the BBB.

One key area of strategy focuses on structural modifications of peptides to improve their properties.

1. Chemical Synthesis and Design: Recent advancements in chemical synthesis and design allow for the production of modified peptides and mimetics with increased resistance to proteolysis and improved bioavailability.
2. N- and C-terminal Modification or Substitution: Modifying the N- and/or C-termini of peptides can enhance their metabolic stability.
3. D-Amino Acid or Unnatural Amino Acid Substitution: Incorporating D-amino acids or unnatural amino acids can make peptides less susceptible to enzymatic degradation (Jin-Feng et al., 2018).
4. Cyclization: Cyclization of peptides can improve stability and resistance to proteolysis. Perfluoroarene-based peptide macrocycles, for instance, have shown increased uptake and

improved proteolytic stability, leading to enhanced penetration of the brain parenchyma in mice (Fadzen et al., 2017).

5. Backbone Modification: Modifying the peptide backbone is primarily done to improve proteolytic stability (Wang et al., 2022).
6. Isomeric Amino Acid Surrogates: Using isomeric amino acid surrogates, where the peptide bond is displaced by isosters, is another strategy to enhance stability (Lamers, 2022).
7. Glycosylation and Lipidation: Glycosylation and lipidation are effective strategies for improving peptide stability and penetration efficiency through the BBB. Glycosylation, in particular, has shown promise for small peptides. Increasing lipid solubility can enhance the ability of compounds to cross cell membranes that form the BBB. However, the relationship between lipid solubility and brain entry is biphasic, peaking at an octanol/water partition coefficient of 10–100 (Banks et al., 2024).
8. Increased Molecular Mass: Increasing the molecular mass of peptides can also contribute to improved stability and longevity in vivo (McGonigle, 2012).

Another set of strategies involves advanced delivery systems and methods to bypass the BBB.

1. Nanoparticle Formulations: Nanoparticle formulations, including liposomes and polymer nanoparticles, are widely used to enhance drug delivery across the BBB. These systems can encapsulate drugs, improve their stability, prolong circulation time, and reduce non-specific adsorption. Liposome drug carriers can be surface-modified, for example, through PEGylation or ligand modification, to enhance their penetration across the BBB. Smaller nanoparticles (typically less than 100 nm) are more likely to pass through the BBB. Polymer nanoparticles with tailored physicochemical properties, such as size, shape, and surface charge, can efficiently cross the BBB (Zhang et al., 2025).
2. Exosomes and Viral Vectors: Exosomes, being natural, cell-secreted vesicles, can pass through biological barriers and are less likely to trigger immune responses, making them promising nanocarriers. Viral vectors also possess natural transmembrane transport capabilities and can achieve brain-targeted drug delivery by mimicking viral infection mechanisms.
3. Cell-Penetrating Peptides (CPPs): CPPs are short peptide sequences capable of translocating across biomembranes with superior permeability and low cytotoxicity, offering a promising solution for delivering therapeutics into the CNS. Cationic CPPs can directly penetrate the BBB via adsorptive-mediated transcytosis through electrostatic interactions (Blades et al., 2023).
4. Ligand-Mediated Targeted Modification: This active targeting strategy uses specific ligands (e.g., antibodies, peptides, small molecules) to bind with highly expressed receptors on BBB endothelial cells (e.g., transferrin receptor (TfR), lactoferrin receptor (LfR), LRP-1), triggering receptor-mediated endocytosis or transport. For example, peptides targeting LRP-1, such as Angiopep-2, mimic endogenous peptide sequences to facilitate receptor-mediated endocytosis across the BBB. Chemical coupling of ligands to carriers and functional optimization, potentially using flexible connection tools like PEG, can enhance targeting efficiency.
5. Focused Ultrasound (FUS): FUS, often combined with intravenous microbubbles (MBs), offers a non-invasive method for the reversible opening of the BBB. This technique can temporarily loosen tight junctions, upregulate integrated membrane proteins, and downregulate efflux pumps like P-gp, thereby enhancing drug delivery.

6. Intranasal Delivery: This method leverages anatomical connections between the nasal cavity and the CNS to bypass the BBB, allowing drugs to reach the brain via olfactory nerves or cerebrospinal fluid. Nanocarriers such as polymers, liposomes, and micelles are utilized to improve delivery efficiency and reduce systemic toxicity.
7. Trojan Horse Approach: This involves conjugating an agent that does not cross the BBB well to one that does, such as antibodies targeted to transferrin receptors or CD98, which are highly expressed at the BBB (Banks et al., 2024).

Despite these advances, challenges remain, including the stability of drug delivery systems, long-term safety, and the feasibility of clinical translation. Species differences between preclinical models and humans, production bottlenecks, and a lack of long-term safety data for nanoparticles in the brain are significant obstacles to clinical approval. The specific choice of immunosuppressive therapy is tailored to the type and severity of the neurological disorder.

6. Innovative delivery approaches

6.1 Chemical modifications for enhanced properties

Chemical modifications are crucial for improving the therapeutic properties of peptides, addressing issues such as poor membrane permeability and instability in vivo. Peptides, due to their natural amino acid composition, possess inherent advantages but also face significant structural challenges as therapeutics. Their size and amino acid makeup can impede their ability to cross cell membranes to reach intracellular targets. Additionally, peptides are vulnerable to enzymatic degradation and hydrolysis of their amide bonds because they lack stable secondary and tertiary structures, leading to short half-lives and rapid elimination in the body. To overcome these limitations, structural modifications are widely used to enhance stability against enzymatic cleavage, improve bioavailability by crossing biological barriers, and refine specificity for target interactions (Li et al., 2025). Examples of such modifications include N-terminal acetylation, which is a common method to increase peptide stability. PEGylation is another effective technique that masks peptides from the immune system and increases their solubility, thereby enhancing their therapeutic properties. Other strategies involve altering the peptide backbone by substituting D-amino acids for L-amino acids, inserting N-alkylated amino acids, or incorporating β-amino acids, all of which aim to improve proteolytic stability. Furthermore, replacing peptide bonds with isosteric or isoelectronic substitutes, such as azapeptides, retro-inverso peptides, and peptoids, introduces diverse modifications with unique functionalities (Tarchoun et al., 2022). Side chain modifications also contribute to enhanced stability and bioavailability by replacing natural amino acids with analogs like β-phenylalanine, benzyloxytyrosine, and homoarginine, which can increase binding affinity and target selectivity. Peptide cyclization is another strategy for improving physicochemical properties. These chemical modifications are essential for developing peptide analogs with desired structures, improved stability, and enhanced activity.

6.2 Nanoparticle encapsulation and drug delivery systems

Nanoparticle encapsulation offers a promising strategy to overcome the challenges associated with peptide drug delivery, particularly in neurological disorders. Nano-drug delivery systems (NDDs) involve assembling various excipients into nanoparticles that encapsulate therapeutic drugs. This method not only increases the half-life of peptides in vivo but also aids in targeted delivery, including efficient transport across the blood-brain barrier (BBB) (Tang et al., 2025). Nanomaterials are utilized for the targeted delivery of both therapeutic peptides and proteins, with properties such as particle size and shape influencing their effectiveness. Encapsulation within nanocarriers provides sustained release and protects unreleased proteins from degradation, which is crucial given the instability of proteins. Various natural and synthetic nanocarriers are employed for encapsulating proteins and peptides, with the choice of method depending on the peptide's physicochemical activity and its intended application. Recent advances in nanotechnology are boosting research into delivery systems for treating neurological diseases more specifically and efficiently.

6.3 Intranasal and other non-invasive delivery methods

Intranasal (IN) delivery is emerging as a significant non-invasive method for administering peptides, offering advantages such as less invasiveness, rapid absorption, and the ability to bypass initial liver metabolism (Maeng & Lee, 2022). This route allows for local, systemic, and central nervous system (CNS) delivery of protein and peptide drugs, effectively bypassing the blood-brain barrier (BBB) and minimizing systemic exposure. Despite the nasal cavity being a major barrier due to enzymes that degrade proteins and peptides, advancements in formulation technologies, nanocarriers, and permeation enhancers are improving the efficiency of nasal peptide delivery. Mucoadhesive polymers are also being explored to enhance nasal retention and increase peptide transport across the nasal mucosa. For example, a CGRP inhibitor peptide prepared as chitosan microparticles was delivered intranasally, preventing degradation and offering migraine relief (Ding et al., 2022). Nanocarriers conjugated with peptides represent another significant approach for brain targeting, as they can recognize transcytosis receptors on the BBB for effective drug delivery. Oral delivery of peptides, traditionally hindered by rapid degradation in the gastrointestinal tract and low bioavailability (often less than 1%), is also being addressed through innovative drug delivery approaches like drug entrapment within small vesicles or enhancing passage through the intestinal paracellular pathway.

7. Translational potential: Preclinical studies and clinical trials

Translational research in neurological diseases is actively exploring new therapeutic avenues, with peptides holding significant promise. Cell-penetrating peptides (CPPs) are being investigated as sophisticated drug delivery mechanisms that can transport therapeutic cargo, including proteins, peptides, nucleic acids, and nanocarriers, into cells Table 5.1. This is particularly relevant for neurodegenerative diseases, where CPPs facilitate transport across the blood-brain barrier (BBB). While challenges exist in translating preclinical success to clinical efficacy, advancements are being made in areas like early diagnosis and biomarker identification. For example, the brain-targeted peptide-drug conjugate (PDC) SNG1005 has shown promising clinical efficacy in treating breast cancer brain metastases and is currently in Phase 3 clinical trials (Jafari et al., 2019). Such studies highlight the ongoing effort to bridge experimental and clinical findings, emphasizing the importance of biomarkers for successful translation.

7.1 Peptides in multiple sclerosis

Multiple sclerosis (MS) is an autoimmune neurological disorder characterized by chronic inflammatory demyelination of the central nervous system (CNS). The immune system mistakenly attacks

Table 5.1 A comprehensive overview of peptide categories, mechanisms, and outcomes in the treatment of neurological conditions.

Neurological condition	Peptide category/ Approach	Target/ Mechanism	Examples/ Compounds	Key findings/ Outcomes
Multiple sclerosis (MS)	Myelin peptides	Mimic immunodominant regions of myelin proteins to induce tolerance	MBP85–99, MOG35–55, PLP139–155 (transdermal patch)	Reduced gadolinium-enhanced lesions, lowered relapse rate, safe and well-tolerated
			Synthetic MBP peptide (residues 82–98) (MBP-8298)	Delayed disease progression in HLA-DR2/DR4-positive patients
	Immune modulating peptides	Regulate T-cell activation and cytokine release	dNP2-ctCTLA-4	Reduced demyelination and CNS infiltration in EAE model
		Inhibit endothelial migration of T-cells	PEPITEM	Delayed EAE onset, reduced severity
	Nanoparticle encapsulation	Enhance stability and CNS delivery	PLGA nanoparticles with glycosylated MOG35–55	Reduced EAE clinical scores and CNS inflammation
	Other peptides	Promote remyelination and immunoregulation	Plant/worm-derived peptides, TIMP-1 peptide	Anti-inflammatory, remyelination-promoting potential
Parkinson's disease (PD)	Neuroprotective peptides	Prevent apoptosis, upregulate BDNF	Synthetic tetrapeptide	Improved motor impairment, low cytotoxicity
	Alpha-synuclein targeting peptides	Prevent or reverse alpha-synuclein aggregation	AmyP53, PQK7, peptide "switch"	Blocked neurotoxicity, stabilized healthy protein form, restored movement in worm models
	GLP-1 analogs	Neuroprotection, anti-inflammatory, improve dopaminergic signaling	Lixisenatide, dual GLP-1/GIP agonists	Reduced progression of motor disability, superior BBB penetration
	Intranasal peptides	Direct CNS delivery bypassing BBB	HLDF-6-H peptide	Improved both motor and non-motor symptoms in PD

Table 5.1 A comprehensive overview of peptide categories, mechanisms, and outcomes in the treatment of neurological conditions.—cont'd

Neurological condition	Peptide category/ Approach	Target/ Mechanism	Examples/ Compounds	Key findings/ Outcomes
Alzheimer's disease (AD)	Aβ aggregation inhibitors	Block amyloid-beta aggregation and fibrillation	OR1 (RGKLVFFGR), OR2 (RGKLVFFGR-NH2), D-peptides (KKLVFFA), AP90	Prevented fibril formation, improved proteolytic stability
	BACE1 Inhibitory peptides	Inhibit beta-site APP cleaving enzyme 1 (BACE1) to block Aβ formation	BACE1-derived peptides	Reduced APP processing, halted Aβ generation
	GAPDH/STEP modulators	Prevent amyloidogenesis and neuronal death	GHK-Cu, GPE peptides	Neuroprotective, improved neuronal survival
	Kv1.3 channel inhibitors	Target potassium channel overexpression	ADWX-1, OsK1–K16-D20	Reduced neuroinflammation in AD
	CDK5 Inhibitory peptides	Block hyperactive CDK5–p25 complex	CDK5 T-loop peptide (12 aa)	Reversed neurodegeneration, improved cognition in mice
	Diagnostic/Imaging peptides	Bind amyloid plaques for early AD detection	ACI-80 derivatives (ACI-87-Kφ, ACI-89-Kφ), C-FRHMTEQ-C	Enabled MRI/PET imaging of amyloid plaques
	Intranasal peptides	Enhance delivery and delay cognitive decline	Intranasal peptide drug (unnamed)	Improved cognition and delayed disease onset in AD mice
Other neurological disorders	Huntington's & ALS	Study misfolded protein aggregation	Peptides for aggregation studies	Insights into protein misfolding and toxicity
	Neuropathic pain/ Spinal cord injury	Reduce glutamate excitotoxicity and amyloid toxicity	Peptide compositions (unspecified)	Promising neuroprotective effects
	Epilepsies & Neurodevelopmental disorders	Restore chloride homeostasis by modulating KCC2	KCC2-upmodulating peptides	Restored neuronal excitation/ inhibition balance
	Brain tumors	Improve BBB drug delivery	Peptide-based nanoparticles	Enhanced brain targeting and therapeutic efficiency

Continued

Table 5.1 A comprehensive overview of peptide categories, mechanisms, and outcomes in the treatment of neurological conditions.—cont'd

Neurological condition	Peptide category/ Approach	Target/ Mechanism	Examples/ Compounds	Key findings/ Outcomes
	Stroke	Neuroprotective, BBB-penetrant peptides	Various synthetic peptides	Reduced neuronal damage post-stroke
	Neuroinflammation	Target CNS inflammation	ApoE-derived peptides	Reduced neuroinflammatory responses
	General neurodegeneration	Antioxidant and neuroprotective peptides	Carnosine, bioactive peptides	Improved cognition, neuroprotection

the myelin sheath, disrupting communication between the brain and body. Peptide-based research has been crucial in understanding the molecular mechanisms of MS and developing immunomodulating therapies (Zoupanou et al., 2024).

Several peptide-based approaches are being investigated for MS treatment:

Myelin Peptides: The myelin basic protein (MBP) is a primary target for autoreactive lymphocytes in MS. Synthetic peptides mimicking immunodominant regions of myelin proteins, such as MBP85-99, MOG35-55, and PLP139-155, have been used in transdermal therapy. A skin patch containing a mixture of these myelin peptides significantly reduced active gadolinium-enhanced lesions and lowered the annual relapse rate in patients with relapsing-remitting MS, proving safe and well-tolerated. MBP-8298, a synthetic peptide corresponding to amino acid residues 82-98 of human MBP, has been shown to delay disease progression in MS patients with HLA-DR2 and/or HLA-DR4 haplotypes (Juryńczyk et al., 2010).

Immune Modulating Peptides: Novel peptides have been developed to modulate T-cell functions, aiming to regulate immune cells more specifically than general immunosuppressants (Kammona & Kiparissides, 2020). For instance, a BBB-permeable peptide called dNP2, conjugated with the cytoplasmic domain of cytotoxic T lymphocyte antigen 4 (dNP2-ctCTLA-4), downregulated cytokine production in activated T cells and inhibited experimental autoimmune encephalomyelitis (EAE), a mouse model of MS. This approach reduced demyelination and infiltration of T helper one and T helper 17 cells in the CNS. PEPITEM, a peptide inhibitor of trans-endothelial migration, demonstrated prophylactic potential by delaying EAE onset, reducing disease severity, and mitigating inflammatory responses in mice.

Nanoparticle Encapsulation: To overcome the short lifespan and rapid hydrolysis of peptides, encapsulation in nanospheres is used to improve pharmacokinetics and bioavailability. Poly(lactic-co-glycolic) acid (PLGA) nanoparticles loaded with glycosylated myelin oligodendrocyte glycoprotein epitope (MOG35-55) conjugated with glucosamine showed efficacy in reducing EAE clinical scores and CNS inflammation in a therapeutic protocol.

Other Peptides: Researchers are exploring various other peptides, including plant-derived cyclotides that prevent the progression of MS symptoms, and peptides from intestinal worms that could treat autoimmune diseases like MS and rheumatoid arthritis. Additionally, studies on TIMP-1 peptide therapy aim to boost remyelination in MS (Zoupanou et al., 2024).

7.2 Peptides in Parkinson's disease

Parkinson's disease (PD) is a progressive neurodegenerative disorder characterized by motor symptoms such as bradykinesia, tremor, rigidity, and postural instability, along with non-motor features like cognitive impairment. Current treatments primarily focus on restoring dopaminergic tone and do not alter the disease course. Peptide-based therapeutics are showing promise in addressing the underlying pathology and improving symptoms in PD.

Key areas of peptide research in PD include:

Neuroprotective Peptides: Many brain-gut peptides exhibit neuroprotective effects in vivo and in vitro, improving motor impairment in PD. Neuropeptides, in particular, play a significant neuroprotective role by preventing caspase-3 activation. Synthetic peptides are being developed to serve as a basis for multifunctional drugs for PD, including those that can upregulate brain-derived neurotrophic factor (BDNF) expression, pass the BBB due to low molecular weight, and show minimal cytotoxicity. A tetrapeptide effectively counteracted Parkinsonian symptoms in a 6-hydroxydopamine model (Tang et al., 2025).

Alpha-Synuclein Targeting: Aggregated alpha-synuclein plays a crucial role in PD pathogenesis. Peptide-based approaches are being developed to directly engage with alpha-synuclein, inhibiting its oligomer formation. For example, AmyP53, an adaptive peptide, blocks the neurotoxic cascade triggered by oligomers in both Alzheimer's and Parkinson's diseases. A novel peptide inhibitor, PQK7, shows potential as a therapeutic agent by targeting early alpha-synuclein aggregates without promoting fibril formation. Scientists have also designed a peptide "switch" to keep the Parkinson's protein in its healthy form, which is stable, penetrates brain-like cells, and restores movement in worm models.

Glucagon-Like Peptide-1 (GLP-1) Analogs: GLP-1 class drugs, originally for diabetes, have demonstrated significant neuroprotective activity in preclinical studies of PD. They inhibit inflammation, improve neuronal survival, maintain synapses, and enhance dopaminergic transmission. Clinical Phase II trials have shown impressive improvements. Dual GLP-1/GIP agonists, which can penetrate the BBB, have shown superior effects in animal models compared to single GLP-1 drugs. A clinical trial using lixisenatide, a GLP-1 receptor agonist, showed less progression of motor disability in early PD patients compared to placebo over 12 months (Khan et al., 2024).

Intranasal Delivery: Intranasal administration of the HLDF-6-H peptide has shown neuroprotective activity in experimental PD models and effectively overcomes motor and non-motor symptoms when chronically administered to patients.

7.3 Peptides in Alzheimer's disease

Alzheimer's disease (AD) is the most common progressive neurodegenerative disease, characterized by extracellular amyloid plaques and intracellular neurofibrillary tangles from hyperphosphorylated tau protein. Amyloid-beta (Aβ) aggregation is a central target for AD management, and peptide-based compounds are being developed for early diagnosis and treatment.

Key applications of peptides in AD include:

Inhibitors of Amyloid-Beta (Aβ) Aggregation: The inhibition of Aβ aggregation and fibrillation is a major research focus. Peptides are designed to bind to Aβ regions critical for aggregation, preventing fibril formation or Aβ elongation. Examples include RGKLVFFGR (OR1) and RGKLVFFGR-NH2 (OR2), which effectively inhibit Aβ fibril formation. Other inhibitors, like those based on modifications of the hydrophobic KLVFF amino acid sequence, have been developed to improve lipophilicity and proteolytic stability. D-enantiomeric peptides, such as KKLVFFA, have shown superior inhibition of Aβ aggregation and neurotoxic effects compared to their L-peptide counterparts (Perugini & Santin, 2022). A 23-residue long hairpin peptide (AP90) with alternating D- and L-amino acids has also been reported to inhibit Aβ aggregation (Kellock et al., 2016). Gold-nanoparticle-based Aβ peptide conjugates (AuNPs@POMD-pep) are also being explored as multifunctional inhibitors.

Targeting BACE1: Beta-site APP cleaving enzyme 1 (BACE1) is believed to play a primary role in Aβ peptide generation. BACE1 levels are elevated in AD patients' brain tissues, and its inhibition halts Aβ formation. Peptides derived from the BACE1 sequence have been shown to inhibit APP processing (Smith Patel et al., 2022).

Modulating GAPDH and Tyrosine Phosphatase: Glyceraldehyde-3-phosphate dehydrogenase (GAPDH) aggregates can accelerate Aβ amyloidogenesis and neuronal cell death. Naturally occurring peptides like Glycyl-L-histidyl-L-lysine-Copper (GHK-Cu) and Gly-Pro-Glu (GPE) are being investigated for their neuroprotective effects. Striatal-Enriched tyrosine phosphatase (STEP), which is overactive in AD, is another potential target, with neuroprotective peptides like GPE and its analogs being evaluated.

Potassium Channel KV1.3 Inhibitors: Overexpression of potassium channel KV1.3 in the frontal cortices of AD patients suggests it as a therapeutic target. Peptides such as BmKTX-R11-T28-H33 (ADWX-1) and OsK1–K16-D20 are designed to target Kv1.3.

CDK5 Overactivation Inhibition: MIT neuroscientists have discovered a peptide that can reverse neurodegeneration and other AD symptoms by blocking a hyperactive brain enzyme called CDK5. This peptide, identical in sequence to a segment of CDK5's T loop (critical for binding to P25), dramatically reduced neurodegeneration and DNA damage and improved cognitive tasks in mouse models (Pao et al., 2023). The peptide, which is 12 amino acids long, does not interfere with essential enzymes like CDK1 or the normal CDK5-P35 complex.

Diagnostic Probes: Peptides are vital tools for early AD detection, as amyloid plaque appears years before cognitive symptoms. Amyloid ligands, such as D-enantiomeric peptides like ACI-80 and its derivatives (ACI-87-Kφ, ACI-88-Kφ, ACI-89-Kφ), bind specifically to Aβ1–42 and can be used as molecular probes for in vivo imaging of amyloid plaque load. Phage display techniques have also identified peptide ligands with high affinity for Aβ42, such as C-FRHMTEQ-C and C-IPLPFYN-C, which showed promise as MRI contrast agents in transgenic mouse models.

Intranasal Delivery: An intranasally delivered peptide drug has been shown to ameliorate cognitive decline in Alzheimer's transgenic mice, offering an efficient and clinically amenable treatment to delay the onset of the disease.

7.4 Other neurological conditions

Peptide-based therapies are gaining traction in addressing a diverse range of neurological conditions beyond Alzheimer's, Parkinson's, and Multiple Sclerosis. The central nervous system (CNS) presents significant challenges due to its complexity and the restrictive blood-brain barrier (BBB), which limits drug entry. However, advances in medicinal chemistry and drug design are leading to novel therapeutic approaches (Szeto, 2008).

Some other neurological conditions where peptides show potential include:

Huntington's Disease and Amyotrophic Lateral Sclerosis (ALS): These are among other fatal neurodegenerative diseases that share characteristics of misfolded protein aggregation with AD. Peptides are proving to be valuable tools for studying the properties of misfolded proteins in these conditions (Marelli & Maschat, 2016).

Neuropathic Pain and Spinal Cord Injury: New combination therapies involving compositions and methods for treating neurological diseases associated with glutamate excitotoxicity and β-amyloid toxicity are being explored for conditions like neuropathic pain and spinal cord injury (Feigin, 1998).

Epilepsies and Neuro-developmental/-traumatic/-degenerative/-psychiatric Disorders: KCC2 (potassium-chloride cotransporter 2), a CNS neuron-specific chloride extruder, has been identified as a genetically validated target for these disorders. KCC2 hypofunction contributes to neuronal excitation/inhibition imbalances, and KCC2-upmodulating drugs are being developed to restore physiological CNS inhibition and address drug resistance (Hruby et al., 2017).

Brain Tumors: Nanoparticle applications are gaining importance in addressing drug delivery to the brain for conditions like brain tumors, offering promising results (Wijesinghe et al., 2022).

Stroke: Peptide drugs have emerged as promising candidates for treating stroke, offering high specificity, low toxicity, and efficient blood-brain barrier penetration.

Neuroinflammation: Neuroinflammation is a recognized factor in acute and chronic neurological disorders, suggesting it as a potential therapeutic target for peptide-based treatments. Apolipoprotein E-derived peptides have been shown to reduce CNS inflammation (Harding & Tong, 2018).

General Neurodegenerative Disorders: Synthetic and natural peptides, such as carnosine, are under research for treating neurodegenerative disorders. Bioactive peptides with neuroprotective effects can improve cognitive decline through various mechanisms.

Despite the potential, the instability of peptides in vivo and their inadequate capacity to cross cell membranes pose difficulties in clinical settings for many neurological disorders. However, research continues to focus on overcoming these barriers and developing effective delivery methods.

8. Future perspectives and conclusion

Peptide therapeutics are advancing rapidly, driven by innovations in design, synthesis, delivery, and artificial intelligence. Their high potency, specificity, and favorable safety make them attractive for treating diverse conditions, including diabetes, cancer, osteoporosis, and neurological disorders.

Key emerging trends include improved stability and bioavailability through structural modifications and controlled-release strategies; advanced delivery systems such as peptide-drug conjugates, brain shuttle peptides, and non-invasive routes like intranasal delivery; peptide-based vaccines with superior specificity; AI-assisted drug discovery; and novel methods for targeting intracellular proteins (Bates & Hockly, 2003).

Personalized medicine is reshaping peptide therapeutics, with genomics, pharmacogenomics, and multiomics guiding individualized treatment. Stem cell models enable patient-specific drug screening, while technologies like RNA editing and interference peptides expand precision therapies for neurological and systemic diseases. These approaches minimize off-target effects and optimize efficacy by tailoring interventions to each patient's genetic and molecular profile.

Impact on neurological diseases is particularly significant. Peptides offer high specificity, low toxicity, and the ability to cross the blood–brain barrier, providing new opportunities for disease-modifying therapies in neurodegenerative and psychiatric disorders. They address many limitations of small molecules and biologics while maintaining low immunogenicity and favorable safety.

Although challenges remain in stability and delivery, ongoing research is delivering creative solutions that are transforming the therapeutic landscape. By combining peptide innovation with precision medicine, the future promises safer, more effective, and more personalized treatments, ultimately improving outcomes and quality of life for patients with complex neurological conditions (Muttenthaler et al., 2021).

References

Abid, S. R., Mousavi, S., & Checco, J. W. (2021). Identifying receptors for neuropeptides and peptide hormones: Challenges and recent progress. *ACS Chemical Biology, 16*(2), 251–263. https://doi.org/10.1021/acschembio.0c00950

Adessi, C., & Soto, C. (2002). Converting a peptide into a drug: Strategies to improve stability and bioavailability. *Current Medicinal Chemistry, 9*, 963–978.

Anna, R., Sara, L. M., Giancarlo, M., Ettore, N., & Daniela, M. (2015). Peptide agonists and antagonists with potential application in neurological disorders. *Recent Patents on CNS Drug Discovery, 10*(2), 76–89. https://doi.org/10.2174/1574889810666160425121833

Ashraf, H., Solla, P., & Sechi, L. A. (2022). Current advancement of immunomodulatory drugs as potential pharmacotherapies for autoimmunity based neurological diseases. *Pharmaceuticals, 15*(9). https://doi.org/10.3390/ph15091077

Azam, S., Haque, M. E., Jakaria, M., Jo, S.-H., Kim, I.-S., & Choi, D.-K. (2020). G-Protein-Coupled receptors in CNS: A potential therapeutic target for intervention in neurodegenerative disorders and associated cognitive deficits. *Cells, 9*(2). https://doi.org/10.3390/cells9020506

Badawi, A. H., & Siahaan, T. J. (2012). Immune modulating peptides for the treatment and suppression of multiple sclerosis. *Clinical Immunology, 144*(2), 127–138. https://doi.org/10.1016/j.clim.2012.05.010

Banks, W. A., Rhea, E. M., Reed, M. J., & Erickson, M. A. (2024). The penetration of therapeutics across the blood-brain barrier: Classic case studies and clinical implications. *Cell Reports Medicine, 5*(11). https://doi.org/10.1016/j.xcrm.2024.101760

Barca, C., Foray, C., Hermann, S., Ulrich, H., Remory, I., Laoui, D., Schäfers, M., Grauer, O. M., Zinnhardt, B., & Jacobs, A. H. (2021). The colony stimulating Factor-1 receptor (CSF-1R)-Mediated regulation of microglia/macrophages as a target for neurological disorders (glioma, stroke). *Frontiers in Immunology, 12*(2021).

Bates, G. P., & Hockly, E. (2003). Experimental therapeutics in huntington's disease: Are models useful for therapeutic trials? *Current Opinion in Neurology, 16*(4).

Berry, M. D. (2004). Mammalian central nervous system trace amines. pharmacologic amphetamines, physiologic neuromodulators. *Journal of Neurochemistry, 90*(2), 257–271. https://doi.org/10.1111/j.1471-4159.2004.02501.x

Birgül Iyison, N., Abboud, C., Abboud, D., Abdulrahman, A. O., Bondar, A.-N., Dam, J., Georgoussi, Z., Giraldo, J., Horvat, A., Karoussiotis, C., Paz-Castro, A., Scarpa, M., Schihada, H., Scholz, N., Güvenc Tuna, B., & Vardjan, N. (2025). ERNEST COST action overview on the (patho)physiology of GPCRs and orphan GPCRs in the nervous system. *British Journal of Pharmacology, 182*(14), 3178–3210. https://doi.org/10.1111/bph.16389

Blades, R., Ittner, L. M., & Tietz, O. (2023). Peptides for trans-blood–brain barrier delivery. *Journal of Labelled Compounds and Radiopharmaceuticals, 66*(9), 237–248. https://doi.org/10.1002/jlcr.4023

Brown, M. R., & Fisher, L. A. (1984). Brain peptides as intercellular messengers: Implications for medicine. *JAMA, 251*(10), 1310–1315. https://doi.org/10.1001/jama.1984.03340340050027

Caetano-Silva, M. E., Rund, L. A., Vailati-Riboni, M., Pacheco, M. T. B., & Johnson, R. W. (2021). Copper-binding peptides attenuate microglia inflammation through suppression of NF-kB pathway. *Molecular Nutrition & Food Research, 65*(22), Article 2100153. https://doi.org/10.1002/mnfr.202100153

Carniglia, L., Ramírez, D., Durand, D., Saba, J., Turati, J., Caruso, C., Scimonelli, T. N., & Lasaga, M. (2017). Neuropeptides and microglial activation in inflammation, pain, and neurodegenerative diseases. *Mediators of Inflammation, 2017*(1), Article 5048616. https://doi.org/10.1155/2017/5048616

Carriba, P., & Comella, J. X. (2015). Neurodegeneration and neuroinflammation: Two processes, one target. *Neural Regeneration Research, 10*(10).

Casello, S. M., Flores, R. J., Yarur, H. E., Wang, H., Awanyai, M., Arenivar, M. A., Jaime-Lara, R. B., Bravo-Rivera, H., & Tejeda, H. A. (2022). Neuropeptide system regulation of prefrontal cortex circuitry: Implications for neuropsychiatric disorders. *Frontiers in Neural Circuits, 16*(2022).

Cohen, J., Mathew, A., Dourvetakis, K. D., Sanchez-Guerrero, E., Pangeni, R. P., Gurusamy, N., Aenlle, K. K., Ravindran, G., Twahir, A., Isler, D., Sosa-Garcia, S. R., Llizo, A., Bested, A. C., Theoharides, T. C., Klimas, N. G., & Kempuraj, D. (2024). Recent research trends in neuroinflammatory and neurodegenerative disorders. *Cells, 13*(6). https://doi.org/10.3390/cells13060511

Crawley, J. N. (1990). Coexistence of neuropeptides and "classical" neurotransmitters. *Annals of the New York Academy of Sciences, 579*(1), 233–241. https://doi.org/10.1111/j.1749-6632.1990.tb48365.x

De Souza Oliveira Carneiro, J. A., Teixeira, G. P., Leandro, R., & Faria, R. X. (2025). Activity of peptides modulating the action of p2x receptors: Focus on the p2x7 receptor. *Pharmaceuticals, 18*(10). https://doi.org/10.3390/ph18101452

DeMaio, A., Mehrotra, S., Sambamurti, K., & Husain, S. (2022). The role of the adaptive immune system and T cell dysfunction in neurodegenerative diseases. *Journal of Neuroinflammation, 19*(1), 251. https://doi.org/10.1186/s12974-022-02605-9

Di, L. (2015). Strategic approaches to optimizing peptide ADME properties. *The AAPS Journal, 17*(1), 134–143. https://doi.org/10.1208/s12248-014-9687-3

Ding, C., Wu, Y., Chen, X., Chen, Y., Wu, Z., Lin, Z., Kang, D., Fang, W., & Chen, F. (2022). Global, regional, and national burden and attributable risk factors of neurological disorders: The global burden of disease study 1990–2019. *Frontiers in Public Health, 10*(2022).

Disha, N. S. (2025). Nanoparticles as game-changers in drug delivery for neurological disorders. *South Eastern European Journal of Public Health*, 3692–3706. https://doi.org/10.70135/seejph.vi.5813

Dong, D., Xie, J., & Wang, J. (2019). Neuroprotective effects of brain-gut peptides: A potential therapy for parkinson's disease. *Neuroscience Bulletin, 35*(6), 1085–1096. https://doi.org/10.1007/s12264-019-00407-3

Eybalin, M. (1993). Neurotransmitters and neuromodulators of the mammalian cochlea. *Physiological Reviews, 73*(2), 309–373. https://doi.org/10.1152/physrev.1993.73.2.309

Fadzen, C. M., Wolfe, J. M., Cho, C.-F., Antonio Chiocca, E., Lawler, S. E., & Pentelute, B. L. (2017). Perfluoroarene–based peptide macrocycles to enhance penetration across the blood–brain barrier. *Journal of American Chemical Society, 139*(44), 15628–15631. https://doi.org/10.1021/jacs.7b09790

Feigin, A. (1998). Advances in Huntington's disease: Implications for experimental therapeutics. *Current Opinion in Neurology, 11*(4).

Firdaus, Z., & Li, X. (2024). Unraveling the genetic landscape of neurological disorders: Insights into pathogenesis, techniques for variant identification, and therapeutic approaches. *International Journal of Molecular Sciences, 25*(4). https://doi.org/10.3390/ijms25042320

Fornari Laurindo, L., Dias, J. A., Araújo, A. C., Torres Pomini, K., Machado Galhardi, C., Detregiachi, C. R. P., de Argollo Haber, L. S., Roque, D. D., Bechara, M. D., de Castro, M. V. M., de Pereira, E. S. B. M., Tofano, R. J.,

Jasmin Santos German Borgo, I., & Barbalho, S. M. (2024). Immunological dimensions of neuroinflammation and microglial activation: Exploring innovative immunomodulatory approaches to mitigate neuro-inflammatory progression. *Frontiers in Immunology, 14*.

García-Domínguez, M. (2025). Neuroinflammation: Mechanisms, dual roles, and therapeutic strategies in neurological disorders. *Current Issues in Molecular Biology, 47*(6). https://doi.org/10.3390/cimb47060417

Gemma, C., Neuroimmunomodulation and aging. Aging and Disease 3 169 –172.

Gokhale, A. S., & Satyanarayanajois, S. (2014). Peptides and peptidomimetics as immunomodulators. *Immunotherapy, 6*(6), 755–774. https://doi.org/10.2217/imt.14.37

Grabon, W., Gasmi, N., Lang, A., Ruiz, A., Georges, B., Blot, V., Ogier, M., Rheims, S., Navarro, F. P., & Bezin, L. (2025). *Brain infiltrated monocyte-macrophages in a rat model of temporal lobe epilepsy: Revisiting the pro-inflammatory paradigm. 2025*. bioRxiv. https://doi.org/10.1101/2025.01.02.631083

Harding, R. J., & Tong, Y.-F. (2018). Proteostasis in huntington's disease: Disease mechanisms and therapeutic opportunities. *Acta Pharmacologica Sinica, 39*(5), 754–769. https://doi.org/10.1038/aps.2018.11

Hisa, Y., Bamba, H., Koike, S., Shogaki, K., Tadaki, N., & Uno, T. (1999). Neurotransmitters and neuromodulators involved in laryngeal innervation. *Annals of Otology, Rhinology & Laryngology, 108*(7_Suppl. 1), 3–14. https://doi.org/10.1177/00034894991080S702

Holzmann, B. (2013). Modulation of immune responses by the neuropeptide CGRP. *Amino Acids, 45*(1), 1–7. https://doi.org/10.1007/s00726-011-1161-2

Hruby, V. J., Lee, Y. S., Cai, M., Olson, K., & Remesic, M. (2017). Peptide therapeutics: Neuropeptides peptide-based drug discovery: Challenges and new therapeutics. *The Royal Society of Chemistry*. https://doi.org/10.1039/9781788011532-00391

Hu, X., Leak, R. K., Thomson, A. W., Yu, F., Xia, Y., Wechsler, L. R., & Chen, J. (2018). Promises and limitations of immune cell-based therapies in neurological disorders. *Nature Reviews Neurology, 14*(9), 559–568. https://doi.org/10.1038/s41582-018-0028-5

Ijaz, M. U., Akbar, A., Ashraf, A., Karatas Yeni, D., Naz, H., & Shahid, M. (2024). *Microbiome and neurological disorders* (pp. 273–301). Singapore: Singapore Springer. https://doi.org/10.1007/978-981-97-3790-1_9

Jafari, B., Pourseif, M. M., Barar, J., & Rafi, M. A. (2019). Yadollah omidi, peptide-mediated drug delivery across the blood-brain barrier for targeting brain. *Expert Opinion on Drug Delivery, 16*(6), 583–605. https://doi.org/10.1080/17425247.2019.1614911

Jessop, D. S. (1998). Neuropeptides, modulators of the immune system. *Current Opinion in Endocrinology Diabetes and Obesity, 5*(1).

Jin-Feng, Y., Hong, Y., Yan-Zhi, Z., & Ming, X. (2018). *Metabolism of peptide drugs and strategies to improve their metabolic stability, 19* (pp. 892–901). https://doi.org/10.2174/1389200219666180628171531

Juryńczyk, M., Walczak, A., Jurewicz, A., Jesionek-Kupnicka, D., Szczepanik, M., & Selmaj, K. (2010). Immune regulation of multiple sclerosis by transdermally applied myelin peptides. *Annals of Neurology, 68*(5), 593–601. https://doi.org/10.1002/ana.22219

Kammona, O., & Kiparissides, C. (2020). Recent advances in antigen-specific immunotherapies for the treatment of multiple sclerosis. *Brain Sciences, 10*(6). https://doi.org/10.3390/brainsci10060333

Kaspar, A. A., & Reichert, J. M. (2013). Future directions for peptide therapeutics development. *Drug Discovery Today, 18*(17), 807–817. https://doi.org/10.1016/j.drudis.2013.05.011

Kaushik, D. K., & Basu, A. (2013). A friend in need may not be a friend indeed: Role of microglia in neuro-degenerative diseases. *CNS & Neurological Disorders - Drug Targets, 12*(6), 726–740. https://doi.org/10.2174/18715273113126660170

Kellock, J., Hopping, G., Caughey, B., & Daggett, V. (2016). Peptides composed of alternating L- and D-Amino acids inhibit amyloidogenesis in three distinct amyloid systems independent of sequence. *Journal of Molecular Biology, 428*(11), 2317–2328. https://doi.org/10.1016/j.jmb.2016.03.013

Khan, T. T. S., Sheikh, Z., Maleknia, S., Oveissi, F., Fathi, A., Abrams, T., Ong, H. X., & Traini, D. (2024). Intranasal delivery of glucagon-like peptide-1 to the brain for obesity treatment: Opportunities and challenges. *Expert Opinion on Drug Delivery, 21*(7), 1081–1101. https://doi.org/10.1080/17425247.2024.2387110

Kim, M. E., & Lee, J. S. (2025). Mechanisms and emerging regulators of neuroinflammation: Exploring new therapeutic strategies for neurological disorders. *Current Issues in Molecular Biology, 47*. https://doi.org/10.3390/cimb47010008

Klopak, E. T., & Crimmins, E. M. (2023). Neurodegeneration biomarkers help explain association between inflammation and cognitive dysfunction. *Innovation in Aging, 7*(Supplment_1), 101–102. https://doi.org/10.1093/geroni/igad104.0329

Krieger, D. T. (1979). Physiological significance of hypophysiotrophic and pituitary hormones on brain. *European Journal of Clinical Investigation, 9*(2), 107–110. https://doi.org/10.1111/j.1365-2362.1979.tb01675.x

Kumar, P., Zelena, D., & Gautam, A. (2024). Neurological disorders and challenges in their theranostics. In *Theranostic applications of nanotechnology in neurological disorders* (pp. 1–29). Hungary: Springer. https://doi.org/10.1007/978-981-99-9510-3_1

Lalatsa, A., Schatzlein, A. G., & Uchegbu, I. F. (2014). Strategies to deliver peptide drugs to the brain. *Molecular Pharmaceutics, 11*(4), 1081–1093. https://doi.org/10.1021/mp400680d

Lamers, C. (2022). Overcoming the shortcomings of peptide-based therapeutics . future drug discovery. *Null, 4*(2), Article FDD75. https://doi.org/10.4155/fdd-2022-0005

Lemus-Conejo, A., Millan-Linares, M.del C., Toscano, R., Millan, F., Pedroche, J., & Muriana, F. J. G. (2022). Sergio Montserrat-de la Paz, GPETAFLR, a peptide from Lupinus angustifolius L. prevents inflammation in microglial cells and confers neuroprotection in brain. *Nutritional Neuroscience, 25*(3), 472–484. https://doi.org/10.1080/1028415X.2020.1763058

Li, K. W. (2012). Peptide neurotransmitters and hormones. *eLS*. https://doi.org/10.1002/9780470015902.a0000063.pub2

Li, Y., Jin, T., Liu, N., Wang, J., Qin, Z., Yin, S., Zhang, Y., Fu, Z., Wu, Y., Wang, Y., Liu, Y., Yang, M., Pang, A., Sun, J., Wang, Y., & Yang, X. (2023). A short peptide exerts neuroprotective effects on cerebral ischemia–reperfusion injury by reducing inflammation via the miR-6328/IKKβ/NF-κB axis. *Journal of Neuroinflammation, 20*(1), 53. https://doi.org/10.1186/s12974-023-02739-4

Li, Q., Wen, C., & Qiu, L. (2025). Therapeutic peptides: Chemical strategies fortify peptides for enhanced disease treatment efficacy. *Amino Acids, 57*(1), 25. https://doi.org/10.1007/s00726-025-03454-5

Lima, C., Luis Almeida Maleski, A., Thiago Gonçalves Bernardo, J., Cataldi Zelli, V., Naname Komegae, E., & Lopes-Ferreira, M. (2022). TnP peptide suppresses experimental autoimmune encephalomyelitis (EAE) in a preclinical mouse model. *Frontiers in Immunology, 13*.

Lipton, J. M., Catania, A., & Delgado, R. (1998). Peptide modulation of inflammatory processes within the brain. *Neuroimmunomodulation, 5*(3–4), 178–183. https://doi.org/10.1159/000026335

Liu, C., Yang, S.-Y., Wang, L., & Zhou, F. (2022). The gut microbiome: Implications for neurogenesis and neurological diseases. *Neural Regeneration Research, 17*(1).

Ma, Z., Zuo, T., Frey, N., & Yusuf Rangrez, A. (2024). A systematic framework for understanding the microbiome in human health and disease: From basic principles to clinical translation. *Signal Transduction and Targeted Therapy, 9*(1), 237. https://doi.org/10.1038/s41392-024-01946-6

Maeng, J., & Lee, K. (2022). Systemic and brain delivery of antidiabetic peptides through nasal administration using cell-penetrating peptides. *Frontiers in Pharmacology, 13*.

Marelli, C., & Maschat, F. (2016). The P42 peptide and peptide-based therapies for Huntington's disease. *Orphanet Journal of Rare Diseases, 11*(1), 24. https://doi.org/10.1186/s13023-016-0405-3

McGonigle, P. (2012). Peptide therapeutics for CNS indications. *Biochemical Pharmacology, 83*(5), 559–566. https://doi.org/10.1016/j.bcp.2011.10.014

McGowan, J. W. D., Bidwell, G. L., III, & Vig, P. J. S. (2015). Challenges and new strategies for therapeutic peptide delivery to the CNS. *Therapeutic Delivery, 6*(7), 841–853. https://doi.org/10.4155/tde.15.30

Mengr, A., Šmotková, Z., Pačesová, A., Železná, B., Kuneš, J., & Maletínská, L. (2025). Reduction of neuroinflammation as a common mechanism of action of anorexigenic and orexigenic peptide analogues in the triple transgenic mouse model of alzheimer's disease. *Journal of Neuroimmune Pharmacology, 20*(1), 18. https://doi.org/10.1007/s11481-025-10174-w

Metaxakis, A., Petratou, D., & Tavernarakis, N. (2020). Molecular interventions towards multiple sclerosis treatment. *Brain Sciences, 10*(5). https://doi.org/10.3390/brainsci10050299

Mignini, F., Streccioni, V., & Amenta, F. (2003). Autonomic innervation of immune organs and neuroimmune modulation. *Autonomic and Autacoid Pharmacology, 23*(1), 1–25. https://doi.org/10.1046/j.1474-8673.2003.00280.x

Muttenthaler, M., King, G. F., Adams, D. J., & Alewood, P. F. (2021). Trends in peptide drug discovery. *Nature Reviews Drug Discovery, 20*(4), 309–325. https://doi.org/10.1038/s41573-020-00135-8

Nath, A., & Berger, J. R. (2012). Complications of immunosuppressive/immunomodulatory therapy in neurological diseases. *Current Treatment Options in Neurology, 14*(3), 241–255. https://doi.org/10.1007/s11940-012-0172-y

Nimmerjahn, A., Kirchhoff, F., & Helmchen, F. (2005). Resting microglial cells are highly dynamic surveillants of brain parenchyma in vivo. *Science, 308*(5726), 1314–1318. https://doi.org/10.1126/science.1110647

Pao, P.-C., Seo, J., Lee, A., Kritskiy, O., Patnaik, D., Penney, J., Raju, R. M., Geigenmuller, U., Catarina Silva, M., Lucente, D. E., Gusella, J. F., Dickerson, B. C., Loon, A., Yu, M. X., Bula, M., Yu, M., Haggarty, S. J., & Tsai, L.-H. (2023). A Cdk5-derived peptide inhibits Cdk5/p25 activity and improves neurodegenerative phenotypes. *Proceedings of the National Academy of Sciences, 120*(16), Article e2217864120. https://doi.org/10.1073/pnas.2217864120

Patel, S., Ankush, V., Bansoad, R., & Singh Gopal, L. K. (2022). *BACE1: A key regulator in alzheimer's disease progression and current, 20.*

Perugini, V., & Santin, M. (2022). The real-time validation of the effectiveness of third-generation hyperbranched poly(ε-lysine) dendrons-modified KLVFF sequences to bind Amyloid-β1-42 peptides using an optical waveguide light-mode spectroscopy system. *Sensors, 22*(23). https://doi.org/10.3390/s22239561

Qin, H., Fang, Y., Di, L., & Jian, X. (2020). Microbiota-immune system interactions in human neurological disorders. *Current Drug Targets - CNS & Neurological Disorders, 19*(7), 509–526. https://doi.org/10.2174/1871527319666200726222138

Reich, N., & Hölscher, C. (2022). The neuroprotective effects of glucagon-like peptide 1 in Alzheimer's and Parkinson's disease: An in-depth review. *Frontiers in Neuroscience*, 16–2022.

Russo, A., Manna, S. L., Morelli, G., Novellino, E., & Marasco, D. (2016). Peptide agonists and antagonists with potential application in. *Recent Patents on CNS Drug Discovery, 10*(2), 76–89.

Savinetti, I., Papagna, A., & Foti, M. (2021). Human monocytes plasticity in neurodegeneration. *Biomedicines, 9*(7). https://doi.org/10.3390/biomedicines9070717

Schäfer, C., Ascui, G., Ribeiro, C. H., López, M., Prados-Rosales, R., González, P. A., Bueno, S. M., Riedel, C. A., Baena, A., Kalergis, A. M., & Carreño, L. J. (2017). Innate immune cells for immunotherapy of autoimmune and cancer disorders. *International Reviews of Immunology, 36*(6), 315–337. https://doi.org/10.1080/08830185.2017.1365145

Shashi, K., & Tiwari Rajnish, K. C. (2014). *Peptide therapeutics in neurodegenerative disorders, 21.* https://doi.org/10.2174/0929867321666140217125857

Silva-Reis, S. C., Sampaio-Dias, I. E., Costa, V. M., Correia, X. C., Costa-Almeida, H. F., García-Mera, X., & Rodríguez-Borges, J. E. (2023). Concise overview of glypromate neuropeptide research: From chemistry to pharmacological applications in neurosciences. *ACS Chemical Neuroscience, 14*(4), 554–572. https://doi.org/10.1021/acschemneuro.2c00675

Singh, K., Jeetendra, K., Gupta, A., Shrivastava, D., Jain, A., Pratap, Y., Sumeet, D., Anubhav, D., & Shivendra, K. (2025). Exploring the pharmacological effects of bioactive peptides on human nervous disorders: A comprehensive review. *Current Drug Targets - CNS & Neurological Disorders, 24*(1), 32–46. https://doi.org/10.2174/0118715273316382240807120241

Song, X.-Y., Fan, C.-X., Muhammad, A.-R., Choudhary, I., & Wang, X.-P. (2024). Neuro-regeneration or repair: Cell therapy of neurological disorders as away forward. *Current Neuropharmacology, 22*. https://doi.org/10.2174/1570159X22666240509092903

Souza-Moreira, L., Campos-Salinas, J., Caro, M., & Gonzalez-Rey, E. (2011). Neuropeptides as pleiotropic modulators of the immune response. *Neuroendocrinology, 94*(2), 89–100. https://doi.org/10.1159/000328636

Strzelec, M., Detka, J., Mieszczak, P., Katarzyna Sobocińska, M., & Majka, M. (2023). Immunomodulation-a general review of the current state-of-the-art and new therapeutic strategies for targeting the immune system. *Frontiers in Immunology, 14*. https://doi.org/10.3389/fimmu.2023.1127704

Sun, B., Sawant, H., Borthakur, A., & Chen Bihl, J. (2023). Emerging therapeutic role of gut microbial extracellular vesicles in neurological disorders. *Frontiers in Neuroscience, 17*.

Szeto, H. H. (2008). Development of mitochondria-targeted aromatic-cationic peptides for neurodegenerative diseases. *Annals of the New York Academy of Sciences, 1147*(1), 112–121. https://doi.org/10.1196/annals.1427.013

Tang, S., Han, E. L., & Mitchell, M. J. (2025). Peptide-functionalized nanoparticles for brain-targeted therapeutics. *Drug Delivery and Translational Research*. https://doi.org/10.1007/s13346-025-01840-w

Tarchoun, K., Yousef, M., & Bánóczi, Z. (2022). Azapeptides as an efficient tool to improve the activity of biologically effective peptides. *Future Pharmacology, 2*(3). https://doi.org/10.3390/futurepharmacol2030020

Tsai, Y.-L., Song, J., Shi, R., Knöll, B., & Synatschke, C. V. (2025). A roadmap of peptide-based materials in neural regeneration. *Advanced Healthcare Materials, 14*(2), Article 2402939. https://doi.org/10.1002/adhm.202402939

Tuominen, M., & Leppäluoto, J. (1987). Peptides and neurotransmission in the central nervous system. *Medical Biology, 65*(2–3), 137–142.

Ulevitch, R. J. (2004). Therapeutics targeting the innate immune system. *Nature Reviews Immunology, 4*(7), 512–520. https://doi.org/10.1038/nri1396

Vrbnjak, K., & Sewduth, R. N. (2024). Recent advances in peptide drug discovery: Novel strategies and targeted protein degradation. *Pharmaceutics, 16*. https://doi.org/10.3390/pharmaceutics16111486

Wang, T.-W., Chang, K.-C., Chen, L.-H., Liao, S.-Y., Yeh, C.-W., & Chuang, Y.-J. (2017). Effects of an injectable functionalized self-assembling nanopeptide hydrogel on angiogenesis and neurogenesis for regeneration of the central nervous system. *Nanoscale, 9*(42), 16281–16292. https://doi.org/10.1039/C7NR06528K

Wang, L., Wang, N., Zhang, W., Cheng, X., Yan, Z., Shao, G., Wang, X., Wang, R., & Fu, C. (2022). Therapeutic peptides: Current applications and future directions. *Signal Transduction and Targeted Therapy, 7*(1), 48. https://doi.org/10.1038/s41392-022-00904-4

Waschek, J. A. (2013). VIP and PACAP: Neuropeptide modulators of CNS inflammation, injury, and repair. *British Journal of Pharmacology, 169*(3), 512–523. https://doi.org/10.1111/bph.12181

Weiner, H. L. (2025). Immune mechanisms and shared immune targets in neurodegenerative diseases. *Nature Reviews Neurology, 21*(2), 67–85. https://doi.org/10.1038/s41582-024-01046-7

Wijesinghe, A., Kumari, S., & Booth, V. (2022). Conjugates for use in peptide therapeutics: A systematic review and meta-analysis. *PLoS One, 17*(3), Article e0255753.

Wolkow, C. A., Kimura, K. D., Lee, M.-S., Ruvkun, G., & Regulation, of C. (2000). Elegans life-span by insulinlike signaling in the nervous system. *Science, 290*(5489), 147–150. https://doi.org/10.1126/science.290.5489.147

Xie, C., Chen, Y., Wang, L., Liao, K., Xue, B., Han, Y., Li, L., & Jiang, Q. (2024). Recent research of peptide-based hydrogel in nervous regeneration. *Bioactive Materials, 40*, 503–523. https://doi.org/10.1016/j.bioactmat.2024.06.013

Yadav, A., Pandey, D., & Ashraf Rachana, G. M. (2021). *Peptide based therapy for neurological disorders, 22* (pp. 656–665). https://doi.org/10.2174/1389203722666210920151810

Yang, F., Luo, Z., Chu, Z., He, Z., Hu, Z., Qu, G., Zhou, Y., Tang, Y., Sun, S., & Luo, F. (2025). Comprehensive analysis of yak milk residue peptides for anti-hypoxic functional foods: Targeting neuroinflammation and apoptosis in hypoxic mice. *Food & Function, 16*(13), 5632–5651. https://doi.org/10.1039/D5FO01223F

Yeo, X. Y., Cunliffe, G., Ho, R. C., Lee, S. S., & Jung, S. (2022). Potentials of neuropeptides as therapeutic agents for neurological diseases. *Biomedicines, 10*(2). https://doi.org/10.3390/biomedicines10020343

Zhang, L., & Eiden, L. E. (2019). Progress in regulatory peptide research. *Annals of the New York Academy of Sciences, 1455*(1), 5–11. https://doi.org/10.1111/nyas.14260

Zhang, X., Fu, M., Wang, Y., & Wu, T. (2025). Strategies for delivering drugs across the blood-brain barrier for the treatment of neurodegenerative diseases. *Frontiers in Drug Delivery, 5.*

Zoupanou, N., Georgiou, N., Moschovou, K., Chasapis, C. T., Kelaidonis, K., Chavda, V. P., Mavromoustakos, T., Matsoukas, J. M., Apostolopoulos, V., Chavda, V. P., Vora, L. K., & Apostolopoulos, V. (2024). Chapter 5 - Peptide-Based vaccines and altered peptide ligands: Multiple sclerosis paving the way. In *Developments in immunology* (pp. 63–72). Academic Press. https://doi.org/10.1016/B978-0-443-18564-9.00010-2

CHAPTER

Vaccines for neurological disorders: Preventive strategies

6

Harshit Saxena[1], **Akhilesh Kumar**[2], **Rohit Kumar Rohit**[2] **and Pooja Solanki Pooja**[2]
[1]*ICAR-IVRI, Izatnagar, Division of Medicine, Bareilly, Uttar Pradesh, India;* [2]*Division of Medicine, ICAR-Indian Veterinary Research Institute, Bareilly, Uttar Pradesh, India*

1. Introduction

The toll of mortality and disability resulting from neurological illnesses is widely acknowledged as a global public health issue, and this burden is projected to escalate in the coming decades. The substantial and escalating burden of neurological disorders is influenced by global population growth and aging; comprehending the impact of neurological diseases has, consequently, been complicated by rapid demographic shifts and alterations in risk factors (e.g., overweight, obesity) in both high-income countries (HICs) and low- and middle-income countries (LMICs) (Kumar et al., 2024). Conditions can impact the nervous system throughout life by hindering brain development, injuring the brain, spinal cord, or peripheral nerves, and altering cognitive, sensory, socioemotional, and motor functions and behaviors. In May 2022, the World Health Assembly endorsed the Intersectoral Global Action Plan on Epilepsy and Other Neurological Disorders 2022–2031 (IGAP) to address the increasing prevalence of nervous system disorders globally. The action plan seeks to mitigate the stigma, impact, and burden of neurological disorders, encompassing their related mortality, morbidity, and disability, while enhancing the quality of life for individuals with neurological disorders, their caregivers, and families (Steinmetz et al., 2024).

Furthermore, the COVID-19 pandemic has revealed that new and re-emerging infectious diseases pose an increasing worldwide threat. Vector-borne viruses, including Zika virus, Japanese encephalitis virus, and West Nile virus, are expanding their geographic distribution due to climate change, posing a significant worldwide public health hazard (Vos et al., 2022). Neuroinfection and neuroimmunology are expanding specialisms within neurology. Notwithstanding significant diagnostic and therapeutic progress over the past 3 decades, including the prevention of infectious diseases via vaccination and the creation of safe, effective antimicrobial agents, neurological infections continue to be a leading cause of permanent neurological disability globally (Millichap & Epstein, 2009).

Managing these disorders entails substantial economic costs, including those for diagnosis, treatment, rehabilitation, and long-term care. Historically, vaccinations have focused on infectious agents; however, advancements in immunology have enabled novel applications, such as therapeutic vaccines for chronic illnesses (Simonsen & Snowden, 2024). Recent investigations have examined the

Immunotherapies for Neurological Disorders. https://doi.org/10.1016/B978-0-443-44631-3.00004-4

efficacy of vaccinations in the treatment of cancer, autoimmune diseases, and neurological disorders such as Alzheimer's and Parkinson's disease (Chumakov et al., 2021).

This chapter focuses on the epidemiology of infectious neurological illnesses, vaccination strategies targeting neurotropic pathogens, immunological approaches to neural protection, vaccine-related safety concerns, and emerging mechanisms in vaccine development. This chapter aims to examine vaccines available for neurologically significant pathogens, assess their field efficacy, evaluate potential adverse neurological effects, and investigate future research directions in vaccine development for controlling neurological disorders.

2. Neurological disorders: an overview classification

Neurological disorders comprise a diverse group of conditions that affect the central nervous system (CNS) and peripheral nervous system (PNS) and can arise from multiple underlying causes. Traditionally, these disorders are classified based on etiology, pathological mechanisms, anatomical involvement, and clinical manifestations, which helps in understanding disease progression and identifying preventive strategies. Among the major categories are neurodegenerative disorders, such as Alzheimer's disease, Parkinson's disease, Huntington's disease, and amyotrophic lateral sclerosis (ALS). These conditions are characterized by progressive neuronal degeneration, abnormal protein accumulation, and gradual impairment of cognitive or motor functions. Another important group includes demyelinating disorders, particularly multiple sclerosis and neuromyelitis optica, where immune-mediated damage to the myelin sheath disrupts nerve impulse transmission. Vascular neurological disorders, including stroke and vascular dementia, occur due to compromised blood supply to the brain, resulting in neuronal injury and long-term neurological deficits.

From a preventive and immunological perspective, neurological disorders may also be categorized into infectious, inflammatory, genetic, metabolic, and traumatic conditions, many of which have direct or indirect implications for vaccine development. Infectious neurological diseases, such as rabies, Japanese encephalitis, poliomyelitis, meningitis, and encephalitis, are caused by microbial pathogens and represent some of the most important targets for vaccination strategies. Autoimmune and inflammatory disorders, including multiple sclerosis and Guillain–Barré syndrome, involve dysregulated immune responses that damage neural tissues, highlighting the importance of understanding immune mechanisms when designing vaccines or immunotherapies. Genetic and congenital neurological disorders, such as spinal muscular atrophy and certain hereditary neuropathies, arise from inherited mutations affecting neural development or function.

Additionally, metabolic and nutritional neurological disorders may occur due to biochemical imbalances that impair neuronal metabolism, while traumatic neurological conditions result from physical injury to the brain or spinal cord. Understanding this broad classification provides essential context for exploring how vaccination and immunological interventions can prevent or mitigate certain neurological diseases, particularly those caused by infectious agents. Neurological disorders are frequently caused by infectious agents, including bacteria, viruses, and protozoa. Bacterial pathogens such as Listeria monocytogenes cause encephalitis (circling disease) in ruminants, while Clostridium tetani and Clostridium botulinum are implicated in tetanus and botulism, respectively, leading to neuromuscular paralysis (Radostits et al., 2007). Organisms such as Streptococcus species, Escherichia coli in neonates, Mycoplasma bovis in cattle, and Borrelia burgdorferi in canines and equines may provoke bacterial meningitis and encephalitis, potentially leading to neurological diseases.

Nervous system illnesses are primarily caused by viruses, including the rabies virus, canine distemper virus, equine herpesvirus-1, and arboviruses such as the West Nile virus, which can result in myelitis or encephalitis. Protozoan pathogens, including Toxoplasma gondii, Neospora caninum, and Sarcocystis neurona, are associated with inflammatory neurological disorders in small animals, livestock, and horses.

Autoimmune illnesses, or immune-mediated diseases, occur when the immune system mistakenly attacks its own cells. Autoimmune and inflammatory neurological disorders in animals arise from immune-mediated attacks on the brain, spinal cord, and peripheral nerves, driven by T-cells, autoantibodies, and chronic neuroinflammation. In dogs, immune-mediated encephalitides, including granulomatous meningoencephalitis and necrotizing encephalitis, are notable non-infectious causes of seizures and paralysis (Vitale & Foss, 2019). Neurodegenerative disorders are conditions marked by the progressive degradation of neurons, leading to neurological disability and often, death. In animals, as in humans, these illnesses may be hereditary, spontaneous, infectious, or age-related, and may affect either the central nervous system (CNS) or the peripheral nervous system (PNS) (Sisó et al., 2006).

Neurodegenerative diseases in animals represent a class of progressive disorders marked by neuronal loss and declining nervous system function. This encompasses prion diseases (transmissible spongiform encephalopathies) including scrapie in ovines, feline spongiform encephalopathy in felines, bovine spongiform encephalopathy in bovines, and chronic wasting disease in cervids, all characterized by spongiform brain degeneration and the aggregation of misfolded prion proteins (Orge et al., 2021).

Nerves possess a complicated structure with characteristics of significant importance to nerve injury and regeneration. Neuronal damage in neurological illnesses results from a convergence of metabolic, inflammatory, ischemic, and degenerative factors that gradually impair normal neuronal structure and function. There are two classifications of nerve injury based on the characteristics of the lesions, rather than their etiology. The first classification encompasses neurapraxia, axonotmesis, and neurotmesis to address conduction block and axonal continuity loss, while the second classification is predicated on the histological architecture of a nerve trunk, delineating 5° of nerve damage with escalating severity, commencing with conduction block and subsequently progressing to the loss of axonal continuity, followed by nerve fibers, fasciculi, and ultimately the entire nerve trunk (Sir Sydney Sunderland, 1990). Acute and chronic compression injuries disrupt nerve microcirculation, hinder axonal transport, and induce edema, ultimately compromising normal nerve function. Anesthesia-related injuries, particularly from intrafascicular injections or prolonged exposure to local anesthetics, can increase intracellular calcium levels and directly damage axons (HOGAN, 2008). Alongside these structural injuries, abnormal regeneration may ensue, resulting in axonal misfiring or neuroma formation, which perpetuates signaling alterations that contribute to chronic neuropathic pain (Rugnath et al., 2024).

Neurological illnesses constitute a complex global burden that impacts healthcare systems, economic productivity, and population health. In 2021, nearly 3.4 billion individuals—exceeding 40% of the global population—were afflicted with at least one neurological disorder, resulting in more than 11 million fatalities globally. The economic ramifications of neurological illnesses stem from direct healthcare expenditures and indirect productivity declines. Chronic diseases such as multiple sclerosis, migraine, and epilepsy markedly diminish labor engagement, elevate absenteeism, and exacerbate presenteeism, cumulatively costing businesses billions of dollars each year. In affluent countries, annual per-capita healthcare spending may surpass USD 12,000, with neurological illnesses classified as high-cost conditions due to their extended treatment, rehabilitation, and long-term care needs. Health systems experience a significant burden during outbreaks of neuroinvasive infectious illnesses, as emergency actions frequently reallocate resources from standard care.

Neurological injury is intricately linked to mental health outcomes, especially after neuro-inflammatory or viral events. Elevated levels of depression, anxiety, and cognitive impairment have been documented in survivors of viral encephalitis and other central nervous system illnesses, with prevalence estimates varying from 20% to over 50% in certain groups. A multitude of developing neurological concerns are zoonotic, stemming from human-animal interactions and environmental alterations. Occupational exposure is a substantial risk factor, especially for agricultural workers and animal handlers, who exhibit markedly elevated infection rates for infections that can induce serious neurological consequences, including encephalitis and autoimmune neuropathies. Neurotropic infections continue to pose a significant global public health threat. Rabies results in roughly 59,000 fatalities each year and is nearly always lethal once clinical signs manifest. The West Nile virus often progresses to neuroinvasive conditions, such as encephalitis and acute flaccid paralysis, accounting for approximately 50% of reported infections in certain areas. The Nipah virus, transmitted via bat and animal reservoirs, has a fatality rate of 40%–75% and induces severe neuroinflammation. Enhancing preventive measures, refining clinical management, and implementing integrated One Health frameworks are crucial to alleviating the growing worldwide burden of neurological diseases.

3. Neuroimmunology and vaccine principles

Neuroimmunology integrates fundamental and applied biology, immunology, chemistry, neurology, pathology, psychiatry, and virology pertaining to the central nervous system (CNS). The interaction between the immune system and the central nervous system is illustrated by the discovery that numerous immune-related chemicals are widely expressed and function within both systems (Fig. 6.1). The interaction between microglia and neurons is crucial for homeostasis, and similar interactions occur between oligodendrocytes and microglia (Peferoen et al., 2014).

The blood-brain barrier (BBB) is crucial for safeguarding the central nervous system (CNS) from potentially detrimental circulating infections. The BBB comprises brain microvascular endothelial cells (BMECs) encircled by pericytes and astrocytes, and is enveloped by two basement membranes: the vascular basement membrane and the glia limitans. The primary physiological functions of the intact blood-brain barrier (BBB) include limiting the entry of plasma macromolecules into the brain, preserving ionic homeostasis, absorbing cerebral nutrients, modulating neurotransmitter levels, and removing substances from the brain. The disruption of the BBB is linked to various neuro-immunological disorders, such as multiple sclerosis (MS), neuromyelitis optica (NMO), myelin oligodendrocyte glycoprotein antibody-associated disease (MOGAD), autoimmune encephalitis (AE), and neuropsychiatric systemic lupus erythematosus (NPSLE) (Brimberg et al., 2015). Disruptions in this communication, generated by peripheral infections, are acknowledged to trigger microglial activation and worsen neurodegeneration.

Microglia, the brain's intrinsic immune cells, react to peripheral signals, whereas cytokines and chemokines may traverse the blood-brain barrier or be synthesized locally in response to systemic immune activation. Pathogens can directly infiltrate the central nervous system or provoke systemic

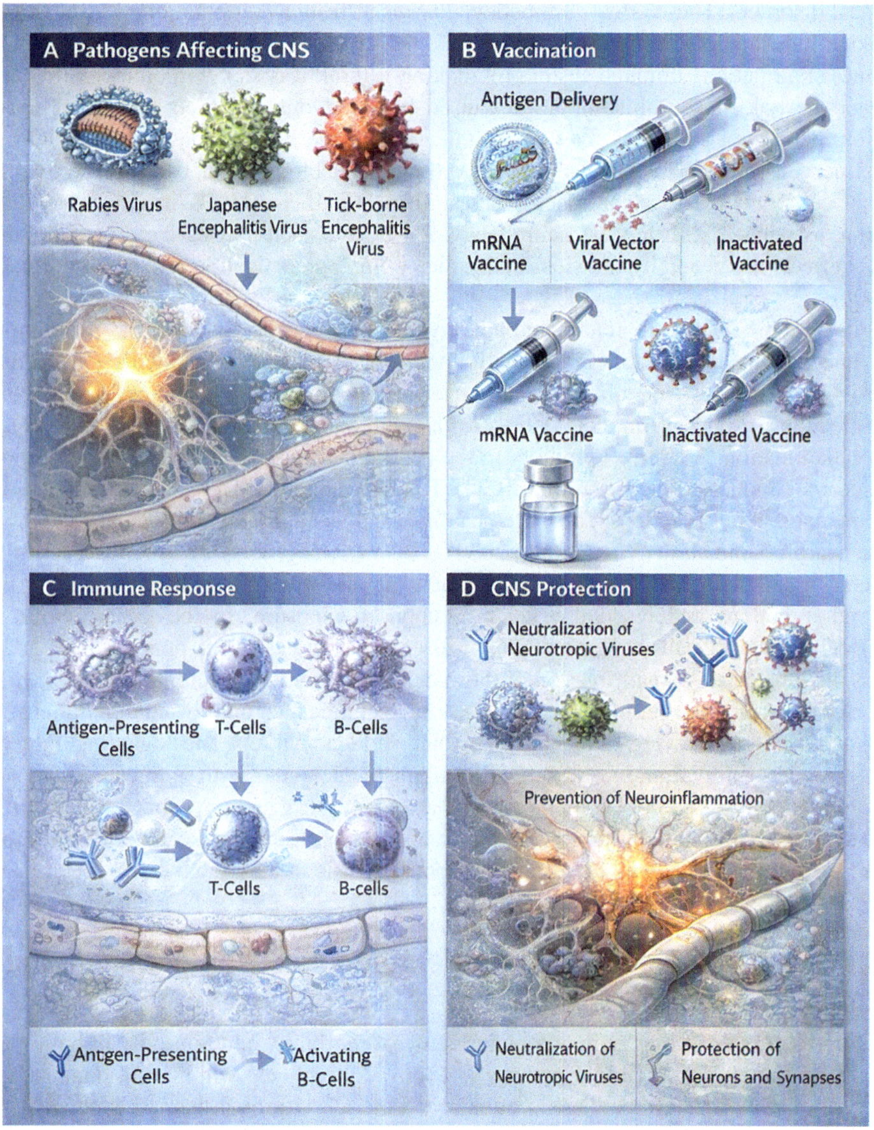

FIGURE 6.1 Mechanisms of neuroprotection by vaccines.

Systematic view of steps involved in providing the neuroprotection by vaccines during different neurological disorders.

inflammation that compromises the blood-brain barrier and activates microglia. This may lead to increased concentrations of pro-inflammatory cytokines such as IL-6, TNF-α, and IL-1β in the brain, which can cause symptoms including fatigue, cognitive impairment, and mood disorders. Several researchers are investigating vaccinations that regulate neuroimmune pathways for the treatment of neurological disorders. These effects are believed to result from a combination of viral neuroinvasion and cytokine-induced neuroinflammation.

Vaccines stimulate the immune system by making it think it is sick without actually getting sick. They lower the risk of neuroinflammation caused by infections and their long-term effects. Post-vaccination, peripheral cytokines may communicate with the brain through neural pathways (e.g., the vagus nerve), humoral mechanisms (e.g., crossing the blood-brain barrier), or by stimulating endothelial cells and perivascular macrophages. IL-6 and IFN-γ levels increase transiently post-vaccination, associated with modest neurobehavioral effects such as weariness or irritability. However, these effects are generally transient and indicate immune activation rather than disease (Heller et al., 2008).

The interaction between the innate and adaptive immune systems is essential for comprehensive immune function. Innate immunity in the central nervous system provides a swift, nonspecific defense via microglia, astrocytes, the blood-brain barrier, and complement proteins. These components identify infections or injury, eliminate debris, restrict infection, and preserve CNS homeostasis while reducing inflammation. Adaptive immunity in the central nervous system provides protection against antigen-specific, enduring defense, primarily via T cells, regulatory T cells, and restricted B cell activity. It regulates viral infections, facilitates healing, and sustains immunological tolerance to avert excessive neuroinflammation (Wang et al., 2024).

Immunological memory is the adaptive capacity of the immune system to identify previously encountered infections and respond efficiently upon re-exposure. In the first immune response, antigen-specific B and T cells undergo clonal proliferation, increasing the population of effector cells to address the infection. A small fraction of these cells concurrently differentiates into memory cells, which persist for prolonged periods. Memory cells have unique phenotypic and functional attributes in contrast to naïve lymphocytes. They have distinct surface markers and signaling molecules that facilitate extended survival and swift activation upon re-encounter with antigens. Upon subsequent exposure to the identical pathogen, memory cells are rapidly triggered. Memory B cells differentiate into plasma cells, which rapidly produce specific antibodies. Memory T cells undergo rapid proliferation and activation, enhancing an immune response that is more effective and specific.

4. Vaccines against neurotropic infectious diseases of human and veterinary importance

Neurotropic infectious diseases remain a major cause of morbidity and mortality in both humans and animals due to the ability of certain pathogens to invade, replicate within, and damage the central nervous system (CNS). These pathogens often reach the CNS through hematogenous spread or via peripheral nerves, ultimately causing encephalitis, meningitis, or myelitis. Vaccination represents one of the most effective preventive strategies against these diseases. Over the past several decades, the development of vaccines against neurotropic pathogens has significantly reduced the incidence of several fatal neurological infections in humans and animals Table 6.1. The integration of vaccination programs into public health and veterinary medicine has been particularly important for controlling zoonotic pathogens that circulate among wildlife, domestic animals, and humans. Modern vaccines employ a variety of platforms, including inactivated viruses, live attenuated strains, recombinant vectors, and subunit antigens, designed to induce strong humoral and cellular immune responses

Table 6.1 Important vaccines for under use/trial for neurological disorders.

Category	Disease	Target/ Pathogen	Vaccine type/ Candidate	Status	References
Neurodegenerative disorders	Alzheimer's disease	Amyloid-β peptide	AN1792 peptide vaccine	Phase I–II trials (discontinued due to inflammatory reactions)	Wisniewski and Goñi (2014)
	Alzheimer's disease	Tau protein	AADvac1, ACI-35 vaccines	Phase I–II clinical trials	Wisniewski and Goñi (2014)
	Parkinson's disease	α-synuclein	Peptide vaccines (e.g., PD01A)	Early clinical trials	Jankovic and Tan (2020)
	Multiple sclerosis	Myelin antigens (MBP, MOG)	Tolerogenic peptide vaccines	Experimental/ early trials	Compston and Coles (2008)
Infectious neurological diseases	Rabies	Rabies virus	Inactivated cell-culture vaccines	Widely used in humans and animals	Plotkin et al. (2018)
	Japanese encephalitis	Japanese encephalitis virus	Live attenuated SA14-14-2 vaccine	Widely used in endemic regions	Solomon et al. (2000)
	Poliomyelitis	Poliovirus	Oral polio vaccine (OPV) and inactivated polio vaccine (IPV)	Global eradication programs	Minor (2009)
	Equine encephalitis (EEE/WEE/ VEE)	Alphaviruses	Inactivated equine vaccines	Used in horses in endemic regions	
	Tetanus	*Clostridium tetani* toxin	Tetanus toxoid vaccine	Routine human and veterinary vaccination	Plotkin et al., (2018)
	Meningococcal meningitis	*Neisseria meningitidis*	Conjugate vaccines	Human vaccination programs	Stephens et al. (2007)

capable of preventing viral invasion of neural tissues (Plotkin et al., 2018). *Plotkin's Vaccines (seventh ed.). Elsevier.*, no date; Barrett & Stanberry, 2009).

4.1 Viral neurological diseases

Among viral neurotropic infections, rabies remains one of the most well-known and deadly diseases affecting both humans and animals. Caused by a neurotropic virus belonging to the genus Lyssavirus in the family Rhabdoviridae, rabies is transmitted primarily through bites of infected animals such as dogs, bats, and other wildlife reservoirs. Following peripheral replication, the virus travels through peripheral nerves via retrograde axonal transport to the brain, leading to fatal encephalitis. Vaccination has played a pivotal role in rabies control. In humans, cell-culture–derived vaccines such as purified chick embryo cell vaccine (PCECV) and human diploid cell vaccine (HDCV) are widely used for both pre-exposure and post-exposure prophylaxis. In animals, particularly dogs and wildlife, mass vaccination campaigns using inactivated or recombinant vaccines have significantly reduced transmission and human mortality in many regions.

Japanese encephalitis (JE) is another important mosquito-borne neurotropic viral disease prevalent in Asia. The causative agent, Japanese encephalitis virus (JEV), belongs to the genus Flavivirus. The virus circulates in a zoonotic cycle involving mosquitoes, pigs, and water birds, with humans and horses acting as incidental hosts. Severe infections can result in encephalitis, characterized by inflammation of the brain parenchyma, neurological deficits, and high case fatality rates. Vaccines against JEV include inactivated mouse brain–derived vaccines, Vero cell-derived inactivated vaccines, and live attenuated vaccines such as the SA14-14-2 strain, which are widely used in endemic regions to prevent disease (Solomon et al., 2000).

West Nile virus (WNV), another flavivirus, has emerged as a significant cause of viral encephalitis in humans, horses, and birds. The virus is transmitted by mosquitoes and maintained in an enzootic cycle between birds and mosquito vectors. While most human infections are asymptomatic, severe cases can lead to meningitis, encephalitis, and acute flaccid paralysis. In veterinary medicine, several equine vaccines, including inactivated whole-virus vaccines, recombinant canarypox-vectored vaccines, and DNA vaccines, have been developed and successfully used to prevent neurological disease in horses. Although human vaccines are still under development, veterinary vaccination programs have proven highly effective in reducing equine morbidity and mortality (Sejvar, 2014).

Poliomyelitis is a classic example of a viral disease that causes neurological impairment by destroying motor neurons in the spinal cord. Caused by poliovirus, a member of the family Picornaviridae, the disease can result in irreversible paralysis. The development of two effective vaccines—the inactivated polio vaccine (IPV) developed by Jonas Salk and the oral polio vaccine (OPV) developed by Albert Sabin—has dramatically reduced global disease incidence. Extensive vaccination campaigns coordinated by the Global Polio Eradication Initiative have brought the world close to complete eradication of poliomyelitis (Minor, 2009). In veterinary medicine, similar neurotropic viral infections, such as louping ill virus in sheep, are controlled using inactivated vaccines.

Other viral infections that can cause neurological complications include measles-associated encephalitis. Although measles is primarily a systemic viral disease caused by Morbillivirus, severe neurological manifestations such as acute disseminated encephalomyelitis and subacute sclerosing panencephalitis can occur as rare complications. Widespread immunization with the live attenuated measles vaccine has significantly reduced both the incidence of measles and its neurological complications (Griffin, 2014).

Equine encephalitides caused by alphaviruses—including Eastern equine encephalitis (EEE), Western equine encephalitis (WEE), and Venezuelan equine encephalitis (VEE)—are important mosquito-borne neurological diseases affecting horses and occasionally humans. These viruses are capable of causing severe encephalitis characterized by neuronal degeneration, inflammation, and high mortality. Vaccines for horses typically consist of inactivated viral preparations or attenuated strains, which are widely used in endemic regions to prevent outbreaks.

In companion animals, viral infections such as feline panleukopenia virus (FPV) and canine distemper virus (CDV) are important neurological pathogens. Canine distemper virus, a member of the genus Morbillivirus, can invade the central nervous system and cause demyelinating encephalitis in dogs and wildlife species. Vaccination using modified live virus vaccines has been highly effective in preventing disease. Similarly, vaccines against feline panleukopenia virus are routinely administered to cats to prevent systemic and neurological complications associated with infection (Sykes, 2022,).

4.2 Bacterial neurological diseases

Bacterial infections can also produce severe neurological disease, often through toxin production or direct invasion of the CNS. Tetanus, caused by Clostridium tetani, is characterized by the production of a potent neurotoxin known as tetanospasmin. This toxin blocks inhibitory neurotransmitter release in the central nervous system, leading to generalized muscle rigidity and spasms. Vaccination with tetanus toxoid is highly effective and forms a core component of human and veterinary immunization programs. In animals such as horses, sheep, and cattle, routine vaccination significantly reduces mortality from the disease.

Listeriosis, caused by Listeria monocytogenes, is another important neurological disease in animals and, occasionally, in humans. The bacterium can invade the brainstem via cranial nerves, resulting in meningoencephalitis, often referred to as "circling disease" in ruminants. Although vaccines are not widely used in humans, experimental vaccines targeting listerial antigens have been investigated in livestock to reduce disease incidence in endemic areas.

Meningococcal meningitis, caused by Neisseria meningitidis, is a serious bacterial infection that leads to inflammation of the meninges surrounding the brain and spinal cord. Conjugate vaccines targeting multiple meningococcal serogroups have been developed and widely implemented in vaccination programs, resulting in significant reductions in disease incidence worldwide (Stephens et al., 2007).

Similarly, pneumococcal meningitis caused by Streptococcus pneumoniae remains a major cause of bacterial meningitis globally. Vaccines such as pneumococcal conjugate vaccines (PCVs) and pneumococcal polysaccharide vaccines (PPSVs) have been highly effective in preventing invasive pneumococcal disease, including meningitis, particularly among children and the elderly (O'Brien et al., 2009).

5. Vaccination strategies for neurodegenerative and immune-mediated neurological disorders

Recent advances in neuroimmunology have expanded the traditional concept of vaccination beyond the prevention of infectious diseases to include immunotherapeutic strategies targeting chronic neurological disorders. Neurodegenerative diseases such as Alzheimer's disease, Parkinson's disease, and amyotrophic lateral sclerosis, along with immune-mediated neurological conditions such as multiple sclerosis, involve complex pathological processes including abnormal protein aggregation, chronic neuroinflammation, and dysregulated immune responses within the central nervous system (CNS). These pathophysiological mechanisms have prompted the development of vaccine-based approaches designed either to stimulate protective immune responses against disease-associated proteins or to induce immune tolerance against autoantigens implicated in neurological damage (Plotkin et al., 2018; Murphy & Weaver, 2022).

One of the most extensively investigated vaccine strategies targets pathological protein aggregates associated with neurodegenerative diseases. In Alzheimer's disease, accumulation of extracellular amyloid-β plaques and intracellular neurofibrillary tangles composed of hyperphosphorylated tau protein are considered central pathological hallmarks. Immunization strategies directed against amyloid-β were first demonstrated in experimental models where active vaccination with amyloid peptides stimulated antibody production and promoted clearance of amyloid plaques from the brain. Early human trials using the AN1792 vaccine showed evidence of plaque reduction but were discontinued due to inflammatory adverse events, highlighting the importance of carefully modulating immune responses in CNS immunotherapy. Consequently, newer vaccine formulations employ epitope-specific antigens and improved adjuvants to enhance humoral immunity while minimizing potentially harmful T-cell–mediated inflammatory responses (Wisniewski & Goñi, 2014; Plotkin et al., 2018).

In addition to amyloid-targeted vaccines, tau-directed immunization strategies are gaining increasing attention. Tau protein aggregation contributes to neuronal dysfunction and propagation of neurodegeneration in Alzheimer's disease and other tauopathies. Experimental vaccines designed to generate antibodies against pathological tau epitopes have shown promising results in reducing tau accumulation and limiting neuronal damage in animal models. These findings suggest that targeting intracellular protein-propagation pathways may represent an effective strategy for slowing disease progression (Jankovic & Tan, 2020).

Vaccination approaches are also being investigated in Parkinson's disease, where α-synuclein aggregation plays a central role in neuronal degeneration in the substantia nigra. Misfolded α-synuclein proteins can spread between neurons, triggering neuroinflammatory responses that contribute to disease progression. Immunotherapeutic vaccines targeting α-synuclein aim to stimulate antibodies capable of neutralizing extracellular protein aggregates and promoting their clearance through microglial phagocytosis. Both peptide-based and recombinant protein vaccines have demonstrated reductions in α-synuclein pathology and neurodegeneration in experimental models, suggesting a potential disease-modifying role for immunization strategies in synucleinopathies (Jankovic & Tan, 2020).

In parallel with protein-targeted vaccines, nucleic acid-based vaccine platforms have emerged as promising tools for neurological immunotherapy. DNA and messenger RNA vaccines encode specific antigenic proteins that are produced by host cells following administration, thereby inducing targeted immune responses. These platforms offer several advantages, including rapid development, high antigen specificity, and the ability to induce both humoral and cellular immune responses. Advances in lipid nanoparticle delivery systems have further improved the stability and cellular uptake of nucleic acid vaccines, making them attractive candidates for targeting antigens associated with neurological diseases.

Vaccination strategies for immune-mediated neurological disorders differ fundamentally from those for neurodegenerative diseases, as the therapeutic objective is not to stimulate immunity but to induce immune tolerance. Multiple sclerosis (MS), for example, is characterized by immune-mediated destruction of myelin sheaths within the CNS, resulting in demyelination and progressive neurological dysfunction. Autoreactive T lymphocytes directed against myelin proteins such as myelin basic protein, proteolipid protein, and myelin oligodendrocyte glycoprotein play a critical role in disease pathogenesis. Peptide-based tolerogenic vaccines containing fragments of these myelin proteins have been investigated as a strategy to retrain the immune system and suppress pathogenic immune responses. These vaccines aim to promote regulatory T-cell responses that reduce inflammation and prevent further demyelination (Murphy & Weaver, 2022; Compston & Coles, 2008).

Another emerging strategy involves dendritic cell-based vaccines designed to promote immune tolerance. In this approach, patient-derived dendritic cells are exposed to specific antigens under tolerogenic conditions and then reintroduced into the body to modulate immune responses. These modified dendritic cells can induce regulatory immune pathways and suppress autoreactive lymphocytes that contribute to neurological damage. Experimental studies in animal models of multiple sclerosis have demonstrated that tolerogenic dendritic cell vaccines can significantly reduce CNS inflammation and disease severity.

Nanotechnology-based delivery systems are also increasingly being explored to enhance vaccine efficacy in neurological disorders. Nanoparticles, liposomes, and virus-like particles can serve as carriers for vaccine antigens and facilitate targeted delivery to antigen-presenting cells. These systems can improve antigen stability, prolong immune stimulation, and potentially help overcome biological barriers, such as the blood–brain barrier. Nanoparticle-based vaccine platforms also allow controlled antigen release and improved immunogenicity while reducing systemic toxicity (Zhao et al., 2014).

Despite these advances, several challenges remain in developing vaccines for neurological disorders. The blood–brain barrier restricts the entry of immune cells and therapeutic molecules into the CNS, potentially limiting vaccine effectiveness. Furthermore, excessive immune activation could potentially trigger neuroinflammation or autoimmune reactions that exacerbate neurological injury. Therefore, vaccine development for neurological diseases requires precise antigen design, careful selection of adjuvants, and controlled modulation of immune responses to ensure both safety and efficacy.

Recent developments in biomarker research and neuroimaging technologies have significantly improved the evaluation of vaccine-based therapies in neurological diseases. Biomarkers such as cerebrospinal fluid concentrations of amyloid-β, tau proteins, and neurofilament light chain provide valuable indicators of neuronal damage and disease progression. When combined with advanced imaging techniques such as magnetic resonance imaging and positron emission tomography, these biomarkers enable researchers to monitor the effects of immunization strategies on CNS pathology and assess therapeutic outcomes in clinical trials (Jankovic & Tan, 2020).

6. Adverse neurological events following vaccination

Although vaccines are among the most effective public health interventions for preventing infectious diseases, rare adverse neurological events have occasionally been reported following immunization. These events include a range of neurological conditions, including encephalitis, acute disseminated encephalomyelitis (ADEM), Guillain–Barré syndrome (GBS), transverse myelitis, febrile seizures, and peripheral neuropathies. Such events are rare and often coincidental; however, careful scientific evaluation is necessary to determine whether a causal relationship exists between vaccination and the neurological outcome. Understanding vaccine-associated neurological complications is essential for maintaining public confidence in immunization programs and for ensuring that vaccination strategies continue to be safe and effective. Importantly, extensive epidemiological evidence indicates that the risk of severe neurological complications from natural infections is far greater than the risk associated with vaccination.

6.1 Epidemiology and causality assessment

Epidemiological studies play a critical role in identifying and evaluating potential adverse neurological events following vaccination. Large population-based studies, case-control analyses, and post-marketing surveillance data are commonly used to estimate the incidence of neurological complications and determine whether they occur more frequently among vaccinated individuals than in the general population. For example, Guillain–Barré syndrome has historically been investigated in association with influenza vaccines, particularly following the 1976 swine influenza vaccination campaign in the United States. Subsequent studies have shown that the risk of GBS following modern influenza vaccines is extremely low—approximately one to two additional cases per million vaccinations—while the risk of GBS following natural influenza infection is significantly higher (Vellozzi et al., 2014).

Establishing causality between vaccination and neurological events requires careful evaluation using standardized frameworks. Organizations such as the World Health Organization (WHO) and the Institute of Medicine have developed criteria for assessing adverse events following immunization (AEFI). These frameworks consider factors such as temporal association, biological plausibility, consistency of evidence across studies, exclusion of alternative causes, and the strength of epidemiological data. Many reported neurological events occurring after vaccination are ultimately classified as coincidental rather than causally related to the vaccine itself.

6.2 Risk–benefit analysis

Risk–benefit analysis is a fundamental component of vaccine safety evaluation. Even when rare adverse events are identified, the overall benefits of vaccination in preventing severe disease, disability, and death must be carefully weighed against potential risks. For most vaccines, the protective benefits vastly outweigh the risks of adverse events. For example, measles infection can lead to severe neurological complications such as encephalitis and subacute sclerosing panencephalitis, whereas the measles vaccine is associated only with extremely rare cases of febrile seizures or transient neurological symptoms. Similarly, rabies vaccination prevents a nearly universally fatal neurological disease, making the benefits of vaccination overwhelmingly greater than the minimal risk of adverse reactions (Plotkin et al., 2018).

Modern vaccine development incorporates rigorous safety testing through multiple phases of clinical trials before regulatory approval. These trials evaluate both common and rare adverse effects and help establish the safety profile of vaccines across diverse populations. After licensure, ongoing surveillance systems continue to monitor vaccine safety to detect any unexpected adverse neurological outcomes that might occur during widespread use.

6.3 Surveillance systems and pharmacovigilance

Post-licensure vaccine safety monitoring relies on comprehensive surveillance systems and pharmacovigilance programs designed to detect, investigate, and respond to adverse events following immunization. Several national and international surveillance systems have been established to ensure vaccine safety. In the United States, the Vaccine Adverse Event Reporting System (VAERS) collects reports of suspected adverse events from healthcare providers, vaccine manufacturers, and the public. Additional systems, such as the Vaccine Safety Datalink (VSD) and the Clinical Immunization Safety Assessment (CISA) project, provide more detailed epidemiological analyses using large healthcare databases (Shimabukuro et al., 2015).

Globally, the World Health Organization coordinates vaccine safety monitoring through the Global Advisory Committee on Vaccine Safety and the Global Vaccine Safety Initiative. These programs facilitate international data sharing and provide guidance for evaluating adverse events following immunization. Pharmacovigilance systems are essential for identifying potential safety signals, conducting rapid investigations, and implementing appropriate regulatory actions when necessary. Continuous monitoring and transparent communication regarding vaccine safety help maintain trust in immunization programs and ensure that vaccines remain one of the safest and most effective tools for disease prevention.

7. Challenges in developing vaccines for neurological disorders blood blood-brain barrier limitations

Neuroinflammation and safety concerns- The brain's capillary microvessels have evolved to limit the passage of cells and chemicals between the blood and the brain, thereby protecting the brain from hazardous or infectious compounds circulating in the body. The blood-brain barrier (BBB) is relatively impermeable because cell adhesion molecules create tight junctions and adherens junctions between capillary endothelial cells. The BBB preserves critical brain homeostasis; however, it constitutes a significant barrier to the efficient treatment of many brain disorders (Pardridge, 1998).

Antibody-dependent enhancement- Antibodies can enhance viral infection. They utilize specific antibodies to enhance entrance into target cells, resulting in heightened infectivity. This effect is referred to as antibody-dependent enhancement (Takada & Kawaoka, 2003).

Genetic and host variability- The genetic variation in vaccination response is crucial for public health and clinical management. Host genetic diversity is a major factor in variation in vaccination response across recipients. The vaccine response is modulated by host genes at every stage, encompassing pathogen recognition, antigen uptake, antigen processing and presentation by natural killer cells, dendritic cells, and macrophages, as well as genes related to B and T cell functionality, immune regulation, and the roles of effector or accessory cells (Kimman et al., 2007). Variations in genes that code for TLRs, HLA molecules, cytokines, and cytokine receptors make people's immune systems different (Newport, 2015). TLRs are proteins with one transmembrane domain that do not act as enzymes. They identify compounds that are conserved and derived from microbes (Kawai & Akira, 2006). TLR3 detects double-stranded RNA, which is produced when many viruses replicate. TLRs play a crucial role in initiating the vaccination response, and various vaccine adjuvants have been recognized as TLR ligands. HLA is a central subject of immunogenetics research aimed at elucidating the genetic and environmental determinants linked to inter-individual variability in vaccine-induced immunity. Most somatic cells express HLA class I genes; however, expression levels vary from tissue to tissue. HLA class II genes are predominantly expressed by certain populations of immune cells, including B cells, activated T cells, thymic epithelial cells, dendritic cells, and macrophages. Allergic responses to vaccines are not rare. It can cause type I hypersensitivity reactions, leading mast cells to release histamine in response to an antigen in the vaccine (Stone et al., 2019). Symptoms appear quickly and can include itching, nausea, vomiting, diarrhea, shortness of breath, hives, and even death in severe cases (McNeil & DeStefano, 2018).

Ethical and regulatory issues- The swift advancement of vaccine research, alongside the progression of various vaccine types into the third phase of clinical trials and the granting of emergency licenses for worldwide application, has prompted numerous ethical dilemmas, primarily rooted in the four principles of bioethics: justice, nonmaleficence, benefit, and autonomy (Kumar et al., 2021). The obstacles can be categorized into four primary domains: (1) secure and standardized manufacturing alongside adherence to scientific and ethical protocols, (2) assessment and surveillance of safety and efficacy, (3) large-scale production and equitable distribution, and (4) societal acceptance (Malekzadeh et al., 2023). Ethical governance in vaccine development and production is typically centered on the concepts of justice, beneficence, non-maleficence, and autonomy. Justice requires fair global access to affordable vaccines, the prevention of exploitative research practices in low-income settings, uniform ethical standards across nations, post-trial access for participants, and adaptable intellectual property regulations during public health crises. Beneficence mandates that manufacturers conduct inclusive trials involving diverse populations, maintain stringent safety and efficacy standards, fulfill social responsibilities—especially toward underprivileged areas—and thoroughly evaluate the risks and long-term consequences of new vaccine technologies. Non-maleficence underscores the necessity of autonomous ethical supervision, the judicious and warranted application of placebos, with assured access to effective vaccinations thereafter, transparency in research and production methodologies, and safeguarding vulnerable groups from harm or exploitation. Autonomy emphasizes stringent informed consent protocols, safeguarding participant privacy and data confidentiality, as well as the right to voluntary participation and withdrawal without compulsion.

8. Future directions: personalized and precision vaccines

Advances in molecular biology, immunology, and biomedical technology are transforming the landscape of vaccine development, particularly in the context of neurological disorders. Traditional vaccines were designed primarily to induce broad protective immunity against infectious agents; however, emerging approaches are increasingly focused on personalized and precision vaccination strategies tailored to individual genetic, immunological, and disease characteristics. Precision vaccines aim to optimize immune responses by targeting specific molecular pathways involved in neurological diseases while minimizing adverse reactions. In neurological disorders, where complex interactions between the immune system and the central nervous system (CNS) contribute to disease pathogenesis, personalized vaccine strategies hold promise for improving therapeutic efficacy and safety. The integration of genomics, systems biology, and advanced computational tools is expected to facilitate the development of next-generation vaccines capable of preventing or modifying neurological diseases at an early stage.

8.1 Neuroprotective and tolerance-inducing vaccines

One promising future direction in neurological vaccine development is the design of neuroprotective vaccines that prevent neuronal damage and promote long-term neural survival. Such vaccines aim to stimulate immune mechanisms that enhance clearance of toxic protein aggregates, reduce oxidative stress, and modulate neuroinflammatory responses within the CNS. For example, vaccines targeting pathological proteins such as amyloid-β, tau, and α-synuclein are being investigated for neurodegenerative disorders including Alzheimer's disease and Parkinson's disease. By inducing antibodies that recognize and neutralize these proteins, neuroprotective vaccines may help prevent the accumulation of toxic aggregates that contribute to neuronal degeneration (Wisniewski & Goñi, 2014).

In addition to neuroprotective strategies, tolerance-inducing vaccines are being explored for immune-mediated neurological disorders. Diseases such as multiple sclerosis are characterized by autoimmune responses against myelin proteins in the CNS. Tolerogenic vaccines containing specific myelin-derived peptides are designed to retrain the immune system, suppress autoreactive T-cell responses, and promote regulatory immune pathways. Such approaches aim to restore immune tolerance and prevent progressive demyelination without broadly suppressing immune function. Experimental studies and early clinical trials suggest that antigen-specific tolerance induction may offer a safer, more targeted alternative to conventional immunosuppressive therapies (Steinman, 2014; Murphy & Weaver, 2022).

8.2 Nanotechnology-based vaccine delivery

Nanotechnology is emerging as a powerful tool for improving vaccine delivery and immunogenicity. Nanoparticle-based vaccine systems can enhance antigen stability, protect vaccine components from degradation, and facilitate targeted delivery to antigen-presenting cells. These platforms include lipid nanoparticles, polymeric nanoparticles, liposomes, and virus-like particles, all of which can be engineered to optimize immune responses. In the context of neurological diseases, nanotechnology-based vaccines may also help overcome biological barriers such as the blood–brain barrier, which limits the entry of therapeutic molecules into the CNS. Nanoparticle carriers can be modified with targeting ligands that enable selective transport across endothelial barriers or enhance uptake by immune cells involved in CNS surveillance (Zhao et al., 2014).

Furthermore, nanotechnology enables the co-delivery of antigens and immunomodulatory molecules, such as adjuvants or cytokines, within a single carrier system. This approach enables precise control over the magnitude and type of immune response generated by the vaccine. Such strategies may be particularly useful for neurological vaccines, where excessive immune activation must be avoided to prevent neuroinflammation.

8.3 AI-guided antigen design

Artificial intelligence (AI) and machine learning technologies are increasingly being applied to vaccine research and development. AI-driven algorithms can analyze large datasets derived from genomic sequencing, structural biology, and immunological studies to identify optimal antigenic targets for vaccine design. In neurological disorders, where disease-associated proteins often have complex structures and multiple pathological variants, AI-guided antigen design can help identify specific epitopes capable of eliciting protective immune responses while minimizing cross-reactivity with healthy tissues.

Computational models can also predict antigen stability, immunogenicity, and potential safety concerns before laboratory testing, thereby accelerating vaccine development. Additionally, AI-based platforms can assist in the design of personalized vaccines by integrating individual genetic information, immune profiles, and disease biomarkers. This approach may enable the development of vaccines tailored to the unique immunological characteristics of individual patients, representing a significant advancement in precision medicine.

8.4 Vaccines for neurodegenerative disorders

The development of vaccines targeting neurodegenerative diseases represents one of the most promising areas of future research in neurological therapeutics. Unlike traditional treatments that primarily alleviate symptoms, vaccine-based immunotherapies aim to target the underlying pathological mechanisms driving neuronal degeneration. Current research is focused on vaccines targeting amyloid-β and tau proteins in Alzheimer's disease, α-synuclein in Parkinson's disease, and other misfolded proteins associated with neurodegeneration. Both active immunization and passive immunotherapy approaches are being explored, with several candidate vaccines currently undergoing clinical evaluation.

In addition to protein-targeted strategies, future vaccines may also focus on modulating neuroinflammatory pathways that contribute to disease progression. Chronic activation of microglia and other immune cells within the CNS plays a key role in many neurodegenerative disorders. Vaccines designed to regulate these immune responses could potentially slow disease progression and protect neuronal integrity. Continued progress in immunology, molecular biology, and translational neuroscience is expected to accelerate the development of such vaccines in the coming years (Jankovic & Tan, 2020).

9. Conclusion

Vaccination remains one of the most effective strategies for preventing diseases that affect the nervous system. Historically, vaccines have played a crucial role in controlling or eliminating several infectious neurological diseases, such as poliomyelitis, rabies, and Japanese encephalitis, thereby significantly reducing global morbidity and mortality. Recent advances in immunology and molecular medicine have broadened the scope of vaccination to include strategies targeting neurodegenerative and immune-mediated neurological disorders. By stimulating immune mechanisms capable of neutralizing pathogens, clearing pathological protein aggregates, or modulating dysregulated immune responses, vaccines offer promising opportunities for preventing neurological damage and improving long-term neurological health. The successful translation of vaccine research into clinical practice requires integration of basic science, clinical trials, and advanced technologies. Emerging platforms such as mRNA vaccines, viral vectors, and nanoparticle-based delivery systems are accelerating the development of next-generation vaccines for neurological diseases. In addition, biomarker-guided clinical trials and advanced neuroimaging are improving the evaluation of vaccine efficacy and safety in neurological conditions (Pardi et al., 2018). Continued investment in vaccination programs and surveillance systems is essential to control neurotropic infectious diseases worldwide. At the same time, expanded research efforts are needed to develop vaccines for neurodegenerative and immune-mediated neurological disorders. International collaboration, improved regulatory frameworks, and advances in precision medicine will play important roles in translating these emerging vaccine strategies into effective preventive and therapeutic interventions.

AI disclosure

During the preparation of this work the author(s) used Gemini AI in order to todraw Fig. 6.1, by providing the proper input/prompt to the AI tool. After using this tool/service, the author(s) reviewed and edited the content as needed and take(s) full responsibility for the content of the publication.

References

Barrett, A. D. T., & Stanberry, L. R. (2009). *Vaccines for biodefense and emerging and neglected diseases vaccines for biodefense and emerging and neglected diseases*. United States: Elsevier Inc.

Brimberg, L., Mader, S., Fujieda, Y., Arinuma, Y., Kowal, C., Volpe, B. T., & Diamond, B. (2015). Antibodies as mediators of brain pathology. *Trends in Immunology, 36*(11), 709–724. https://doi.org/10.1016/j.it.2015.09.008

Chumakov, K., Avidan, M. S., Benn, C. S., Bertozzi, S. M., Blatt, L., Chang, A. Y., Jamison, D. T., Khader, S. A., Kottilil, S., Netea, M. G., Sparrow, A., & Gallo, R. C. (2021). Old vaccines for new infections: Exploiting innate immunity to control COVID-19 and prevent future pandemics. *Proceedings of the National Academy of Sciences of the United States of America, 118*(21). https://doi.org/10.1073/pnas.2101718118

Compston, A., & Coles, A. (2008). Multiple sclerosis. *The Lancet, 372*(9648), 1502–1517. https://doi.org/10.1016/s0140-6736(08)61620-7

Griffin, D. E. (2014). Measles virus and the nervous system. *Handbook of Clinical Neurology, 123*, 577–590. https://doi.org/10.1016/B978-0-444-53488-0.00027-4

Heller, F., Fromm, A., Gitter, A. H., Mankertz, J., & Schulzke, J.-D. (2008). Epithelial apoptosis is a prominent feature of the epithelial barrier disturbance in intestinal inflammation: Effect of pro-inflammatory interleukin-13 on epithelial cell function. *Mucosal Immunology*, (1), S58. https://doi.org/10.1038/mi.2008.46

Hogan, Q. (2008). Pathophysiology of peripheral nerve injury during regional anesthesia. *Regional Anesthesia and Pain Medicine, 33*(5), 435–441. https://doi.org/10.1016/j.rapm.2008.03.002

Jankovic, J., & Tan, E. K. (2020). Parkinson's disease: Etiopathogenesis and treatment. *Journal of Neurology, Neurosurgery and Psychiatry, 91*(8), 795–808. https://doi.org/10.1136/jnnp-2019-322338

Kawai, T., & Akira, S. (2006). TLR signaling. *Cell Death & Differentiation, 13*(5), 816–825. https://doi.org/10.1038/sj.cdd.4401850

Kimman, T. G., Vandebriel, R., & Hoebee, B. (2007). Genetic variation in the response to vaccination. *Public Health Genomics, 10*(4), 201–217.

Kumar, V., Aranha, V., Rajgarhia, R., Royal, A., & Mehta, K. (2021). Expanded principles of ethics and its implementation during COVID-19 vaccine trials: A scoping evidence based research synthesis. *Human Vaccines & Immunotherapeutics, 17*(11), 3843–3849. https://doi.org/10.1080/21645515.2021.1947101

Kumar, P., Zelena, D., & Gautam, A. (2024). *Neurological disorders and challenges in their theranostics theranostic applications of nanotechnology in neurological disorders* (pp. 1–29). Hungary: Springer. https://doi.org/10.1007/978-981-99-9510-3_1

Malekzadeh, R., Abedi, G., Ziapour, A., Yıldırım, M., & Amirkhanlou, A. (2023). Analysis of ethical considerations of COVID-19 vaccination: Lessons for future. *BMC Medical Ethics, 24*(1). https://doi.org/10.1186/s12910-023-00969-y

McNeil, M. M., & DeStefano, F. (2018). Vaccine-associated hypersensitivity. *Journal of Allergy and Clinical Immunology, 141*(2), 463–472. https://doi.org/10.1016/j.jaci.2017.12.971

Millichap, J. J., & Epstein, L. G. (2009). Emerging subspecialties in neurology: Neuroinfectious diseases. *Neurology, 73*(4), e14. https://doi.org/10.1212/WNL.0b013e3181af7a46

Minor, P. (2009). Vaccine-derived poliovirus (VDPV): Impact on poliomyelitis eradication. *Vaccine, 27*(20), 2649–2652. https://doi.org/10.1016/j.vaccine.2009.02.071

Murphy, K., & Weaver, C. (2022). *Janeway's Immunobiology* (10th ed.). Garland Science.

Newport, M. J. (2015). The genetic regulation of infant immune responses to vaccination. *Frontiers in Immunology, 6*. https://doi.org/10.3389/fimmu.2015.00018

O'Brien, K. L., Wolfson, L. J., Watt, J. P., Henkle, E., Deloria-Knoll, M., McCall, N., Lee, E., Kim, M., Levine, O. S., & Cherian, T. (2009). Burden of disease caused by Streptococcus pneumoniae in children younger than 5 years: Global estimates. *The Lancet, 374*(9693), 893–902. https://doi.org/10.1016/S0140-6736(09)61204-6

Orge, L., Lima, C., Machado, C., Tavares, P., Mendonça, P., Carvalho, P., Silva, J., Pinto, M.de L., Bastos, E., Pereira, J. C., Gonçalves-Anjo, N., Gama, A., Esteves, A., Alves, A., Matos, A. C., Seixas, F., Silva, F., Pires, I., Figueira, L., & Sargo, R. (2021). Maria dos anjos pires, neuropathology of animal prion diseases. *Biomolecules, 11*(3), 466. https://doi.org/10.3390/biom11030466

Pardridge, W. M. (1998). CNS drug design based on principles of blood-brain barrier transport. *Journal of Neurochemistry, 70*(5), 1781–1792. https://doi.org/10.1046/j.1471-4159.1998.70051781.x

Peferoen, L., Kipp, M., van der Valk, P., van Noort, J. M., & Amor, S. (2014). Oligodendrocyte-microglia cross-talk in the central nervous system. *Immunology, 141*(3), 302–313. https://doi.org/10.1111/imm.12163

Plotkin, S. A., Orenstein, W. A., Offit, P. A., & Edwards, K. (2018). *Plotkin's vaccines* (7th ed.). Elsevier.

Radostits, O. M., Gay, C. C., Hinchcliff, K. W., & Constable, P. D. (2007). *Veterinary medicine: A textbook of the diseases of cattle, horses, sheep, pigs and goats*. Saunders Elsevier.

Rugnath, R., Orzechowicz, C., Newell, C., Carullo, V., & Rugnath, A. (2024). A literature review: The mechanisms and treatment of neuropathic pain—A brief discussion. *Biomedicines, 12*(1), 204. https://doi.org/10.3390/biomedicines12010204

Sejvar, J. J. (2014). Clinical manifestations and outcomes of west nile virus infection. *Viruses, 6*(2), 606–623. https://doi.org/10.3390/v6020606

Shimabukuro, T. T., Nguyen, M., Martin, D., & DeStefano, F. (2015). Safety monitoring in the vaccine adverse event reporting system (VAERS). *Vaccine, 33*(36), 4398–4405. https://doi.org/10.1016/j.vaccine.2015.07.035

Simonsen, K. A., & Snowden, J. (2024). *Smallpox*. Treasure Island (FL): StatPearls Publishing [Updated 2023 Aug 8]. StatPearls.

Sir Sydney Sunderland. (1990). The anatomy and physiology of nerve injury. *Muscle & Nerve, 13*(9), 771–784. https://doi.org/10.1002/mus.880130903

Sisó, S., Hanzlicek, D., Fluehmann, G., Kathmann, I., Tomek, A., Papa, V., & Vandevelde, M. (2006). Neurodegenerative diseases in domestic animals: A comparative review. *The Veterinary Journal, 171*(1), 20–38. https://doi.org/10.1016/j.tvjl.2004.08.015

Solomon, T., Dung, N. M., Kneen, R., Gainsborough, M., Vaughn, D. W., & Khanh, V. T. (2000). Japanese encephalitis. *Journal of Neurology Neurosurgery and Psychiatry, 68*(4), 405–415. https://doi.org/10.1136/jnnp.68.4.405

Steinmetz, J. D., Maria Seeher, K., Schiess, N., Nichols, E., Cao, B., Servili, C., Cavallera, V., Cousin, E., Hagins, H., Moberg, M. E., Mehlman, M. L., Habtegiorgis Abate, Y., Abbas, J., Akram Abbasi, M., Abbasian, M., Abbastabar, H., Abdelmasseh, M., Abdollahi, M., Abdollahi, M., & Dua, T. (2024). Global, regional, and national burden of disorders affecting the nervous system, 1990–2021: A systematic analysis for the global burden of disease study 2021. *The Lancet Neurology, 23*(4), 344–381. https://doi.org/10.1016/s1474-4422(24)00038-3

Stephens, D. S., Greenwood, B., & Brandtzaeg, P. (2007). Epidemic meningitis, meningococcaemia, and Neisseria meningitidis. *The Lancet, 369*(9580), 2196–2210.

Stone, C. A., Rukasin, C. R. F., Beachkofsky, T. M., & Phillips, E. J. (2019). Immune-mediated adverse reactions to vaccines. *British Journal of Clinical Pharmacology, 85*(12), 2694–2706. https://doi.org/10.1111/bcp.14112

Sykes, J. E. (2022). *Greene's infectious diseases of the dog and cat, fifth edition greene's infectious diseases of the dog and cat* (5th ed., pp. 1–1802). https://doi.org/10.1016/C2014-0-03934-2

Takada, A., & Kawaoka, Y. (2003). Antibody-dependent enhancement of viral infection: Molecular mechanisms and in vivo implications. *Reviews in Medical Virology, 13*(6), 387–398. https://doi.org/10.1002/rmv.405

Vellozzi, C., Iqbal, S., & Broder, K. (2014). Guillain-Barre syndrome, influenza, and influenza vaccination: The epidemiologic evidence. *Clinical Infectious Diseases, 58*(8), 1149–1155.

Vitale, S., & Foss, K. (2019). Immune-mediated central nervous system disease—current knowledge and recommendations. *Topics in Companion Animal Medicine, 34*, 22–29. https://doi.org/10.1053/j.tcam.2018.11.003

Vos, T., Hanson, S. W., Abbafati, C., Aerts, J. G., Al-Aly, Z., Ashbaugh, C., Ballouz, T., Blyuss, O., Bobkova, P., Bonsel, G., Borzakova, S., Buonsenso, D., Butnaru, D., Carter, A., Chu, H., De Rose, C., Diab, M. M., Ekbom, E., Tantawi, M. E., … Murray, C. J. L. (2022). Estimated global proportions of individuals with persistent fatigue, cognitive, and respiratory symptom clusters following symptomatic COVID-19 in 2020 and 2021. *JAMA, 328*(16), 1604–1615. https://doi.org/10.1001/jama.2022.18931

Wang, R., Lan, C., Benlagha, K., Camara, N. O. S., Miller, H., Kubo, M., Heegaard, S., Lee, P., Yang, L., Forsman, H., Li, X., Zhai, Z., & Liu, C. (2024). The interaction of innate immune and adaptive immune system. *MedComm, 5*(10). https://doi.org/10.1002/mco2.714

Wisniewski, T., & Goñi, F. (2014). Immunotherapy for alzheimer's disease. *Biochemical Pharmacology, 88*(4), 499–507. https://doi.org/10.1016/j.bcp.2013.12.020

Zhao, L., Seth, A., Wibowo, N., Zhao, C. X., Mitter, N., Yu, C., & Middelberg, A. P. J. (2014). Nanoparticle vaccines. *Vaccine, 32*(3), 327–337. https://doi.org/10.1016/j.vaccine.2013.11.069

Further reading

Habib, J., Amraei, M., Javanshir, E., Jamebozorgi, K., & Faraji-Khiavi, F. (2023). Ethical considerations of the vaccine development process and vaccination: A scoping review. *BMC Health Services Research, 23*(1). https://doi.org/10.1186/s12913-023-09237-6

Ian, R. M., Rosen, F. S., Klein, J., & Sato, A. (2000). The HLA system. *New England Journal of Medicine, 343*(10), 702–709. https://doi.org/10.1056/NEJM200009073431006

Lawrence, S. (2014). Immunology of relapse and remission in multiple sclerosis. *Annual Review of Immunology, 32*, 257–281. https://doi.org/10.1146/annurev-immunol-032713-120227

CHAPTER

7 Nucleic acid drug therapies for CNS diseases: Present status and future perspectives

Yanying Chen[1], Diji Kuriakose[2] and Zhicheng Xiao[1,2]

[1]*Center for Life Sciences, Shaoxing Institute, Zhejiang University, Shaoxing, China;* [2]*Department of Anatomy and Developmental Biology, Monash University, Clayton, VIC, Australia*

1. Introduction

CNS diseases encompass a broad spectrum of conditions affecting the CNS, including neurodegenerative, vascular degenerative, infectious, and structural degenerative disorders. Representative examples include Parkinson's disease (PD), Alzheimer's disease (AD), spinal muscular atrophy (SMA), multiple sclerosis (MS), encephalitis, meningitis, brain or spinal cord injury, epilepsy, and migraine, among others. With increasing human life expectancy, population aging, and heightened social pressures, the prevalence of CNS diseases has risen steadily in recent years, imposing a substantial burden on society (Steinmetz et al., 2024). Despite this growing impact, the development of therapeutics for CNS disorders has lagged behind that for tumors and autoimmune diseases, and most CNS conditions remain incurable. Current pharmacological interventions primarily aim to relieve symptoms rather than provide definitive treatment.

Several major factors contribute to the challenges in CNS drug development: (1) the BBB restricts drug penetration into the CNS (Pardridge, 1998); (2) the underlying pathological mechanisms remain incompletely understood and exhibit high heterogeneity (Badhwar et al., 2020; Carceles-Cordon et al., 2023; Lázaro & Lee, 2024); (3) there is a lack of effective disease models (McGonigle, 2014); (4) clinical trial design is challenging, compounded by the scarcity of reliable disease biomarkers and the reliance on subjective outcome measures (Cummings, 2020; Schneider et al., 2014); and (5) CNS-targeted drugs carry a high risk of significant toxic side effects, necessitating rigorous risk-benefit assessment (Mahase, 2021). Nevertheless, recent years have seen the approval of novel mechanism-based drugs for specific CNS indications, including AD, schizophrenia, and migraine. Notable examples are the Aβ monoclonal antibodies Lecanemab and Donanemab for AD, KarXT for schizophrenia (Horan et al., 2024), and Zuranolone for postpartum depression in adults (Slomski, 2021), among others.

NADs, representing a new generation of therapeutic modalities, have emerged as one of the most promising avenues for drug development in the treatment of CNS disorders. Currently approved NADs for CNS-related diseases include Upstaza for the treatment of human aromatic L-amino acid decarboxylase (AADC) deficiency (Keam, 2022), Luxturna for inherited retinal disease (IRD)

Immunotherapies for Neurological Disorders. https://doi.org/10.1016/B978-0-443-44631-3.00006-8

(Johnson et al., 2019), Zolgensma for treating SMA (Hoy, 2019), and Tofersen for amyotrophic lateral sclerosis (ALS) (Cerillo & Parmar, 2025), among others. Compared with conventional small-molecule chemotherapeutic agents and monoclonal antibody therapies, NADs offer multiple advantages. The most fundamental of these is their ability to directly target genes to modulate cellular activities, rather than binding to specific proteins. Moreover, when combined with suitable delivery systems, NADs can penetrate cells to exert their therapeutic effects. This property enables them to circumvent the limitations associated with "undruggable" targets encountered by traditional small-molecule and antibody-based drugs, allowing the regulation of intracellular, extracellular, and membrane-associated components. Because NADs act directly on genes, they have the potential to fundamentally prevent or reverse disease progression, in contrast to conventional therapeutics, which primarily alleviate symptoms.

Furthermore, stable transgene expression or permanent genomic modification achieved by certain NADs may enable single-dose treatments (Blair, 2022; Katzmann et al., 2020). NADs function on the principle of complementary base pairing, with sequences designed according to the nucleotide sequence of the target gene. This confers a substantial advantage for precision medicine, particularly in CNS diseases characterized by complex pathogenic mechanisms and high heterogeneity (Cheng et al., 2025). Nevertheless, several challenges hinder their clinical translation. NADs are prone to degradation by ubiquitous nucleases, and their negatively charged, macromolecular nature limits their ability to traverse cell membranes. They also generally lack inherent tissue or cell specificity, making delivery strategies and carrier systems critical determinants of therapeutic success (Miao et al., 2024). Additionally, small NADs may cause notable toxicities, including off-target effects and immunogenic responses (Alhamadani et al., 2022; Goyenvalle et al., 2023). For CNS indications, a major obstacle is their inability to efficiently cross the BBB (Zhang et al., 2022). To overcome these limitations, ongoing research focuses on enhancing the physicochemical properties of NADs through chemical modifications, alongside the development of diverse delivery vectors to improve their stability, safety, and therapeutic efficacy (Matsuda et al., 2023; Tan et al., 2020). The subsequent section will provide an overview of the major classes of NADs and their current applications in CNS diseases, followed by a discussion of strategies aimed at improving NAD delivery to brain tissue, thereby advancing translational research on NAD-based therapies for CNS disorders.

2. Overview of nucleic acid therapies for CNS diseases

NADs can be broadly classified into three principal categories. The first category encompasses NADs that directly target nucleic acids, modulating their activity through diverse mechanisms to either promote or suppress protein expression; notable examples include antisense oligonucleotides (ASOs), small interfering RNAs (siRNAs), microRNAs (miRNAs), and the CRISPR/Cas genome-editing system. The second category comprises NADs designed to express proteins, such as DNA plasmids, messenger RNA (mRNA), and self-amplifying RNA (saRNA) molecules, which facilitate the upregulation of gene expression. The third category consists of NADs that primarily regulate proteins, including aptamers with high binding specificity. Owing to their capacity to directly target disease-associated genes or proteins, NADs hold substantial promise for precision medicine and sustained therapeutic interventions. However, unlike conventional small-molecule drugs, the unique physicochemical properties of NADs, combined with the body's intrinsic biological barriers, necessitate the integration of specialized delivery strategies to enable their effective administration and therapeutic action (Kulkarni et al., 2021).

In recent years, substantial advances have been achieved in both NADs and drug delivery technologies. This review provides a comprehensive overview of the current research landscape and recent progress in mainstream NADs and their therapeutic applications in CNS disorders. Furthermore, it examines the key challenges and outlines future directions for their development. A schematic summary of the principal topics discussed is presented in Fig. 7.1.

2.1 Antisense oligonucleotides therapies

ASOs are short synthetic nucleic acid sequences, typically 8–50 base pairs (bp) in length, designed to selectively modulate the expression of disease-associated RNA, including both protein-coding messenger RNA (mRNA) and non-coding RNA (ncRNA). By regulating transcription or translation of target genes, ASOs can upregulate or downregulate gene expression through three primary mechanisms: (i) RNase-mediated mRNA degradation, (ii) steric hindrance of mRNA translation, and (iii) modulation of protein expression via alternative splicing of precursor mRNA (pre-mRNA) (Dhuri et al., 2020). To enhance therapeutic efficacy, safety, and long-term stability, ASOs are commonly subjected to chemical modifications during development. First-generation modifications involve incorporating thiophosphate (PS) linkages into the nucleic acid backbone, which prolong serum half-life, improve cellular uptake, and increase nuclease resistance (DeVos & Miller, 2013). However, PS linkages may also reduce target-binding affinity and activate immune receptors, potentially inducing non-specific pro-inflammatory toxicity. Second-generation modifications build upon PS chemistry by introducing substituents at the ribose 2′position, such as 2′-O-methyl (2′-OMe), 2′-O-methoxyethyl (2′-MOE), and 2′-fluoro (2′-F), at the terminal "wings" or central region of the ASO, thereby improving target specificity and further protecting against enzymatic degradation (Holm et al., 2022). Third-generation chemistries include bridged nucleic acids (BNAs), peptide nucleic acids (PNAs), and phosphoramidite morpholino oligonucleotides (PMOs). Among BNAs, the most widely used are locked nucleic acids (LNAs), constrained ethyl BNAs (cEt), and 2′-O,4′-C-ethylene-bridged nucleic acids (ENAs), which confer enhanced nuclease resistance, improved binding affinity, and greater target-site specificity (Liang et al., 2021; Quemener et al., 2022).

Despite advances in chemical modifications, challenges in ASO delivery, particularly tissue-specific targeting and endosomal escape-remain unresolved. Consequently, the development of specialized delivery systems is critical to improving ASO targeting and bioavailability. Current delivery strategies fall into two main categories: (1) direct covalent conjugation of bioactive moieties to the ASO termini, such as GalNAc, peptides, lipids, antibodies, and aptamers; and (2) nanoparticle-based carriers, including cationic liposomes, exosomes, and spherical nucleic acids (Gagliardi & Ashizawa, 2021). Among these, GalNAc conjugation is the most widely adopted and the only ASO delivery approach approved for clinical use, exemplified by Eplontersen for treating adult hereditary transthyretin amyloid polyneuropathy (ATTR-PN) (Nie, 2024). GalNAc achieves targeted delivery to hepatocytes via specific binding to the asialoglycoprotein receptor (ASGPR) (Coelho et al., 2023). However, effective extrahepatic delivery, particularly to the CNS, remains a major unmet need.

NADs currently approved by the FDA or EMA for CNS disorders are summarized in Table 7.1, with ASOs comprising the largest group. These agents are typically administered via direct injection, such as intrathecal delivery, to enable penetration into brain tissue. SMA, a rare neuromuscular

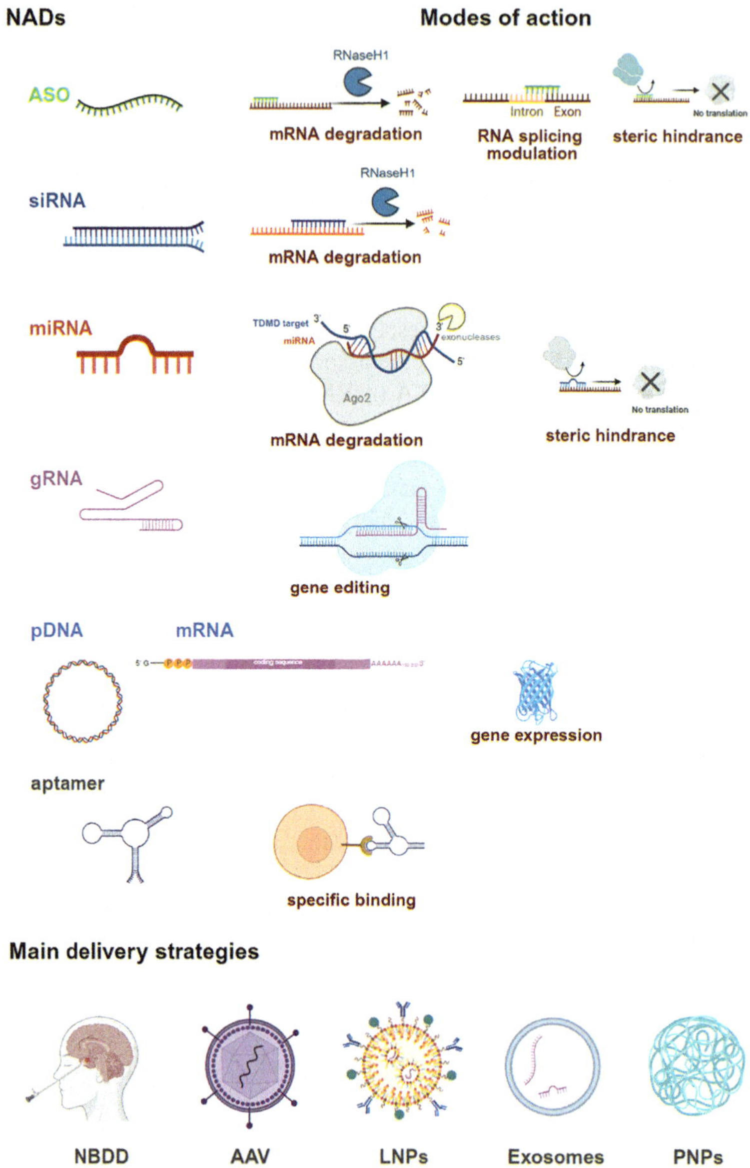

FIGURE 7.1

Overview of types, modes of action, and delivery strategies of NADs for CNS diseases.
AAV, adeno-associated virus; *ASO*, antisense oligonucleotide; *gRNA*, guide RNA; *LNPs*, lipid nanoparticles; *miR*, microRNA; *mRNA*, messenger RNA; *NBDD*, nasal-brain drug delivery route; *pDNA*, plasmid DNA; *PNPs*, polymeric nanoparticles; *siRNA*, small interfering RNA.

Created with Biorender.com.

Table 7.1 FDA/EMA-approved NADs for treating CNS diseases.

Drug name	Drug type	Condition	Target	Delivery method	Year approved
Nusinersen	ASO	SMA	SMN2	IT	2016
Milasen	ASO	Batten disease	CLN7	IT	2018
Tofersen	ASO	ALS	SOD1	IT	2024
Zolgensma	Gene therapies	SMA	SMN1	IV	2019
Skysona	HSC gene therapies	CALD	ABCD1	IV	2021
Upstaza	Gene therapies	AADC	DDC	ICM	2022

AADC, *aromatic L-amino acid decarboxylase;* ALS, *amyotrophic lateral sclerosis;* CALD, *cerebral adrenoleukodystrophy;* ICM, *intracerebral injection;* IT, *intrathecal;* IV, *intravenous;* SMA, *spinal muscular atrophy.*

disorder, is most often caused by homozygous deletion of the SMN1 gene on chromosome 5. Although the SMN2 gene can produce limited amounts of full-length survival motor neuron (SMN) protein, exon 7 skipping predominantly yields truncated, unstable forms, resulting in SMN deficiency in spinal motor neurons and consequent progressive muscle atrophy and motor function loss. Nusinersen, an ASO, promotes exon 7 inclusion in SMN2 precursor mRNA, restoring full-length SMN protein production and serving as a key therapeutic for SMA (Hoy, 2017). Milasen is a personalized ASO, developed within eight months, for a patient with neuronal ceroid lipofuscinosis 7 (NCL; Batten disease). By targeting a cryptic splice site in CLN7 pre-mRNA, Milasen normalizes exon 6-7 splicing (Kim et al., 2019). This case underscores the transformative potential of NADs in precision medicine. ALS is characterized by progressive muscle weakness and wasting, typically spreading from a focal onset and culminating in respiratory muscle failure. In April 2023, the FDA granted accelerated approval to Tofersen, an ASO for SOD1-related ALS. Tofersen induces RNase H-mediated degradation of SOD1 mRNA, reducing SOD1 protein synthesis, lowering cerebrospinal fluid (CSF) SOD1 concentrations, and decreasing plasma neurofilament light chain levels released from damaged neurons, thereby slowing the decline in respiratory function and muscle strength (Miller et al., 2022).

NADs currently in clinical development for CNS diseases are summarized in Table 7.2, with ASO drugs being the most numerous. Intrathecal injection remains the primary administration route, highlighting the persistent challenge of systemic delivery for ASO drugs. Cell-penetrating peptides (CPPs) have been shown to enhance NAD delivery across the BBB by conjugation with ASOs or formation of non-covalent nanoparticle complexes, positioning them as potential drug carriers (Ghorai et al., 2023). However, clinical translation is limited by unclear mechanisms of action and toxicity concerns (Leckie & Yokota, 2024). Yuting Sun et al. developed ZAAM, an ASO-loaded, Apt 19S-conjugated, neural stem cell membrane (NSCM)-coated nanoparticle, which demonstrates therapeutic efficacy by overcoming the BBB (Sun et al., 2023). Similarly, Amirah et al. designed apolipoprotein A-I nanodisks (apoA-I NDs) encapsulating mHTT-lowering ASOs capable of brain entry via intranasal administration to treat Huntington's disease (Aly et al., 2023). Despite growing clinical evidence supporting ASO efficacy in neurological disorders, off-target effects, high organ-specific toxicity, and immune stimulation remain significant challenges (Goyenvalle et al., 2023). Therefore, optimizing ASOs for high silencing efficiency with minimal CNS toxicity is critical for safe and effective CNS therapies. Notably, Taiki et al. demonstrated that BNAP-AEO-modified ASOs exhibit potent gene silencing with low acute CNS toxicity, suggesting a promising new modification strategy for CNS-targeted ASO drugs (Matsubayashi et al., 2024).

2.2 Small interfering RNA (siRNA) and microRNA (miRNA) therapies

RNAi-mediated gene silencing primarily utilizes two classes of nucleic acids: exogenously introduced double-stranded RNA (siRNA) and endogenous small non-coding microRNA (miRNA). siRNAs promote target mRNA degradation, whereas miRNAs either degrade mRNA or inhibit its translation (Rana, 2007). A key advantage of miRNA therapy is its ability to modulate multiple mRNA targets, offering potential for comprehensive treatment of CNS diseases with complex pathogenesis. However, this broad targeting also carries a higher risk of off-target effects (Brennan & Henshall, 2020; Lam et al., 2015). emphasizing the need for a thorough understanding of miRNAs' physiological and pathological roles in CNS disorders. Several miRNA-based therapies have been explored: AMT-130, an AAV-mediated delivery system administered via striatal infusion for Huntington's disease, demonstrated favorable safety and preliminary efficacy (Estevez-Fraga et al., 2024), while nanotechnology-based miRNA interventions have shown promise in AD, neuroblastoma, stroke, and other CNS conditions (Kadir et al., 2022; Ouyang et al., 2022; Pottoo et al., 2021).

Nevertheless, only a few miRNA drugs have advanced to clinical trials, with none reaching Phase III, highlighting the challenges in miRNA drug development. In contrast, siRNAs are synthetically produced NADs with high target specificity, making them clinically valuable for precise interventions. The approval of Patisiran in 2018 marked the advent of RNAi therapeutics; delivered via lipid nanoparticles (LNP), Patisiran silences thyroxine-binding transferrin (TTR) mRNA, reducing both wild-type and mutant TTR protein deposits in peripheral tissues and restoring function (Garber, 2018). Beyond LNPs, GalNAc conjugation has emerged as the main strategy for liver-specific siRNA delivery (Scott, 2020). Developing efficient delivery platforms for diverse organs and tissues remains a critical area for advancement.

In the development of siRNA therapeutics for targeted CNS applications, Alnylam Pharmaceuticals established a C16-siRNA conjugation strategy, enabling effective extrahepatic tissue delivery, including the brain (Brown et al., 2022). ALN-APP is the first siRNA drug incorporating a proprietary 2′-O-hexadecyl (C16) lipophilic conjugate, targeting mRNA encoding beta-amyloid precursor protein (APP) in neurons, for the treatment of AD and Cerebral Amyloid Angiopathy (Thirumalai, Patani and Hung, 2024). Arrowhead Pharmaceuticals has developed two generations of the CNS-targeting TRiMTM platform. The first generation combines lipid-conjugated siRNA with intrathecal administration, achieving sustained gene knockdown with a single dose; ARO-ATXN2, for spinocerebellar ataxia type 2 (SCA2), exemplifies this approach (Table 7.2). The second-generation platform employs transferrin receptor (TfR1)-targeted ligands for subcutaneous delivery across the BBB, exemplified by ARO-MAPT, which reduces MAPT expression and pathological tau aggregation throughout the CNS (https://lifescievents.com/event/arrowheadsummerseries5/). Kumthekar et al. reported NU-0129, spherical nucleic acids with gold nanoparticle cores conjugated to siRNA targeting Bcl2L12, capable of BBB penetration and tumor localization following intravenous infusion for glioblastoma (GBM) (Kumthekar et al., 2021). Similarly, ER2001 utilizes intravenous delivery via self-assembled exosomes labeled with rabies virus glycoprotein (RVG) to encapsulate mHTT siRNA, targeting the brain and reducing HTT levels in Huntington's disease (HD) (Zhang et al., 2021).

Table 7.2 Clinical-stage NADs for the treatment of CNS diseases.

Drug type	Drug name	Target	Condition	Delivery method	Phase	ClinicalTrials.gov ID
ASO	Elsunersen	Nav1.2	Pediatric SCN2A-DEE	IT	III	NCT07019922
	ION363	FUS	FUS-ALS	IT	III	NCT04768972
	Zilganersen	GFAP	AxD	IT	III	NCT04849741
	GTX-102	UBE3A	AS	IT	III	NCT06415344
	Zorevunersen	SCN1A	DS		III	NCT06872125
	ION582	UBE3A	AS	IT	III	NCT06914609
	PYC-001	OPA1	ADOA	IVT	I/II	NCT06970106
	WVE-003	HTT	HD	IT	I/II	NCT05032196
	Tominersen (RG6042)	HTT	HD	IT	II	NCT05686551
	RG6042	HTT	HD	IT	I	NCT04000594
	VP-001	PRPF31	RP11	IVT	I	NCT05902962
	AMX0114	Calpain-2	ALS	IT	I	NCT06665165
	QRL-201	STMN2	ALS	IT	I	NCT05633459
	IONIS-MAPTRx	TAU	AD	IT	I	NCT03186989
	BIIB094	LRRK2	PD	IT	I	NCT03976349
	ION464	Alpha-synuclein	MSA	IT	I	NCT04165486
	NIO752	TAU	AD	IT	I	NCT05469360
	RO7248824	UBE3A	AS	IT	I	NCT04428281
siRNA	RAG-17	SOD1	ALS	IT	I	NCT05903690
	ALN-HTT02	HTT	HD	IT	I	NCT06585449
	ALN-APP	APP	AD	IT	I	NCT05231785
	ER2001	HTT	HD	IV	I	NCT06024265
	ARO-ATXN2	ATXN2	SCA2	IT	I	NCT06672445
AAV-mediated gene therapy	GC101	SMN1	SMA2	IT	I/II	NCT05901987
	AMT-130	HTT	HD	ICM	I/II	NCT05243017
	AXO-AAV-GM1	GLB1	GM1 gangliosidosis	IV	I/II	NCT03952637
	AVXS-101	SMN	SMA1	IV	I	NCT02122952
	VGN-RO8b	GBA1	GD2	ICV	I	NCT06272149
	RGL-193	DDC	PD	ICM	I	NCT06195124
Aptamers	ApTOLL	TLR4	AIS	IV	I/II	NCT04734548
DNA vaccines	AV-1959D	Aβ	AD	ID	I	NCT05642429

AD, *Alzheimer's disease;* ADOA, *autosomal sominant optic atrophy;* AIS, *acute ischemic stroke;* AIS, *acute ischemic stroke;* ALS, *amyotrophic lateral sclerosis;* AS, *Angelman syndrome;* AxD, *Alexander disease;* DS, *Dravet syndrome;* FUS-ALS, *fused in Sarcoma mutations in amyotrophic lateral sclerosis;* GD2, *Type II Gaucher disease;* HD, *Huntington's disease;* ICM, *intracerebral injection;* ICV, *intra-cerebroventricular injection;* ID, *intradermal injection;* IT, *intrathecal;* IV, *intravenous;* IVT, *intravitreal injections;* MSA, *multiple system atrophy;* PD, *Parkinson's disease;* RP11, *retinitis pigmentosa type 11;* SCA2, *spinocerebellar Ataxia Type 2;* SCN2A-DEE, *SCN2A developmental and epileptic encephalopathy;* SMA1, *spinal muscular atrophy Type 1;* SMA2, *spinal muscular atrophy type 2.*
Data sourced from www.clinicaltrials.gov.

siRNA and ASO therapeutics offer notable advantages, including high target specificity, the ability to modulate "undruggable" targets, prolonged activity, and potential curative effects, making them highly promising for CNS diseases driven by gene mutations or dysregulated gene expression. Given the complex pathogenic mechanisms of many CNS disorders, such as AD, single-target drugs may be insufficient for effective treatment, highlighting the emerging importance of multi-target strategies. In this context, ASO and siRNA drugs—with their straightforward design, rapid development, and broad target repertoire—represent powerful tools for addressing such multifactorial diseases. Nonetheless, overcoming the BBB limitations, enhancing delivery efficiency, minimizing off-target effects, and reducing immunogenicity remain critical challenges for future research and development.

2.3 CRISPR/Cas9 sgRNA (gene therapies)

CRISPR/Cas9, the third-generation gene editing technology following ZFNs and TALENs, is currently the most widely used platform for gene modification (Dunbar et al., 2018). Cas9, guided by sgRNA, locates specific DNA sequences and introduces double-strand breaks, enabling homologous recombination with inserted DNA fragments to correct mutations or achieve gene knockout, insertion, or replacement (Moreno-Mateos et al., 2015). Recent studies highlight its therapeutic potential for neurological disorders associated with genetic mutations, including PD, ALS, AD, and HD (Aronin & DiFiglia, 2014; Chacko et al., 2023; Duan et al., 2020; Yoon et al., 2022). CRISPR delivery typically relies on three vector types: viral, viral-like, and non-viral, with adeno-associated virus (AAV) being the most extensively studied viral vector. Notably, AAV9, first identified in 2009, crosses the BBB and efficiently transduces astrocytes and endothelial cells in the CNS (Foust et al., 2009). In 2019, Zolgensma became the first FDA-approved AAV9-based gene therapy for SMA, delivering functional full-length SMN genes to motor neurons via a single intravenous infusion (Hoy, 2019). However, AAV9 exhibits significant peripheral tissue tropism, particularly in the liver, underscoring the need for CNS-specific variants (Chen et al., 2021). Similarly, Upstaza, approved in the EU in July 2022 for AADC deficiency, is delivered directly to the brain via a single stereotactic injection (Keam, 2022). Beyond these approved therapies, numerous gene therapies for CNS diseases are currently in active clinical trials (Table 7.2).

AAV-mediated gene therapy has shown remarkable potential for fundamentally treating CNS diseases caused by gene mutations; however, several challenges limit its broader application. The capsid's limited packaging capacity ($\leq$4.8 kb) remains a major constraint on its use in gene therapy (Kolesnik et al., 2024). Additionally, AAV immunogenicity complicates repeated administration and poses risks of potential genomic integration and off-target effects (Greig et al., 2024; Xiong et al., 2025). Consequently, virus-like particles (VLPs) have emerged as promising alternative delivery systems. VLPs are replication-deficient and lack viral genomes, substantially reducing risks associated with viral replication in vivo (An et al., 2024; Geilenkeuser et al., 2025). Their utility is further enhanced by the ability to exploit diverse viral tropisms to target specific cells or tissues (Rohovie, Nagasawa and Swartz, 2017). Moreover, VLPs' high immunogenicity has been leveraged in vaccine development, including vaccines against neurodegenerative diseases (Lim et al., 2025; Mohsen and Bachmann, 2022).

2.4 mRNA/DNA vaccine therapy

There is a complex, bidirectional relationship between CNS diseases and the immune system. Traditionally, the CNS was considered "immune privileged", protected by the BBB and largely isolated from systemic immunity. However, it is now clear that the immune system critically regulates both physiological and pathological CNS processes. Immune responses can protect the CNS but may also contribute to the pathogenesis or progression of various CNS disorders (Smyth and Kipnis, 2025). Dysregulated or excessive inflammation is a hallmark of many CNS diseases, including AD. Insights into CNS immunity have driven the development of diverse immunotherapies (Hanif et al., 2020), which are broadly classified as active or passive (Brody & Holtzman, 2008). Active immunotherapy, in particular, extends beyond infectious disease prevention to induce beneficial immune responses that counter pathological processes, including those underlying CNS disorders.

MS is an autoimmune demyelinating disease of the CNS, characterized by the immune system targeting myelin, a complex of proteins and fatty acids forming the protective myelin sheath around axons (Blaylock, 2025; Föttinger et al., 2025). Therapeutic vaccines that restore antigen tolerance offer a promising treatment strategy for MS. BHT-3009, a DNA vaccine encoding full-length human myelin basic protein (MBP), has been shown in clinical trials that low-dose administration effectively induces immune tolerance and downregulates pathogenic myelin-specific autoantibodies (Correale & Fiol, 2009; Garren et al., 2008). Similarly, vaccines designed to elicit neutralizing antibodies against pathogenic targets provide an approach for treating CNS diseases, exemplified by the Aβ vaccine for AD (Morgan et al., 2000). While autologous antigen-based vaccines hold therapeutic potential, they risk provoking inflammatory autoimmune reactions (Lambracht-Washington & Rosenberg, 2013; Panza et al., 2012).

Learning from the failure of the AN-1792 peptide vaccine, AC Immune developed ACI-24, which removes the self-T epitope and combines the B epitope (Aβ1-15) with an exogenous universal T epitope to elicit a safe Th2-type immune response in patients with sporadic AD and Down syndrome (Rafii et al., 2022; Sol et al., 2023). Armine et al. have developed DNA vaccines for multiple neurodegenerative diseases using their proprietary MultiTEP platform, including AV-1959D, a DNA vaccine targeting pathological Aβ. AV-1959D is currently being evaluated in early-stage Alzheimer's disease patients for safety and tolerability (Table 7.2, NCT05642429). Its mRNA counterpart, AV-1959LR, has demonstrated stronger immunogenicity than AV-1959D in both mice and non-human primates, suggesting that it may ultimately replace DNA-based vaccines (Hovakimyan et al., 2024). In parallel, earlier work with a DNA vaccine targeting tau protein showed robust immune responses and significantly reduced tau pathology in THY-Tau22 mice (Davtyan et al., 2017). Complementing these efforts, Professor Colin Pouton and Dr. Rebecca Nisbet are advancing an mRNA vaccine targeting tau for AD, with results anticipated by late 2025 (https://research.monash.edu/en/projects/developing-an-mrna-vaccine-for-the-treatment-of-alzheimers-diseas).

For CNS disorders with complex pathogenic mechanisms, such as AD, multitarget vaccines hold promise for improved clinical outcomes. Xuejian Feng et al. developed a dual AD vaccine combining Aβ and pTau antigens, which induced simultaneous antibody production against pathological Aβ and pTau in mice and significantly enhanced cognitive performance (Feng, Hou, et al., 2024). A DNA vaccine targeting multiple axonal regeneration-inhibitory factors has also shown therapeutic potential in diverse animal models (Nie et al., 2007), including AD (Zhang et al., 2013), spinal cord injury (Zhang et al., 2009), and traumatic brain injury (Zhang et al., 2008). Despite their promise, multitarget vaccines face significant challenges. Epitope conflict or immune interference may occur when multiple antigens interact physically or chemically, altering conformation and stability. Achieving correct folding and native epitope presentation of all target antigens remains a major design hurdle. Furthermore, highly immunogenic epitopes can dominate immune responses, suppressing weaker epitopes and resulting in imbalanced protection. Epitope selection must also ensure effective presentation across prevalent HLA alleles in the target population. Finally, the inclusion of multiple antigens may increase the risk and complexity of immune-related adverse events—such as excessive inflammation or autoimmune reactions—underscoring the need for rigorous safety monitoring.

Vaccine type, administration route, adjuvant, and dosage are key determinants of vaccine efficacy (Zimmermann and Curtis, 2019). The predominant delivery method, such as intramuscular injection and intradermal injection, has limitations, as antibodies generated through peripheral immunity must reach high systemic concentrations to cross the BBB and access the CNS. This underscores the need for alternative delivery routes that enhance antibody penetration into brain tissue. Historically, the CNS was considered an immune-privileged site; however, the discovery of meningeal lymphatic vessels (mLVs) has redefined brain immunology (Castellani et al., 2023). Acting as a critical interface between central and peripheral immunity, mLVs facilitate CSF drainage to cervical deep lymph nodes (dCLNs) and clearance of metabolic waste and senescent cells (Patel et al., 2019; Wen et al., 2018), while also contributing to immune surveillance and homeostasis (Frederick & Louveau, 2020). Dysfunction of mLVs is implicated in various neurological disorders, including traumatic brain injury (Bolte et al., 2020), AD (Guo et al., 2023), CNS infections (Feng, Ren, et al., 2024) and brain tumors (Hu et al., 2020). Elucidating the interplay between central and peripheral immune systems is therefore essential for understanding CNS disease pathogenesis.

Known anatomical hubs mediating mLV-peripheral immune interactions include the mLV-CLN axis, the cribriform plate, and cranial bone marrow (Xie et al., 2024). Zachary et al. identified a beak-nose lymphatic hub at the sinus junction containing B cell germinal centers that support somatic hypermutation in response to nasal pathogens (Fitzpatrick et al., 2024), suggesting intranasal vaccination as a promising approach for CNS-targeted immunization (Kehagia et al., 2023). Similarly, CLNs, as the link between mLVs and peripheral immunity, highlight the potential of subcutaneous neck vaccination (Qi et al., 2023). Nevertheless, immunization strategies with enhanced CNS access require rigorous safety assessment. Advancing such approaches will depend on a deeper mechanistic understanding of central-peripheral immune crosstalk to optimize nucleic acid vaccine efficacy while minimizing potential risks.

2.5 Aptamers

Aptamers are single-stranded nucleic acids with defined three-dimensional structures, developed using Systemic Evolution of Ligands by Exponential Enrichment (SELEX) technology, which enables them to selectively bind various target molecules and cells. They act similarly to antibodies but offer distinct advantages over monoclonal antibodies and small-molecule drugs, such as high specificity and affinity, straightforward synthesis, ease of modification, smaller size, low immunogenicity, and cost-effective production. Consequently, aptamers have been extensively explored for both therapeutic and diagnostic applications in CNS diseases (Zhuo et al., 2017).

The pathogenic mechanisms of numerous CNS disorders are thought to be closely linked to pathological protein aggregation, and aptamers are anticipated to provide therapeutic benefits by inhibiting such aggregation in the brain. For instance, pathological β-amyloid (Aβ) is a major pathological target in Alzheimer's disease (AD), and aptamers targeting Aβ are expected to serve as potential treatments for AD (Bloom, 2014; Zheng et al., 2022). Xin Feng et al. developed a circular RNA aptamer that suppresses abnormal PKR activation and significantly ameliorates the AD phenotype in mouse models(Feng et al., 2025). Calcineurin regulatory factor 1 (RCAN1) has been identified as a novel RNA-binding protein, and its corresponding RNA aptamer shows promise for treating Down syndrome and AD (Yun et al., 2021). α-Synuclein is a key pathogenic protein in Parkinson's disease, and a DNA aptamer targeting α-synuclein can specifically bind to it, effectively preventing aggregation, promoting degradation, and rescuing mitochondrial dysfunction and cellular defects caused by α-synuclein overexpression (Zheng et al., 2018).

Toll-like receptor 4 (TLR4) plays a role in the innate immune response during CNS inflammation. The DNA aptamer ApTOLL, which targets TLR4, can inhibit inflammation triggered by TLR4 activation, representing a potential therapeutic strategy for various CNS disorders, including demyelinating diseases (e.g., MS), acute ischemic stroke (AIS), and other stroke-related conditions (Fernández et al., 2018; Fernández-Gómez et al., 2024). Clinical studies have demonstrated ApTOLL's safety and favorable pharmacokinetics in healthy individuals (ApTOLL-FIH-01 trial, NCT04742062). A Phase I/IIa trial (Table 7.2, NCT04734548) evaluating ApTOLL in acute ischemic stroke patients showed that a 0.2 mg/kg dose effectively reduced infarct volume and neurological deficits within 72 h post-stroke, providing a promising treatment option.

Beyond therapy, aptamers also hold considerable promise as diagnostic tools, applicable to both solid tissue staining and liquid biopsy diagnostics. For CNS diseases that are challenging to diagnose, aptamers can improve detection sensitivity and accuracy. For example, combining antibody-aptamer molecular recognition with DNA amplification technology enables efficient detection of AD biomarkers in human serum and CSF samples (Chan et al., 2019). Holly et al. employed a novel RNA aptamer, TDP-43APT, which markedly enhances early detection of TDP-43 pathology and may play a key role in the early prevention of ALS (Spence et al., 2024).

Despite these advantages, clinical application of aptamers faces several challenges. Unmodified aptamers are inherently unstable and prone to degradation by plasma nucleases, while chemical modifications may introduce toxicity; for example, a Phase III study reported severe immune reactions with polyethylene glycol-modified aptamer drugs (Lincoff et al., 2016). Moreover, as an emerging class of therapeutics, information on aptamer pharmacokinetics—including absorption, distribution, metabolism, elimination, and toxicity—is limited. Potential off-target effects, polyionic interactions, unintended tissue accumulation, and non-specific immune activation further complicate their clinical development (Amero et al., 2020).

3. CNS delivery strategies

Drug therapy for CNS disorders is critically limited by the BBB. As shown in Fig. 7.2, the BBB is constituted by neurovascular units comprising pericytes, endothelial cells, astrocytes, and other CNS-supporting cells (Liu et al., 2025). It restricts over 98% of small-molecule drugs and virtually all macromolecular agents, including NADs, thereby representing the principal challenge to effective CNS drug delivery (Abbott, 2013). Drug transport across the BBB occurs via adsorptive-mediated transcytosis(ATM), carrier-mediated transport (CMT), cell-mediated transcytosis, and receptor-mediated transcytosis (RMT). Of these, RMT has been the most extensively investigated for facilitating drug delivery to the CNS (Terstappen et al., 2021).

CNS drug delivery can be achieved via invasive local administration (e.g., intrathecal, intracerebral, intraventricular injections), systemic administration (e.g., intravenous injection), or alternative routes such as nasal delivery. Invasive local administration remains the primary approach for bypassing

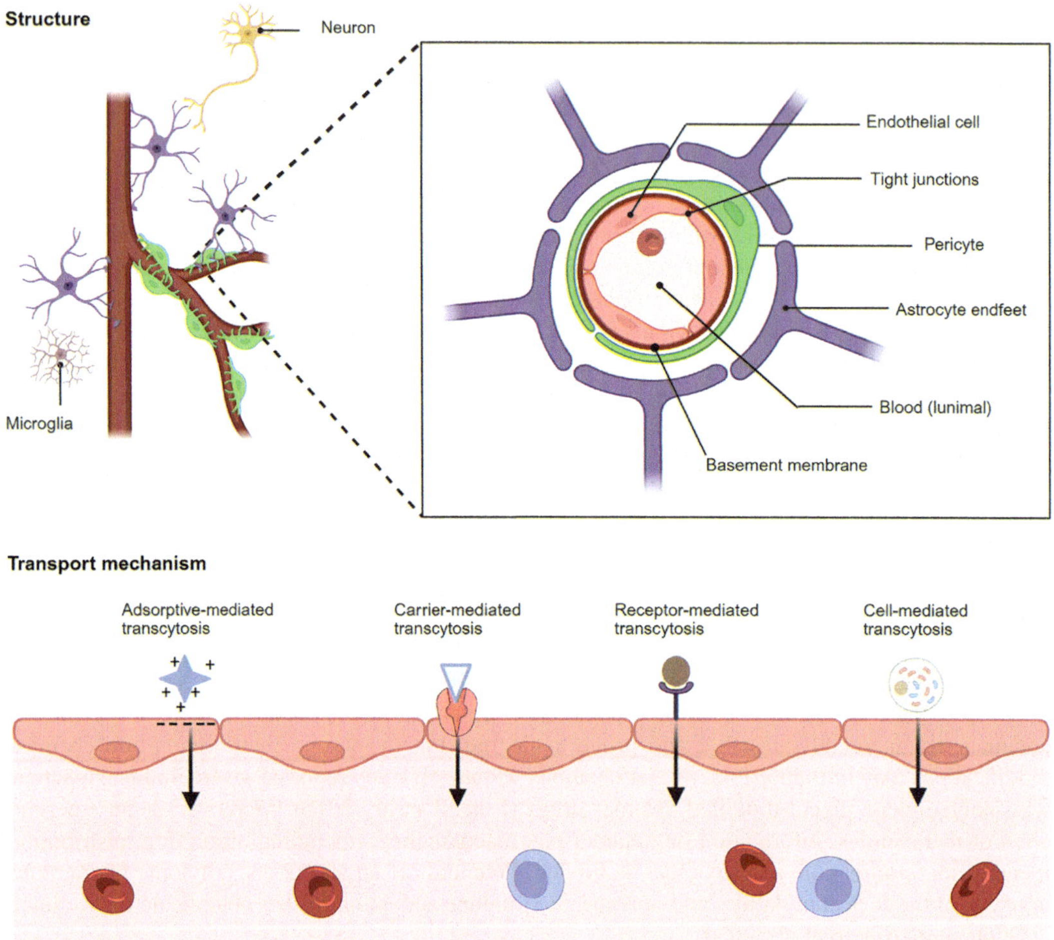

FIGURE 7.2 Structural diagram of the BBB and transport routes of the drug molecules across the BBB.

Brain capillaries are surrounded by tightly connected endothelial cells. On the brain side, the endothelial cells are covered by a continuous basement membrane extracellular matrix, pericytes, and astrocyte terminal processes. The innervation of neuronal synapses and adjacent microglia (and other immune cells, not shown) constitutes the neurovascular unit. Nucleic acid drugs are transported across adsorptive-mediated transcytosis, carrier-mediated transcytosis, receptor-mediated transcytosis and cell-mediated transcytosis.

Created with Biorender.com.

the BBB, enabling precise drug targeting and reducing peripheral toxicity. Approved therapies such as Nusinersen and Tofersen employ intrathecal injection, while the AAV-based gene therapy Upstaza is delivered intracerebrally. However, this route carries substantial drawbacks, including post-puncture headache, back pain, infection, bleeding, and low patient compliance with repeated dosing (Delhaas & Huygen, 2020; Stolte et al., 2018). Consequently, systemic delivery strategies are under active investigation. One approach combines transient BBB disruption with intravenous administration; for instance, Rezai et al. employed MRI-guided low-intensity focused ultrasound to reversibly open the BBB in AD patients, improving drug efficacy with minimal adverse events (Rezai et al., 2024). Despite promise, this method requires stringent parameter control, lacks robust predictive models, and presents potential safety concerns (Dai et al., 2025; Todd et al., 2020). These limitations have driven growing interest in specialized delivery routes such as the Nasal-Brain Drug Delivery Route (NBDD), which offers direct CNS access. Concurrently, nanoparticles (NPs) and exosomes have emerged as leading NADs carriers due to their favorable physicochemical and biological properties (Kim et al., 2024; Liu et al., 2025). The above section discussed commonly used AAV and the next section will discuss NBDD and highlight the most promising non-viral vehicle for CNS-targeted NAD delivery.

3.1 NBDD

NBDD has gained considerable attention as a strategy to bypass the BBB and deliver therapeutics directly to the brain. This approach accommodates a wide range of cargo, from large molecules to cells, and offers several advantages, including rapid onset, non-invasiveness, avoidance of first-pass metabolism, enhanced brain targeting, and reduced systemic exposure(Qiu et al., 2025).NBDD operates through two main routes: direct and indirect. Direct delivery involves the respiratory and olfactory zones of the upper nasal cavity, where the olfactory nerve pathways in the olfactory zone and trigeminal nerve pathways in the respiratory zone transport drugs directly to the brain (Bahadur et al., 2020; Semyachkina-Glushkovskaya et al., 2023). The indirect route entails drug transport to the CSF via olfactory/nasal lymphatic pathways around the olfactory nerve and the nasopharyngeal lymphatic system, followed by distribution into the brain parenchyma (Sun et al., 2018). Several CNS-targeting drugs, predominantly small molecules, have already been developed using NBDD (Alabsi et al., 2022). However, challenges such as limited nasal absorption surface area, mucociliary clearance, enzymatic degradation, and incomplete understanding of nasal-brain delivery mechanisms limit drug deposition in the olfactory region and hinder precise targeting of specific brain regions.

Moreover, prolonged or frequent use of absorption enhancers may facilitate pathogen or toxin entry into the CNS. Consequently, optimized delivery devices and formulations are critical (Chen et al., 2024; Xi et al., 2016). Clinically, bidirectional breathing-powered devices have been shown to increase deposition at target sites and improve pharmacokinetic profiles (Silberstein, 2017). Recent innovations to enhance transnasal brain delivery include nanocarriers, viral vectors, extracellular vesicle (EV) carriers, and stimuli-responsive systems (Qiu et al., 2025). Among these, LNPs offer notable benefits in improving drug bioavailability in the brain (Hathout & El-Marakby, 2022), and are widely used for conditions such as neurodegenerative diseases and gliomas. Exosomes also represent a promising platform. For example, Minkyung et al. developed a receptor for advanced glycation end-products (RAGE)-binding peptide-modified exosome carrying miR-181a, which specifically targeted ischemic brain regions via intranasal delivery (Kim et al., 2021). Additionally, Haosheng Shen et al. reported that Lactobacillus plantarum, a commensal microorganism that selectively binds the olfactory mucosa, could be engineered as a nasal-targeted delivery vehicle, offering a novel avenue for brain disease therapy (Shen et al., 2025).

NBDD-based NADs hold significant potential to revolutionize the treatment of CNS diseases. While nucleic acid drug therapy can achieve substantial therapeutic effects with a single low-dose administration, the complex pathogenic mechanisms of CNS disorders make multitargeted drug delivery an emerging priority. The NBDD approach offers the dual advantage of enhancing drug efficacy and minimizing peripheral side effects associated with multitargeted delivery. Nonetheless, key challenges remain for clinical translation, including administration accuracy, patient compliance, formulation stability, and long-term safety concerns (Qiu et al., 2025). Advances in formulation technology, particularly the development of biocompatible nanocarriers, novel safe permeation enhancers, improved understanding of transport mechanisms, and precision delivery devices are expected to overcome these barriers. Ultimately, NBDD could provide an efficient, non-invasive delivery platform with broad therapeutic value for CNS diseases using NADs.

3.2 Lipid nanoparticles

LNPs are currently the only approved nanocarriers for nucleic acid drug (NAD) delivery and possess inherent liver-targeting properties (Garber, 2018). Classical LNPs typically comprise four components: ionizable (cationic) lipids, helper lipids, cholesterol, and polyethylene glycol (PEG)-modified lipids. The ionizable lipid is the pivotal element, conferring structural stability, mediating interactions with cell membranes, and facilitating endosomal escape. Helper lipids such as DOPE and DSPC influence biodistribution; cholesterol stabilizes the particle and modulates targeting; and PEG-lipids enable ligand or biomolecule conjugation through surface functionalization (Eygeris et al., 2022). To achieve extrahepatic targeting, compositional and chemical modifications have yielded novel LNP systems, including a three-component formulation for lung delivery (Fei et al., 2024). In 2020, Ma et al. introduced neurotransmitter-derived lipidoids (NT-lipidoids) that, when incorporated into LNPs, overcame the BBB to deliver cargo to neuronal cells for functional gene silencing or recombination (Ma et al., 2020). In 2023, Mitchell and Peranteau developed a C3-LNP platform capable of mRNA delivery to the fetal CNS (Palanki et al., 2023). Surface functionalization with bioactive ligands offers another strategy for CNS targeting via receptor or transporter-mediated transcytosis in brain endothelial cells. For example, Arora et al. engineered RVG and mannose-modified targeted liposomes encapsulating an ApoE2 plasmid to deliver therapeutics to the brain for AD treatment (Arora et al., 2021). Similarly, Marcos-Contreras et al. conjugated LNPs with an anti-VCAM-1 antibody, enabling targeted mRNA delivery to inflamed brain tissue and significantly reducing TNFα-induced cerebral edema (Marcos-Contreras et al., 2020).

Extensive evidence indicates that LNP-based delivery of NADs holds significant potential for treating CNS diseases. However, translation from laboratory research to clinical application faces substantial challenges. These include the intricate design and rigorous quality control required for preparing antibody-modified LNPs; limitations in circulation, biodistribution, and brain targeting; off-target effects; suboptimal cellular uptake and endosomal escape; immunogenicity and associated inflammatory risks within the CNS; and potential neurotoxicity from lipid accumulation or their metabolic byproducts (Chatterjee et al., 2024; Wang et al., 2024; Zhang et al., 2024). The development of LNP delivery platforms is inherently interdisciplinary, integrating materials science, nanotechnology, pharmacology, molecular biology, immunology, and physiology. Ongoing research must refine LNP architectures to enhance brain-targeting efficiency while minimizing toxicity, thereby enabling safe and effective clinical translation for CNS therapeutics.

3.3 Exosomes

Compared with LNP systems, biological carriers such as exosomes offer a safer and more efficient delivery strategy. Exosomes are 40–160 nm nanovesicles secreted by diverse cell types that mediate intercellular communication and naturally transport nucleic acids and proteins (Wang et al., 2022). Their intrinsic biocompatibility, low immunogenicity and toxicity, and innate ability to cross the BBB make them an ideal drug delivery platform for the CNS.

Exosome transport across the BBB relies on non-brain-specific mechanisms, including clathrin-mediated endocytosis (CME), ligand-receptor interactions on endothelial cells, integrin binding, and membrane fusion. Consequently, systemic administration often results in off-target accumulation in peripheral organs such as the liver and spleen (Salimi et al., 2023). To enhance CNS-targeted delivery, two main approaches are under investigation: surface engineering and cell-derived targeting (Liang et al., 2021). Surface engineering can be achieved via (i) genetic modification of donor cells to produce exosomes with specific ligands, as demonstrated by RVG-modified exosomes from human embryonic kidney 293T (HEK 293T) cells delivering MOR siRNA for morphine addiction therapy (Wang et al., 2021), or (ii) post-isolation biochemical functionalization through covalent or non-covalent modification, exemplified by quercetin-loaded exosomes conjugated with anti-GAP43 monoclonal antibodies for targeted delivery to ischemic neurons in cerebral ischemia (Guo et al., 2021). Cell-derived targeting leverages the intrinsic brain tropism of exosomes originating from specific CNS cell types, which are rapidly recognized, internalized, and activated by corresponding receptor cells. Neurons and glial cells release exosomes enriched in bioactive components that can be transferred to adjacent or distant cells, mediating neuroprotective, anti-inflammatory, reparative, and regenerative effects (Frühbeis et al., 2012). Among these, neural stem cell-derived extracellular vesicles (NSC-EVs) have gained particular interest due to their prolonged circulation time, high stability, strong permeability, and low immunogenicity, making them promising candidates for the treatment of neurological disorders (Li et al., 2020).

Clinically, ER2001 (Table 7.2, NCT06024265) is the first investigational siRNA drug globally administered intravenously to deliver siRNA across the BBB via self-assembled exosomes for targeted CNS delivery. Currently in Phase 1 trials, it has demonstrated favorable safety and efficacy, notably reducing CSF NfL levels in patients with early-stage Huntington's disease. Despite the immense potential of exosome-based therapies, their clinical translation faces significant challenges, including immunogenicity, regulatory hurdles, and scalable production. Immunogenicity and biocompatibility are critical considerations, yet few studies have examined unintended immune recognition of exosomes. A comprehensive understanding of exosome-induced immunogenicity and clearance is essential, particularly when surface modifications may alter immunogenic profiles, necessitating immune-evasion strategies to enhance therapeutic feasibility (Li et al., 2024). Regulatory and production challenges further complicate clinical application. Common isolation methods, such as ultracentrifugation and size exclusion chromatography, are labor-intensive and yield heterogeneous exosome populations, compromising product consistency and efficacy. Moreover, low exosome yield limits current large-scale production, restricting broader clinical implementation. Continuous technological advancements are expected to overcome these barriers, positioning exosome-based drug delivery to redefine CNS disease treatment (Lee et al., 2024).

3.4 Polymeric nanoparticles

Polymeric nanoparticles (PNPs) are formed through electrostatic, hydrophobic, and/or hydrogen bonding between polymers and NADs, offering diverse and highly tunable designs. Their size, shape, surface charge, and modifications critically influence functional properties, including in vivo circulation and tissue targeting (Beach et al., 2024). For CNS-targeted PNPs, biocompatible, non-toxic, and non-immunogenic polymers are essential to ensure safety. Poly (lactic-co-glycolic acid) (PLGA), an FDA-approved copolymer, has been widely employed in disease treatment and tissue engineering (Martins et al., 2018). Although PLGA nanoparticles possess a natural, yet limited, ability to cross the BBB, surface modification can enhance penetration via active endocytosis. For instance, Wen Li et al. engineered PLGA nanoparticles loaded with siRNA, optimizing surface ligand density to maximize BBB transport (Li et al., 2021). Chitosan, a cationic polymer with excellent biocompatibility and biodegradability, is a safe organic material that can improve nanoparticle biological and physicochemical properties, enabling brain delivery via intranasal administration (Haroon et al., 2021). Nevertheless, high production costs and complex preparation limit the clinical translation of chitosan nanoparticle (Obeidat and Lahlouh, 2025). Overall, significant challenges remain in developing safe, effective, and scalable PNPs for CNS therapies (Annu et al., 2022). Despite this, the structural versatility of PNPs positions them as promising platforms for "smart" drug delivery systems capable of precise targeting and responsive controlled release in clinical applications.

3.5 Other delivery vehicles

Inorganic nanoparticles are increasingly explored for nucleic acid delivery. To traverse the BBB, they are often conjugated with brain-targeting peptides. Jinmyoung et al. demonstrated that biodegradable mesoporous silicon nanoparticles (pSiNPs) encapsulating siRNA, coupled with the RVG peptide, enabled targeted delivery to brain tissue and effectively treated brain injury via intravenous injection (Joo et al., 2016). A major limitation for clinical translation remains the potential toxicity from nanoparticle accumulation (Enea et al., 2019).

DNA nanoparticles represent a promising platform for nucleic acid drug delivery in CNS disorders. Unlike inorganic or polymer-based nanoparticles, DNA nanomaterials are biocompatible, biodegradable, readily modifiable for targeted delivery, and capable of controlled payload release (Guan et al., 2021). Nonetheless, their clinical translation is constrained by susceptibility to nuclease-mediated degradation, potential immunogenicity, and challenges in large-scale production (Kashani et al., 2024).

Spherical nucleic acids (SNAs) are an emerging and highly promising delivery system, comprising a nanoparticle core densely coated with oligonucleotides. The nanoparticle core can be constructed from diverse organic or inorganic materials (Song et al., 2022). SNAs offer rapid cellular transfection and efficient penetration of biological barriers, including the BBB, while demonstrating high nuclease stability, minimal toxicity, and low immunogenicity (Valatabar et al., 2024).NU-0129, currently in clinical development, is an siRNA-based SNA arranged on gold nanoparticles (AuNPs) and represents the first SNA drug to cross the BBB and enter brain tissue via intravenous administration (Kumthekar et al., 2021). Despite their potential as CNS drug carriers, SNAs face challenges before widespread clinical use. Future studies must elucidate factors influencing their metabolism, distribution, and stability in vivo, as well as explore additional biological functions and long-term safety as a novel molecular polymer.

4. Future roadmap & industry pipeline trends

Multi-Antigen and Self-Amplifying Platforms: Next-generation immunotherapies will migrate from single-antigen constructs to multivalent "string-of-beads" mRNA and DNA platforms that simultaneously target amyloid, tau, and neurite-outgrowth inhibitors (NOIs). saRNA and circular RNA formats promise lower dose requirements and prolonged antigen expression, reducing manufacturing costs and enhancing immunogenicity in chronic CNS indications such as AD.

Advanced Delivery Technologies: Clinical pipelines increasingly embrace engineered lipid nanoparticles (LNPs) with NT-lipidoids for efficient BBB penetration (Ma et al., 2020), as well as ligand-decorated exosomes and virus-like particles for cell-specific targeting (Guo et al., 2021). Intranasal mRNA formulations that harness meningeal lymphatic routes are entering early-stage studies, offering non-invasive, direct nose-to-brain delivery with rapid onset and minimal systemic exposure (Qiu et al., 2025).

AI-Driven Design and Decentralized Validation: Artificial intelligence will streamline antigen selection through in silico immunogenicity and epitope mapping, accelerating candidate screening and optimizing HLA coverage. Parallel adoption of open-science, milestone-based pipelines—inspired by DeSci governance models—will de-risk early preclinical stages via community-sourced replication bounties and transparent data sharing, tightening feedback loops between industry and academia.

Personalized and Precision Immunotherapy: DNA and mRNA vaccine platforms are poised to enable truly individualized CNS immunotherapies by leveraging patient-specific genomic and transcriptomic data. High-throughput sequencing combined with advanced epitope prediction algorithms can rapidly identify neoantigens associated with distinct neurodegenerative or autoimmune subtypes, facilitating the design of bespoke vaccine constructs that target disease-relevant epitopes while minimizing off-target responses (Li et al., 2023). Multi-antigen formulations with adjustable immunogenicity profiles can address epitope dominance and immune interference, and when paired with tolerogenic DNA backbones or checkpoint modulators, these personalized approaches hold promise for restoring immune tolerance in disorders such as MS (Mannie & Curtis, 2013).

Regulatory & Commercial Outlook: With LNP-based mRNA vaccines already approved for non-infectious indications, regulators are drafting adaptive pathways for CNS immunotherapies. Industry consortia and public–private partnerships are funding pivotal Phase I/II trials of mRNA immunogens in Alzheimer's disease, spinal cord injury, and ALS. By 2030, modular mRNA platforms are expected to enter late-stage studies across multiple neurodegenerative and neurotraumatic disorders, setting the stage for first-in-class regenerative vaccines.

5. Conclusion and future prospects

CNS diseases represent a significant medical challenge due to their complexity and heterogeneity. These disorders, including SCA2, AD, PD, MS, HD, and others, have profound impacts on human health and are difficult to treat. In this context, nucleic acid precision-targeted therapies have emerged, prompting a shift from traditional small-molecule approaches. Given the CNS's vulnerability, drug safety is paramount, and developing multitarget NADs offers a promising strategy for addressing complex CNS disorders. Furthermore, elucidating how mLVs mediate communication between central and peripheral immune systems is essential for understanding the pathogenesis of CNS immune-related diseases and for guiding the development of novel therapeutics, including vaccine-based interventions.

As a novel therapeutic approach, the long-term safety of nucleic acid therapies remains to be fully evaluated. Nucleic acid molecules may exhibit off-target effects and, as bioactive entities, can disrupt normal cellular processes upon entry into host cells. For instance, evidence suggests that COVID-19 mRNA vaccines may induce adverse reactions by interfering with endogenous miRNA pathways (Stati et al., 2023). Safe delivery vehicles must be biodegradable, biocompatible, and non-immunogenic; however, most current carriers exhibit significant immunogenicity, posing a particular challenge for the "sensitive and fragile" CNS. LNP systems, widely studied for nucleic acid delivery, are constrained by immune activation-related toxicity (Shiraishi and Yokoyama, 2019), prompting efforts to employ machine learning and high-throughput screening to identify safer, more effective LNP formulations (Xu et al., 2024). Beyond safety, efficacy is critically dependent on carrier properties, including targeting specificity, in vivo circulation stability, efficient cellular uptake, and intracellular release, which collectively determine whether nucleic acids reach their intended targets (Lu et al., 2023). CNS therapeutics currently rely largely on invasive local administration, whereas systemic delivery capable of crossing the BBB represents a key future direction. No single carrier yet achieves both safe and efficient systemic delivery, highlighting the need for hybrid carriers that combine multiple advantages with ligand-specific modifications for precise, effective, and safe targeting. Moreover, integrating nasal-to-brain administration technologies with delivery systems offers a promising avenue for direct and efficient CNS therapy.

In summary, advances in BBB-penetrating technologies, precision drug delivery design, and mechanistic understanding of neuropathology are critical for effective CNS disease therapies. Looking forward, clinical translation combined with multidimensional technological innovations—including novel ligand screening, AI-driven target prediction, and optimization of delivery vehicles and NBDD may shift neurodegenerative disease treatment from a "symptom-delaying" approach to one enabling single-dose administration with sustained reversal, offering transformative solutions for currently intractable CNS disorders.

References

Abbott, N. J. (2013). Blood-brain barrier structure and function and the challenges for CNS drug delivery. *Journal of Inherited Metabolic Disease, 36*(3), 437–449. https://doi.org/10.1007/s10545-013-9608-0

Alabsi, W., Eedara, B. B., Encinas-Basurto, D., Polt, R., & Mansour, H. M. (2022). Nose-to-brain delivery of therapeutic peptides as nasal aerosols. *Pharmaceutics, 14*(9). https://doi.org/10.3390/pharmaceutics14091870

Alhamadani, F., Zhang, K., Parikh, R., Wu, H., Rasmussen, T. P., Bahal, R., Zhong, X. B., & Manautou, J. E. (2022). Adverse drug reactions and toxicity of the food and drug administration–approved antisense oligonucleotide drugs. *Drug Metabolism and Disposition, 50*(6), 879–887. https://doi.org/10.1124/dmd.121.000418

Aly, A. E. E., Caron, N. S., Black, H. F., Schmidt, M. E., Anderson, C., Ko, S., Baddeley, H. J. E., Anderson, L., Casal, L. L., Rahavi, R. S. M., Martin, D. D. O., & Hayden, M. R. (2023). Delivery of mutant huntingtin-lowering antisense oligonucleotides to the brain by intranasally administered apolipoprotein A-I nanodisks. *Journal of Controlled Release, 360*, 913–927. https://doi.org/10.1016/j.jconrel.2023.07.027

Amero, P., Khatua, S., Rodriguez-Aguayo, C., & Lopez-Berestein, G. (2020). Aptamers: Novel therapeutics and potential role in neuro-oncology. *Cancers, 12*(10), 2889. https://doi.org/10.3390/cancers12102889

An, M., Raguram, A., Du, S. W., Banskota, S., Davis, J. R., Newby, G. A., Chen, P. Z., Palczewski, K., & Liu, D. R. (2024). Engineered virus-like particles for transient delivery of prime editor ribonucleoprotein complexes in vivo. *Nature Biotechnology, 42*(10), 1526–1537. https://doi.org/10.1038/s41587-023-02078-y

Annu, Sartaj, A., Qamar, Z., Alhakamy, S. N. A., Baboota, S., & Ali, J. (2022). An insight to brain targeting utilizing polymeric nanoparticles: Effective treatment modalities for neurological disorders and brain tumor. *Frontiers in Bioengineering and Biotechnology, 10*. https://doi.org/10.3389/fbioe.2022.788128

Aronin, N., & DiFiglia, M. (2014). Huntingtin-lowering strategies in huntington's disease: Antisense oligonucleotides, small RNAs, and gene editing. *Movement Disorders, 29*(11), 1455–1461. https://doi.org/10.1002/mds.26020

Arora, S., Layek, B., & Singh, J. (2021). Design and validation of liposomal ApoE2 gene delivery system to evade blood–brain barrier for effective treatment of Alzheimer's disease. *Molecular Pharmaceutics, 18*(2), 714–725. https://doi.org/10.1021/acs.molpharmaceut.0c00461

Badhwar, A. P., McFall, G. P., Sapkota, S., Black, S. E., Chertkow, H., Duchesne, S., Masellis, M., Li, L., Dixon, R. A., & Bellec, P. (2020). A multiomics approach to heterogeneity in Alzheimer's disease: Focused review and roadmap. *Brain, 143*(5), 1315–1331. https://doi.org/10.1093/brain/awz384

Bahadur, S., Pardhi, D. M., Rautio, J., Rosenholm, J. M., & Pathak, K. (2020). Intranasal nanoemulsions for direct nose-to-brain delivery of actives for cns disorders. *Pharmaceutics, 12*(12), 1–27. https://doi.org/10.3390/pharmaceutics12121230

Beach, M. A., Nayanathara, U., Gao, Y., Zhang, C., Xiong, Y., Wang, Y., & Such, G. K. (2024). Polymeric nanoparticles for drug delivery. *Chemical Reviews, 124*(9), 5505–5616. https://doi.org/10.1021/acs.chemrev.3c00705

Blair, H. A. (2022). Valoctocogene roxaparvovec: First approval. *Drugs, 82*(14), 1505–1510. https://doi.org/10.1007/s40265-022-01788-y

Blaylock, R. L. (2025). Immunoexcitoxicity as the possible major pathophysiology behind multiple sclerosis and other autoimmune disorders. *Surgical Neurology International, 16*, 26. https://doi.org/10.25259/SNI_1114_2024

Bloom, G. S. (2014). Amyloid-β and tau: The trigger and bullet in alzheimer disease pathogenesis. *JAMA Neurology, 71*(4), 505–508. https://doi.org/10.1001/jamaneurol.2013.5847

Bolte, A. C., Dutta, A. B., Hurt, M. E., Smirnov, I., Kovacs, M. A., McKee, C. A., Ennerfelt, H. E., Shapiro, D., Nguyen, B. H., Frost, E. L., Lammert, C. R., Kipnis, J., & Lukens, J. R. (2020). Meningeal lymphatic dysfunction exacerbates traumatic brain injury pathogenesis. *Nature Communications, 11*(1). https://doi.org/10.1038/s41467-020-18113-4

Brennan, G. P., & Henshall, D. C. (2020). MicroRNAs as regulators of brain function and targets for treatment of epilepsy. *Nature Reviews Neurology, 16*(9), 506–519. https://doi.org/10.1038/s41582-020-0369-8

Brody, D. L., & Holtzman, D. M. (2008). Active and passive immunotherapy for neurodegenerative disorders. *Annual Review of Neuroscience, 31*, 175–193. https://doi.org/10.1146/annurev.neuro.31.060407.125529

Brown, K. M., Nair, J. K., Janas, M. M., Anglero-Rodriguez, Y. I., Dang, L. T. H., Peng, H., Theile, C. S., Castellanos-Rizaldos, E., Brown, C., Foster, D., Kurz, J., Allen, J., Maganti, R., Li, J., Matsuda, S., Stricos, M., Chickering, T., Jung, M., Wassarman, K., … Jadhav, V. (2022). Expanding RNAi therapeutics to extrahepatic tissues with lipophilic conjugates. *Nature Biotechnology, 40*(10), 1500–1508. https://doi.org/10.1038/s41587-022-01334-x

Carceles-Cordon, M., Weintraub, D., & Chen-Plotkin, A. S. (2023). Cognitive heterogeneity in parkinson's disease: A mechanistic view. *Neuron, 111*(10), 1531–1546. https://doi.org/10.1016/j.neuron.2023.03.021

Castellani, G., Croese, T., Peralta Ramos, J. M., & Schwartz, M. (2023). Transforming the understanding of brain immunity. American association for the advancement of science. *Israel Science, 380*(6640). https://doi.org/10.1126/SCIENCE.ABO7649

Cerillo, J. L., & Parmar, M. (2025). *Tofersen*.

Chacko, L., Chaudhary, A., Singh, B., Dewanjee, S., & Kandimalla, R. (2023). CRISPR-Cas9 in Alzheimer's disease: Therapeutic trends, modalities, and challenges. *Drug Discovery Today, 28*(8), 103652. https://doi.org/10.1016/j.drudis.2023.103652

Chan, H. N., Xu, D., Ho, S. L., He, D., Wong, M. S., & Li, H. W. (2019). Highly sensitive quantification of alzheimer's disease biomarkers by aptamer-assisted amplification. *Theranostics, 9*(10), 2939–2949. https://doi.org/10.7150/thno.29232

Chatterjee, S., Kon, E., Sharma, P., & Peer, D. (2024). Endosomal escape: A bottleneck for LNP-Mediated therapeutics. *Proceedings of the National Academy of Sciences, 121*(11). https://doi.org/10.1073/pnas.2307800120

Chen, J., Finlay, W. H., Vehring, R., & Martin, A. R. (2024). Characterizing regional drug delivery within the nasal airways. *Expert Opinion on Drug Delivery, 21*(4), 537–551. https://doi.org/10.1080/17425247.2024.2336494

Chen, W., Yao, S., Wan, J., Tian, Y., Huang, L., Wang, S., Akter, F., Wu, Y., Yao, Y., & Zhang, X. (2021). , BBB-Crossing adeno-associated virus vector: An excellent gene delivery tool for CNS disease treatment. *Journal of Controlled Release, 333*, 129–138. https://doi.org/10.1016/j.jconrel.2021.03.029

Cheng, X., Wang, Y., Zhang, T., Cao, Y., Cheng, H., Du, Y., Ge, X., Ren, B., Lu, J., & Li, L. (2025). Emergence of small nucleic acids as drugs in precision medicine. *Clinical Pharmacology and Therapeutics, 118*(2), 308–323. https://doi.org/10.1002/cpt.3678

Coelho, T., Marques, W., Dasgupta, N. R., Chao, C. C., Parman, Y., França, M. C., Guo, Y. C., Wixner, J., Ro, L. S., Calandra, C. R., Kowacs, P. A., Berk, J. L., Obici, L., Barroso, F. A., Weiler, M., Conceição, I., Jung, S. W., Buchele, G., Brambatti, M., … Waddington Cruz, M. (2023). Eplontersen for hereditary transthyretin amyloidosis with polyneuropathy. *JAMA, 330*(15), 1448–1458. https://doi.org/10.1001/jama.2023.18688

Correale, J., & Fiol, M. (2009). Bht-3009, a myelin basic protein-encoding plasmid for the treatment of multiple sclerosis. *Current Opinion in Molecular Therapeutics, 11*(4), 463–470.

Cummings, J. (2020). The role of clinical trials in preclinical alzheimer's disease drug development programs. *The Journal of Prevention of Alzheimer's Disease, 7*(4), 288–290. https://doi.org/10.14283/jpad.2020.28

Dai, H., Li, W., Wang, Q., & Cheng, B. (2025). Multiple instance learning-based prediction of blood-brain barrier opening outcomes induced by focused ultrasound. *IEEE Transactions on Biomedical Engineering, 72*(4), 1465–1472. https://doi.org/10.1109/tbme.2024.3509533

Davtyan, H., Chen, W. W., Zagorski, K., Davis, J., Petrushina, I., Kazarian, K., Cribbs, D. H., Agadjanyan, M. G., Blurton-Jones, M., & Ghochikyan, A. (2017). MultiTEP platform-based DNA epitope vaccine targeting N-terminus of tau induces strong immune responses and reduces tau pathology in THY-Tau22 mice. *Vaccine, 35*(16), 2015–2024. https://doi.org/10.1016/j.vaccine.2017.03.020

Delhaas, E. M., & Huygen, F. J. P. M. (2020). Complications associated with intrathecal drug delivery systems. *BJA Education, 20*(2), 51–57. https://doi.org/10.1016/j.bjae.2019.11.002

DeVos, S. L., & Miller, T. M. (2013). Antisense oligonucleotides: Treating neurodegeneration at the level of RNA. *Neurotherapeutics, 10*(3), 486–497. https://doi.org/10.1007/s13311-013-0194-5

Dhuri, K., Bechtold, C., Quijano, E., Pham, H., Gupta, A., Vikram, A., & Bahal, R. (2020). Antisense oligonucleotides: An emerging area in drug discovery and development. *Journal of Clinical Medicine, 9*(6), 2004. https://doi.org/10.3390/jcm9062004

Duan, W., Guo, M., Yi, Le, Liu, Y., Li, Z., Ma, Y., Zhang, G., Liu, Y., Bu, H., Song, X., & Li, C. (2020). The deletion of mutant SOD1 via CRISPR/Cas9/sgRNA prolongs survival in an amyotrophic lateral sclerosis mouse model. *Gene Therapy, 27*(3–4), 157–169. https://doi.org/10.1038/s41434-019-0116-1

Dunbar, C. E., High, K. A., Joung, J. K., Kohn, D. B., Ozawa, K., & Sadelain, M. (2018). Gene therapy comes of age. American association for the advancement of science. *United States Science, 359*(6372). https://doi.org/10.1126/science.aan4672

Enea, M., Peixoto de Almeida, M., Eaton, P., Dias da Silva, D., Pereira, E., Soares, M. E., Bastos, M.d. L., & Carmo, H. (2019). A multiparametric study of gold nanoparticles cytotoxicity, internalization and permeability using an in vitro model of blood–brain barrier. Influence of size, shape and capping agent. *Nanotoxicology, 13*(7), 990–1004. https://doi.org/10.1080/17435390.2019.1621398

Estevez-Fraga, C., Tabrizi, S. J., & Wild, E. J. (2024). Huntington's disease clinical trials corner: march 2024. *Journal of Huntington's Disease, 13*(1), 1–14. https://doi.org/10.3233/JHD-240017

Eygeris, Y., Gupta, M., Kim, J., & Sahay, G. (2022). Chemistry of lipid nanoparticles for RNA delivery. *Accounts of Chemical Research, 55*(1), 2–12. https://doi.org/10.1021/acs.accounts.1c00544

Föttinger, F., Krajnc, N., Riedl, K., Leutmezer, F., Ponleitner, M., Rommer, P., Kornek, B., Macher, S., Schmied, C., Zebenholzer, K., Zulehner, G., Zrzavy, T., Berger, T., & Bsteh, G. (2025). Autoimmune screening panel in patients with multiple sclerosis: A Vienna multiple sclerosis database study. *European Journal of Neurology, 32*(1). https://doi.org/10.1111/ene.16558

Fei, Y., Yu, X., Liu, P., Ren, H., Wei, T., & Cheng, Q. (2024). Simplified lipid nanoparticles for Tissue- and cell-targeted mRNA delivery facilitate precision tumor therapy in a lung metastasis mouse model. *Advanced Materials, 36*(48). https://doi.org/10.1002/adma.202409812

Feng, X., Hou, Y., Liu, J., Yan, F., Dai, M., Chen, Mo, Wang, J., Li, J., Liu, Z., Sun, D., Zhang, Y., Yu, X., Kong, W., & Wu, H. (2024). A multi-targeting immunotherapy ameliorates multiple facets of Alzheimer's disease in 3xTg mice. *Npj Vaccines, 9*(1). https://doi.org/10.1038/s41541-024-00942-9

Feng, X., Jiang, B. W., Zhai, S. N., Liu, C. X., Wu, H., Zhu, B. Q., Wei, M. Y., Wei, J., Yang, L., & Chen, L. L. (2025). Circular RNA aptamers targeting neuroinflammation ameliorate alzheimer disease phenotypes in mouse models. *Nature Biotechnology.* https://doi.org/10.1038/s41587-025-02624-w

Feng, J., Ren, Y., Wang, X., Li, X., Zhu, X., Zhang, B., Zhao, Q., Sun, X., Tian, X., Liu, H., Dong, F., Li, X.-L., Qi, L., & Wei, B. (2024). Impaired meningeal lymphatic drainage in Listeria monocytogenes infection. *Frontiers in Immunology, 15.* https://doi.org/10.3389/fimmu.2024.1382971

Fernández, G., Moraga, A., Cuartero, M. I., García-Culebras, A., Peña-Martínez, C., Pradillo, J. M., Hernández-Jiménez, M., Sacristán, S., Ayuso, M. I., Gonzalo-Gobernado, R., Fernández-López, D., Martín, M. E., Moro, M. A., González, V. M., & Lizasoain, I. (2018). TLR4-Binding DNA aptamers show a protective effect against acute stroke in animal models. *Molecular Therapy, 26*(8), 2047–2059. https://doi.org/10.1016/j.ymthe.2018.05.019

Fernández-Gómez, B., Marchena, M. A., Piñeiro, D., Gómez-Martín, P., Sánchez, E., Laó, Y., Valencia, G., Nocera, S., Benítez-Fernández, R., Castaño-León, A. M., Lagares, A., Hernández-Jiménez, M., & de Castro, F. (2024). ApTOLL: A new therapeutic aptamer for cytoprotection and (re)myelination after multiple sclerosis. *British Journal of Pharmacology, 181*(17), 3263–3281. https://doi.org/10.1111/bph.16399

Fitzpatrick, Z., Ghabdan Zanluqui, N., Rosenblum, J. S., Tuong, Z. K., Lee, C. Y. C., Chandrashekhar, V., Negro-Demontel, M. L., Stewart, A. P., Posner, D. A., Buckley, M., Allinson, K. S. J., Mastorakos, P., Chittiboina, P., Maric, D., Donahue, D., Helmy, A., Tajsic, T., Ferdinand, J. R., Portet, A., … McGavern, D. B. (2024). Venous-plexus-associated lymphoid hubs support meningeal humoral immunity. Nature research. *United States Nature, 628*(8008), 612–619. https://doi.org/10.1038/s41586-024-07202-9

Foust, K. D., Nurre, E., Montgomery, C. L., Hernandez, A., Chan, C. M., & Kaspar, B. K. (2009). Intravascular AAV9 preferentially targets neonatal neurons and adult astrocytes. *Nature Biotechnology, 27*(1), 59–65. https://doi.org/10.1038/nbt.1515

Frühbeis, C., Fröhlich, D., & Krämer-Albers, E.-M. (2012). Emerging roles of exosomes in neuron–glia communication. *Frontiers in Physiology, 3.* https://doi.org/10.3389/fphys.2012.00119

Frederick, N., & Louveau, A. (2020). Meningeal lymphatics, immunity and neuroinflammation. *Current Opinion in Neurobiology, 62*, 41–47. https://doi.org/10.1016/j.conb.2019.11.010

Gagliardi, M., & Ashizawa, A. T. (2021). The challenges and strategies of antisense oligonucleotide drug delivery. *Biomedicines, 9*(4). https://doi.org/10.3390/biomedicines9040433

Garber, K. (2018). Alnylam launches era of RNAi drugs. *Nature Biotechnology, 36*(9), 777–778. https://doi.org/10.1038/nbt0918-777

Garren, H., Robinson, W. H., Krasulová, E., Havrdová, E., Nadj, C., Selmaj, K., Losy, J., Nadj, I., Radue, E. W., Kidd, B. A., Gianettoni, J., Tersini, K., Utz, P. J., Valone, F., Steinman, L., Milanov, I., Georgiev, D.,

Shotekov, P., Stamenova, P., … Kasper, L. (2008). Phase 2 trial of a DNA vaccine encoding myelin basic protein for multiple sclerosis. *Annals of Neurology, 63*(5), 611–620. https://doi.org/10.1002/ana.21370

Geilenkeuser, J., Armbrust, N., Steinmaßl, E., Du, S. W., Schmidt, S., Binder, E. M. H., Li, Y., Warsing, N. W., Wendel, S. V., von der Linde, F., Schiele, E. M., Niu, X., Stroppel, L., Berezin, O., Santl, T. H., Orschmann, T., Nelson, K., Gruber, C., Palczewska, G., … Truong, D. J. J. (2025). Engineered nucleocytosolic vehicles for loading of programmable editors. *Cell, 188*(10), 2637. https://doi.org/10.1016/j.cell.2025.03.015

Ghorai, S. M., Deep, A., Magoo, D., Gupta, C., & Gupta, N. (2023). Cell-penetrating and targeted peptides delivery systems as potential pharmaceutical carriers for enhanced delivery across the blood–brain barrier (BBB). multidisciplinary digital publishing institute (MDPI). *India Pharmaceutics, 15*(7). https://doi.org/10.3390/pharmaceutics15071999

Goyenvalle, A., Jimenez-Mallebrera, C., Van Roon, W., Sewing, S., Krieg, A. M., Arechavala-Gomeza, V., & Andersson, P. (2023). Considerations in the preclinical assessment of the safety of antisense oligonucleotides. *Nucleic Acid Therapeutics, 33*(1), 1–16. https://doi.org/10.1089/nat.2022.0061

Greig, J. A., Martins, K. M., Breton, C., Lamontagne, R. J., Zhu, Y., He, Z., White, J., Zhu, J. X., Chichester, J. A., Zheng, Q., Zhang, Z., Bell, P., Wang, L., & Wilson, J. M. (2024). Integrated vector genomes May contribute to long-term expression in primate liver after AAV administration. *Nature Biotechnology, 42*(8), 1232–1242. https://doi.org/10.1038/s41587-023-01974-7

Guan, C., Zhu, X., & Feng, C. (2021). DNA nanodevice-based drug delivery systems. *Biomolecules, 11*(12), 1855. https://doi.org/10.3390/biom11121855

Guo, L., Huang, Z., Huang, L., Liang, J., Wang, P., Zhao, L., & Shi, Y. (2021). Surface-modified engineered exosomes attenuated cerebral ischemia/reperfusion injury by targeting the delivery of Quercetin towards impaired neurons. *Journal of Nanobiotechnology, 19*(1). https://doi.org/10.1186/s12951-021-00879-4

Guo, X., Zhang, G., Peng, Q., Huang, L., Zhang, Z., & Zhang, Z. (2023). Emerging roles of meningeal lymphatic vessels in Alzheimer's disease. *Journal of Alzheimer's Disease, 94*(s1), S355. https://doi.org/10.3233/jad-221016

Hanif, S., Muhammad, P., Chesworth, R., & Rehman, F. U. (2020). R.j. qian, M. Zheng, B.y. shi, Nanomedicine-based immunotherapy for central nervous system disorders. *Acta Pharmacologica Sinica, 41*(7), 936–953. https://doi.org/10.1038/s41401-020-0429-z

Haroon, H. B., Mukherjee, D., Anbu, J., & Teja, B. V. (2021). Thiolated chitosan-centella asiatica nanocomposite: A potential brain targeting strategy through nasal route. *AAPS PharmSciTech, 22*(8). https://doi.org/10.1208/s12249-021-02131-6

Hathout, R. M., & El-Marakby, E. M. (2022). Meta-analysis: A convenient tool for the choice of nose-to-brain nanocarriers. *Bioengineering, 9*(11). https://doi.org/10.3390/bioengineering9110647

Holm, A., Hansen, S. N., Klitgaard, H., & Kauppinen, S. (2022). Clinical advances of RNA therapeutics for treatment of neurological and neuromuscular diseases. *RNA Biology, 19*(1), 594–608. https://doi.org/10.1080/15476286.2022.2066334

Horan, W. P., Targum, S. D., Claxton, A., Kaul, I., Yohn, S. E., Marder, S. R., Miller, A. C., & Brannan, S. K. (2024). Efficacy of KarXT on negative symptoms in acute schizophrenia: A post hoc analysis of pooled data from 3 trials. *Schizophrenia Research, 274*, 57–65. https://doi.org/10.1016/j.schres.2024.08.001

Hovakimyan, A., Chilingaryan, G., King, O., Kai Capocchi, J., Paul Chadarevian, J., Davtyan, H., Kniazev, R., Agadjanyan, M. G., & Ghochikyan, A. (2024). mRNA vaccine for Alzheimer's disease: Pilot study. *Vaccines, 12*(6), 659. https://doi.org/10.3390/vaccines12060659

Hoy, S. M. (2017). Nusinersen: First global approval. *Drugs, 77*(4), 473–479. https://doi.org/10.1007/s40265-017-0711-7

Hoy, S. M. (2019). Onasemnogene abeparvovec: First global approval. *Drugs, 79*(11), 1255–1262. https://doi.org/10.1007/s40265-019-01162-5

Hu, X., Deng, Q., Ma, L., Li, Q., Chen, Y., Liao, Y., Zhou, F., Zhang, C., Shao, L., Feng, J., He, T., Ning, W., Kong, Y., Huo, Y., He, A., Liu, B., Zhang, J., Adams, R., He, Y., … Luo, J. (2020). Meningeal lymphatic vessels regulate brain tumor drainage and immunity. *Cell Research, 30*(3), 229–243. https://doi.org/10.1038/s41422-020-0287-8

Johnson, S., Buessing, M., O'Connell, T., Pitluck, S., & Ciulla, T. A. (2019). Cost-effectiveness of voretigene neparvovec-rzyl vs standard care for RPE65 -Mediated inherited retinal disease. *JAMA Ophthalmology, 137* (10), 1115–1123. https://doi.org/10.1001/jamaophthalmol.2019.2512

Joo, J., Kwon, E. J., Kang, J., Skalak, M., Anglin, E. J., Mann, A. P., Ruoslahti, E., Bhatia, S. N., & Sailor, M. J. (2016). Porous silicon-graphene oxide core-shell nanoparticles for targeted delivery of siRNA to the injured brain. *Nanoscale Horizons, 1*(5), 407–414. https://doi.org/10.1039/c6nh00082g

Kadir, R. R. A., Alwjwaj, M., & Bayraktutan, U. (2022). MicroRNA: An emerging predictive, diagnostic, prognostic and therapeutic strategy in ischaemic stroke. *Cellular and Molecular Neurobiology, 42*(5), 1301–1319. https://doi.org/10.1007/s10571-020-01028-5

Kashani, G. K., Naghib, S. M., Soleymani, S., & Mozafari, M. R. (2024). A review of DNA nanoparticles-encapsulated drug/gene/protein for advanced controlled drug release: Current status and future perspective over emerging therapy approaches. *International Journal of Biological Macromolecules, 268*. https://doi.org/10.1016/j.ijbiomac.2024.131694

Katzmann, J. L., Packard, C. J., Chapman, M. J., Katzmann, I., & Laufs, U. (2020). Targeting RNA with antisense oligonucleotides and small interfering RNA: JACC state-of-the-art review. *Journal of the American College of Cardiology, 76*(5), 563–579. https://doi.org/10.1016/j.jacc.2020.05.070

Keam, S. J. (2022). Eladocagene exuparvovec: First approval. *Drugs, 82*(13), 1427–1432. https://doi.org/10.1007/s40265-022-01775-3

Kehagia, E., Papakyriakopoulou, P., & Valsami, G. (2023). Advances in intranasal vaccine delivery: A promising non-invasive route of immunization. *Vaccine, 41*(24), 3589–3603. https://doi.org/10.1016/j.vaccine.2023.05.011

Kim, J., Hu, C., El Achkar, C. M., Black, L. E., Douville, J., Larson, A., Pendergast, M. K., Goldkind, S. F., Lee, E. A., Kuniholm, A., Soucy, A., Vaze, J., Belur, N. R., Fredriksen, K., Stojkovska, I., Tsytsykova, A., Armant, M., DiDonato, R. L., Choi, J., … Yu, T. W. (2019). Patient-customized oligonucleotide therapy for a rare genetic disease. *New England Journal of Medicine, 381*(17), 1644–1652. https://doi.org/10.1056/NEJMoa1813279

Kim, M., Lee, Y., & Lee, M. (2021). Hypoxia-specific anti-RAGE exosomes for nose-to-brain delivery of anti-miR-181a oligonucleotide in an ischemic stroke model. *Nanoscale, 13*(33), 14166–14178. https://doi.org/10.1039/d0nr07516g

Kim, H. I., Park, J., Zhu, Y., Wang, X., Han, Y., & Zhang, D. (2024). Recent advances in extracellular vesicles for therapeutic cargo delivery. *Experimental and Molecular Medicine, 56*(4), 836–849. https://doi.org/10.1038/s12276-024-01201-6

Kolesnik, V. V., Nurtdinov, R. F., Sola Oloruntimehin, E., Karabelsky, A. V., & Malogolovkin, A. S. (2024). Optimization strategies and advances in the research and development of AAV-based gene therapy to deliver large transgenes. *Clinical and Translational Medicine, 14*(3). https://doi.org/10.1002/ctm2.1607

Kulkarni, J. A., Witzigmann, D., Thomson, S. B., Chen, S., Leavitt, B. R., Cullis, P. R., & der Meel, R.van (2021). Author correction: The current landscape of nucleic acid therapeutics. *Nature Nanotechnology, 16*(7), 841. https://doi.org/10.1038/s41565-021-00937-w

Kumthekar, P., Ko, C. H., Paunesku, T., Dixit, K., Sonabend, A. M., Bloch, O., Tate, M., Schwartz, M., Zuckerman, L., Lezon, R., Lukas, R. V., Jovanovic, B., McCortney, K., Colman, H., Chen, S., Lai, B., Antipova, O., Deng, J., Li, L., … Stegh, A. H. (2021). A first-in-human phase 0 clinical study of RNA interference-based spherical nucleic acids in patients with recurrent glioblastoma. *Science Translational Medicine, 13*(584). https://doi.org/10.1126/scitranslmed.abb3945

Lázaro, D. F., & Lee, V. M.-Y. (2024). Navigating through the complexities of synucleinopathies: Insights into pathogenesis, heterogeneity, and future perspectives. *Neuron, 112*(18), 3029–3042. https://doi.org/10.1016/j.neuron.2024.05.017

Lam, J. K. W., et al. (2015). siRNA versus miRNA as therapeutics for gene silencing. *Molecular Therapy - Nucleic Acids, 4*(9), e252. https://doi.org/10.1038/mtna.2015.23

Lambracht-Washington, D., & Rosenberg, R. N. (2013). Advances in the development of vaccines for Alzheimer's disease. *Discovery Medicine, 15*(84), 319–326.

Leckie, J., & Yokota, T. (2024). Potential of cell-penetrating peptide-conjugated antisense oligonucleotides for the treatment of SMA. *Molecules, 29*(11), 2658. https://doi.org/10.3390/molecules29112658

Lee, K. W. A., Chan, L. K. W., Hung, L. C., Phoebe, L. K. W., Park, Y., & Yi, K. H. (2024). Clinical applications of exosomes: A critical review. *International Journal of Molecular Sciences, 25*(14). https://doi.org/10.3390/ijms25147794

Li, W., Qiu, J., Li, X. L., Aday, S., Zhang, J., Conley, G., Xu, J., Joseph, J., Lan, H., Langer, R., Mannix, R., Karp, J. M., & Joshi, N. (2021). BBB pathophysiology–independent delivery of siRNA in traumatic brain injury. *Science Advances, 7*(1). https://doi.org/10.1126/sciadv.abd6889

Li, G., Zhang, S., Zou, Y., Ai, H., Zheng, X., Qian, K., Lei, C., & Fu, W. (2024). The therapeutic potential of exosomes in immunotherapy. *Frontiers in Immunology, 15*. https://doi.org/10.3389/fimmu.2024.1424081

Li, X., Zhu, Y., Wang, Y., Xia, X., & Zheng, J. C. (2020). Neural stem/progenitor cell-derived extracellular vesicles: A novel therapy for neurological diseases and beyond. *MedComm, 4*, e214. https://doi.org/10.1002/mco2.214

Li, X., Zhu, Y., Wang, Y., Xia, X., & Zheng, J. C. (2023). Neural stem/progenitor cell-derived extracellular vesicles: A novel therapy for neurological diseases and beyond. *MedComm, 4*(1). https://doi.org/10.1002/mco2.214

Liang, Y., Duan, L., Lu, J., & Xia, J. (2021). Engineering exosomes for targeted drug delivery. *Theranostics, 11*(7), 3183–3195. https://doi.org/10.7150/thno.52570

Lim, L. W. C., Lee, J. Y., Chen, C. H., Voon, K. G. L., Koh, R. Y., & Chye, S. M. (2025). Virus-like particles-based vaccine to combat neurodegenerative diseases. *Current Pharmaceutical Biotechnology*. https://doi.org/10.2174/0113892010331763241002122854

Lincoff, A. M., Mehran, R., Povsic, T. J., Zelenkofske, S. L., Huang, Z., Armstrong, P. W., Steg, P. G., Bode, C., Cohen, M. G., Buller, C., Laanmets, P., Valgimigli, M., Marandi, T., Fridrich, V., Cantor, W. J., Merkely, B., Lopez-Sendon, J., Cornel, J. H., Kasprzak, J. D., … Alexander, J. H. (2016). Effect of the REG1 anticoagulation system versus bivalirudin on outcomes after percutaneous coronary intervention (REGULATE-PCI): A randomised clinical trial. *The Lancet, 387*(10016), 349–356. https://doi.org/10.1016/S0140-6736(15)00515-2

Liu, J., Wang, T., Dong, J., & Lu, Y. (2025). The blood–brain barriers: Novel nanocarriers for central nervous system diseases. *Journal of Nanobiotechnology, 23*(1). https://doi.org/10.1186/s12951-025-03247-8

Lu, Z. G., Shen, J., Yang, J., Wang, J. W., Zhao, R. C., Zhang, T. L., Guo, J., & Zhang, X. (2023). Nucleic acid drug vectors for diagnosis and treatment of brain diseases. *Signal Transduction and Targeted Therapy, 8*(1). https://doi.org/10.1038/s41392-022-01298-z

Ma, F., Yang, L., Sun, Z., Chen, J., Rui, X., Glass, Z., & Xu, Q. (2020). Neurotransmitter-derived lipidoids (NT-lipidoids) for enhanced brain delivery through intravenous injection. *Science Advances, 6*(30). https://doi.org/10.1126/sciadv.abb4429

Mahase, E. (2021). Aducanumab: 4 in 10 high dose trial participants experienced brain swelling or bleeding. *BMJ, 375*, n2975. https://doi.org/10.1136/bmj.n2975

Mannie, M. D., & Curtis, A. D. (2013). Tolerogenic vaccines for multiple sclerosis. *Human Vaccines & Immunotherapeutics, 9*(5), 1032–1038. https://doi.org/10.4161/hv.23685

Marcos-Contreras, O. A., Greineder, C. F., Kiseleva, R. Y., Parhiz, H., Walsh, L. R., Zuluaga-Ramirez, V., Myerson, J. W., Hood, E. D., Villa, C. H., Tombacz, I., Pardi, N., Seliga, A., Mui, B. L., Tam, Y. K., Glassman, P. M., Shuvaev, V. V., Nong, J., Brenner, J. S., Khoshnejad, M., … Muzykantov, V. R. (2020). Selective targeting of nanomedicine to inflamed cerebral vasculature to enhance the blood–brain barrier.

Proceedings of the National Academy of Sciences of the United States of America, 117(7), 3405–3414. https://doi.org/10.1073/pnas.1912012117

Martins, C., Sousa, F., Araújo, F., Sarmento, B., Functionalizing, P. L. G. A., & Derivatives, P. L. G. A. (2018). For drug delivery and tissue regeneration applications. *Advanced Healthcare Materials, 7*(1). https://doi.org/10.1002/adhm.201701035

Matsubayashi, T., Yoshioka, K., Lei Mon, S. S., Katsuyama, M., Jia, C., Yamaguchi, T., Iwata Hara, R., Nagata, T., Nakagawa, O., Obika, S., & Yokota, T. (2024). Favorable efficacy and reduced acute neurotoxicity by antisense oligonucleotides with 2′,4′-BNA/LNA with 9-(aminoethoxy)phenoxazine. *Molecular Therapy - Nucleic Acids, 35*(2), 102161. https://doi.org/10.1016/j.omtn.2024.102161

Matsuda, S., Bala, S., Liao, J. Y., Datta, D., Mikami, A., Woods, L., Harp, J. M., Gilbert, J. A., Bisbe, A., Manoharan, R. M., Kim, M. B., Theile, C. S., Guenther, D. C., Jiang, Y., Agarwal, S., Maganti, R., Schlegel, M. K., Zlatev, I., Charisse, K., … Manoharan, M. (2023). Shorter is better: The α-(l)-Threofuranosyl nucleic acid modification improves stability, potency, safety, and Ago2 binding and mitigates off-target effects of small interfering RNAs. *Journal of the American Chemical Society, 145*(36), 19691–19706. https://doi.org/10.1021/jacs.3c04744

McGonigle, P. (2014). Animal models of CNS disorders. *Biochemical Pharmacology, 87*(1), 140–149. https://doi.org/10.1016/j.bcp.2013.06.016

Miao, Y., Fu, C., Yu, Z., Yu, L., Tang, Y., & Wei, M. (2024). Current status and trends in small nucleic acid drug development: Leading the future. *Acta Pharmaceutica Sinica B, 14*(9), 3802–3817. https://doi.org/10.1016/j.apsb.2024.05.008

Miller, T. M., Cudkowicz, M. E., Genge, A., Shaw, P. J., Sobue, G., Bucelli, R. C., Chiò, A., Van Damme, P., Ludolph, A. C., Glass, J. D., Andrews, J. A., Babu, S., Benatar, M., McDermott, C. J., Cochrane, T., Chary, S., Chew, S., Zhu, H., Wu, F., … Fradette, S. (2022). Trial of antisense oligonucleotide tofersen for SOD1 ALS. *New England Journal of Medicine, 387*(12), 1099–1110. https://doi.org/10.1056/NEJMoa2204705

Mohsen, M. O., & Bachmann, M. F. (2022). Virus-like particle vaccinology, from bench to bedside. *Cellular and Molecular Immunology, 19*(9), 993–1011. https://doi.org/10.1038/s41423-022-00897-8

Moreno-Mateos, M. A., Vejnar, C. E., Beaudoin, J. D., Fernandez, J. P., Mis, E. K., Khokha, M. K., & Giraldez, A. J. (2015). CRISPRscan: Designing highly efficient sgRNAs for CRISPR-Cas9 targeting in vivo. *Nature Methods, 12*(10), 982–988. https://doi.org/10.1038/nmeth.3543

Morgan, D., Diamond, D. M., Gottschall, P. E., Ugen, K. E., Dickey, C., Hardy, J., Duff, K., Jantzen, P., DiCarlo, G., Wilcock, D., Connor, K., Hatcher, J., Hope, C., Gordon, M., & Arendash, G. W. (2000). A β peptide vaccination prevents memory loss in an animal model of Alzheimer's disease. *Nature, 408*(6815), 982–985. https://doi.org/10.1038/35050116

Nie, T. (2024). Eplontersen: First approval. *Drugs, 84*(4), 473–478. https://doi.org/10.1007/s40265-024-02008-5

Nie, D. Y., Xu, G., Ahmed, S., & Xiao, Z. C. (2007). DNA vaccine and the CNS axonal regeneration. *Current Pharmaceutical Design, 13*(24), 2500–2506. https://doi.org/10.2174/138161207781368567Singapore

Obeidat, W. M., & Lahlouh, I. K. (2025). Chitosan nanoparticles: Approaches to preparation, key properties, drug delivery systems, and developments in therapeutic efficacy. *AAPS PharmSciTech, 26*(5). https://doi.org/10.1208/s12249-025-03100-z

Ouyang, Q., Liu, K., Zhu, Q., Deng, H., Le, Y., Ouyang, W., Yan, X., Zhou, W., & Tong, J. (2022). Brain-Penetration and neuron-targeting DNA nanoflowers Co-Delivering miR-124 and rutin for synergistic therapy of Alzheimer's Disease. *Small, 18*(14). https://doi.org/10.1002/smll.202107534

Palanki, R., Bose, S. K., Dave, A., White, B. M., Berkowitz, C., Luks, V., Yaqoob, F., Han, E., Swingle, K. L., Menon, P., Hodgson, E., Biswas, A., Billingsley, M. M., Li, L., Yiping, F., Carpenter, M., Trokhan, A., Yeo, J., Johana, N., … Peranteau, W. H. (2023). Ionizable lipid nanoparticles for therapeutic base editing of congenital brain disease. *ACS Nano, 17*(14), 13594–13610. https://doi.org/10.1021/acsnano.3c02268

Panza, F., Frisardi, V., Solfrizzi, V., Imbimbo, B. P., Logroscino, G., Santamato, A., Greco, A., Seripa, D., & Pilotto, A. (2012). Immunotherapy for Alzheimer's disease: From anti-β-amyloid to tau-based immunization strategies. *Immunotherapy, 4*(2), 213–238. https://doi.org/10.2217/imt.11.170

Pardridge, W. M. (1998). CNS drug design based on principles of blood-brain barrier transport. *Journal of Neurochemistry, 70*(5), 1781–1792. https://doi.org/10.1046/j.1471-4159.1998.70051781.x

Patel, T. K., Habimana-Griffin, L., Gao, X., Xu, B., Achilefu, S., Alitalo, K., McKee, C. A., Sheehan, P. W., Musiek, E. S., Xiong, C., Coble, D., & Holtzman, D. M. (2019). Dural lymphatics regulate clearance of extracellular tau from the CNS. *Molecular Neurodegeneration, 14*(1). https://doi.org/10.1186/s13024-019-0312-x

Pottoo, F. H., Barkat, M. A., Harshita, Ansari, M. A., Javed, M. N., Sajid Jamal, Q. M., & Kamal, M. A. (2021). Nanotechnological based miRNA intervention in the therapeutic management of neuroblastoma. *Seminars in Cancer Biology, 69*, 100–108. https://doi.org/10.1016/j.semcancer.2019.09.017

Qi, Y., Xiong, W., Chen, Q., Ye, Z., Jiang, C., He, Y., & Ye, Q. (2023). New trends in brain tumor immunity with the opportunities of lymph nodes targeted drug delivery. *Journal of Nanobiotechnology, 21*(1). https://doi.org/10.1186/s12951-023-02011-0

Qiu, Y., Huang, S., Peng, L., Yang, L., Zhang, G., Liu, T., Yan, F., & Peng, X. (2025). The nasal–brain drug delivery route: Mechanisms and applications to central nervous System diseases. *MedComm, 6*(6). https://doi.org/10.1002/mco2.70213

Quemener, A. M., Centomo, M. L., Sax, S. L., & Panella, R. (2022). Small drugs, huge impact: The extraordinary impact of antisense oligonucleotides in research and drug development. *Molecules*, (2), 27. https://doi.org/10.3390/molecules27020536

Rafii, M. S., Sol, O., Mobley, W. C., Delpretti, S., Skotko, B. G., Burke, A. D., Sabbagh, M. N., Yuan, S. H., Rissman, R. A., Pulsifer, M., Evans, C., Evans, A. C., Beth, G., Fournier, N., Gray, J. A., Dos Santos, A. M., Hliva, V., Vukicevic, M., Kosco-Vilbois, M., … Feldman, H. H. (2022). Safety, tolerability, and immunogenicity of the ACI-24 vaccine in adults with Down Syndrome: A phase 1b randomized clinical trial. *JAMA Neurology, 79*(6), 565–574. https://doi.org/10.1001/jamaneurol.2022.0983

Rana, T. M. (2007). Illuminating the silence: Understanding the structure and function of small RNAs. *Nature Reviews Molecular Cell Biology, 8*(1), 23–36. https://doi.org/10.1038/nrm2085

Rezai, A. R., D'Haese, P. F., Finomore, V., Carpenter, J., Ranjan, M., Wilhelmsen, K., Mehta, R. I., Wang, P., Najib, U., Vieira Ligo Teixeira, C., Arsiwala, T., Tarabishy, A., Tirumalai, P., Claassen, D. O., Hodder, S., & Haut, M. W. (2024). Ultrasound blood-brain barrier opening and aducanumab in Alzheimer's Disease. *New England Journal of Medicine, 390*(1), 55–62. https://doi.org/10.1056/NEJMoa2308719

Rohovie, M. J., Nagasawa, M., & Swartz, J. R. (2017). Virus-like particles: Next-generation nanoparticles for targeted therapeutic delivery. *Bioengineering & Translational Medicine, 2*(1), 43–57. https://doi.org/10.1002/btm2.10049

Salimi, L., Seyedaghamiri, F., Karimipour, M., Mobarak, H., Mardi, N., Taghavi, M., & Rahbarghazi, R. (2023). Physiological and pathological consequences of exosomes at the blood–brain-barrier interface. *Cell Communication and Signaling, 21*(1). https://doi.org/10.1186/s12964-023-01142-z

Schneider, L. S., Mangialasche, F., Andreasen, N., Feldman, H., Giacobini, E., Jones, R., Mantua, V., Mecocci, P., Pani, L., Winblad, B., & Kivipelto, M. (2014). Clinical trials and late-stage drug development for A lzheimer's disease: An appraisal from 1984 to 2014. *Journal of Internal Medicine, 275*(3), 251–283. https://doi.org/10.1111/joim.12191

Scott, L. J. (2020). Givosiran: First approval. *Adis, New Zealand Drugs, 80*(3), 335–339. https://doi.org/10.1007/s40265-020-01269-0

Semyachkina-Glushkovskaya, O., Shirokov, A., Blokhina, I., Telnova, V., Vodovozova, E., Alekseeva, A., Boldyrev, I., Fedosov, I., Dubrovsky, A., Khorovodov, A., Terskov, A., Evsukova, A., Elovenko, D., Adushkina, V., Tzoy, M., Agranovich, I., Kurths, J., & Rafailov, E. (2023). Intranasal delivery of liposomes to glioblastoma by photostimulation of the lymphatic System. *Pharmaceutics, 15*(1), 36. https://doi.org/10.3390/pharmaceutics15010036

Shen, H., Aggarwal, N., Cui, B., Foo, G. W., He, Y., Srivastava, S. K., Li, S., Seah, M. Z. X., Wun, K. S., Ling, H., Hwang, I. Y., Ho, C. L., Lee, Y. S., & Chang, M. W. (2025). Engineered commensals for targeted nose-to-brain drug delivery. *Cell, 188*(6), 1545. https://doi.org/10.1016/j.cell.2025.01.017

Shiraishi, K., & Yokoyama, M. (2019). Toxicity and immunogenicity concerns related to PEGylated-micelle carrier systems: A review. *Science and Technology of Advanced Materials, 20*(1), 324–336. https://doi.org/10.1080/14686996.2019.1590126

Silberstein, S. (2017). AVP-825: A novel intranasal delivery system for low-dose sumatriptan powder in the treatment of acute migraine. *Expert Review of Clinical Pharmacology, 10*(8), 821–832. https://doi.org/10.1080/17512433.2017.1339600

Slomski, A. (2021). Novel oral drug rapidly treats postpartum depression. *JAMA, 326*(9), 800. https://doi.org/10.1001/jama.2021.14708

Smyth, L. C. D., & Kipnis, J. (2025). Redefining CNS immune privilege. *Nature Reviews Immunology.* https://doi.org/10.1038/s41577-025-01175-0

Sol, O., Le, B., Wagg, J., Delpretti, S., Fiorini, E., Vukicevic, M., MacSweeney, E., Borejko, O., Aarsland, D., Morató Arús, X., Boada, M., Matias-Guiu, J. A., Lleo, A., Fournier, N., Valatsou, E., Feige, A., Rongere, J., Jg Gray, J., Hliva, V., … Streffer, J. (2023). 4. An innovative clinical trial designed to evaluate the effects of ACI-24.060 in Alzheimer's Disease and in Down syndrome (ABATE Study). *Alzheimer's & Dementia, 19*(S21). https://doi.org/10.1002/alz.075830

Song, Y., Song, W., Lan, X., Cai, W., & Jiang, D. (2022). Spherical nucleic acids: Organized nucleotide aggregates as versatile nanomedicine. *Aggregate, 3*(1). https://doi.org/10.1002/agt2.120

Spence, H., Waldron, F. M., Saleeb, R. S., Brown, A. L., Rifai, O. M., Gilodi, M., Read, F., Roberts, K., Milne, G., Wilkinson, D., O'Shaughnessy, J., Pastore, A., Fratta, P., Shneider, N., Tartaglia, G. G., Zacco, E., Horrocks, M. H., & Gregory, J. M. (2024). RNA aptamer reveals nuclear TDP-43 pathology is an early aggregation event that coincides with STMN-2 cryptic splicing and precedes clinical manifestation in ALS. *Acta Neuropathologica, 147*(1). https://doi.org/10.1007/s00401-024-02705-1

Stati, G., Amerio, P., Nubile, M., Sancilio, S., Rossi, F., & Di Pietro, R. (2023). Concern about the effectiveness of mRNA vaccination technology and its long-term safety: Potential interference on miRNA machinery. *International Journal of Molecular Sciences, 24*(2), 1404. https://doi.org/10.3390/ijms24021404

Steinmetz, J. D., et al. (2024). Global, regional, and national burden of disorders affecting the nervous system, 1990–2021: A systematic analysis for the global Burden of Disease Study 2021. *The Lancet Neurology, 23*(4), 344–381. https://doi.org/10.1016/s1474-4422(24)00038-3

Stolte, B., Totzeck, A., Kizina, K., Bolz, S., Pietruck, L., Mönninghoff, C., Guberina, N., Oldenburg, D., Forsting, M., Kleinschnitz, C., & Hagenacker, T. (2018). Feasibility and safety of intrathecal treatment with nusinersen in adult patients with spinal muscular atrophy. *Therapeutic Advances in Neurological Disorders, 11.* https://doi.org/10.1177/1756286418803246

Sun, Y., Kong, J., Ge, X., Mao, M., Yu, H., & Wang, Y. (2023). An antisense oligonucleotide-loaded blood–brain barrier penetrable nanoparticle mediating recruitment of endogenous neural stem cells for the treatment of parkinson's disease. *ACS Nano, 17*(5), 4414–4432. https://doi.org/10.1021/acsnano.2c09752

Sun, B. L., Wang, L.h., Yang, T., Sun, J.y., Mao, L.l., Yang, M.f., Yuan, H., Colvin, R. A., & Yang, X.y. (2018). Lymphatic drainage system of the brain: A novel target for intervention of neurological diseases. *Progress in Neurobiology, 163–164*, 118–143. https://doi.org/10.1016/j.pneurobio.2017.08.007

Tan, X., Jia, F., Wang, P., & Zhang, K. (2020). Nucleic acid-based drug delivery strategies. *Journal of Controlled Release, 323*, 240–252. https://doi.org/10.1016/j.jconrel.2020.03.040

Terstappen, G. C., Meyer, A. H., Bell, R. D., & Zhang, W. (2021). Strategies for delivering therapeutics across the blood–brain barrier. *Nature Reviews Drug Discovery, 20*(5), 362–383. https://doi.org/10.1038/s41573-021-00139-y

Thirumalai, S., Patani, R., & Hung, C. (2024). Therapeutic potential of APP antisense oligonucleotides for Alzheimer's disease and down syndrome-related Alzheimer's disease. *Molecular Neurodegeneration, 19*(1). https://doi.org/10.1186/s13024-024-00745-5

Todd, N., Angolano, C., Ferran, C., Devor, A., Borsook, D., & McDannold, N. (2020). Secondary effects on brain physiology caused by focused ultrasound-mediated disruption of the blood–brain barrier. *Journal of Controlled Release, 324*, 450–459. https://doi.org/10.1016/j.jconrel.2020.05.040

Valatabar, N., Oroojalian, F., Kazemzadeh, M., Mokhtarzadeh, A. A., Safaralizadeh, R., & Sahebkar, A. (2024). Recent advances in gene delivery nanoplatforms based on spherical nucleic acids. BioMed Central Ltd. *Iran Journal of Nanobiotechnology, 22*(1). https://doi.org/10.1186/s12951-024-02648-5

Wang, Q., Cheng, S., Qin, F., Fu, A., & Fu, C. (2021). Application progress of RVG peptides to facilitate the delivery of therapeutic agents into the central nervous system. *RSC Advances, 11*(15), 8505–8515. https://doi.org/10.1039/d1ra00550b

Wang, S., Wang, H., Drabek, A., Sha Smith, W., Liang, F., & Richard Huang, Z. (2024). Unleashing the potential: Designing antibody-targeted lipid nanoparticles for industrial applications with CMC considerations and clinical outlook. *Molecular Pharmaceutics, 21*(1), 4–17. https://doi.org/10.1021/acs.molpharmaceut.3c00735

Wang, J., Yue, B. L., Huang, Y. Z., Lan, X. Y., Liu, W. J., & Chen, H. (2022). Exosomal RNAs: Novel potential biomarkers for Diseases—A review. *International Journal of Molecular Sciences, 23*(5). https://doi.org/10.3390/ijms23052461

Wen, Y. R., Yang, J. H., Wang, X., & Yao, Z. B. (2018). Induced dural lymphangiogenesis facilities soluble amyloid-beta clearance from brain in a transgenic mouse model of Alzheimer's disease. *Neural Regeneration Research, 13*(4), 709–716. https://doi.org/10.4103/1673-5374.230299

Xi, J., Eddie Yuan, J., Zhang, Y., Nevorski, D., Wang, Z., & Zhou, Y. (2016). Visualization and quantification of nasal and olfactory deposition in a sectional adult nasal Airway cast. *Pharmaceutical Research, 33*(6), 1527–1541. https://doi.org/10.1007/s11095-016-1896-2

Xie, L., He, M., Ying, C., & Chu, H. (2024). Mechanisms of inflammation after ischemic stroke in brain-peripheral crosstalk. *Frontiers in Molecular Neuroscience, 17*. https://doi.org/10.3389/fnmol.2024.1400808

Xiong, K., Wang, X., Feng, C., Zhang, K., Chen, Di, & Yang, S. (2025). Vectors in CRISPR gene editing for neurological disorders: Challenges and opportunities. *Advanced Biology, 9*(3). https://doi.org/10.1002/adbi.202400374

Xu, Y., Ma, S., Cui, H., Chen, J., Xu, S., Gong, F., Golubovic, A., Zhou, M., Chang Wang, K., Varley, A., Ze Lu, R. X., Wang, B., & Li, B. (2024). AGILE platform: A deep learning powered approach to accelerate LNP development for mRNA delivery. *Nature Communications, 15*(1). https://doi.org/10.1038/s41467-024-50619-z

Yoon, H. H., Ye, S., Lim, S., Jo, A., Lee, H., Hong, F., Lee, S. E., Oh, S. J., Kim, N. R., Kim, K., Kim, B. J., Kim, H., Lee, C. J., Nam, M. H., Hur, J. W., & Jeon, S. R. (2022). CRISPR-Cas9 gene editing protects from the A53T-SNCA overexpression-induced pathology of Parkinson's disease in vivo. *CRISPR Journal, 5*(1), 95–108. https://doi.org/10.1089/crispr.2021.0025

Yun, Y., Zhang, Y., Zhang, C., Huang, L., Tan, S., Wang, P., Vilariño-Gúell, C., Song, W., & Sun, X. (2021). Regulator of calcineurin 1 is a novel RNA-binding protein to regulate neuronal apoptosis. *Molecular Psychiatry, 26*(4), 1361–1375. https://doi.org/10.1038/s41380-019-0487-0

Zhang, Y., Ang, B. T., Xiao, Z. C., & Ng, I. (2008). DNA vaccination against neurite growth inhibitors to enhance functional recovery following traumatic brain injury. *Acta Neurochirurgica, Supplementum*, (102), 347–351. https://doi.org/10.1007/978-3-211-85578-2_66

Zhang, Z., Conniot, J., Amorim, J., Jin, Y., Prasad, R., Yan, X., Fan, K., & Conde, J. (2022). Nucleic acid-based therapy for brain cancer: Challenges and strategies. *Journal of Controlled Release, 350*, 80–92. https://doi.org/10.1016/j.jconrel.2022.08.014

Zhang, H., Gao, X., Sun, Q., Dong, X., Zhu, Z., & Yang, C. (2024). Incorporation of poly(γ-glutamic acid) in lipid nanoparticles for enhanced mRNA delivery efficiency in vitro and in vivo. *Acta Biomaterialia*, (177), 361–376. https://doi.org/10.1016/j.actbio.2024.02.004

Zhang, Y., Hao, C. G., Hu, L. Q., Dong, J., Wei, P., Xu, D., Xiao, Z. C., & Wang, T. H. (2009). Recombinant DNA vaccine against inhibition of neurite outgrowth promotes functional recovery associated with endogeous ngf expression in spinal cord hemisected adult rats. *Neurochemical Research, 34*(9), 1635–1641. https://doi.org/10.1007/s11064-009-9951-6

Zhang, L., Ma, Q., Yang, W., Qi, X., Yao, Z., Liu, Y., Liang, L., Wang, X., Ma, C., Huang, L., Xu, Y., Zhu, H., Deng, W., Gao, Y., Ruan, L., Xiao, Z., & Qin, C. (2013). Recombinant DNA vaccine against neurite outgrowth inhibitors attenuates behavioral deficits and decreases Abeta in an Alzheimer's disease mouse model. *Neuropharmacology, 70*, 200–210. https://doi.org/10.1016/j.neuropharm.2012.10.023

Zhang, L., Wu, T., Shan, Y., Li, G., Ni, X., Chen, X., Hu, X., Lin, L., Li, Y., Guan, Y., Gao, J., Chen, D., Zhang, Y., Pei, Z., & Chen, X. (2021). Therapeutic reversal of Huntington's disease by in vivo self-assembled siRNAs. *Brain, 144*(11), 3421–3435. https://doi.org/10.1093/brain/awab354

Zheng, Y., Qu, J., Xue, F., Zheng, Y., Yang, B., Chang, Y., Yang, H., & Zhang, J. (2018). Novel DNA aptamers for parkinson's disease treatment inhibit α-Synuclein aggregation and facilitate its degradation. *Molecular Therapy - Nucleic Acids*, (11), 228–242. https://doi.org/10.1016/j.omtn.2018.02.011

Zheng, Y., Zhang, L., Zhao, J., Li, L., Wang, M., Gao, P., Wang, Q., Zhang, X., & Wang, W. (2022). Advances in aptamers against Aβ and applications in Aβ detection and regulation for Alzheimer's disease. *Theranostics, 12*(5), 2095–2114. https://doi.org/10.7150/thno.69465

Zhuo, Z., Yu, Y., Wang, M., Li, J., Zhang, Z., Liu, J., Wu, X., Lu, A., Zhang, G., & Zhang, B. (2017). Recent advances in SELEX technology and aptamer applications in biomedicine. *International Journal of Molecular Sciences, 18*(10), 2142. https://doi.org/10.3390/ijms18102142

Zimmermann, P., & Curtis, N. (2019). Factors that influence the immune response to vaccination. *Clinical Microbiology Reviews, 32*(2). https://doi.org/10.1128/cmr.00084-18

CHAPTER

Therapeutic potential of immune cells for neurological disorders

8

Anisha David[1] and J. Deepa Arul Priya[2]

[1]*Department of Biology, St. Joseph's University, Bengaluru, Karnataka, India;* [2]*Department of Biotechnology, Sri Paramakalyani College, Alwarkurichi, Tamil Nadu, India*

1. Introduction

Neurological disorders like multiple sclerosis (MS), Parkinson's disease (PD), Alzheimer's disease (AD), stroke, and Amyotrophic lateral sclerosis (ALS) collectively affect millions of people worldwide and remain largely incurable with conventional pharmacotherapies (Sheikh et al., 2013). To date, there are more than 600 brain disorders falling into four sets of conditions, like sudden onset, intermittent, progressive and stable (Liu et al., 2021). Some diseases reveal cognitive and memory disability, some affect movements. Some are associated with genetic factors, and some are etiologically unresolved (Pasko et al., 2023). Although there are many conventional therapies available currently, they only alleviate the symptoms and fail to slow or reverse the progression of these diseases (Kumar et al., 2024).

The typical symptom of most of these diseases is the gradual disruption of neural cells and synaptic connections. The mechanism by which the immune system and nervous system mediate as a response to external stimuli, injury or the aggregation of defective proteins is termed neuroinflammation. This process shows a dual nature as a double-edged sword, as detrimental when dysregulated and beneficial when acting as a defense to protect. In defense mode, the immune cells are recruited to get rid of the stimulating factors, clearing the debris and starting repair mechanisms. The initiation of repair to dampen the inflammatory response kicks off with the activation of microglia and astrocytes (Xu, Huang, & Zhou, 2025). This leads to alteration in transcriptional profile, expression of surface molecular markers and secretion of inflammatory mediators (cytokines and chemokines) (Jain & Yong, 2022).

The blood-brain barrier (BBB) endothelial cells are connected with tight junctions and adherens that limit diapedesis due to low expression of adhesion molecules. The inflammatory molecules upregulate the expression and permeabilize the BBB, thus increasing lymphocytic movement (Maurya et al., 2023). The early immune response is stimulated by the infiltration of macrophages, followed by adaptive immune cells (T and B lymphocytes). T cells aid other immune cells in performing immunoregulatory functions to destroy pathogenic or infectious cells. After debris clearance, T cells are restored in the central nervous system (CNS) as memory cells to destroy or dampen, in case of reinfection (Passaro et al., 2021). In neuropathology, this defense mechanism becomes unbalanced and

Immunotherapies for Neurological Disorders. https://doi.org/10.1016/B978-0-443-44631-3.00011-1

persistent due to the secretion of reactive oxygen and pro-inflammatory molecules by activated glial cells in a prolonged process. This turns into a chronic condition where neuronal malfunction is observed with intensified protein aggregation and uncontrolled disease progression (Dash et al., 2025).

The CNS was historically viewed as an immune-privileged site isolated from immune surveillance. This concept emphasizes that the CNS, compared with peripheral organs, is privileged with the presence of the BBB and the absence of lymphatic drainage. Recent studies have revealed that neuroimmune crosstalk, especially at borders, are recognized as immunological sites (Smyth & Kipnis, 2025). These are the meningeal region, choroid plexus, perivascular region and meningeal lymphatic vessels (MLVs) (Masuda et al., 2022; Robert et al., 2023; Rustenhoven et al., 2023; Salvador et al., 2024). These sites are in contact with the cerebrospinal fluid (CSF, immune mediator) to protect the CNS parenchyma from inflammatory damage through controlled immune surveillance. Understanding the mechanism behind immune privilege can give a main focus on targeted immunotherapies (Smyth & Kipnis, 2025).

The regulatory T cells (Tregs), regulatory B cells (Bregs), regulatory Dendritic cells (DCs), macrophages and monocytes act as natural checkpoints of a healthy immune system, mitigating the detrimental inflammation resulting from the immune response. Consequently, these regulatory immune cells hold great potential as novel cell-based therapies for neurological disorders, thereby reducing overdependence on medications that only mask clinical symptoms (Hu et al., 2018; Jie et al., 2026). Therefore, research in immunotherapeutic approaches has gained momentum in the last few years for the treatment of neurological disorders (Weiner, 2025). This chapter focuses on the mechanistic insights, preclinical efficacy, clinical translational efforts and the barriers to therapeutic implementation.

2. Immune system and central nervous system: A bidirectional crosstalk

2.1 Immune-privileged site

The CNS is the command center and a highly specialized system in vertebrates, which mainly includes the brain and spinal cord. The functional complexity of the CNS, with a delicate, organized neural network structure for receiving information, integrating and coordinating the body's responses, requires a homeostatic environment (Rouleau et al., 2023). For decades, the historic view of CNS as an immune-privileged site (organ with tolerance for foreign grafts) implied seclusion from peripheral immunological surveillance for its maintenance and repair. This was explained with perceptions as the presence of BBB to inhibit the efferent arm to restrict immune cell entry and the absence of lymphatic vessels to inhibit the afferent arm to drain antigens. But the conflation between isolation and privilege led to refining the neuro-immune mechanisms (Galea et al., 2007; Medawar, 1948).

2.2 Immune surveillance

In the early 20th century, a study revealed that access to CSF, which is associated with CNS borders, is critical for immune surveillance (Fig. 8.1). This was further supported by the 'glymphatic hypothesis' which described, CSF and Interstitial fluid (ISF) get exchanged for waste removal (Iliff et al., 2012). The epithelial cells present in the choroid plexus secrete CSF, which circulates into the subarachnoid space (SAS) between the leptomeninges layers (pia mater and arachnoid mater). The pia mater

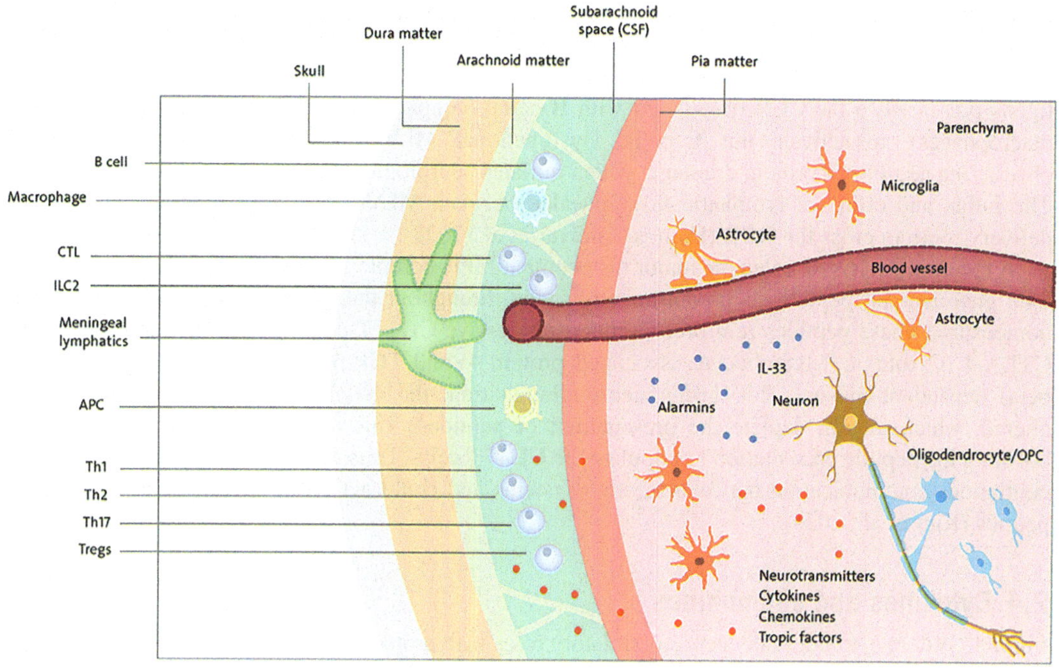

FIGURE 8.1 Neuroimmune Interfaceat CNS Borders.

Immune surveillance by innate and adaptive immune cells with mediators like cytokines, chemokines, neurotransmitters and tropic factors.

From Matejuk, A., Vandenbark, A.A., & Offner, H. (2021). Cross-talk of the CNS with immune cells and functions in health and disease. Frontiers in Neurology, 12 (672455), 1-19. 10.3389/fneur.2021.672455.

(innermost layer) facilitates exchange between the fluids and adhesion of immune cells, but arachnoid barrier cells present in the arachnoid mater (outer layer) limit the exchange and repel adhesion. The CSF and associated antigens from SAS cross the arachnoid cuff exits around the bridging veins and enter the dura mater. The dura mater (outermost layer), which borders the arachnoid barrier, contains molecules that also repel adhesion and regulate ISF composition to validate immune cell trafficking. The CSF mixes with the ISF and gets drained by MLVs. These lymphatics merge into collecting vessels, which end up draining into cervical lymph nodes (CLN), which behave as hubs for the neuroimmune communication (Smyth & Kipnis, 2025).

2.3 Meningeal lymphatic vessels (MLVs)

MLVs existence and their vital part in carrying metabolic wastes to the CLN were confirmed in 2015 (Louveau et al., 2015). MLVs require constant VEGF-C (Vascular endothelial growth factor C, lymphatic marker) signaling for its development, maintenance and modulation. The function of MLVs can be summarized in two aspects: waste drainage and immune surveillance. During drainage, MLVs maintain fluid dynamics in the brain by regulating the release of waste metabolites, enabling normal cognitive function. The drainage capacity of basal MLVs is more compared to dorsal MLVs due to their capillary mechanism. During immune cell drainage, MLVs regulate both (pro and anti) inflammatory responses to maintain homeostasis. The drainage efficiency decides the quantity of antigens presented to the CLN (populated with B cells) compared to the dura mater (populated with macrophages), to activate the T cells. Dysfunctional MLVs modulate neuroinflammation by obstructing neurotoxic protein drainage, which initiates neurological disorders (Salvador et al., 2024). The influx and efflux of lymphatic flow revealed between MLVs and CLN suggested a new drug delivery route to cross the BBB (Ramos-Zaldívar et al., 2024).

A recent work has revealed the major histocompatibility complex (MHC-II) peptidome of the CNS with guardian self-peptides is predominantly found throughout the lymphatic drainage pathway. In homeostasis, these peptides reinforce immunosuppressive $CD4^{+}$T cells to spur up suppression in a CTLA-4 (Cytotoxic T-lymphocyte associated protein 4) and TGF-β (Transforming Growth Factor-beta) dependent manner. But during neuroinflammation, the antigen processing mechanisms are altered, which in turn deplete the presentation of peptides. This condition can be overturned by boosting the peptide presentation to populate the $CD4^{+}$T cells. Thus, regulatory self-peptides ensure a continuous communication between the two systems and could act as an attractive route for therapeutics (Kim et al., 2025).

2.4 Cytokines and chemokines

Immune system cytokines play neuromodulatory roles with protective mechanisms in homeostasis and persistent neuroinflammation in disorders. Varied sets of signaling molecules, such as IFNs (Interferons), ILs (Interleukins), TNFs (Tumor necrosis factors), chemokines and cognate receptors, regulate the neural circuit system. Pro-inflammatory cytokines like IL-1β, IL-6 and TNF-α are linked with many neurological diseases. These cytokines activate NF-κB (Nuclear Factor kappa B) and JAK/STAT (Janus Kinase/Signal Transducer and Activator of Transcription) signaling pathways by disrupting the BBB. The tight junction proteins' expression is lowered with an increase in MMPs (Matrix metalloproteinases) expression that weakens the BBB by permitting the influx of molecules, thereby aggravating inflammation (Mallick et al., 2025).

Chemokines are small proteins (8–12 kDa) with three or four conserved cysteine residues. Their role in the interplay between the nervous and immune system is mediated by biased signaling (ligand bias, receptor bias, tissue bias) to activate molecular signaling pathways. Chemokines are regulated by post-translational modification for activation and binding affinity (ligand-receptor bonding). Chemokine receptors are involved in signaling cascades like G-protein pathway, PKC-β (Protein Kinase C beta, regulates cytosolic Ca^{2+} levels), MAPK (Mitogen-Activated Protein Kinase, affects neuronal loss), p38 MAPK (regulates synaptic plasticity), PI3K/AKT/ERK ½ (Phosphoinositide 3-kinase/Protein kinase B/Extracellular signal-regulated kinase ½, regulates apoptosis and neuroprotection) and NF-κB and JAKs. The complicated interplay of signaling molecules in the CNS emphasizes the need for combination therapies to restore normal function (Sowa & Tokarski, 2021).

Despite the CNS being shielded with anatomical barriers to protect from pathogens, circulating immune cells and blood factors, it is not fully obscured from the immune system. Under homeostatic conditions, the brain plasticity, cognition and neuroprotection are promoted by the immune system through short-range or long-range interactions. Thus, the CNS have a unique bidirectional communication between the wired neuronal circuits and the wireless immune system, which differs from other peripheral organs. The immune privilege principles thus govern the CNS from immune-mediated damage with controlled immune surveillance (Smyth et al., 2024).

3. Pathophysiological role of immune cells in neurological disorders

The role of neuro-immune crosstalk in shaping the brain from the developmental stage to maintaining homeostasis till aging involves several innate and adaptive immune responses (Fig. 8.2). Inflammation is a natural defense mechanism to protect the body from injury, pathogens and infection. In pathological conditions, the inflammatory damage of neural structures by internal or external factors is irreversible, which leads to acute or chronic infections in the CNS. But in a beneficial role, the resident immune cells release signaling molecules to recruit adaptive cells. These cells differentiate functionally based on the degree of infection and phagocytose to carry out the repair mechanism. The role can turn out to be detrimental if the overexpression of immune cells is not suppressed. So understanding the molecular mechanisms of macrophages, glial cells, lymphocytes and killer cells in neuro-immune communication would lead us to find effective immunotherapies for neurological disorders (Xu et al., 2022).

3.1 Microglia

Microglia are resident macrophages and primary innate cells found abundantly in the brain parenchyma, exerting functions which are region-specific either in the neonatal or adult brain. They serve as immune sentinels while patrolling and participate in brain health by modulating brain development, synaptic pruning, repair mechanisms by secreting anti-inflammatory cytokines, debris clearance by phagocytosis, neurotrophic factors secretion and supporting metabolism of neurons and other glial cells. Microglia display interchangeable and coexisting activation states (M1, M2) according to the stimuli or course of a disease. M1 (classical activation) is a pro-inflammatory phenotype with neurotoxic effect and secretes IL-1β, IL-6, TNF-α and ROS (Reactive Oxygen Species). M2 (alternative activation) is an anti-inflammatory phenotype with neuroprotective effect, secreting IL-10, TGF-β, IL-4 and IL-13. In case of injury, microglia release pro-inflammatory molecules to initiate an inflammatory response, which recruits lymphocytes to assist phagocytosis. In case of tissue regeneration, anti-inflammatory molecules are released to revoke inflammation (Paolicelli et al., 2022). When activated during neuroinflammation, they become detrimental due to excessive restoration of protein aggregates, a condition observed in neurodegeneration. The specific phenotypic markers expressed at steady-state are TMEM119 (Transmembrane protein 119) and P2RY12 (Purinergic receptor). The rapid transition in morphology during disease conditions downregulates these markers along with other homeostatic markers (Holtman et al., 2017).

3.2 Border-associated macrophages

BAMs are non-parenchymal macrophages found in the borders between the brain and the peripheral tissues with diversified subsets. Each subset with a unique morphological signature and transcriptomic profile carries out specialized functions in immune surveillance and homeostasis regulation. The meningeal macrophages act as the first line of defense against microbial infection and the entry portal for infiltrating immune cells. Based on location, they are classified as dural and leptomeningeal macrophages. In adults, they can be further subdivided into two based on MHC II expression (Utz et al., 2020). Dural vasculature is enriched with immune cells due to high expression of adhesion molecules, which enables dural macrophages to serve as APCs (Antigen-presenting cells). Leptomeningeal macrophages

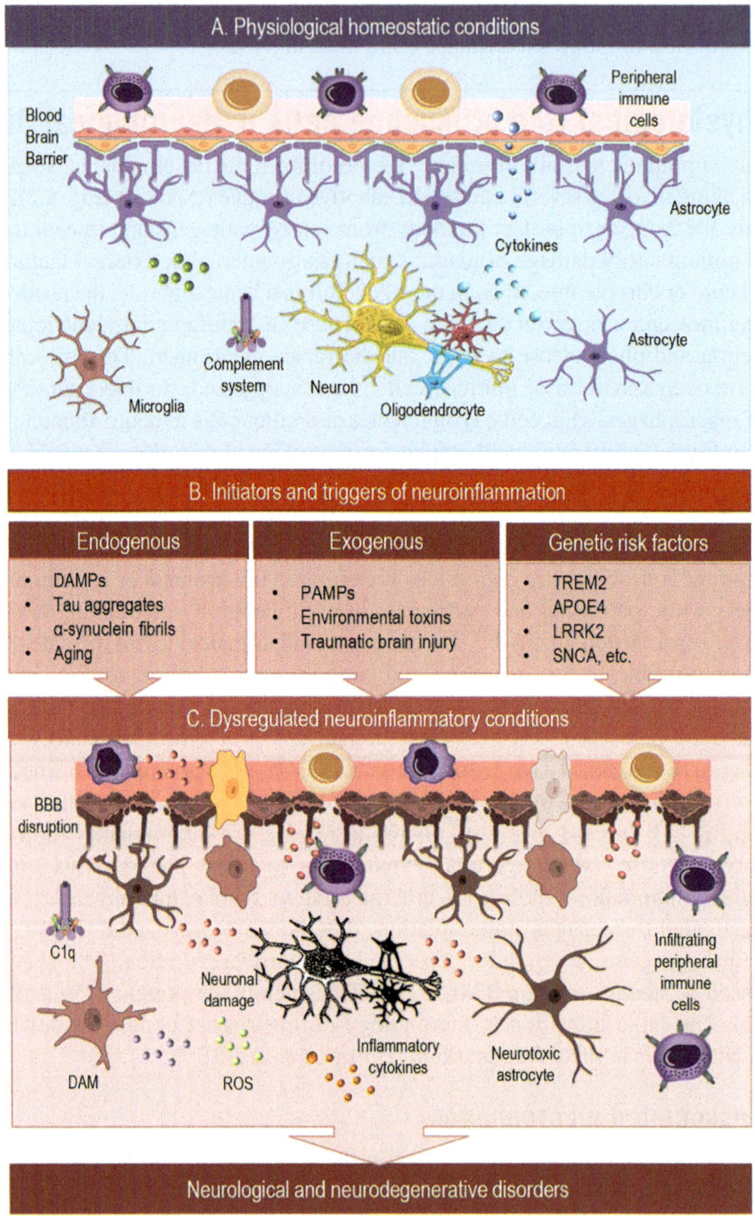

FIGURE 8.2 CNS in Health and Disease.

(A) – Under homeostatic conditions, role of resident cells by releasing signaling molecules to maintain balanced immune surveillance and prevent excessive immune activity. (B) – Triggering agents which leads to neuroinflammation. (C) – Under pathological conditions, resident cells are activated, BBB is disrupted, infiltration of peripheral immune cells leads to disease progression.

From Müller, L., Di Benedetto, S., & Müller, V. (2025). The dual nature of neuroinflammation in networked brain. Frontiers in Immunology, 16(1659947), 1-13. 10.3389/fimmu.2025.1659947.

are found more in SAS, which limits their contact with peripheral immune cells. Even then, autoantigen presentation is more efficient compared to dural, which leads to more T cell infiltration (Zhan et al., 2024). Perivascular macrophages, a subset of BAM, depending on the perivascular localization fulfill functions like sustaining CNS homeostasis, antigen presentation, phagocytosis, maintaining BBB integrity and neuroprotection (Zhan et al., 2025). Choroid plexus macrophages (epiplexus cells and stromal) play an active role in choroid plexus immunity, clearing cellular debris and barrier functioning. Epiplexus cells are mobile and show saltatory movements, whereas stromal cells are stationary and non-motile (Shipley et al., 2020). BAMs express specific markers [LYVE 1 (Lymphatic Vessel Endothelial Hyaluronan Receptor 1), CD38, CD206, MHC II] that help them to differentiate from microglia. During infections, BAMs sustain long-term transcriptional alterations and are replaced by inflammatory monocytes, which overturn their beneficial role (Mrdjen et al., 2018).

3.3 Astrocytes

Astrocytes (star-like cells) (Lenhossék, 1895), a subtype of glial cells, populate the brain from embryogenesis to parenchymal astrocytes in adulthood through symmetric division. Astrocytes provide crucial support for brain health by participating in ion signal transmission between neurons, pH homeostasis, structural support, regulation of metabolic processes, synaptogenesis modulation, neurotransmitter uptake and recycling, neuroprotection, axon myelination, maintaining BBB integrity and secretion of neurotrophic factors to promote neurogenesis (Verkhratsky et al., 2021). They display two distinct reactive states, A1 - inflammatory/neurotoxic and A2 - neuroprotective (Reid & Kuipers, 2021). Astrocytes produce and respond to inflammatory mediators (IL-6, TNF-α, TNF-β), such as cytokines and chemokines, as an early immune defense mechanism, to promote debris clearance and repair. Astrogliosis is a phenotypic shift undergone in response to inflammation, where reactive astrocytes form a fibrous scar to envelope the injured site in a beneficial role. The outcome can become detrimental if astrocyte dysfunction leads to metabolic disruption, glutamate excitotoxicity and synaptic function alteration, which inhibits regenerative processes (Hart & Karimi-Abdolrezaee, 2021). Among the multifaceted roles in neuroinflammation, the upregulation of GFAP (Glial Fibrillary Acidic Protein), a cytochemical marker, is characterized by morphological changes (Hol & Pekny, 2015).

3.4 Lymphocytes

T cells are vital components of the adaptive immune system, which play key roles in CNS immunity. Hematopoietic stem cells after maturation produce T cell precursors, which shift to the thymus, where T cell receptors are developed to recognize specific antigens dispensed by MHC molecules to trigger immune responses against stimuli. This APC activation forms a peptide-MHC complex to multiply and segregate T cells into their subsets according to their functions (Shokr, 2025). $CD4^+$ helper T cells play a significant role in connecting the immune responses to release cytokines to influence other immune cells. Th1 cells secrete TNF-α and IFN-γ to induce cell-mediated immunity in intracellular infections. Th2 cells secrete IL-4, IL-5 and IL-13 to induce humoral immunity. Th17 cells secrete IL-17 and IL-22 to induce inflammation and defense mechanisms against microbial infections. Treg cells, expressed by transcription factor FoxP3, are involved in homeostasis and immunosuppression of activated effector T cells along with other immune cells. $CD8^+$ cytotoxic T cells, when activated, secrete granzymes and perforins, which induce apoptosis and eliminate target cells (Raphael et al., 2015). Hence, these multifunctional T cell subsets, when dysregulated, can lead to immunodeficiency or inflammatory disorders (Shokr, 2025). With the onset of inflammation or injury, the BBB integrity is disturbed, allowing migration of T cells. After the penetration, a dynamic interchange happens in the CNS, which kick-starts a pro-inflammatory response according to the insult. Cytokines and chemokines are released by the resident cells to come into contact with the brain endothelial cells to express adhesion molecules (selectins) (Alcaide, 2022). After adhesion, T cells undergo diapedesis and move into the endothelium paracellularly or transcellularly. The rate of T cell infiltration depends on the severity of the stimuli, BBB permeability and disease condition (Shokr, 2025).

B cells, also a part of the adaptive immune system, develop and differentiate in multiple stages and mature from hematopoietic stem cells. With T follicular helper cells and specific antigen exposure, B cells are activated and differentiated into antibody-producing plasma cells and memory B cells. The primary function of B cells includes antibody production and acting as APCs (Lebien & Tedder, 2008). Breg cells are immunosuppressive in nature and are found along with B cells in every developmental stage (Mauri & Bosma, 2012). Upon injury, B cells act as immune modulators by secreting anti- and pro-inflammatory mediators to reduce inflammation. In healthy conditions, parenchyma B cells are rarely found in the CNS and infiltrating immune cells as a small fraction in CSF. B cells are infiltrated through transmigration, initiated by chemokines for the upregulation of adhesion molecules to undergo diapedesis (Aspden et al., 2023).

3.5 Innate lymphoid cells

ILCs are tissue-resident lymphocytes that react early to inflammatory insults and maintain homeostasis even when lacking antigen receptors. NK cells, ILC1, ILC2, and ILC3 are grouped under the ILC family based on their function, transcription factor expression and cytokine secretion profile (Vivier et al., 2018). In the steady state, ILCs are present significantly in the meninges and the choroid plexus but not in the parenchyma. But during inflammation or infections, ILCs infiltrate into the parenchyma (Kveštak et al., 2024).

3.6 Gamma delta T cells

γδT cells are a subset of T cells found in the meninges, which mainly regulate homeostasis and BBB integrity. These cells are programmed in the thymus and exhibit cytotoxicity and cytokine secretion upon activation. γδT cells respond immediately upon infection or injury to regulate immune responses by bridging innate and adaptive immunity. They are resistant to MHC-mediated antigen presentation but recognize microbial molecules, stress-inducing molecules and phosphoantigens. The two functional subsets are - IFN-γ producing γδT cells (antiviral and antitumoral) and IL-17A producing γδT cells (antifungal or autoimmunity). IL-17A, found in the meninges, gets infiltrated into the parenchyma during inflammation (Park et al., 2022).

3.7 Innate-like T cells

Mucosal-associated invariant T cells (MAIT) and Natural killer T cells (NKT) are innate-like T cells which share similar characteristics. MAIT cells identify microbial-derived vitamin B-derived metabolites presented by the MHC class I-related molecule (MR1), and NKT cells identify lipid antigens presented by the MHC class 1-like CD1d molecule. Both cells exhibit antimicrobial and antitumor properties by releasing anti- and pro-inflammatory cytokines. Their pathophysiological role in neurological disease still remains elusive (Wyatt-Johnson et al., 2024).

3.8 Immune cells in CNS diseases

According to several studies, in MS, the microglial activation downregulates P2RY12 and TMEM119 and upregulates CD68, p22phox (Phagocyte oxidase 22-kDa subunit), APOE (Apolipoprotein E) and MAFB (Musculoaponeurotic Fibrosarcoma Oncogene Homolog B) markers (Zrzavy et al., 2017). In AD, studies suggest that the TREM2 (Triggering receptor expressed on myeloid cells 2) marker in microglia upon activation plays a protective role in early stages of disease, but when mutated, it increases the risk at later stages by responding as a pro-inflammatory phenotype (Onuska, 2020). Microglial activation by NLRP3 (NOD-, LRR- and pyrin domain-containing protein 3) inflammasome and upregulation of CSF1R (Colony-stimulating factor 1 receptor) can also contribute to AD pathology (Akiyama et al., 1994; Saresella et al., 2016).

In ALS, with the disease onset, SOD1 (Superoxide dismutase 1), TDP-43 (TAR-DNA binding protein-43), and C9orf72 (Chromosome 9open reading frame 72) undergo mutations (Clarke & Patani, 2020). Activated microglia act as a pro-inflammatory phenotype, exerting neuron degeneration by secreting cytokines (IL-1β, TNF, IL-6) to suppress homeostatic markers (Liao et al., 2012). In PD, α-synuclein oligomers activate microglia through TLR2 (Toll-like receptor 2) and hinder phagocytosis, thereby reducing clearance of defective α-synuclein (Kim et al., 2013).

In MS, the inflammatory phase starts with the leakage in the BBB, where the effector T cells ($CD4^+$ T cells, Th1, Th17, $CD8^+$ T cells and Tregcells) infiltrate into the CNS and play a crucial role in pathogenesis (Ortiz et al., 2014). $CD8^+$ T cells are found in perivascular lesions and express IL-17, which derails the regulatory function of the cells (Fransen et al., 2020). KIR^+CD8^+ Treg (Killer cell immunoglobulin-like receptors$^+CD8^+$ Treg) cells are expressed more while $CD4^+CD25^+FOXP3^{+-}$ Treg ($CD4^+CD25^+$Forkhead box $P3^+$Treg) cells and Th17 phenotype are expressed in low levels, revealing abnormality in diseased condition (Li et al., 2022; Verma et al., 2021). Dysfunction of Breg is identified by decreased IL-10 production (Knippenberg et al., 2011).

In AD, dysregulated expression of Th1, Th17 and JKAP (Jun N-terminal kinase pathway-associated phosphatase) T cells, declined levels of Th2 and $CDC42^+$ (Cell division cycle 42^+) increased levels of $CD8^+$ T cells and depletion of Treg cells, upon activation, impairs cognitive learning (Unger et al., 2020; Zeng et al., 2022; Zhang & Niu, 2022). $CD3^+$ T cell infiltration levels were correlated with tau but not with Aβ pathology (Merlini et al., 2018).

In ALS, at the initial stage, Th2 and Tregcells respond with a protective role, but gradually they are replaced with Th1, Th17 pro-inflammatory response at a later stage (Jin et al., 2020). Increased level of $CD8^+$ T cells destroyed motor neurons and thereby leading to dysfunction of neuronal function in peripheral nerves (Campisi et al., 2022).

In PD, $CD4^+$ T cell levels were decreased, while HLA-DR^+ (Human Leukocyte Antigen – DR isotype) T cells and $CD45RO^+$ memory T cells levels were increased. Tregcells were reduced in number, which made them insufficient to suppress effector T cell function (Saunders et al., 2012).

4. Immune cell–based therapeutic strategies

4.1 Brief overview of strategies

Promising results from preclinical studies and early clinical trials have generated significant interest in immune cell-based therapies for neurological disorders (Hu et al., 2018) Table 8.1. To enhance the number and function of regulatory immune cells - such as Tregs, Bregs, tolerogenic dendritic cells, and

Table 8.1 List of preclinical and clinical studies using immune-cell–based therapies for neurological disorders.

S. No.	Cell type	Model/Disease	Therapeutic approach	Key outcome	References
1	Anti-CD19 CAR T cells	Refractory myasthenia gravis	Autologous CAR T-cell infusion	Sustained clinical remission, reduced autoantibody titers, manageable CRS; drug-free follow-up up to 12 months	Haghikia et al. (2024)
2	Autologous tregs (adoptive transfer)	Alzheimer's disease (AD)	Intravenous infusion of ex vivo–expanded autologous tregs (GB301)	Phase I trial (NCT03865017); ongoing-preclinical data show reduced amyloid plaques and improved cognition	Jie et al. (2026)
	Low-dose IL-2	AD, ALS, MS	Subcutaneous low-dose IL-2 to expand endogenous tregs	Phase I/II trials (NCT05468073, NCT03039673, NCT05245344); preliminary safety confirmed; increased Treg frequency and IL-10 production	Jie et al. (2026)
3	B-cell depletion (anti-CD20 mAbs)	Relapsing-remitting and primary progressive MS	Rituximab, ocrelizumab, ofatumumab (approved monoclonal antibodies)	>94% reduction in new MRI lesions; 46%–47% reduction in relapse rate; slowed disability in inflammatory PPMS	Kanatas et al. (2023)
	Autologous treg adoptive transfer	Parkinson's disease mice	Co-transplanted with dopaminergic neurons	Feasible and safe; enhanced graft survival	Park et al. (2023)
4	Tregs (adoptive transfer)	Middle cerebral artery occlusion (MCAO) mice (stroke model)	IV injection of $CD4^+CD25^+$ tregs	Enhanced white matter repair, reduced microglial activation, improved motor recovery	Ito et al. (2019a)

Table 8.1 List of preclinical and clinical studies using immune-cell–based therapies for neurological disorders.—cont'd

S. No.	Cell type	Model/Disease	Therapeutic approach	Key outcome	References
5	Tregs (adoptive transfer)	SOD1-G93A mice (ALS model)	IL-2/anti–IL-2 complex to expand tregs	Slowed disease progression, prolonged survival, reduced neuroinflammation	Sheean et al. (2018)
6	Microglia modulation (TREM2 agonism)	AD mice (Alzheimer's model)	TREM2 agonistic antibody that increases TREM2 activity	Enhanced Aβ phagocytosis, reduced plaque burden, shift toward protective microglial phenotype	Xu et al. (2019)

anti-inflammatory macrophages and monocytes - researchers have developed a range of therapeutic strategies.

Adoptive cell transfer (ACT) - This strategy involves the infusion of cultured immune cells to a patient during the therapy. The process involves isolating, expanding and sometimes genetically modifying them (to enhance their function) before infusion. If immune cells are derived from the patient, it is autologous (self), and if the cells are derived from banked umbilical cord blood or from human thymuses (removed during pediatric cardiac surgery), it is referred to as non-autologous (non-self). Depending on how urgently the infusion is required, immune cells can be derived from either of the above-mentioned ways. ACT requires a large number of high-purity immune cells, and it usually takes several weeks to culture them; therefore, while treating patients with abrupt brain injuries like stroke, non-autologous immune cells like Tregs provide an avenue (Jie et al., 2026).

In vivo induction of immune cells - This strategy involves in vivo recruitment and activation of endogenous immune cells to facilitate the expansion of specific immune cells as a therapy for neurological disorders. In recent years, in vivo induction of immune cells has greatly advanced, involving activation of endogenous Tregs, Cell-free engineering strategies and targeted delivery of immunomodulators to convert effector T cells into Tregs (Jie et al., 2026).

(a) In situ recruitment and activation of immune cells - This strategy modulates the local immune microenvironment by selective recruitment and activation of specific immune cells. Such specific activation significantly improves therapeutic outcomes while preserving the host's immune defense against other infections.

(b) Cell-free engineering strategies - Extracellular vesicles (EV), particularly exosomes, represent the key components of cell-free engineering strategies. They are 30–150 nm in diameter, rich in biologically active molecules like proteins, lipids and nucleic acids (like mRNA and miRNA), reflecting the characteristics of the parent cells. Interestingly, when these EVs are delivered to specific cells or tissues, they modulate the functions of the recipient cells. Exosomes derived from Tregs are particularly enriched with various anti-inflammatory molecules and factors, which suppress the activity of effector T cells and promote tissue-specific immune tolerance. The natural biocompatibility and low immunogenicity of the EVs position them as ideal carriers and effectors for cell-free therapies. Moreover, through genetic engineering or chemical modifications, artificially designed bioactive molecules can be delivered to regulate in vivo cell behavior and immune responses without the need for live cells, thus avoiding complexities and risks associated with cell-based therapies (Jie et al., 2026).

The main advantages of immune cell therapy in neurological disorders include avoidance of toxicity associated with the drug regimens and the potential for reversal of the underlying disease processes. Especially, the ACT is considered a 'Living treatment' where the transferred cells continue to proliferate in the patient and continue to provide the benefit from sustained treatment over a long course.

4.2 Microglia-targeted therapies

Microglia, the resident immune cells of the CNS, play dual roles in neurodegenerative diseases - both protective and pathogenic - depending on their activation state, disease stage, and microenvironmental cues. Recent advances have revealed that microglial dysfunction contributes significantly to the progression of AD, PD, ALS, and other neurological disorders. Consequently, therapeutic strategies that selectively modulate or replace dysfunctional microglia have emerged as promising avenues for disease modification. The following three principal approaches are currently under preclinical and clinical investigation.

(a) Microglial transplantation and reprogramming - This involves the transplantation of healthy, exogenously derived microglia-like cells into the CNS to replace or augment impaired endogenous populations. Advances in stem cell biology now allow for the efficient derivation of microglia-like cells from human induced pluripotent stem cells (iPSCs) that closely mimic native microglial functionality, including phagocytosis, cytokine secretion, and response to disease-associated signals (Gao et al., 2023). An alternative to cell transplantation is in situ reprogramming, which involves direct conversion of resident CNS cells (e.g., astrocytes or NG2 glia) into functional microglia-like cells. This approach bypasses the need for invasive delivery and leverages the brain's intrinsic cellular reservoir. While still in early experimental stages, such reprogramming strategies hold potential for restoring homeostatic microglial functions. Notably, in mouse models of neurodegeneration, transplantation of healthy microglia or microglia-like cells has been shown to reduce protein aggregation, dampen neuroinflammation, and improve cognitive or motor outcomes (Abud et al., 2017; Chadarevian et al., 2025). A recent work demonstrated that microglial depletion followed by repopulation attenuated perineuronal net loss in a Huntington's disease model, underscoring their role in synaptic integrity (Crapser et al., 2020; Gao et al., 2023).

(b) Pharmacological modulation - Pharmacological strategies aim to fine-tune microglial activity without eliminating the entire population. Two major therapeutic targets highlighted in recent literature are CSF1R and TREM2. CSF1R inhibitors (e.g., PLX3397/pexidartinib, PLX5622) transiently deplete microglia by blocking survival signaling. Following withdrawal, the CNS is repopulated by microglia exhibiting a rejuvenated, homeostatic phenotype with enhanced phagocytic capacity. In AD mouse models, this "reset" strategy reduced amyloid plaque and improved cognitive function. However, timing is critical; late-stage depletion may fail to rescue neurodegeneration despite reducing inflammation, as seen in models of multiple system atrophy

(MSA) (Gao et al., 2023). TREM2 agonists represent a more nuanced approach. TREM2 is a microglia-specific receptor that promotes phagocytosis, lipid metabolism, and transition to a protective "disease-associated microglia" (DAM) phenotype. Loss-of-function variants (e.g., R47H) increase AD risk, underscoring its neuroprotective role. Agonistic antibodies (e.g., AL002c) that enhance TREM2 signaling have shown efficacy in preclinical models: they boost Aβ clearance, reduce tau pathology, and improve cognition (Schlepckow et al., 2020; Wang et al., 2020; Zhao et al., 2022). AL002c is currently in Phase 2 clinical trials for early AD (NCT04592874), marking a significant translational milestone. Other pharmacological agents under study include NOD-like receptor protein 3 (NLRP3) inflammasome inhibitors (e.g., MCC950/Inzomelid), myeloperoxidase (MPO) inhibitors (e.g., verdiperstat), and Peroxysome proliferator-activated receptors (PPARγ) or AMP-activated protein kinase (AMPK) activators, all of which shift microglia toward an anti-inflammatory, phagocytic state (Gao et al., 2023; Gordon et al., 2018).

(c) Microglial replacement by peripheral monocytes - Although microglia are largely self-renewing and of embryonic yolk sac origin, near complete ablation (via CSF1R inhibition combined with irradiation or genetic models) creates a permissive niche for infiltration and long-term engraftment of bone marrow-derived monocytes, which differentiate into microglia-like cells in the CNS. These monocyte-derived cells can acquire microglial morphology and express key markers (e.g., Ionized calcium-binding adaptor molecule - 1 (Iba1), TMEM119), though their functional equivalence to microglia remains debated. Nevertheless, this plasticity offers a therapeutic window: monocytes can be genetically engineered ex vivo (e.g., to overexpress TREM2, APOE2, or lysosomal enzymes) before reintroduction, enabling targeted correction in monogenic neurodegenerative disorders (Gao et al., 2023).

4.3 Macrophage-based interventions

While microglia constitute the brain's resident immune population, peripheral monocyte-derived macrophages (MDMs) can infiltrate the CNS under pathological conditions and significantly influence the neuro-inflammatory dynamics. MDMs have a higher phagocytic activity than microglia, promote tissue repair and the resolution of inflammation. Unlike microglia, macrophages are accessible to ex vivo manipulation, making them attractive vehicles for cell-based immunotherapies in neurodegenerative disorders. The two principal strategies that are under active investigation have been discussed here.

(a) Adoptive Transfer of M2-like Macrophages - Macrophages exhibit remarkable phenotypic plasticity and can be polarized along a continuum ranging from a pro-inflammatory (M1-like) state to an anti-inflammatory, tissue-reparative (M2-like) phenotype. M2-macrophages secrete trophic factors (e.g., IGF-1, TGF-β) and anti-inflammatory cytokines (e.g., IL-10), that promote clearance of protein aggregates, and dampen chronic neuro-inflammation (Xiao & Yang, 2025). Preclinical studies demonstrate that systemic or intrathecal delivery of ex vivo polarized M2-like macrophages can modulate CNS pathology (Na et al., 2023). In ALS, replacement of peripheral nerve macrophages with exogenously derived M2-like cells at disease onset significantly reduced pro-inflammatory microglial responses, reduced motor neuron degeneration, and prolonged survival in SOD1-G93A mice (Chiot et al., 2020). Similarly, in PD models, adoptive transfer of M2 macrophages reduced dopaminergic neuron loss by suppressing α-synuclein–driven neuroinflammation (Adebowale et al., 2025). Importantly, M2 macrophages may also engraft in the CNS following BBB disruption and acquire microglia-like properties, though they retain distinct transcriptional signatures (Shemer et al., 2018). Their strategic positioning at perivascular and meningeal interfaces further enables them to regulate immune cell trafficking and shape the neuroinflammatory milieu (Chamkouri & Motlagh Mohavi, 2025).

(b) Genetic Engineering for Enhanced Function - To amplify therapeutic efficacy, macrophages can be precisely modified ex vivo to overexpress molecules that enhance their protective functions, like

- Enhanced phagocytosis: Microglia and infiltrating macrophages normally clear the misfolded protein aggregates through phagocytosis, but this capacity is often impaired in disease states. Genetic engineering offers a means to restore or augment this function by overexpression of receptors like TREM2 or CD36, which boost clearance of amyloid-β or myelin debris (Fu et al., 2025).
- Sustained anti-inflammatory signaling: Macrophages transduced to secrete IL-10 or TGF-β can shift the CNS microenvironment toward tissue repair. CRISPR-Cas9 or siRNA-based approaches have been employed to silence pro-inflammatory pathways, while upregulating genes associated with the M2 phenotype, such as IL-10. In murine models of AD, siRNA-loaded nanoparticles targeting TNF-α or IL-1β have significantly attenuated neurotoxic glial activation and synaptic loss (Chamkouri & Motlagh Mohavi, 2025; Wang et al., 2023).
- Targeted antigen recognition: Chimeric antigen receptor (CAR) engineered macrophages represent an emerging frontier. By directing macrophages to disease-specific epitopes (e.g., oligomeric Aβ or phosphorylated tau), such approaches could enable precision clearance of pathological proteins without broad immunosuppression (Chamkouri & Motlagh Mohavi, 2025).

4.4 Regulatory T cell–based approaches

Among the immune cells, Tregs have gained much more attention for immune cell-based therapy, as they naturally suppress the inflammatory response and maintain immunologic homeostasis. Regulatory T cells (Tregs) constitute a specialized subset of $CD4^+$ T lymphocytes defined by the expression of the master transcription factor FOXP3. To exert their suppressive functions, Tregs secrete immunoregulatory cytokines such as TGF-β, IL-10, and IL-35; they consume IL-2 via high-affinity CD25, thereby limiting its availability to effector T cells (Bittner et al., 2023). The therapeutic potential of natural Tregs has been studied in preclinical models for various diseases, which has paved the way for clinical applications. Recent advances, such as engineering Treg cells with antigen-specific T cell receptors (TCRs) or artificial chimeric antigen receptors (CARs), have provided access to antigen-specific Treg (Xu, Huang, & Zhou, 2025).

Tregs have also been induced in vivo by cytokine-mediated activation, especially low-dose IL-2 or complexes of IL-2 and anti-IL-2 antibody and monoclonal antibodies against death receptor-3 (DR3) (Sheean et al., 2018). IL2 selectively binds with Tregs, preferentially activating them to exert immune regulation that plays a critical role in the treatment of neurological disorders. In recent years, strategies such as PEGylated IL2 (chemically modified to improve its half-life and pharmacokinetics) and nanowire-based delivery systems have enhanced Treg expansion and function, while minimising systemic toxicity (Zamecnik et al., 2020). Treg activators like

Pramipexole (a dopamine receptor agonist) used clinically for PD symptom management, have been shown to increase peripheral Treg numbers and enhance their IL-10 mediated neuroprotective capacity (Guevara-Salinas et al., 2024). Similarly, vitamin D_3 supplementation in early-phase trials has demonstrated an elevation in the Treg to Th17 proportion, correlating with improved motor outcomes (Li, Ma, et al., 2025; Li, Sun, et al., 2025). These modified strategies have shown significant improvement in therapeutic outcomes in preclinical studies, but still lack tissue-specific precision (Jie et al., 2026).

In yet another research on the development of new therapies for MS, aminooxy acetic acid (AOA) has been reported to promote the expression of Foxp3, thereby inducing the conversion of Th17 cells into Tregs. The only challenge faced during the preclinical trials was its inability to cross the BBB (Shevach, 2012). To overcome this problem a drug delivery strategy was developed (Shi et al., 2023), wherein AOA was conjugated with Th17 cells (nanocapsules technology) and administered intravenously to MS model mice for preclinical trials. These nanocapsules were reported to cross the BBB and release AOA to induce the conversion of Th17 into Tregs. These Tregs were then shown to reduce the inflammation and exert immune regulation in mice (Jie et al., 2026).

Natural Tregs have been employed in adoptive T-cell therapy in MS and autoimmune encephalitis. Due to their low frequency and properties, Tregs are expanded or activated ex vivo by cross-linking them with anti-CD3 and anti-CD28 antibodies in the presence of TGF-β and IL-2. Although these polyclonal Treg are feasible and show certain clinical benefits, but are reported not to be very effective. Secondly, their nonspecific expansion may aggravate the risk for generalised immunosuppression, which may increase susceptibility to opportunistic infections (Xu, Huang, & Zhou, 2025; Xu, Xu, Lu, et al., 2025). To address the deficiencies of polyclonal Treg cell therapy, protocols for engineering and generating antigen-specific Treg cells have been developed. These cells preferentially localise to the site of antigen presentation, exhibit improved efficiency, and do not compromise general immune defence in certain CNS diseases (Pishesha et al., 2022; Xu, Huang, & Zhou, 2025; Xu, Xu, Lu, et al., 2025).

Preclinical studies in PD mouse models show that infusion of α-synuclein-specific Tregs reduces microglia activation, attenuates dopaminergic neuron degeneration and improves motor function. These antigen-specific suppressive Tregs were prepared by co-culturing $CD4^+$ T cells with α-syn-presenting DCs for 4 days and subsequent isolation and expansion of α-syn-specific $CD4^+CD25^+$ Tregs. This approach is now being explored in early-phase human trials, with protocols for ex vivo expansion and reinfusion of autologous Tregs (Park et al., 2023).

Genetic engineering has paved the way for the generation of two types of antigen-specific Tregs, the TCR Tregs and the CAR Tregs. TCR-engineered Tregs show MHC dependent antigen recognition, whereas CAR Tregs are MHC independent (can directly interact with the antigen) and suppress effector T cell activity in an antigen-specific manner. A chimeric receptor is synthesised by combining the single-chain variable fragment (scFv) derived from the variable regions of an antibody and the intracellular signalling/activation domain CD3ζ (from TCR) connected by a transmembrane domain. The CAR gene is introduced into $FOXP3^+$ Treg cells using viral (lentiviral or retroviral) or non-viral (transposon systems, CRISPR/Cas9) vectors. The CAR-expressing Treg cell now exhibits targeted antigen recognition (Mishra et al., 2025). Additionally, knocking out genes involved in inflammatory responses or overexpressing genes that support neural regeneration, engineered T cells can be tailored to effectively suppress inflammation in targeted cells, while promoting tissue repair (Jie et al., 2026).

4.5 B Cell–targeted therapy

B cells in the CNS contribute to neuroinflammation in disorders like MS, not only by producing antibodies but also through several antibody-independent mechanisms. B cells present myelin-derived antigens to auto-reactive T cells via MHC class II molecules and co-stimulatory proteins such as CD80 and CD86, thereby amplifying T-cell activation. B cells also secrete pro-inflammatory cytokines (such as TNF-α and IL-6) that promote Th17 differentiation, and sustain neuroinflammation. These functions support the formation and maintenance of ectopic lymphoid structures in the meninges, which are linked to cortical demyelination, neurodegeneration, and disease progression in MS (Kanatas et al., 2023; Sabatino et al., 2019). In contrast, regulatory B cells (Bregs) produce anti-inflammatory cytokines like IL-10 and IL-35 that suppress autoimmune responses. These insights have reshaped our understanding of MS and related disorders, once viewed primarily as T cell–mediated condition, MS is now recognised to involve B cells as central driver of pathology. This paradigm shift has led to the development of B–cell–targeted therapies, especially anti-CD20 monoclonal antibodies, that effectively reduce disease activity and are now cornerstone treatments for many of these conditions (Kanatas et al., 2023).

4.5.1 *Anti-CD20 monoclonal antibodies (anti-CD20 mAbs)*

They are the most widely used B-cell targeted therapy, where CD20 acts like a B-cell identity tag. CD20 is a transmembrane protein expressed from the pre-B (early) to mature and memory B-cell stage, but it is turned off in plasma cells (fully mature, antibody-producing) and pro-B cells (very early, precursors). This selectivity allows anti-CD20 mAbs to target pathogenic B-cells without harming CD20-negative plasma cells or pro-B cells, therefore allowing replenishment of peripheral B-cells within 6–9 months of therapy (Miyazaki & Niino, 2022). B-cell depletion through this therapy is believed to dampen antigen presentation and subsequent activation to pathogenic T cell, suppression of the proinflammatory cytokines released by B cells, promotes transition toward a more regulated environment in patients with MS (Cree et al., 2025). It has been recently reported that, not just the B cells, but a subset of T cells (CD4 and CD8 T cells), also expresses low levels of CD20 (de Sèze et al., 2023). These are often termed $CD20^{dim}$ T cells and are correlated with MS disease severity (Von Essen et al., 2019). Thus, treatment effects associated with anti-CD20 mAbs may result from the depletion of both B cells and -$CD20^{+}$ T cells (Cree et al., 2025). Currently, the following four anti-CD20 therapies are used in the treatment of MS (Cree et al., 2025; Kanatas et al., 2023; Miyazaki & Niino, 2022).

(a) Rituximab: It is a first generation chimeric monoclonal antibody (IgG1), engineered by fusing a murine Fab with a human Fc domain (Whittam et al., 2019). It depletes B cells via complement-dependent cytotoxicity (CDC) and antibody-dependent cellular cytotoxicity (ADCC), where CDC predominates over ADCC. It demonstrated a 91% reduction in gadolinium-enhancing (Gd^{+}) MRI lesions in relapsing-remitting MS (RRMS) and showed benefit in younger patients with active primary progressive MS (PPMS) (Hauser et al., 2008).

(b) Ocrelizumab: It is a second generation recombinant humanized anti-CD20 mAb (IgG1) and favors ADCC over CDC (Klein et al., 2013). In phase III trials (OPERA I/II), it reduced annualized relapse rates by 47% and disability progression in RRMS (Hauser et al., 2017). Crucially, it became the first and only therapy to show efficacy in PPMS (ORATORIO trial; hazard ratio for disability progression = 0.76) (Montalban et al., 2017a). This therapy is FDA-approved.

(c) Ofatumumab: It is second generation, fully human IgG1 mAb, which provides rapid and near-complete B cell depletion via CDA and ADCC (Florou et al., 2020). In the ASCLEPIOS trials, it reduced Gd^{+} lesions by 94%–97% and annualized relapse rates to ~0.10 (Hauser et al., 2020). This therapy is FDA-approved.

(d) Ublituximab: It is a third generation anti-CD20 glycoengineered chimeric IgG1 mAb that exerts its action primarily via ADCC facilitated by defucosylation of its Fc region, which enables potent B-cell depletion with a 1-hour infusion time, improving patient convenience (Whittam et al., 2019).

These agents consistently suppress peripheral and CSF B cells, reduce T-cell activation and trafficking into the CNS, and shift the repopulating B-cell pool toward a more regulatory, naïve phenotype, effects that persist beyond B cell recovery and underlie their durable clinical efficacy (Cree et al., 2025).

4.5.2 Anti-CD19 therapies

CD19 is expressed earlier in B-cell development (from pro-B cells) and on plasmablasts but not on long-lived plasma cells (Cree et al., 2025). Inebilizumab, an afucosylated anti-CD19 monoclonal antibody, has been administered in patients with relapsing MS with positive results, but no phase III trials for MS are currently known (Agius et al., 2019; Kanatas et al., 2023). Some of the emerging and Next-Generation strategies have been mentioned below.

(a) CAR T-Cell Therapy - Originally developed for B-cell malignancies, CD19-directed CAR T cells are now being repurposed for the treatment of autoimmune neurological diseases. Unlike monoclonal antibodies, CAR T cells are autonomous, tissue-penetrant, and capable of sustained in vivo expansion, enabling durable depletion of B cells (excluding long-lived plasma cells) (Blache et al., 2023). The CAR T cells, upon recognizing B cells, release inflammatory cytokines, thus depleting them (Cree et al., 2025).

(b) Chimeric Autoantibody Receptor (CAAR) T Cells therapy - Though the B cells depleted during CAR T cell therapy usually recover over time, but there are instances where B cell populations do not return for months to years due to CAR T cell persistence and memory responses against B cells (Mougiakakos et al., 2021). Therefore, to enhance specificity and avoid global B-cell depletion, CAAR T cells are engineered to recognize autoantigen (the targets of harmful autoantibodies) on autoreactive B-cells. These cells selectively eliminate only autoantibody-producing B cells (Sahlolbei et al., 2023).

(c) Brain-Shuttle Antibodies - The transferrin receptor system enables transport of transferrin across the BBB. Leveraging this, fusion of anti-CD20 mAbs to transferrin can enhance their penetration of the BBB, giving rise to brain-shuttle technology. RO7121932, based on this technology, aims to directly target CNS-resident B cells and serve as a treatment for MS (Cree et al., 2025).

4.6 DC-based immunotherapies for neurodegenerative diseases

Dendritic cells are APCs recognized for their central role in initiating and shaping adaptive immune responses in peripheral tissues. Recent research confirms that DCs actively participate in CNS immune surveillance and can be harnessed therapeutically in neurodegenerative conditions. DCs are not abundant in healthy brain parenchyma, but they reside in CNS border regions, which include the meninges, choroid plexus and perivascular spaces. DCs monitor for danger signals, like the misfolded proteins Aβ in AD or α-Syn in PD. Upon detecting these signals, DCs migrate through meningeal and cervical lymphatic drainage pathways, initiating antigen-specific adaptive immunity (Brezovakova et al., 2018; Ugen et al., 2015).

Studies have revealed a decline in both frequency and functionality of circulating myeloid and plasmacytoid DCs in AD and PD patients, suggesting that peripheral immune dysfunction may exacerbate disease progression rather than merely reflect it (Ciaramella et al., 2016). Given their pivotal role in antigen presentation and T-cell polarization, ex vivo generated, antigen-sensitized DCs can be engineered to promote anti-inflammatory, Th2-biased, or Treg responses, thereby enhancing clearance of pathological aggregates without inciting neurotoxic inflammation (Brezovakova et al., 2018).

The general protocol involves isolation of autologous monocytes or bone marrow progenitors; differentiation into immature DCs using granulocyte-macrophage colony-stimulating factor (GM-CSF) and IL-4; antigen loading with disease-relevant peptides (e.g., Aβ, α-Syn); reintroduction into the host via intravenous or subcutaneous routes (Ugen et al., 2015). Once administered, antigen-loaded DCs migrate to draining lymph nodes, where they prime naïve T cells and stimulate B-cell maturation, leading to the production of high-affinity, conformation-specific antibodies that cross the BBB, opsonize pathological aggregates, and facilitate microglial phagocytosis (Brezovakova et al., 2018).

In AD Cao et al. (2008), demonstrated that vaccination with bone marrow-derived DCs sensitized with a mutant Aβ42 peptide induced robust anti-Aβ antibody titers in APP(SW) transgenic mice, reduced amyloid plaque burden, and improved cognitive function without triggering microglial overactivation or T-cell–mediated encephalitis (Cao et al., 2008).

Dendritic cell–based immunotherapy represents a precision immunological platform capable of harnessing the adaptive immune system to target the root causes of neurodegeneration. By generating antigen-specific antibodies and regulatory immune responses, DC vaccines offer a dual benefit: enhanced clearance of pathological proteins and suppression of chronic neuroinflammation. While still in preclinical development for neurological indications, this approach holds transformative potential for altering the trajectory of diseases once deemed incurable.

5. Challenges and limitations

Despite promising preclinical trials, the clinical translation of immune-based therapies for neurological disorders faces significant hurdles. One of the critical factors deciding the success of clinical trials is the timing of the intervention. In most trials, the enrolled patients have mild-to-moderate dementia and exhibit extensive neurodegeneration. This limits the potential for functional recovery, thus missing the therapeutic window for neuroprotection (Heneka et al., 2015). Another major barrier is the heterogeneity of immune responses across patients. Neurological disorders are not uniform; there exists variation in genetics, age, sex, gut microbiota, and comorbidities among patients, which influences the baseline immune status and therapeutic responsiveness. This variability complicates patient stratification and biomarker development, making it difficult to predict the efficacy of immunotherapy.

Other challenges associated with the application of immune cells for neurological disorders are given here.

(a) BBB permeability and cell delivery constraints - It is known that neuroinflammation in AD may increase BBB permeability, but still, the penetration limits are poor. Therefore, Treg access to the CNS needs invasive delivery routes like intrathecal infusion (Yang et al., 2024), advanced delivery platforms (e.g., nanoparticle carriers, intranasal administration), which are still in the experimental phase (Jie et al., 2026).

(b) Target specificity - While T cells and microglia are key players in neuronal pathogenesis, they also perform essential homeostatic functions, and their global immunosuppression or broad inhibition impairs the protective responses. Though engineered Aβ-specific Tregs and α-synuclein–specific Tregs show improved targeting and efficacy in preclinical models, producing clinical-grade, stable, and potent autologous or engineered Tregs at scale remains costly and technically complex (Jie et al., 2026).

(c) Risk of autoimmunity or off-target inflammation - Although immune cell-based therapies hold promise for treating neurological disorders, their potential to provoke autoimmunity or off-target inflammatory responses remains a major concern. Tregs, for instance, are generally immunosuppressive, but their functional plasticity can shift under inflammatory cues. In highly pro-inflammatory environments, such as those rich in IL-6, Tregs may lose Foxp3 expression and convert into pro-inflammatory Th17-like cells, thereby exacerbating neuroinflammation instead of mitigating it (Komatsu et al., 2009; Korn, 2023). Even in autoimmune applications, like CAR-T cell–mediated B-cell depletion for MS, non-selective targeting may eliminate protective B-cell subsets or trigger compensatory immune dysregulation (Baumgarten et al., 2023; Mackensen et al., 2022).

(d) Cell survival, integration, and long-term safety - A major challenge in ACT lies in ensuring the survival, CNS homing, and sustained functionality of transferred cells, particularly Tregs within the hostile microenvironment of the injured or diseased CNS. The CNS milieu in pathological states is characterized by elevated oxidative stress, excitotoxicity, pro-inflammatory cytokine signaling, and a paucity of trophic support, all of which can critically impair the viability and persistence of therapeutic immune cells. For example, systemically administered Tregs typically exhibit only transient residency in the CNS, with detectable populations persisting for approximately 2–4 weeks post transfer unless they encounter their cognate antigen, which can drive in situ clonal expansion and prolong their immunomodulatory activity (Ito et al., 2019b; Liston et al., 2024).

(e) Standardization and reproducibility issues - Reproducible manufacturing of therapeutic immune cells remains a significant hurdle. Treg identity is typically defined by co-expression of CD4, CD25, and Foxp3; however, Foxp3 staining requires cell fixation, which precludes live-cell sorting for therapy (Hu et al., 2018). Although CD127 (IL-7Rα) low expression is used as a surrogate surface marker, heterogeneity persists among isolated populations. Moreover, ex vivo expansion protocols vary, leading to differences in suppressive potency and stability (Hu et al., 2018; Jie et al., 2026). For Breg and dendritic cell therapies, the lack of unique lineage-defining markers further complicates standardization (Hu et al., 2018). Clinical translation is also hindered by batch-to-batch variability, donor-dependent functional differences, and the absence of universally accepted potency assays (Hu et al., 2018; Jie et al., 2026). Another challenge includes insufficient purity, unstable activity, and potential shifts in phenotype or functional loss following expansion (Jie et al., 2022).

Together, these issues highlight the need for precision immunology approaches that are tailored to individual immune phenotypes, delivered at optimal disease stages, and monitored via dynamic biomarkers to realize the full therapeutic potential of immune cell modulation in neurological disorders (Jie et al., 2022).

6. Translational and clinical perspectives

6.1 Ongoing and completed clinical trials

Immune cell targeted therapies have entered mainstream neurology largely through B-cell depletion in RRMS and PPMS. Anti-CD20 monoclonal antibodies - rituximab, ocrelizumab, and ofatumumab - have demonstrated robust efficacy in phase III trials (OPERA I/II, ORATORIO, ASCLEPIOS), but ocrelizumab is the only therapy approved by EMA for inflammatory PPMS (Kanatas et al., 2023; Montalban et al., 2017b). Beyond antibody-mediated depletion, first-in-human trials of CAR T cell-stargeting B-lineage antigens (CD19/CD20) are emerging therapies. A phase I trial (NCT06138132) is now evaluating anti-CD19 CAR T cells in progressive MS. A Phase I clinical trial to study the effect of Treg-based therapy for MS was conducted (Chwojnicki et al., 2021). This trial included 14 people with MS. In this clinical trial, some participants received ex vivo expanded Tregs intravenously while while a few received intrathecally. Interestingly, it was observed that the disease progression was halted in participants who received the Tregs intrathecally, while those who received the Tregs intravenously still experienced relapses and deterioration of their disability.

Clinical trials for the treatment of Alzheimer's disease are under active investigation. One of the approaches is *in vivo* induction of functional Tregs using Low-dose IL-2. Two ongoing Phase 2 trials (NCT05468073 and NCT06096090) are evaluating the safety and cognitive effects of repeated low-dose IL-2 in patients with mild-to-moderate AD (Jie et al., 2026). The other approach is ACT, which includes early-phase trials to test both autologous and allogeneic Treg products. VTBIO Co. Ltd. is conducting Phase 1 studies using intravenous delivery of ex vivo expanded polyclonal Tregs (VT301/GB301). Similarly, Novabio Therapeutics has launched a Phase 1 trial (NCT06671236) assessing NP001, an autologous human polyclonal Treg therapy (Jie et al., 2026). While these initial clinical trials rely on polyclonal Tregs, their success provides a strong rationale for next-level trials incorporating antigen specificity. In recent work, scientists employed Aβ-specific human Tregs (Aβ-hTregs) in preclinical trials and reported a phenotypic shift in microglial cells toward an anti-inflammatory state, thereby modulating neuroinflammation and improving cognitive outcomes (Yang et al., 2024). Phase I clinical trials indicated good tolerability to the immune cell therapy with valuable insights. Moreover, scalable manufacturing of Aβ-hTregs via a simplified culture system offers a practical pathway toward clinical adoption (Yang et al., 2024).

6.2 Biomarkers for immune modulation efficacy

The assessment of therapeutic efficacy in immune cell-based therapies for neurological disorders relies on a multidimensional biomarker framework. These biomarkers can be broadly categorized into three as follows.

(a) Cellular Efficacy Biomarkers-these biomarkers quantify shifts in immune cell populations in peripheral blood and CSF, providing direct evidence for immune cell therapy success. The restoration or expansion of CD4+Foxp3+ Tregs or Treg frequency is a critical indicator of immune re-equilibration post-treatment (Jie et al., 2026). A shift from pathogenic Th1/Th17 profiles toward anti-inflammatory Th2 or Treg phenotypes reflects therapeutic success of MS, and this is referred to as T-cell Polarisation (Ma et al., 2023). In CD19 or CD20 targeted therapies and emerging CAR T-cell approaches, sustained B-cell depletion correlates strongly with reduced MRI lesion activity (Haghikia et al., 2024; Kanatas et al., 2023). Phenotypic switching of microglia and macrophages from pro-inflammatory to reparative states (assessed via single-cell RNA sequencing) is also recognized as a biomarker of CNS immune remodeling (Gao et al., 2023; Jie et al., 2026).

(b) Fluid-Based Protein Biomarkers in CSF and Serum - These biomarkers offer non-invasive, quantifiable metrics of neuronal integrity and glial activation. These include Neurofilament Light Chain (NfL), Glial Fibrillary Acidic Protein (GFAP), Cytokine and Chemokine Signatures. NfL is the most validated biomarker of neuroaxonal injury across neurological disorders, including MS, ALS, and AD. Effective immune cell therapies consistently reduce serum or CSF NfL levels, reflecting diminished inflammatory demyelination or neuronal stress (Bittner et al., 2021; Kanatas et al., 2023). GFAP is a specific marker of astrocytic activation and injury, relevant in progressive MS. Elevated GFAP during acute attacks decreases with successful B-cell depletion or Treg therapy, indicating attenuated astrogliosis and blood–brain barrier stabilization (Bandara et al., 2025; Gao et al., 2023). Decreased levels of pro-inflammatory mediators (e.g., IL-6, TNF-α, GM-CSF, IL-17) and increased anti-inflammatory factors (e.g., IL-10, TGF-β, IL-35) in CSF and serum serve as a good marker for a favorable therapeutic response. Treg-based therapies elevate IL-10 and TGF-β, fostering an immunoregulatory milieu (Jie et al., 2026).

(c) Molecular Markers - Novel biomarkers are enhancing sensitivity and specificity in monitoring advanced cellular therapies. Serum exosomal microRNAs (miRNAs) released by immune and neural cells carry miRNA cargo that reflects disease activity and treatment response. For example, Treg-derived exosomes enriched in miR-142-3p modulate osteogenesis and angiogenesis, suggesting their potential as regenerative biomarkers. In neurodegenerative contexts, exosomal miRNAs linked to synaptic plasticity (e.g., miR-132) or inflammation (e.g., miR-155) are being explored as dynamic indicators of therapeutic efficacy (Jie et al., 2026).

6.3 Regulatory frameworks and ethical issues

Most approved immune-modulating biologics (e.g., ocrelizumab, natalizumab) follow standard FDA/EMA pathways for biologics in chronic autoimmune disease. However, immune cell-based products for neurological disorders, including CAR T cells and Tregs, fall under advanced therapy medicinal product (ATMP) regulations laid by the European Medicines Agency (EMA) and Regenerative Medicine Advanced Therapy (RMAT) products regulations laid by the Food and Drug Administration, US (FDA). This classification imposes stringent requirements for safety, potency, and manufacturing consistency (Haghikia et al., 2024). Good Manufacturing Practice (GMP) compliance is mandatory. All cell preparations must document isolation, expansion, and quality control procedures. For genetically modified cells (e.g., CAR T), a vector copy number (VCN) of less than five per genome is recommended by the FDA to minimize insertional mutagenesis risk. For full approval, randomised controlled trials (RCTs) are required.

There should be no space for therapeutic misconception. Clear communication and structured consent processes are essential. In an early-phase trial, participants may overestimate clinical benefit when the primary goal is safety assessment. In cognitively impaired patients (e.g., AD, advanced ALS), obtaining Proxy consent is ethically complex, keeping in consideration the irreversibility of CNS-targeted cellular interventions (Jayaram et al., 2025). Equitable access is a growing priority: with CAR T-cell therapies often exceeding $400,000 per patient, disparities in geographic and socioeconomic access raise justice concerns (Jayaram et al., 2025; Sainatham et al., 2024). Stem (and immune) cell tourism, the commercial sale of unproven "immune cell" infusions outside clinical trials, is widely condemned as professional misconduct by global ethics bodies (Hwang & Muzammil, 2025).

Together, these frameworks ensure that the remarkable therapeutic promise of immune cell therapies is balanced with rigorous oversight, patient protection, and commitment to equitable translation.

6.4 Personalized immune-cell therapy

Neurological disorders are not uniform across patients; matching the immune phenotype to disease stage aids in providing personalized cellular therapy. For example, in early inflammatory MS, B-cell depletion (anti-CD20) or Treg expansion effectively controls relapses driven by peripheral lymphocyte infiltration and meningeal follicles. Whereas, in progressive MS, where compartmentalized CNS inflammation and microglial activation dominate, therapies targeting microglia (e.g., TREM2 agonists, NLRP3 inhibitors) or CNS-penetrant agents like Bruton's tyrosine kinase inhibitors (e.g., evobrutinib) are more relevant (Gao et al., 2023; Kanatas et al., 2023). Single-cell profiling of CSF reveals patient-specific immune endophenotypes, paving the way for biomarker-guided therapy selection.

7. Future directions

While current immune cell-based therapies for neurological disorders face significant biological and translational hurdles, the convergence of synthetic biology, nanotechnology, systems immunology, and artificial intelligence is opening transformative avenues for next-generation interventions. These emerging strategies aim not only to overcome the limitations of conventional approaches but also to actively reprogram the neuroimmune landscape toward repair and homeostasis. Emerging engineering strategies aim to enhance the specificity, safety, and reparative capacity of immune cells. CAR-Tregs are being designed to home to disease-specific CNS antigens. These cells can deliver localized immunosuppression and neurotrophic support without systemic immune compromise (Baumgarten et al., 2023; Jie et al., 2026). Similarly, CAR T cells, CAAR T cells and microglia-like cells are under investigation (Cree et al., 2025). Reprogramming endogenous microglia using CSF1R inhibitors or CRISPR-based tools to adopt anti-inflammatory, pro-clearance phenotypes represents another frontier (Gao et al., 2023; Pan et al., 2025).

Synergistic approaches that couple immune cells with advanced delivery systems offer enhanced precision. For example, Tregs engineered to secrete IL-10 or brain-derived neurotrophic factor (BDNF) can be augmented with nanoparticle-based payloads that release anti-inflammatory drugs or RNA therapeutics in response to local cues (Cheng et al., 2022). Similarly, Trojan horse strategies, where immune cells carry nanocapsules across the BBB, have already shown promise (Shi et al., 2023). Such hybrid platforms merge cellular tropism with molecular programmability, enabling spatiotemporally controlled interventions. Single-cell RNA sequencing (scRNA-seq) and TCR repertoire analysis are revolutionizing our understanding of neuroimmune heterogeneity. These tools have revealed disease-specific Treg subsets in stroke, aging, and AD, each with distinct transcriptional and functional signatures (Ito et al., 2019b; Jie et al., 2026). Integration of such datasets with machine learning models can predict optimal cell phenotypes for therapy, identify novel targets, and stratify patients based on immune endophenotypes (Xu, Huang, & Zhou, 2025; Xu, Xu, et al., 2025). AI-driven platforms could also simulate immune CNS interactions in silico, accelerating the design of next-generation CAR constructs or combination regimens (Luo et al., 2021; Pan et al., 2025).

The convergence of immune profiling, biomaterials, and gene editing is paving the way for precision neuro-immunotherapy. Such strategies align with the vision of treating neurological disorders not merely by suppressing pathology, but by actively remodeling the CNS toward homeostasis, turning immune cells into "precision construction crews" for neural repair (Boskovic et al., 2024). Future regimens may involve patient-specific T cell receptor Tregs, generated from CSF-derived T-cell clones reactive to disease-relevant neoantigens (Boskovic et al., 2024). We have on-demand immunomodulation, where we can use biomaterial scaffolds that release IL-2 complexes or Treg-recruiting chemokines only at lesion sites (Santos Roballo et al., 2019; Zhang et al., 2021). Moreover, a dynamic feedback system can be designed where engineered cells sense local inflammation and adjust their response in real-time (Choe et al., 2021).

8. Conclusion

Immune cell–based therapies are redefining the therapeutic landscape for neurological disorders. From B-cell depletion in MS to Treg augmentation in neurodegeneration and microglial reprogramming in proteinopathies, these strategies move beyond symptomatic relief towards disease modification. The remarkable efficacy of CAR T cells in autoimmune neuropathies signals a potential paradigm shift - offering durable, possibly curative immune resets. However, significant challenges remain: balancing efficacy with infection risk, overcoming the protective blood-brain barrier, managing therapy-related toxicities (e.g., Cytokine Release Syndrome or CRS), and defining patient subgroups that are most likely to benefit. Regulatory guidelines for approving cell therapies for diseases other than cancer are insufficient, and they must evolve to address these unique complexities. Looking forward, the convergence of single-cell immunophenotyping, gene-editing (e.g., CRISPR-engineered Tregs), and biomaterial-assisted delivery will enable truly personalized immune interventions. The long-term vision is a precision immunology toolkit, where the right immune cell therapy is matched to the right patient at the right disease stage, ultimately halting progression, restoring neurological function and perhaps, one day, curing.

References

Abud, E. M., Ramirez, R. N., Martinez, E. S., Healy, L. M., Nguyen, C. H. H., Newman, S. A., Yeromin, A. V., Scarfone, V. M., Marsh, S. E., Fimbres, C., Caraway, C. A., Fote, G. M., Madany, A. M., Agrawal, A., Kayed, R., Gylys, K. H., Cahalan, M. D., Cummings, B. J., Antel, J. P., … Blurton-Jones, M. (2017). iPSC-derived human microglia-like cells to study neurological diseases. *Neuron, 94*(2), 278. https://doi.org/10.1016/j.neuron.2017.03.042

Adebowale, A., Byun, J. H., Chung, J., Lee, H. J., Gresham, D., Lim, J., & Lee, J.-K. (2025). Adoptive NK cell transfer confers neuroprotection by attenuating neuroinflammation and alpha-synuclein pathology in a mouse model of synucleinopathy. *Molecular Neurodegeneration Advances, 1*(1). https://doi.org/10.1186/s44477-025-00006-9

Agius, M. A., Klodowska-Duda, G., Maciejowski, M., Potemkowski, A., Li, J., Patra, K., Wesley, J., Madani, S., Barron, G., Katz, E., & Flor, A. (2019). Safety and tolerability of inebilizumab (MEDI-551), an anti-CD19 monoclonal antibody, in patients with relapsing forms of multiple sclerosis: Results from a phase 1 randomised, placebo-controlled, escalating intravenous and subcutaneous dose study. *Multiple Sclerosis Journal, 25* (2), 235–245. https://doi.org/10.1177/1352458517740641

Akiyama, H., Nishimura, T., Kondo, H., Ikeda, K., Hayashi, Y., & McGeer, P. L. (1994). Expression of the receptor for macrophage colony stimulating factor by brain microglia and its upregulation in brains of patients with alzheimer's disease and amyotrophic lateral sclerosis. *Brain Research, 639*(1), 171–174. https://doi.org/10.1016/0006-8993(94)91779-5

Alcaide, P. (2022). Mechanisms regulating T cell–endothelial cell interactions. *Cold Spring Harbor Perspectives in Medicine, 12*(7), Article a041170. https://doi.org/10.1101/cshperspect.a041170

Aspden, J. W., Murphy, M. A., Kashlan, R. D., Xiong, Y., Poznansky, M. C., & Sîrbulescu, R. F. (2023). Intruders or protectors – The multifaceted role of B cells in CNS disorders. *Frontiers in Cellular Neuroscience, 17.* https://doi.org/10.3389/fncel.2023.1329823

Bandara, E. M. S., Asih, P. R., Pedrini, S., Hone, E., Fernando, W. M. A. D. B., & Martins, R. N. (2025). The role of glial fibrillary acidic protein in the neuropathology of alzheimer's disease and its potential as a blood biomarker for early diagnosis and progression. *Molecular Neurobiology, 62*(12), 15576–15608. https://doi.org/10.1007/s12035-025-05219-3

Baumgarten, L. V., Stauss, H. J., & Lünemann, J. D. (2023). Synthetic cell-based immunotherapies for neurologic diseases. *Neurology: Neuroimmunology and Neuroinflammation, 10*(5). https://doi.org/10.1212/NXI.0000000000200139

Bittner, S., Hehlgans, T., & Feuerer, M. (2023). Engineered treg cells as putative therapeutics against inflammatory diseases and beyond. *Trends in Immunology, 44*(6), 468–483. https://doi.org/10.1016/j.it.2023.04.005

Bittner, S., Oh, J., Kubala Havrdová, E., Tintoré, M., & Zipp, F. (2021). The potential of serum neurofilament as biomarker for multiple sclerosis. *Brain, 144*(10), 2954–2963. https://doi.org/10.1093/brain/awab241

Blache, U., Tretbar, S., Koehl, U., Mougiakakos, D., & Fricke, S. (2023). CAR T cells for treating autoimmune diseases. *RMD Open, 9*(4). https://doi.org/10.1136/rmdopen-2022-002907

Boskovic, P., Gao, W., & Kipnis, J. (2024). Will cellular immunotherapies end neurodegenerative diseases? *Trends in Immunology, 45*(5), 329–337. https://doi.org/10.1016/j.it.2024.03.006

Brezovakova, V., Valachova, B., Hanes, J., Novak, M., & Jadhav, S. (2018). Dendritic cells as an alternate approach for treatment of neurodegenerative disorders. *Cellular and Molecular Neurobiology, 38*(6), 1207–1214. https://doi.org/10.1007/s10571-018-0598-1

Campisi, L., Chizari, S., Ho, J. S. Y., Gromova, A., Arnold, F., Mosca, L., Mei, X., Fstkchyan, Y., Torre, D., Beharry, C., Garcia-Forn, M., Jiménez-Alcázar, M., Korobeynikov, V. A., Prazich, J., Fayad, Z. A., Seldin, M. M., De Rubeis, S., Bennett, C. L., Ostrow, L. W., … Marazzi, I. (2022). Clonally expanded CD8 T cells characterize amyotrophic lateral sclerosis-4. *Nature, 606*(7916), 945–952. https://doi.org/10.1038/s41586-022-04844-5

Cao, C., Lin, X., Zhang, C., Wahi, M. M., Wefes, I., Arendash, G., & Potter, H. (2008). Mutant amyloid-beta-sensitized dendritic cells as alzheimer's disease vaccine. *Journal of Neuroimmunology, 200*(1–2), 1–10. https://doi.org/10.1016/j.jneuroim.2008.05.017

Chadarevian, J. P., Davtyan, H., Chadarevian, A. L., Nguyen, J., Capocchi, J. K., Le, L., Escobar, A., Chadarevian, T., Mansour, K., Deynega, E., Mgerian, M., Tu, C., Kiani Shabestari, S., Carlen-Jones, W., Eskandari-Sedighi, G., Hasselmann, J., Spitale, R. C., & Blurton-Jones, M. (2025). Harnessing human iPSC-microglia for CNS-wide delivery of disease-modifying proteins. *Cell Stem Cell, 32*(6), 914. https://doi.org/10.1016/j.stem.2025.03.009

Chamkouri, H., & Motlagh Mohavi, S. (2025). Microglia and macrophages in central nervous system homeostasis and disease progression: Guardians and executioners. *Neuroglia, 6*(3), 31. https://doi.org/10.3390/neuroglia6030031

Cheng, P., Cheng, L., Han, H., Li, J., Ma, C., Huang, H., Zhou, J., Feng, J., Huang, Y., Lv, Y., Huang, H., Wang, Y., Hou, L., Chen, Y., & Li, G. (2022). A pH/H 2 O 2/MMP9 time-response gel system with sparc high tregs derived extracellular vesicles promote recovery after acute myocardial infarction. *Advanced Healthcare Materials, 11*(22). https://doi.org/10.1002/adhm.202200971

Chiot, A., Zaïdi, S., Iltis, C., Ribon, M., Berriat, F., Schiaffino, L., Jolly, A., de la Grange, P., Mallat, M., Bohl, D., Millecamps, S., Seilhean, D., Lobsiger, C. S., & Boillée, S. (2020). Modifying macrophages at the periphery has the capacity to change microglial reactivity and to extend ALS survival. *Nature Neuroscience, 23*(11), 1339–1351. https://doi.org/10.1038/s41593-020-00718-z

Choe, J. H., Watchmaker, P. B., Simic, M. S., Gilbert, R. D., Li, A. W., Krasnow, N. A., Downey, K. M., Yu, W., Carrera, D. A., Celli, A., Cho, J., Briones, J. D., Duecker, J. M., Goretsky, Y. E., Dannenfelser, R., Cardarelli, L., Troyanskaya, O., Sidhu, S. S., Roybal, K. T., Okada, H., & Lim, W. A. (2021). SynNotch-CAR T cells overcome challenges of specificity, heterogeneity, and persistence in treating glioblastoma. *Science Translational Medicine, 13*(591). https://doi.org/10.1126/scitranslmed.abe7378

Chwojnicki, K., Iwaszkiewicz-Grześ, D., Jankowska, A., Zieliński, M., Łowiec, P., Gliwiński, M., Grzywińska, M., Kowalczyk, K., Konarzewska, A., Glasner, P., Sakowska, J., Kulczycka, J., Jaźwińska-Curyło, A., Kubach, M., Karaszewski, B., Nyka, W., Szurowska, E., & Trzonkowski, P. (2021). Administration of CD4+CD25highCD127−FoxP3+ regulatory T cells for relapsing-remitting multiple sclerosis: A phase 1 study. *BioDrugs, 35*(1), 47–60. https://doi.org/10.1007/s40259-020-00462-7

Ciaramella, A., Salani, F., Bizzoni, F., Donata Orfei, M., Caltagirone, C., Spalletta, G., & Bossù, P. (2016). Myeloid dendritic cells are decreased in peripheral blood of Alzheimer's disease patients in association with disease progression and severity of depressive symptoms. *Journal of Neuroinflammation, 13*(1). https://doi.org/10.1186/s12974-016-0483-0

Clarke, B. E., & Patani, R. (2020). The microglial component of amyotrophic lateral sclerosis. *Brain, 143*(12), 3526–3539. https://doi.org/10.1093/brain/awaa309

Crapser, J. D., Spangenberg, E. E., Barahona, R. A., Arreola, M. A., Hohsfield, L. A., & Green, K. N. (2020). Microglia facilitate loss of perineuronal nets in the alzheimer's disease brain. *EBioMedicine, 58*. https://doi.org/10.1016/j.ebiom.2020.102919

Cree, B. A. C., Berger, J. R., & Greenberg, B. (2025). Correction: The evolution of Anti-CD20 treatment for multiple sclerosis: Optimization of antibody characteristics and function. *CNS Drugs, 39*(7), 721–724. https://doi.org/10.1007/s40263-025-01187-3

Dash, U. C., Bhol, N. K., Swain, S. K., Samal, R. R., Nayak, P. K., Raina, V., Panda, S. K., Kerry, R. G., Duttaroy, A. K., & Jena, A. B. (2025). Oxidative stress and inflammation in the pathogenesis of neurological disorders: Mechanisms and implications. *Acta Pharmaceutica Sinica B, 15*(1), 15–34. https://doi.org/10.1016/j.apsb.2024.10.004

de Sèze, J., Maillart, E., Gueguen, A., Laplaud, D. A., Michel, L., Thouvenot, E., Zephir, H., Zimmer, L., Biotti, D., & Liblau, R. (2023). Anti-CD20 therapies in multiple sclerosis: From pathology to the clinic. *Frontiers in Immunology, 14*. https://doi.org/10.3389/fimmu.2023.1004795

Florou, D., Katsara, M., Feehan, J., Dardiotis, E., & Apostolopoulos, V. (2020). Anti-CD20 agents for multiple sclerosis: Spotlight on ocrelizumab and ofatumumab. *Brain Sciences, 10*(10), 758. https://doi.org/10.3390/brainsci10100758

Fransen, N. L., Hsiao, C. C., Van Der Poel, M., Engelenburg, H. J., Verdaasdonk, K., Vincenten, M. C. J., Remmerswaal, E. B. M., Kuhlmann, T., Mason, M. R. J., Hamann, J., Smolders, J., & Huitinga, I. (2020). Tissue-resident memory T cells invade the brain parenchyma in multiple sclerosis white matter lesions. *Brain, 143*(6), 1714–1730. https://doi.org/10.1093/brain/awaa117

Fu, J., Huang, S., Zhang, A., Shi, R., Wei, Y., He, S., Huang, S., Lin, L., Sun, X., Gong, T., Zhang, L., Lin, Q., & Zhang, Z. (2025). Therapeutic strategies based on macrophages and their derivatives: Targeted drug delivery platforms and disease treatment. *Journal of Pharmaceutical Analysis, 15*(12), Article 101413. https://doi.org/10.1016/j.jpha.2025.101413

Galea, I., Bechmann, I., & Perry, V. H. (2007). What is immune privilege (not)? *Trends in Immunology, 28*(1), 12–18. https://doi.org/10.1016/j.it.2006.11.004

Gao, C., Jiang, J., Tan, Y., & Chen, S. (2023). Microglia in neurodegenerative diseases: Mechanism and potential therapeutic targets. *Signal Transduction and Targeted Therapy, 8*(1). https://doi.org/10.1038/s41392-023-01588-0

Gordon, R., Albornoz, E. A., Christie, D. C., Langley, M. R., Kumar, V., Mantovani, S., Robertson, A. A. B., Butler, M. S., Rowe, D. B., O'Neill, L. A., Kanthasamy, A. G., Schroder, K., Cooper, M. A., & Woodruff, T. M. (2018). Inflammasome inhibition prevents -synuclein pathology and dopaminergic neurodegeneration in mice. *Science Translational Medicine, 10*(465). https://doi.org/10.1126/scitranslmed.aah4066

Guevara-Salinas, A., Netzahualcoyotzi, C., Álvarez-Luquín, D. D., Pérez-Figueroa, E., Sevilla-Reyes, E. E., Castellanos-Barba, C., Vega-Ángeles, V. T., Terán-Dávila, E., Estudillo, E., Velasco, I., & Adalid-Peralta, L. (2024). Treating activated regulatory T cells with pramipexole protects human dopaminergic neurons from 6-OHDA-induced degeneration. *CNS Neuroscience and Therapeutics, 30*(8). https://doi.org/10.1111/cns.14883

Haghikia, A., Schett, G., & Mougiakakos, D. (2024). B cell-targeting chimeric antigen receptor T cells as an emerging therapy in neuroimmunological diseases. *The Lancet Neurology, 23*(6), 615–624. https://doi.org/10.1016/s1474-4422(24)00140-6

Hart, C. G., & Karimi-Abdolrezaee, S. (2021). Recent insights on astrocyte mechanisms in CNS homeostasis, pathology, and repair. *Journal of Neuroscience Research, 99*(10), 2427–2462. https://doi.org/10.1002/jnr.24922

Hauser, S. L., Bar-Or, A., Cohen, J. A., Comi, G., Correale, J., Coyle, P. K., Cross, A. H., De Seze, J., Leppert, D., Montalban, X., Selmaj, K., Wiendl, H., Kerloeguen, C., Willi, R., Li, B., Kakarieka, A., Tomic, D., Goodyear, A., Pingili, R., … Kappos, L. (2020). Ofatumumab versus teriflunomide in multiple sclerosis. *New England Journal of Medicine, 383*(6), 546–557. https://doi.org/10.1056/NEJMoa1917246

Hauser, S. L., Bar-Or, A., Comi, G., Giovannoni, G., Hartung, H. P., Hemmer, B., Lublin, F., Montalban, X., Rammohan, K. W., Selmaj, K., Traboulsee, A., Wolinsky, J. S., Arnold, D. L., Klingelschmitt, G., Masterman, D., Fontoura, P., Belachew, S., Chin, P., Mairon, N., Garren, H., & Kappos, L. (2017). Ocrelizumab versus interferon beta-1a in relapsing multiple sclerosis. *New England Journal of Medicine, 376*(3), 221–234. https://doi.org/10.1056/NEJMoa1601277

Hauser, S. L., Waubant, E., Arnold, D. L., Vollmer, T., Antel, J., Fox, R. J., Bar-Or, A., Panzara, M., Sarkar, N., Agarwal, S., Langer-Gould, A., & Smith, C. H. (2008). B-cell depletion with rituximab in relapsing-remitting multiple sclerosis. *New England Journal of Medicine, 358*(7), 676–688. https://doi.org/10.1056/NEJMoa0706383

Heneka, M. T., Carson, M. J., Khoury, J. E., Landreth, G. E., Brosseron, F., Feinstein, D. L., Jacobs, A. H., Wyss-Coray, T., Vitorica, J., Ransohoff, R. M., Herrup, K., Frautschy, S. A., Finsen, B., Brown, G. C., Verkhratsky, A., Yamanaka, K., Koistinaho, J., Latz, E., Halle, A., … Kummer, M. P. (2015). Neuroinflammation in alzheimer's disease. *The Lancet Neurology, 14*(4), 388–405. https://doi.org/10.1016/S1474-4422(15)70016-5

Hol, E. M., & Pekny, M. (2015). Glial fibrillary acidic protein (GFAP) and the astrocyte intermediate filament system in diseases of the central nervous system. *Current Opinion in Cell Biology, 32*, 121–130. https://doi.org/10.1016/j.ceb.2015.02.004

Holtman, I. R., Skola, D., & Glass, C. K. (2017). Transcriptional control of microglia phenotypes in health and disease. *Journal of Clinical Investigation, 127*(9), 3220–3229. https://doi.org/10.1172/JCI90604

Hu, X., Leak, R. K., Thomson, A. W., Yu, F., Xia, Y., Wechsler, L. R., & Chen, J. (2018). Promises and limitations of immune cell-based therapies in neurological disorders. *Nature Reviews Neurology, 14*(9), 559–568. https://doi.org/10.1038/s41582-018-0028-5

Hwang, W. Y. K., & Muzammil, E. M. (2025). The current state of cytotherapy and the field of cell and gene therapy. *Cytotherapy, 27*(6), 678–685. https://doi.org/10.1016/j.jcyt.2025.01.017

Iliff, J. J., Wang, M., Liao, Y., Plogg, B. A., Peng, W., Gundersen, G. A., Benveniste, H., Vates, G. E., Deane, R., Goldman, S. A., Nagelhus, E. A., & Nedergaard, M. (2012). A paravascular pathway facilitates CSF flow through the brain parenchyma and the clearance of interstitial solutes, including amyloid β. *Science Translational Medicine, 4*(147). https://doi.org/10.1126/scitranslmed.3003748UnitedStates

Ito, M., Komai, K., Mise-Omata, S., Iizuka-Koga, M., Noguchi, Y., Kondo, T., Sakai, R., Matsuo, K., Nakayama, T., Yoshie, O., Nakatsukasa, H., Chikuma, S., Shichita, T., & Yoshimura, A. (2019). Brain regulatory T cells suppress astrogliosis and potentiate neurological recovery. *Nature, 565*(7738), 246–250. https://doi.org/10.1038/s41586-018-0824-5

Jain, R. W., & Yong, V. W. (2022). B cells in central nervous system disease: Diversity, locations and pathophysiology. *Nature Reviews Immunology, 22*(8), 513–524. https://doi.org/10.1038/s41577-021-00652-6

Jayaram, P., Danilkowicz, R. M., & Yuan, X. (2025). Ethical and regulatory considerations related to regenerative medicine. *HSS Journal®: The Musculoskeletal Journal of Hospital for Special Surgery, 21*(4), 463–468. https://doi.org/10.1177/15563316251361511

Jie, J., Mao, D., Cao, J., Feng, P., & Yang, P. (2022). Customized multifunctional peptide hydrogel scaffolds for CAR-T-Cell rapid proliferation and solid tumor immunotherapy. *ACS Applied Materials and Interfaces, 14*(33), 37514–37527. https://doi.org/10.1021/acsami.2c10727

Jie, J., Yao, X., Deng, H., Zhou, Y., Jiang, X., Dai, X., Yang, Y., & Yang, P. (2026). Regulatory T cells in neurological disorders and tissue regeneration: Mechanisms of action and therapeutic potentials. *Neural Regeneration Research, 21*(4), 1277–1291. https://doi.org/10.4103/NRR.NRR-D-24-01363

Jin, M., Günther, R., Akgün, K., Hermann, A., & Ziemssen, T. (2020). Peripheral proinflammatory Th1/Th17 immune cell shift is linked to disease severity in amyotrophic lateral sclerosis. *Scientific Reports, 10*(1). https://doi.org/10.1038/s41598-020-62756-8

Kanatas, P., Stouras, I., Stefanis, L., & Stathopoulos, P. (2023). B-Cell-Directed therapies: A new era in multiple sclerosis treatment. *Canadian Journal of Neurological Sciences/Journal Canadien des Sciences Neurologiques, 50*(3), 355–364. https://doi.org/10.1017/cjn.2022.60

Kim, M. W., Gao, W., Lichti, C. F., Gu, X., Dykstra, T., Cao, J., Smirnov, I., Boskovic, P., Kleverov, D., Salvador, A. F. M., Drieu, A., Kim, K., Blackburn, S., Crewe, C., Artyomov, M. N., Unanue, E. R., & Kipnis, J. (2025). Endogenous self-peptides guard immune privilege of the central nervous system. *Nature, 637*(8044), 176–183. https://doi.org/10.1038/s41586-024-08279-y

Kim, C., Ho, D. H., Suk, J. E., You, S., Michael, S., Kang, J., Lee, S. J., Masliah, E., Hwang, D., Lee, H. J., & Lee, S. J. (2013). Neuron-released oligomeric α-synuclein is an endogenous agonist of TLR2 for paracrine activation of microglia. *Nature Communications, 4*. https://doi.org/10.1038/ncomms2534

Klein, C., Lammens, A., Schäfer, W., Georges, G., Schwaiger, M., Mössner, E., Hopfner, K. P., Umaña, P., & Niederfellner, G. (2013). Epitope interactions of monoclonal antibodies targeting CD20 and their relationship to functional properties. *Monoclonal antibodies, 5*(1), 22–33. https://doi.org/10.4161/mabs.22771 Switzerland

Knippenberg, S., Peelen, E., Smolders, J., Thewissen, M., Menheere, P., Cohen Tervaert, J. W., Hupperts, R., & Damoiseaux, J. (2011). Reduction in IL-10 producing B cells (breg) in multiple sclerosis is accompanied by a reduced naïve/memory breg ratio during a relapse but not in remission. *Journal of Neuroimmunology, 239*(1–2), 80–86. https://doi.org/10.1016/j.jneuroim.2011.08.019

Komatsu, N., Mariotti-Ferrandiz, M. E., Wang, Y., Malissen, B., Waldmann, H., & Hori, S. (2009). Heterogeneity of natural Foxp3+ T cells: A committed regulatory T-cell lineage and an uncommitted minor population retaining plasticity. *Proceedings of the National Academy of Sciences of the United States of America, 106*(6), 1903–1908. https://doi.org/10.1073/pnas.0811556106Japan

Korn, T. (2023). Foxp3 + regulatory T cells in the central nervous system and other nonlymphoid tissues. *European Journal of Immunology, 53*(8). https://doi.org/10.1002/eji.202250227

Kumar, P., Zelena, D., & Gautam, A. (2024). *Neurological disorders and challenges in their theranostics Theranostic applications of Nanotechnology in neurological disorders* (pp. 1–29). Hungary: Springer. https://doi.org/10.1007/978-981-99-9510-3_1

Kveštak, D., Mihalić, A., Jonjić, S., & Brizić, I. (2024). Innate lymphoid cells in neuroinflammation. *Frontiers in Cellular Neuroscience, 18*. https://doi.org/10.3389/fncel.2024.1364485

Lebien, T. W., & Tedder, T. F. (2008). B lymphocytes: How they develop and function. *Blood, 112*(5), 1570–1580. https://doi.org/10.1182/blood-2008-02-078071

Li, D., Ma, X., Zhang, W., Zhong, P., Mei, L., & Liu, S. (2025a). Impact of vitamin D3 supplementation on motor functionality and the immune response in Parkinson's disease patients with vitamin D deficiency. *Scientific Reports, 15*(1). https://doi.org/10.1038/s41598-025-10821-5

Li, X., Sun, W., Chen, W., Wang, N., & Wang, S. (2025b). Neuroimmune crosstalk in Parkinson's disease: The pivotal role of microglia and infiltrating T cells. *Molecular Biology Reports, 52*(1). https://doi.org/10.1007/s11033-025-11067-0

Li, J., Zaslavsky, M., Su, Y., Guo, J., Sikora, M. J., van Unen, V., Christophersen, A., Chiou, S. H., Chen, L., Li, J., Ji, X., Wilhelmy, J., McSween, A. M., Palanski, B. A., Mallajosyula, V. V. A., Bracey, N. A., Dhondalay, G. K. R., Bhamidipati, K., Pai, J., … Davis, M. M. (2022). KIR+CD8+ T cells suppress pathogenic T cells and ar active in autoimmune diseases and COVID-19. *Science, 376*(6590). https://doi.org/10.1126/science.abi9591

Liao, B., Zhao, W., Beers, D. R., Henkel, J. S., & Appel, S. H. (2012). Transformation from a neuroprotective to a neurotoxic microglial phenotype in a mouse model of ALS. *Experimental Neurology, 237*(1), 147–152. https://doi.org/10.1016/j.expneurol.2012.06.011

Liston, A., Pasciuto, E., Fitzgerald, D. C., & Yshii, L. (2024). Brain regulatory T cells. *Nature Reviews Immunology, 24*(5), 326–337. https://doi.org/10.1038/s41577-023-00960-z

Liu, D., Bobrovskaya, L., & Zhou, X. F. (2021). Cell therapy for neurological disorders: The perspective of promising cells. *Biology, 10*(11). https://doi.org/10.3390/biology10111142

Louveau, A., Smirnov, I., Keyes, T. J., Eccles, J. D., Rouhani, S. J., Peske, J. D., Derecki, N. C., Castle, D., Mandell, J. W., Lee, K. S., Harris, T. H., & Kipnis, J. (2015). Structural and functional features of central nervous system lymphatic vessels. *Nature, 523*(7560), 337–341. https://doi.org/10.1038/nature14432

Luo, Y., Xu, C., Wang, B., Niu, Q., Su, X., Bai, Y., Zhu, S., Zhao, C., Sun, Y., Wang, J., Liu, M., Sun, X., Song, G., Cui, H., Chen, X., Huang, H., Wang, H., Han, M., Jiang, E., Shi, L., & Feng, X. (2021). Single-cell transcriptomic analysis reveals disparate effector differentiation pathways in human treg compartment. *Nature Communications, 12*(1). https://doi.org/10.1038/s41467-021-24213-6

Mackensen, A., Müller, F., Mougiakakos, D., Böltz, S., Wilhelm, A., Aigner, M., Völkl, S., Simon, D., Kleyer, A., Munoz, L., Kretschmann, S., Kharboutli, S., Gary, R., Reimann, H., Rösler, W., Uderhardt, S., Bang, H., Herrmann, M., Ekici, A. B., … Schett, G. (2022). Anti-CD19 CAR T cell therapy for refractory systemic lupus erythematosus. *Nature Medicine, 28*(10), 2124–2132. https://doi.org/10.1038/s41591-022-02017-5

Mallick, R., Basak, S., Chowdhury, P., Bhowmik, P., Das, R. K., Banerjee, A., Paul, S., Pathak, S., & Duttaroy, A. K. (2025). Targeting cytokine-mediated inflammation in brain disorders: Developing new treatment strategies. *Pharmaceuticals, 18*(1). https://doi.org/10.3390/ph18010104

Masuda, T., Amann, L., Monaco, G., Sankowski, R., Staszewski, O., Krueger, M., Gaudio, F. Del, He, L., Paterson, N., Nent, E., Fernández-Klett, F., Yamasaki, A., Frosch, M., Fliegauf, M., Bosch, L. F. P., Ulupinar, H., Hagemeyer, N., Schreiner, D., Dorrier, C., … Prinz, M. (2022). Specification of CNS macrophage subsets occurs postnatally in defined niches. *Nature, 604*(7907), 740–748. https://doi.org/10.1038/s41586-022-04596-2

Matejuk, A., Vandenbark, A. A., & Offner, H. (2021). Cross-talk of the CNS with immune cells and functions in health and disease. *Frontiers in Neurology, 12*(672455), 1–19. https://doi.org/10.3389/fneur.2021.672455

Mauri, C., & Bosma, A. (2012). Immune regulatory function of B cells. *Annual Review of Immunology, 30*(1), 221–241. https://doi.org/10.1146/annurev-immunol-020711-074934

Maurya, S. K., Baghel, M. S., Gaurav, Chaudhary, V., Kaushik, A., & Gautam, A. (2023). Putative role of mitochondria in SARS-CoV-2 mediated brain dysfunctions: A prospect. *Biotechnology & Genetic Engineering Reviews, 39*(2), 167–192. https://doi.org/10.1080/02648725.2022.2108998

Medawar, P. B. (1948). Immunity to homologous grafted skin; the fate of skin homografts transplanted to the brain, to subcutaneous tissue, and to the anterior chamber of the eye. *British Journal of Experimental Pathology, 29*(1), 58–69.

Merlini, M., Kirabali, T., Kulic, L., Nitsch, R. M., & Ferretti, M. T. (2018). Extravascular CD3+ T cells in brains of alzheimer disease patients correlate with tau but not with amyloid pathology: An immunohistochemical study. *Neurodegenerative Diseases, 18*(1), 49–56. https://doi.org/10.1159/000486200

Mishra, A. P., Singh Meena, V., Ukey, P., Kumar, M., & Babu Gosipatala, S. (2025). Modulating autoimmune diseases with CAR-tregs: A cutting-edge therapeutic strategy. *Nature Cell and Science, 3*(3), Article e00022. https://doi.org/10.61474/ncs.2025.00022

Miyazaki, Y., & Niino, M. (2022). B-cell depletion therapy for multiple sclerosis. *Immunological Medicine, 45*(2), 54–62. https://doi.org/10.1080/25785826.2021.1952543

Montalban, X., Hauser, S. L., Kappos, L., Arnold, D. L., Bar-Or, A., Comi, G., De Seze, J., Giovannoni, G., Hartung, H. P., Hemmer, B., Lublin, F., Rammohan, K. W., Selmaj, K., Traboulsee, A., Sauter, A., Masterman, D., Fontoura, P., Belachew, S., Garren, H., … Wolinsky, J. S. (2017). Ocrelizumab versus placebo in primary progressive multiple sclerosis. *New England Journal of Medicine, 376*(3), 209–220. https://doi.org/10.1056/NEJMoa1606468

Mougiakakos, D., Krönke, G., Völkl, S., Kretschmann, S., Aigner, M., Kharboutli, S., Böltz, S., Manger, B., Mackensen, A., & Schett, G. (2021). CD19-Targeted CAR T cells in refractory systemic lupus erythematosus. *New England Journal of Medicine, 385*(6), 567–569. https://doi.org/10.1056/nejmc2107725

Mrdjen, D., Pavlovic, A., Hartmann, F. J., Schreiner, B., Utz, S. G., Leung, B. P., Lelios, I., Heppner, F. L., Kipnis, J., Merkler, D., Greter, M., & Becher, B. (2018). High-dimensional single-cell mapping of central nervous system immune cells reveals distinct myeloid subsets in health, aging, and disease. *Immunity, 48*(2), 380. https://doi.org/10.1016/j.immuni.2018.01.011

Müller, L., Di Benedetto, S., & Müller, V. (2025). The dual nature of neuroinflammation in networked brain. *Frontiers in Immunology, 16*(1659947), 1–13. https://doi.org/10.3389/fimmu.2025.1659947

Na, Y. R., Kim, S. W., & Seok, S. H. (2023). A new era of macrophage-based cell therapy. *Experimental and Molecular Medicine, 55*(9), 1945–1954. https://doi.org/10.1038/s12276-023-01068-z

Onuska, K. M. (2020). The dual role of microglia in the progression of alzheimer's disease. *Journal of Neuroscience, 40*(8), 1608–1610. https://doi.org/10.1523/JNEUROSCI.2594-19.2020

Ortiz, G. G., Pacheco-Moisés, F. P., Macías-Islas, M.Á., Flores-Alvarado, L. J., Mireles-Ramírez, M. A., González-Renovato, E. D., Hernández-Navarro, V. E., Sánchez-López, A. L., & Alatorre-Jiménez, M. A. (2014). Role of the blood-brain barrier in multiple sclerosis. *Archives of Medical Research, 45*(8), 687–697. https://doi.org/10.1016/j.arcmed.2014.11.013

Pan, J., Zhong, J., Geng, J., Oberhauser, J., Shi, S., & Wan, J. (2025). Microglial Lyzl4 facilitates β-Amyloid clearance in alzheimer's disease. *Advanced Science, 12*(2). https://doi.org/10.1002/advs.202412184

Paolicelli, R. C., Sierra, A., Stevens, B., Tremblay, M. E., Aguzzi, A., Ajami, B., Amit, I., Audinat, E., Bechmann, I., Bennett, M., Bennett, F., Bessis, A., Biber, K., Bilbo, S., Blurton-Jones, M., Boddeke, E., Brites, D., Brône, B., Brown, G. C., … Wyss-Coray, T. (2022). Microglia states and nomenclature: A field at its crossroads. *Neuron, 110*(21), 3458–3483. https://doi.org/10.1016/j.neuron.2022.10.020

Park, J. H., Kang, I., & Lee, H. K. (2022). γδ T cells in brain homeostasis and diseases. *Frontiers in Immunology, 13*. https://doi.org/10.3389/fimmu.2022.886397

Park, S.-Y., Yang, H. J., Kim, S., Yang, J., Go, H., & Bae, H. (2023). Alpha-synuclein-specific regulatory T cells ameliorate parkinson's disease progression in mice. *International Journal of Molecular Sciences, 24*(20), Article 15237. https://doi.org/10.3390/ijms242015237

Pasko, V. I., Churkina, A. S., Shakhov, A. S., Kotlobay, A. A., & Alieva, I. B. (2023). Modeling of neurodegenerative diseases: 'Step by Step' and 'Network' organization of the complexes of model systems. *Federation International Journal of Molecular Sciences, 24*(1). https://doi.org/10.3390/ijms24010604

Passaro, A. P., Lebos, A. L., Yao, Y., & Stice, S. L. (2021). Immune response in neurological pathology: Emerging role of central and peripheral immune crosstalk. *Frontiers in Immunology, 12*. https://doi.org/10.3389/fimmu.2021.676621

Pishesha, N., Harmand, T. J., & Ploegh, H. L. (2022). A guide to antigen processing and presentation. *Nature Reviews Immunology, 22*(12), 751–764. https://doi.org/10.1038/s41577-022-00707-2

Ramos-Zaldívar, H. M., Polakovicova, I., Salas-Huenuleo, E., Yefi, C. P., Silva-Ancahuail, D., Jara-Guajardo, P., Oyarzún, J. E., Neira-Troncoso, Á., Burgos, P. V., Cavieres, V. A., Arias-Muñoz, E., Martínez, C., Riveros, A. L., Corvalán, A. H., Kogan, M. J., & Andia, M. E. (2024). The cervical and meningeal lymphatic network as a pathway for retrograde nanoparticle transport to the brain. *International Journal of Nanomedicine, 19*, 10725–10743. https://doi.org/10.2147/IJN.S477159

Raphael, I., Nalawade, S., Eagar, T. N., & Forsthuber, T. G. (2015). T cell subsets and their signature cytokines in autoimmune and inflammatory diseases. *Cytokine, 74*(1), 5–17. https://doi.org/10.1016/j.cyto.2014.09.011

Reid, J. K., & Kuipers, H. F. (2021). She doesn't Even Go here: The role of inflammatory astrocytes in CNS disorders. *Frontiers in Cellular Neuroscience, 15*. https://doi.org/10.3389/fncel.2021.704884

Robert, S. M., Reeves, B. C., Kiziltug, E., Duy, P. Q., Karimy, J. K., Mansuri, M. S., Marlier, A., Allington, G., Greenberg, A. B. W., DeSpenza, T., Singh, A. K., Zeng, X., Mekbib, K. Y., Kundishora, A. J., Nelson-Williams, C., Hao, L. T., Zhang, J., Lam, T. K. T., Wilson, R., … Kahle, K. T. (2023). The choroid plexus links innate immunity to CSF dysregulation in hydrocephalus. *Cell, 186*(4), 764. https://doi.org/10.1016/j.cell.2023.01.017

Rouleau, N., Murugan, N. J., & Kaplan, D. L. (2023). Functional bioengineered models of the central nervous system. *Nature Reviews Bioengineering, 1*(4), 252–270. https://doi.org/10.1038/s44222-023-00027-7

Rustenhoven, J., Pavlou, G., Storck, S. E., Dykstra, T., Du, S., Wan, Z., Quintero, D., Scallan, J. P., Smirnov, I., Kamm, R. D., & Kipnis, J. (2023). Age-related alterations in meningeal immunity drive impaired CNS lymphatic drainage. *Journal of Experimental Medicine, 220*(7). https://doi.org/10.1084/JEM.20221929

Sabatino, J. J., Pröbstel, A. K., & Zamvil, S. S. (2019). B cells in autoimmune and neurodegenerative central nervous system diseases. *Nature Reviews Neuroscience, 20*(12), 728–745. https://doi.org/10.1038/s41583-019-0233-2

Sahlolbei, M., Azangou-Khyavy, M., Khanali, J., Khorsand, B., Shiralipour, A., Ahmadbeigi, N., Madjd, Z., Ghanbarian, H., Ardjmand, A., Hashemi, S. M., & Kiani, J. (2023). Engineering chimeric autoantibody receptor T cells for targeted B cell depletion in multiple sclerosis model: An in-vitro study. *Heliyon, 9*(9), Article e19763. https://doi.org/10.1016/j.heliyon.2023.e19763

Sainatham, C., Yadav, D., Dilli Babu, A., Tallapalli, J. R., Kanagala, S. G., Filippov, E., Murillo Chavez, F., Ahmed, N., & Lutfi, F. (2024). The current socioeconomic and regulatory landscape of immune effector cell therapies. *Frontiers of Medicine, 11*. https://doi.org/10.3389/fmed.2024.1462307

Salvador, A. F. M., Abduljawad, N., & Kipnis, J. (2024). Meningeal lymphatics in central nervous system diseases. *Annual Review of Neuroscience, 47*(1), 323–344. https://doi.org/10.1146/annurev-neuro-113023-103045

Santos Roballo, K. C., Dhungana, S., Jiang, Z., Oakey, J., & Bushman, J. S. (2019). Localized delivery of immunosuppressive regulatory T cells to peripheral nerve allografts promotes regeneration of branched segmental defects. *Biomaterials, 209*, 1–9. https://doi.org/10.1016/j.biomaterials.2019.04.015

Saresella, M., La Rosa, F., Piancone, F., Zoppis, M., Marventano, I., Calabrese, E., Rainone, V., Nemni, R., Mancuso, R., & Clerici, M. (2016). The NLRP3 and NLRP1 inflammasomes are activated in alzheimer's disease. *Molecular Neurodegeneration, 11*(1). https://doi.org/10.1186/s13024-016-0088-1

Saunders, J. A. H., Estes, K. A., Kosloski, L. M., Allen, H. E., Dempsey, K. M., Torres-Russotto, D. R., Meza, J. L., Santamaria, P. M., Bertoni, J. M., Murman, D. L., Ali, H. H., Standaert, D. G., Mosley, R. L., & Gendelman, H. E. (2012). CD4+ regulatory and effector/memory T cell subsets profile motor dysfunction in parkinson's disease. *Journal of Neuroimmune Pharmacology, 7*(4), 927–938. https://doi.org/10.1007/s11481-012-9402-z

Schlepckow, K., Monroe, K. M., Kleinberger, G., Cantuti-Castelvetri, L., Parhizkar, S., Xia, D., Willem, M., Werner, G., Pettkus, N., Brunner, B., Sülzen, A., Nuscher, B., Hampel, H., Xiang, X., Feederle, R., Tahirovic, S., Park, J. I., Prorok, R., Mahon, C., … Haass, C. (2020). Enhancing protective microglial activities with a dual function TREM2 antibody to the stalk region. *EMBO Molecular Medicine, 12*(4). https://doi.org/10.15252/emmm.201911227

Sheean, R. K., McKay, F. C., Cretney, E., Bye, C. R., Perera, N. D., Tomas, D., Weston, R. A., Scheller, K. J., Djouma, E., Menon, P., Schibeci, S. D., Marmash, N., Yerbury, J. J., Nutt, S. L., Booth, D. R., Stewart, G. J., Kiernan, M. C., Vucic, S., & Turner, B. J. (2018). Association of regulatory T-Cell expansion with progression of amyotrophic lateral sclerosis a study of humans and a transgenic mouse model. *JAMA Neurology, 75*(6), 681–689. https://doi.org/10.1001/jamaneurol.2018.0035

Sheikh, S., Safia, E. H., & Snober, S. (2013). Mir, neurodegenerative diseases: Multifactorial conformational diseases and their therapeutic interventions. *Journal of Neurodegenerative Diseases, 2013*, 1–8. https://doi.org/10.1155/2013/563481

Shemer, A., Grozovski, J., Tay, T. L., Tao, J., Volaski, A., Sub, P., Ardura-Fabregat, A., Gross-Vered, M., Kim, J. S., David, E., Chappell-Maor, L., Thielecke, L., Glass, C. K., Cornils, K., Prinz, M., & Jung, S. (2018). Engrafted parenchymal brain macrophages differ from microglia in transcriptome, chromatin landscape and response to challenge. *Nature Communications, 9*(1). https://doi.org/10.1038/s41467-018-07548-5

Shevach, E. M. (2012). Application of IL-2 therapy to target T regulatory cell function. *Trends in Immunology, 33*(12), 626–632. https://doi.org/10.1016/j.it.2012.07.007

Shi, C., Zhang, J., Wang, H., Chen, C., Han, M., Gao, L., Tang, C., Sun, P., Zhao, X., Guo, F., Wang, Z., Abdalla, M., Yang, Z., Liu, Y., Li, A., Zhang, C., & Jiang, X. (2023). Trojan horse nanocapsule enabled in situ modulation of the phenotypic conversion of Th17 cells to treg cells for the treatment of multiple sclerosis in mice. *Advanced Materials, 35*(11). https://doi.org/10.1002/adma.202210262

Shipley, F. B., Dani, N., Xu, H., Deister, C., Cui, J., Head, J. P., Sadegh, C., Fame, R. M., Shannon, M. L., Flores, V. I., Kishkovich, T., Jang, E., Klein, E. M., Goldey, G. J., He, K., Zhang, Y., Holtzman, M. J., Kirchhausen, T., Wyart, C., … Lehtinen, M. K. (2020). Tracking calcium dynamics and immune surveillance at the choroid plexus blood-cerebrospinal fluid interface. *Neuron, 108*(4), 623. https://doi.org/10.1016/j.neuron.2020.08.024

Shokr, M. M. (2025). Beyond the blood–brain barrier: Unraveling T cell subsets in CNS immunity and disease. *Inflammopharmacology, 33*(10), 5799–5818. https://doi.org/10.1007/s10787-025-01955-z

Smyth, L. C. D., & Kipnis, J. (2025). Redefining CNS immune privilege. *Nature Reviews Immunology, 25*(10), 766–775. https://doi.org/10.1038/s41577-025-01175-0

Smyth, L. C. D., Xu, D., Okar, S. V., Dykstra, T., Rustenhoven, J., Papadopoulos, Z., Bhasiin, K., Kim, M. W., Drieu, A., Mamuladze, T., Blackburn, S., Gu, X., Gaitán, M. I., Nair, G., Storck, S. E., Du, S., White, M. A., Bayguinov, P., Smirnov, I., … Kipnis, J. (2024). Identification of direct connections between the dura and the brain. *Nature, 627*(8002), 165–173. https://doi.org/10.1038/s41586-023-06993-7

Sowa, J. E., & Tokarski, K. (2021). Cellular, synaptic, and network effects of chemokines in the central nervous system and their implications to behavior. *Pharmacological Reports, 73*(6), 1595–1625. https://doi.org/10.1007/s43440-021-00323-2

Ugen, K. E., Lin, X., Bai, G., Liang, Z., Cai, J., Li, K., Song, S., Cao, C., & Sanchez-Ramos, J. (2015). Evaluation of an α synuclein sensitized dendritic cell based vaccine in a transgenic mouse model of parkinson disease. *Human Vaccines and Immunotherapeutics, 11*(4), 922–930. https://doi.org/10.1080/21645515.2015.1012033

Unger, M. S., Li, E., Scharnagl, L., Poupardin, R., Altendorfer, B., Mrowetz, H., Hutter-Paier, B., Weiger, T. M., Heneka, M. T., Attems, J., & Aigner, L. (2020). CD8+ T-cells infiltrate alzheimer's disease brains and regulate neuronal- and synapse-related gene expression in APP-PS1 transgenic mice. *Brain, Behavior, and Immunity, 89*, 67–86. https://doi.org/10.1016/j.bbi.2020.05.070

Utz, S. G., See, P., Mildenberger, W., Thion, M. S., Silvin, A., Lutz, M., Ingelfinger, F., Rayan, N. A., Lelios, I., Buttgereit, A., Asano, K., Prabhakar, S., Garel, S., Becher, B., Ginhoux, F., & Greter, M. (2020). Early fate defines microglia and non-parenchymal brain macrophage development. *Cell, 181*(3), 557. https://doi.org/10.1016/j.cell.2020.03.021

Verkhratsky, A., Parpura, V., Li, B., & Scuderi, C. (2021). Astrocytes: The housekeepers and guardians of the CNS. *Advances in Neurobiology, 26*, 21–53. https://doi.org/10.1007/978-3-030-77375-5_2

Verma, N. D., Lam, A. D., Chiu, C., Tran, G. T., Hall, B. M., & Hodgkinson, S. J. (2021). Multiple sclerosis patients have reduced resting and increased activated CD4+CD25+FOXP3+T regulatory cells. *Scientific Reports, 11*(1). https://doi.org/10.1038/s41598-021-88448-5

Vivier, E., Artis, D., Colonna, M., Diefenbach, A., Di Santo, J. P., Eberl, G., Koyasu, S., Locksley, R. M., McKenzie, A. N. J., Mebius, R. E., Powrie, F., & Spits, H. (2018). Innate lymphoid cells: 10 years on. *Cell, 174*(5), 1054–1066. https://doi.org/10.1016/j.cell.2018.07.017

Von Essen, M. R., Ammitzbøll, C., Hansen, R. H., Petersen, E. R. S., McWilliam, O., Marquart, H. V., Damm, P., & Sellebjerg, F. (2019). Proinflammatory CD20+ T cells in the pathogenesis of multiple sclerosis. *Brain, 142*(1), 120–132. https://doi.org/10.1093/brain/awy301

Wang, H. L., Cheng, Y. C., Yeh, T. H., Liu, H. F., Weng, Y. H., Chen, R. S., Chen, Y. C., Lu, J. C., Hwang, T. L., Wei, K. C., Liu, Y. C., Wang, Y. T., Hsu, C. C., Chiu, T. J., & Chiu, C. C. (2023). HCH6-1, an antagonist of formyl peptide receptor-1, exerts anti-neuroinflammatory and neuroprotective effects in cellular and animal models of parkinson's disease. *Biochemical Pharmacology, 212*. https://doi.org/10.1016/j.bcp.2023.115524

Wang, S., Mustafa, M., Yuede, C. M., Viveros Salazar, S., Kong, P., Long, H., Ward, M., Siddiqui, O., Paul, R., Gilfillan, S., Ibrahim, A., Rhinn, H., Tassi, I., Rosenthal, A., Schwabe, T., & Colonna, M. (2020). Anti-human TREM2 induces microglia proliferation and reduces pathology in an alzheimer's disease model. *Journal of Experimental Medicine, 217*(9). https://doi.org/10.1084/jem.20200785

Weiner, H. L. (2025). Immune mechanisms and shared immune targets in neurodegenerative diseases. *Nature Reviews Neurology, 21*(2), 67–85. https://doi.org/10.1038/s41582-024-01046-7

Whittam, D. H., Tallantyre, E. C., Jolles, S., Huda, S., Moots, R. J., Kim, H. J., Robertson, N. P., Cree, B. A. C., & Jacob, A. (2019). Rituximab in neurological disease: Principles, evidence and practice. *Practical Neurology, 19*(1), 5–20. https://doi.org/10.1136/practneurol-2018-001899

Wyatt-Johnson, S. K., Afify, R., & Brutkiewicz, R. R. (2024). The immune system in neurological diseases: What innate-like T cells have to say. *Journal of Allergy and Clinical Immunology, 153*(4), 913–923. https://doi.org/10.1016/j.jaci.2024.02.003

Xiao, H., & Yang, K. (2025). Role of macrophages in neuroimmune regulation. *Frontiers in Immunology, 16*. https://doi.org/10.3389/fimmu.2025.1573174

Xu, W., Huang, Y., & Zhou, R. (2025a). NLRP3 inflammasome in neuroinflammation and central nervous system diseases. *Cellular and Molecular Immunology, 22*(4), 341–355. https://doi.org/10.1038/s41423-025-01275-w

Xu, J., Ma, C., Hua, M., Li, J., Xiang, Z., & Wu, J. (2022). CNS and CNS diseases in relation to their immune system. *Frontiers in Immunology, 13*. https://doi.org/10.3389/fimmu.2022.1063928

Xu, Q., Xu, W., Cheng, H., Yuan, H., & Tan, X. (2019). Efficacy and mechanism of cGAMP to suppress alzheimer,' s disease by elevating TREM2. *Brain, Behavior, and Immunity, 81*, 495–508. https://doi.org/10.1016/j.bbi.2019.07.004

Xu, Z., Xu, Z., Lu, J., Zhang, J., & Shi, L. (2025b). Regulatory T cells as novel cell-based therapy for ischemic stroke. *Journal of Cerebral Blood Flow and Metabolism, 45*(10), 1859–1876. https://doi.org/10.1177/0271678X251366071

Yang, H., Soo Byun, M., Ha, N.-Y., Yang, J., Park, S.-Y., Jee, E. P., Yi, D., Chang, Y.-T., Jung, W. S., Kim, J. Y., Kim, J., Dong, Y. L., & Bae, H. (2024). A preclinical and phase i clinical study of ex vivo-expanded amyloid beta-specific human regulatory T cells in alzheimer's disease. *Biomedicine and Pharmacotherapy, 181*, Article 117721. https://doi.org/10.1016/j.biopha.2024.117721

Zamecnik, C. R., Levy, E. S., Lowe, M. M., Zirak, B., Rosenblum, M. D., & Desai, T. A. (2020). An injectable cytokine trap for local treatment of autoimmune disease. *Biomaterials, 230.* https://doi.org/10.1016/j.biomaterials.2019.119626

Zeng, J., Liu, J., Qu, Q., Zhao, X., & Zhang, J. (2022). JKAP, Th1 cells, and Th17 cells are dysregulated and intercorrelated, among them JKAP and Th17 cells relate to cognitive impairment progression in alzheimer's disease patients. *Irish Journal of Medical Science, 191*(4), 1855–1861. https://doi.org/10.1007/s11845-021-02749-2

Zhan, T., Tian, S., & Chen, S. (2024). Border-associated macrophages: From embryogenesis to immune regulation. *CNS Neuroscience and Therapeutics, 30*(11). https://doi.org/10.1111/cns.70105

Zhan, X., Wang, S., Bèchet, N., Gouras, G., & Wen, G. (2025). Perivascular macrophages in the central nervous system: Insights into their roles in health and disease. *Cell Death & Disease, 16*(1). https://doi.org/10.1038/s41419-025-07592-2

Zhang, Y., & Niu, C. (2022). Relation of CDC42, Th1, Th2, and Th17 cells with cognitive function decline in alzheimer's disease. *Annals of Clinical and Translational Neurology, 9*(9), 1428–1436. https://doi.org/10.1002/acn3.51643

Zhang, B., Sun, J., Wang, Y., Ji, D., Yuan, Y., Li, S., Sun, Y., Hou, Y., Li, P., Zhao, L., Yu, F., Ma, W., Cheng, B., Wu, L., Hu, J., Wang, M., Song, W., Li, X., Li, H., … Zhang, X. (2021). Site-specific PEGylation of interleukin-2 enhances immunosuppression via the sustained activation of regulatory T cells. *Nature Biomedical Engineering, 5*(11), 1288–1305. https://doi.org/10.1038/s41551-021-00797-8

Zhao, P., Xu, Y., Jiang, L. L., Fan, X., Li, L., Li, X., Arase, H., Zhao, Y., Cao, W., Zheng, H., Xu, H., Tong, Q., Zhang, N., & An, Z. (2022). A tetravalent TREM2 agonistic antibody reduced amyloid pathology in a mouse model of alzheimer's disease. *Science Translational Medicine, 14*(661). https://doi.org/10.1126/scitranslmed.abq0095

Zrzavy, T., Hametner, S., Wimmer, I., Butovsky, O., Weiner, H. L., & Lassmann, H. (2017). Loss of 'homeostatic' microglia and patterns of their activation in active multiple sclerosis. *Brain, 140*(7), 1900–1913. https://doi.org/10.1093/brain/awx113

CHAPTER

Genetherapy in neurological disorders

9

Victor Bushlyar[1], Bhaskar Roy[1] and Atri Chatterjee[2]

[1]*Department of Neurology, Yale School of Medicine, New Haven, CT, United States;* [2]*Department of Neurology, Varshman Mahavir Medical College & Safdarjung Hospital, New Delhi, Delhi, India*

1. Introduction

Genetic disorders affect approximately 10 per 1000 live births worldwide (Blencowe et al., 2018). Nearly 10,000 monogenic disorders have been identified so far, out of which 17% are neurologic disorders (Devinsky et al., 2025). Although genetic disorders vary widely in clinical manifestations, most of them are devastating, causing lifelong suffering to affected patients and families. Gene therapy attempts to correct the effects of genetic mutations by introducing novel genetic material into the affected host or by altering the genetic sequence of the host. Gene therapy applications have extended beyond inherited genetic disorders into cancer treatment, as cancer cells frequently harbour genetic mutations. The European Medicines Agency (EMA) defines gene therapy as "therapeutic agents that contain genes that lead to a therapeutic, prophylactic or diagnostic effect(EMA definition, n.d.)." The United States Food and Drug Administration (US FDA) defines gene therapy as a technique that "seeks to modify or manipulate the expression of a gene or to alter the biological properties of living cells for therapeutic use" through one of the following approaches: (1) replacing a disease causing gene with a healthy copy of the gene, (2) inactivating a disease causing gene and (3) introducing a new or modified gene into the body to cure a disease (*USFDA definition*, 2018). In this chapter, we provide an overview of the development of gene therapy, current approaches and clinical applications in neurologic disorders.

2. Development of gene therapy

The first genetic mutation causing a human disease was identified in the beta globin gene, where mutations lead to a haemoglobinopathy like thalassemia. The first neurologic disorder with an identified genetic locus was Huntington's disease, which was linked to chromosome 4(MacDonald et al., 1993). The advent of positional cloning and polymerase chain reaction rapidly accelerated the pace of discovery of disease-causing genetic mutations. Dystrophin, the gene associated with Duchenne muscular dystrophy (DMD), was one of the first genes identified by positional cloning in 1986 (van Ommen et al., 1986). By 2000, the Online Mendelian Inheritance in Man (OMIM) database recorded 1000 genes with disease-causing variants. Some major successes included identifying the *SMN1* gene

Immunotherapies for Neurological Disorders. https://doi.org/10.1016/B978-0-443-44631-3.00001-9

responsible for spinal muscular atrophy and presenilin1 (*PSEN1*), responsible for familial Alzheimer's disease. Since the turn of the century, next-generation sequencing technology has radically reduced the cost and time required to perform genetic sequencing. As a result, nearly 3000 disease-causing genetic variants were discovered during the first 2 decades of the 21st century.

In 1944, Avery, McLeod and McCarthy demonstrated that pneumococci can accept and express foreign DNA (Averyet al., 1944). In mammalian cells, Polyomavirus and Simian virus 40 (SV40) were shown to be able to integrate their genome into the host DNA and cause neoplasia. This discovery opened up the possibilities of modifying the human genome using foreign DNA. In 1972, Friedmann and Roblin published a seminal paper in Science proposing the possible treatment of genetic disease in humans by genetic modification (Friedmann & Roblin, 1972). In one of the first attempts at gene therapy, Rogers and colleagues injected wild-type Shope papilloma virus into two girls diagnosed with hyperargininemia, with the hope of expressing arginine in vivo (Friedmann, 2001). Unfortunately, genetic and immunological principles of gene therapy were unknown then, and the experiment failed.

The calcium phosphate chemical transfection process was discovered in the 1970s, which enabled researchers to introduce large amounts of cloned DNA into mammalian cells (Friedmann, 1992). In an HPRT-deficient cell culture model of Lesch-Nyhan syndrome, murine GPT enzyme was introduced into the cells to correct their enzyme deficiency. Using the calcium phosphate transfection method, Cline and colleagues introduced the beta globin gene into murine bone marrow cells. The modified cells were introduced into the animals after irradiating the bone marrow. The same group of researchers attempted to treat two patients of severe beta thalassemia with recombinant plasmids containing the beta globin gene without proper institutional approvals (Beutler, 2001). The attempt was unsuccessful and laid bare the need for ethical regulations in an emerging frontier of medicine. In response to the Cline experiments, the National Institute of Health (NIH) of the United States of America (USA) established a Gene Therapy Subcommittee to regulate the use of genetic tools in humans (Sun, 1981). In 1983, researchers came together at the Banbury conference centre of the Cold Spring Harbour Laboratory on Long Island, New York and charted future directions in the development of gene therapy (Greenberg et al., 2011).

In the 1980s, the replication and gene transcription processes of retroviruses were discovered. Temin and colleagues developed techniques to use retroviruses as vectors by inserting mammalian genes into the retroviral DNA (Shimotohno & Temin, 1981). The retroviral vectors proved far more efficient than the chemical transfection method. In Lesch-Nyhan cells, a retroviral vector with the HPRT gene insert induced stable expression of the deficient enzyme. Despite the breakthrough, the limitations of the early retroviral vectors soon became apparent. These vectors could insert a limited genetic payload in the host genome, and in the process, may integrate at random sites in the host DNA, running the risk of insertional mutagenesis due to enhancers in the vector DNA. They could only integrate into the host genome during cell division and could not be used for neurological diseases, as neurons are post-mitotic cells. As a next step, researchers engineered lentiviral vectors from the human immunodeficiency virus (HIV) by replacing the env protein with the capsid protein of the vesicular stomatitis virus (Naldini et al., 1996). Further modifications of the HIV produced a self-inactivating strain, reducing the risk of infection. Lentiviral vectors could deliver genes to the central nervous system of experimental animals (Milone & O'Doherty, 2018). In mouse models of neurological disorders like metachromatic leukodystrophy and Parkinson's disease, lentivirus vectors proved effective.

In a quest for better vectors, adenovirus strains were modified by substituting the E1 and E3 regions of their DNA with an expression cassette (Muravyeva & Smirnikhina, 2024). The early generation adenovirus vectors generated a strong immunological response, and their tropism to a wide variety of host cells proved a disadvantage. In September 1999, Jesse Gelsinger, participating in a gene therapy trial at the University of Pennsylvania, received a second-generation adenovirus factor to treat ornithine transcarbamylase deficiency(Sibbald, 2001). Gelsinger developed symptoms of liver injury and disseminated intravascular coagulation within hours of receiving the treatment and died 4 days later. An autopsy revealed that the adenovirus vector had reached the spleen, bone marrow and lymph nodes and triggered a severe inflammatory response. In response to the unfortunate death of Gelsinger, the US Food and Drug Administration (US FDA) halted ongoing gene therapy clinical trials and initiated two new programs: the Gene Therapy Clinical Trial Monitoring Plan and the Gene Transfer Safety Symposium (Sibbald, 2001). This incident remains a stark reminder of ethical and practical challenges in the field of gene therapy.

Adeno-associated viruses (AAV) were first discovered as contaminants in cell culture preparations. The lifecycle of AAV is dependent on a helper virus, hence its name. Following the sequencing of the AAV genome, it was considered a potential vector because of its widespread tissue tropism and lack of pathogenicity. Recombinant AAV vectors became the leading candidate for therapeutic use because of their safety and efficiency. In 2012, the European Medicines Agency (EMA) approved the first recombinant AAV gene therapy, alipogenetiparvovec (Glybera), for lipoprotein lipase deficiency (Ylä-Herttuala, 2012). In 2017, the USFDA approved voretigenenivarcin (Luxturna) for RPE65-associated blindness (*USFDA Luxturna*, 2017). The AAV9 serotype showed the ability to cross the blood-brain barrier and was considered a candidate for gene delivery to the central nervous system. The AAV9 vector was used to develop onasemnogeneabeparvovec (Zolgensma) for the treatment of spinal muscular atrophy (SMA). This breakthrough drug significantly improved the ability of the affected children to reach developmental milestones and received US FDA approval for the treatment of children under 2 years of age diagnosed with SMA in 2019 (Blair, 2022).

Herpesviruses can infect the nervous system and remain latent for prolonged periods. This property, and the ability to carry large genetic payloads of 30–40 kilobases, makes herpes viruses interesting candidates as vectors for neurological disorders. Early clinical trials leveraged the ability of the herpes simplex virus to infect dorsal root ganglion cells, leading to the successful treatment of intractable cancer-associated pain. The first viral gene therapy for cancer was based on a modified herpes simplex virus 1 (HSV-1); the US FDA approved talimogene laherparepvec for the treatment of unresectable melanoma in 2015 (Pol et al., 2016). Further developments led to the approval of beremagenegeperpavec in 2022, a topical gene therapy for the devastating skin disease recessive dystrophic epidermolysis bullosa(Koutsoukos & Bilousova, 2024).

Due to concerns about the immunological response to viral vectors and the limitations of the genetic payload size, a parallel strand of research focused on developing non-viral delivery systems for gene therapy. In 1972, Nobel Laureate Har Govind Khorana published a series of papers describing the synthesis of an artificial DNA sequence corresponding to a yeast RNA sequence (Kresge et al., 2009). In 1978, Stephenson and colleagues synthesized an oligonucleotide to bind and inhibit rod sarcoma virus in a wheat embryo cell-free system (Stephenson & Zamecnik, 1978). Stephenson's work became the foundation for developing antisense oligonucleotides (ASOs), short synthetic nucleic acid sequences that bind cellular RNAs to modify gene expression. The ASOs are susceptible to degradation by nucleases, limiting their utility. To prevent nuclease-mediated degradation, Joseph Walder developed gapmers, a short DNA nucleotide core flanked by a segment of nucleic acids. Gapmers bind a target RNA transcript, and the DNA-RNA hybrid activates RNAase H, which degrades the target RNA

(Lauffer et al., 2024). In the 1990s, the first clinical trials of ASOs commenced, targeting p53 transcription in leukaemia. In 1998, fomivirsen became the first ASO approved for clinical use to treat cytomegalovirus retinitis (Roehr, 1998). In 2002, tricycloDNA oligonucleotides were synthesized by modifying the nucleosides (Renneberg & Leumann, 2002). In 2013, Mendell et al. demonstrated the efficacy of eteplirsen in children with DMD. This ASO directed the cellular machinery to skip exon 51 of the dystrophin gene harbouring mutations, which leads to the production of a truncated but functional proteins (Mendell et al., 2013). In 2016, the US FDA approved eteplirsen for treating DMD (Stein, 2016). In the same year, nusinersen was approved for spinal muscular atrophy (SMA) treatment. Subsequently, golodirsen and viltolarsen were also approved for the treatment of DMD by the US FDA in 2019 and 2020, respectively.

RNA-associated interference (RNAi), a natural defence mechanism found in plants against foreign nucleic acids, was discovered in 1998 (Fire et al., 1998). In 2001, Tuschl and colleagues used an siRNA to silence gene expression in mammalian cells (Elbashir et al., 2001). This opened up the possibility of using siRNAs as therapeutic agents, but several hurdles remained. For clinical use, siRNAs had to be stable, bind specific targets with minimal off-target binding and avoid eliciting a strong immune response. Over the next 2 decades, several technical developments enabled researchers to overcome these hurdles. For example, conjugation of siRNA with N-acetylgalactosamine (GalNAc) improved cellular uptake of therapeutic siRNAs, particularly in hepatocytes (Zhang et al., 2022). Givosiran, a GalNAc-siRNA conjugate developed for treating acute hepatic porphyria, received US FDA approval in 2019 (Dickey & Leaf, 2024). Lipid nanoparticles have been under development for efficient delivery of macromolecules like siRNAs into cells; the development of ionizable cationic lipids finally enabled clinical translation of lipid nanoparticles into viable drug delivery vehicles. The lipid encapsulates the RNA and enables cellular uptake via the low-density lipoprotein receptor. Based on this technology, patisiran was developed to treat hereditary transthyretin amyloidosis, which was approved for clinical use in 2018.

In 1987, Ishino et al. from Osaka University discovered an interesting feature in the Escherichia coli genome, later named clustered regularly interspersed short palindromic repeats (CRISPR) (Ishino et al., 1987). Although the biological function of the CRISPR sequences was unknown, as different strains of bacteria possessed specific CRISPR sequences, scientists proposed that CRISPR sequences may be utilized to detect bacterial strains. In 1995, Mojica identified similar sequences in the genome of Haloferax mediterranei (Mojica et al., 1995). He hypothesized that the CRISPR sequences may represent a bacterial defence against viral infections. In 2007, Barrangou and Horvath, working with yoghurt cultures, demonstrated that Streptococcus thermophilus acquired new spacer sequences at the CRISPR locus in response to bacteriophage infections (Barrangou et al., 2007). It was also observed that the bacterial genes for Cas nucleases were located in close proximity to the CRISPR loci. In 2005, Bolotin et al. described the function of the Cas9 nuclease, which worked like a pair of genetic scissors against foreign DNA entering the bacterial cell (Bolotin et al., 2005). Emmanuelle Charpentier's research discovered the trans-activating CRISPR RNA in 2011, which proved to be essential for the use of the CRISPR-Cas9 system as a tool for genetic modification (Deltcheva et al., 2011). In 2013, five groups, including Jennifer Doudna's research group, reported the first use of CRISPR-Cas9 to edit the genome in human cells. Doudna published the structure of the Cas9 nuclease the following year (Jinek et al., 2014). The enormous clinical potential of the CRISPR-Cas9 system was immediately apparent, and a lengthy battle for intellectual property rights ensued between research groups and institutes. The scientific community was also concerned about the ethical use of gene editing in humans, particularly in germline cells. Doudna organized a scientific meeting focused on different aspects of CRISPR-Cas9 use, and the report was published in Science in 2015 (Baltimore et al., 2015). The first report on clinical use of CRISPR-Cas9 emerged from China in the same year, when a group of scientists edited the genome of human embryos resulting from in vitro fertilization (IVF) (Gostimskaya, 2022). In 2017, the first human clinical trials using CRISPR-Cas9 commenced in parallel in the USA and China. The trials utilized an ex vivo approach to modify the PD-1 gene of cancer patients in an attempt to reprogram the immune system against tumours. In a shocking development, scientist and startup founder Jiankui He modified and recruited couples undergoing IVF treatment for a clinical trial. He edited the CCR5 gene in the embryos in an attempt to develop resistance to HIV infection. He reported the birth of twin girls in 2018, the world's first CRISPR-edited babies (Gostimskaya, 2022). His work resulted in worldwide furore, and he was put under house arrest in China. A historic milestone was achieved in 2023, when exagamglogeneautotemcel (exa-cel) became the first CRISPR therapy approved for clinical use in sickle cell disease (Singh et al., 2024). Neurological disorders associated with point mutations have become a focus of therapeutic development using the CRISPR-Cas9 system. Treatments of neurodegenerative disorders like Alzheimer's disease, Parkinson's disease, amyotrophic lateral sclerosis, muscular dystrophies like DMD and genetic epilepsies are presently under investigation. Despite some successes in preclinical models, CRISPR therapy for neurological disorders faces crucial barriers, such as efficient delivery across the blood-brain barrier.

The culmination of gene therapy from a theoretical concept to reality took decades and involved multiple strands of research. As our understanding of the biology of gene expression and mechanisms of genetic disorders has evolved, gene therapy tools and techniques have become increasingly sophisticated and specific. The field continues to move apace with many clinical trials testing emerging therapeutics. These techniques and their applications are discussed in the following sections. An overview of different types of gene therapies has been shown in Figs. 9.1 and 9.2.

3. Approaches to gene therapy

There are approximately 1700 known genetic disorders affecting the nervous system. Due to the heterogeneity of the pathophysiology of neurogenic disorders, gene therapy in neurologic diseases involves several considerations. First, whether the disorder is monogenic or polygenic. Early successes in gene therapy were achieved in monogenic disorders like SMA and DMD, where genetic modification lead to durable treatment effects. On the other hand, for polygenic disorders like sporadic Alzheimer's disease, a significant risk factor like *APOE4* may be modified, but a curative effect may not be possible. Second, the type of causative genetic mutation dictates the gene therapy solutions that may be available. Genetic mutations can range from subtle changes like point mutations and copy number variations to large-scale abnormalities such as chromosomal aneuploidy. Most genetic therapies approved for clinical use target point mutations. Recently, Hashizume et al. developed a method to remove the extra copy of chromosome 21 in Down syndrome from pluripotent stem cells and fibroblasts using CRISPR-Cas9 (Hashizume et al., 2025). Third, the effect of a genetic mutation may lead to either a toxic gain of function or a loss of function. Depending upon the pathophysiology, gene therapy may target suppression of the mutant gene or supplementation of the protein transcribed from the mutant gene.

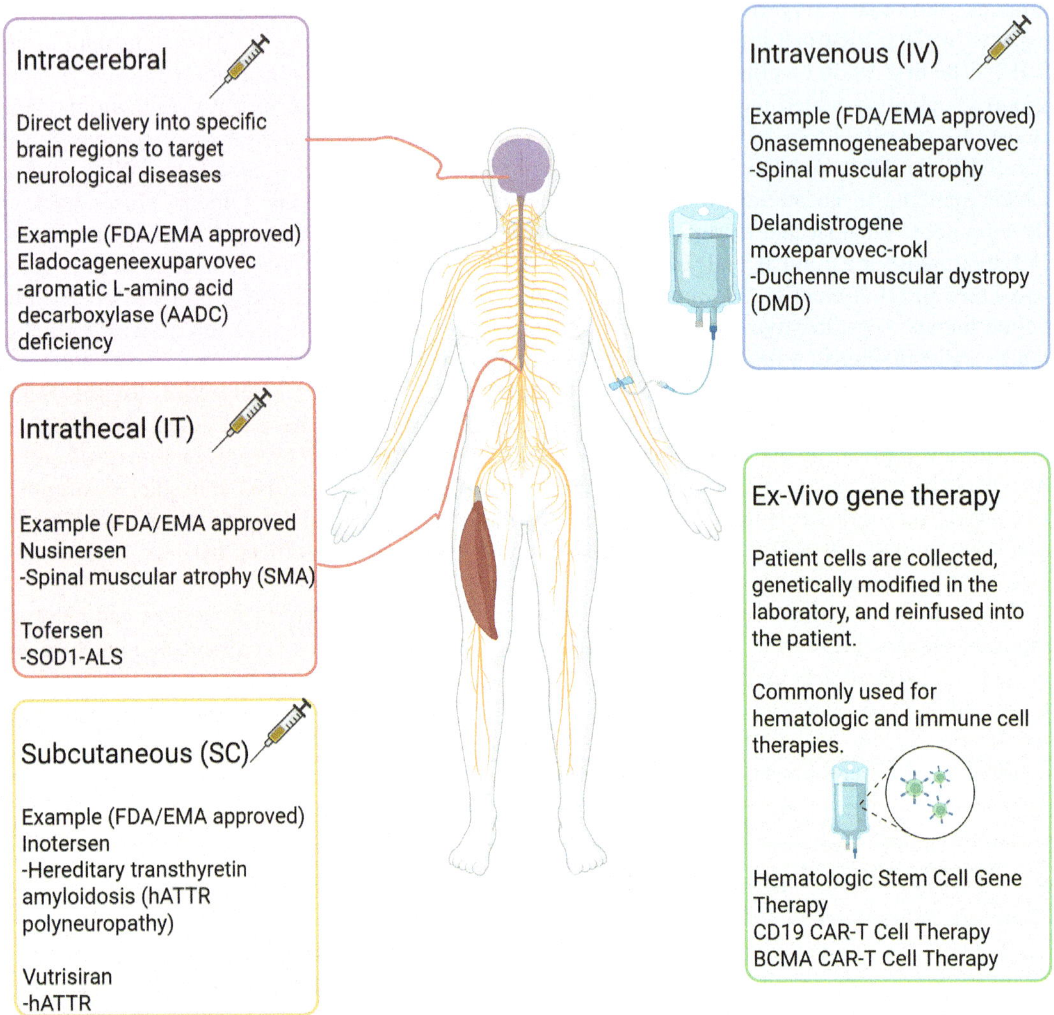

FIGURE 9.1

Common methods of gene therapy, including RNA interference therapy, gene replacement therapy, and genome and epigenome editing.

Figure generated using artificial intelligence and adapted from Coller et al., Trends in Molecular Medicine, 2025. https://doi.org/10.1016/j.molmed.2025.01.015.

There are two major approaches to gene therapy at present: ex-vivo and in-vivo genetic modification of host cells. In the ex-vivo approach, cells from the patient are collected, modified and transferred back to the host. For example, $CD34^+$ cells from the bone marrow of patients with severe combined immune deficiency due to a lack of adenosine deaminase were transfected with a retroviral vector containing a functional *ADA* gene. The treatment resulted in the recovery of immune function in

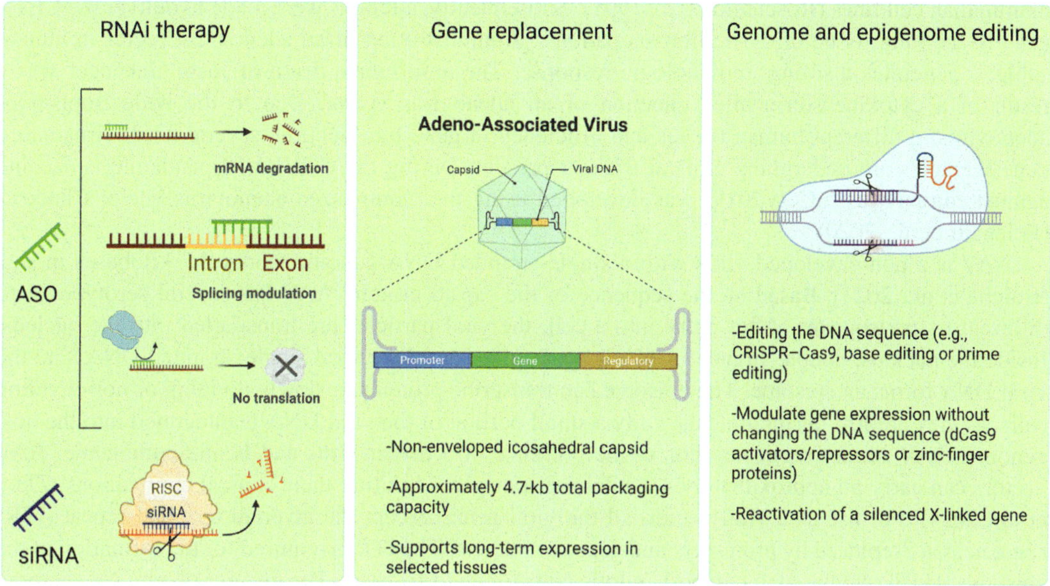

FIGURE 9.2

Different administration routes and some examples in gene therapy. Figure generated using artificial intelligence.

nine out of 10 patients (Griesenbach, 2007). In chimeric antigen receptor (CAR) T cell therapy, T cells from a patient are transduced ex-vivo to express a CAR targeting a specific cancer-associated antigen. Several CAR T cell therapies have received approval for clinical use in hematological malignancies.

In the in-vivo approach, the therapeutic genetic material is injected into the host, preferably into the affected tissue. Luxturna is administered as a subretinal injection in each eye in patients affected by *RPE65*-associated blindness. For therapies targeting the CNS, adequate dose delivery across the BBB remains an important concern. Zolgensma demonstrates therapeutic effects after intravenous administration. On the other hand, eladocageneexuparvovec-tneq (Kebilidi), a gene replacement therapy approved for aromatic L-amino acid decarboxylase deficiency, is required to be administered into the brain by a stereotactic procedure (Zhang et al., 2025).

Adenovirus is a non-enveloped virus with a 26–45 kilobase linear, double-stranded DNA genome. It commonly causes respiratory tract infections in humans (Bulcha et al., 2021). There are seven subgroups of adenovirus, named A to G, that cause infection in humans. The virus binds to different cell surface receptors, such as the Coxsackie virus – Ad receptor and sialic acid. Binding to the cell surface receptor is followed by endocytosis of the virus particle. Inside the cell, the capsule is dismantled, and the viral DNA enters the nucleus through nuclear pores. The viral DNA remains in the nucleus without integrating into the host genome, forming an episome. Adenovirus vectors are able to transduce genes efficiently in mitotic and post-mitotic cells. They can be used for a broad range of target tissues, and the episome persists in the host cell for a prolonged period. Third-generation adenovirus vectors are prepared by deleting all the viral genes except the inverted terminal repeats and a packaging signal. Adenovirus vectors were first used to express the α1-antitrypsin enzyme in mammalian cell lines (Rosenfeld et al., 1991). Subsequently, attempts were made to deliver the CFTR gene to the lung tissue of cystic fibrosis patients. Administration of an adenovirus vector in human subjects generates a strong immunologic response. The unfortunate death of Jesse Gelsinger was a result of a cytokine storm after injection of an adenovirus vector. Due to the wide tropism of adenovirus in different human tissues and efficiency in gene transduction, several adenovirus-based gene therapies are undergoing clinical trials at present. During the COVID-19 pandemic, a vaccine against coronavirus (nCOV2019) was developed using the chimpanzee adenovirus vector Chadox1 (Folegatti et al., 2020).

AAV is a non-enveloped virus with a single-stranded DNA genome, about 4.7 kilobases in size (Bulcha et al., 2021). Based on the sequence of the capsid protein, AAV has several serotypes with different tissue tropisms. After entry into a cell, the viral particles are transported into the nucleus. Inside the nucleus, double-stranded DNA is synthesized from the viral single-stranded DNA, and the viral DNA forms an episome. The episome can transcribe proteins in slowly dividing or non-dividing cells, as they are lost during mitosis. Only a small portion of the viral DNA is integrated into the host genome. AAV cannot replicate without the presence of a helper virus and is non-pathogenic. AAV vectors can carry an approximately 4.7-kilobase transgene, limiting their clinical applications (Zhou et al., 2024). For use as a viral vector, all the viral genes except the inverted terminal repeat (ITR) sequences are replaced by promoters and genes of interest. The ITR is required for the formation of the episome, which remains stable in post-mitotic cells for up to 10 years. The first use of an AAV vector in humans was reported in 1995, when the *CFTR* gene was packaged in an AAV2 vector and administered to a patient with cystic fibrosis (Flotte et al., 1996). Subsequently, voretigeneneparvovec was developed using an AAV2 vector for delivery of the *RPE65* gene to the retina. AAV9 can cross the blood-brain barrier (BBB) and reach the central nervous system (CNS) after an intravenous infusion (Zhou et al., 2024). It can transduce both neurons and astrocytes in the CNS. Due to these advantages, AAV9 has become the most widely used vector for gene delivery to the CNS. Based on the AAV9 vector, Zolgensma was developed for clinical use in SMA. Although AAV has low immunogenicity, recombinant AAV-based gene therapies elicit an adaptive immune response to viral capsids. In addition, there may be an innate immune response, which is not well-studied. Determination of the correct dose remains a challenge to avoid eliciting a strong immunological response. In addition to immune activation, severe adverse effects to AAV gene therapy have been reported, which include hepatic and renal toxicity, myocarditis and death.

Lentiviruses are single-stranded RNA viruses belonging to the family Retroviridae. Lentiviruses bind to glycoprotein receptors on the surface of host cells and deliver the viral genome into the cytoplasm. The viral RNA induces reverse transcription into DNA, which is integrated into the host genome. Lentivirus vectors are derived from HIV. The vectors can carry a genetic cargo of approximately nine kilobases. A single vector can carry several genes, both in mitotic and post-mitotic cells (Bulcha et al., 2021). To mitigate the risk of generation of replication-competent viruses inside the host, most native viral genes are deleted, along with part of the 3′ LTR sequence. The lentivirus vector was first used in HIV seropositive patients, where autologous CD4 T cells were transduced with an anti-sense sequence against the viral envelope gene of HIV. When the modified T cells were transfused back into the patients, the viral load was significantly lowered (Levine et al., 2006). Using a similar approach, hematopoietic stem cells and progenitor cells from patients suffering from sickle cell anemia were transduced with a lentiviral vector BB305 encoding a modified β globin(Thompson et al.,

2018) gene. This gene therapy, known as lovotibeglogeneautotemcel, resulted in a significant increase in hemoglobin and resolution of vaso-occlusive crises in treated patients (Kanter NEJM 2022). In a clinical trial, autologous $CD34^+$ cells from patients of X-linked adrenoleukodystrophy were transduced with a lentiviral vector containing the ABCD1 gene and infused back into the patients (Eichler et al., 2017). The STARBEAM study demonstrated functional and radiological stabilization of patients after treatment and Elivaldogeneautotemcel (Skysona), as approved for clinical use in 2022 (Scott et al., 2023).

Herpes simplex virus (HSV) is an enveloped virus with a double-stranded DNA. The virus can infect neurons, particularly sensory neurons in the dorsal root ganglia and remain dormant for years. Three types of HSV vectors have been developed for gene therapy. First, amplicon HSV vectors can carry a large genetic payload of approximately 100 kilobases. Second, replication-deficient HSV vectors do not possess genes necessary for replication. Third, replication-competent HSV vectors can replicate in vitro but not in vivo. Due to the ability of HSV vectors to induce cellular lysis, most HSV vector clinical trials are focused on cancer therapy. An HSV-based gene therapy, talimogene laherparepvec (Imlygic), was approved for the treatment of unresectable melanoma by the US FDA. Imlygic is undergoing further clinical trials for use in other cancers such as breast cancer and hepatocellular carcinoma. In the CNS, HSV-based gene therapy is under development for the treatment of recurrent glioma. Use of HSV as a vector is fraught with the risk of disseminated herpes infection and serious inflammatory reactions such as glomerulonephritis.

While the majority of gene therapy clinical trials have employed viral vectors, this approach continues to face significant challenges. Viral vectors are difficult to manufacture at scale and fraught with the risk of immunological reactions upon administration. Therefore, non-viral delivery methods for gene therapy have been an active field of research. Non-viral vectors include polymers, lipids, peptides and inorganic materials. Polyethylenimine (PEI) was the first synthetic polymer invented for gene therapy in 1995 (Casper et al., 2023). Although PEI has the ability to efficiently transfect cells with a genetic cargo, it is a non-biodegradable polymer that gradually accumulates within a cell. To avoid cellular toxicity from the vector after repeated administrations, biodegradable polymers were designed. For example, chitosan is a bio-degradable, carbohydrate-based polymer that can enter cells through tight junctions (Antoniou et al., 2024). Chitosan nanoparticles are being developed for gene therapy in cancer. Lipids can bind nucleic acids to form lipoplexes, which can be formulated as lipid nanoparticles, liposomes or lipid emulsions. Lipid nanoparticles are used for mRNA and siRNA delivery, as the lipid protects the RNA from degradation by nucleases. Onpattro, an anti-transthyretin siRNA contained in liposomes, was approved for clinical use in hereditary transthyretin amyloidosis (Adams et al., 2018).

ASOs are a novel class of therapeutic agents that target mRNAs. ASOs are generally 15 to 20 base pairs in length and bind RNAs with complementary sequence (Collotta et al., 2023). The binding results in interference with RNA function, either by arrest of translation of the RNA into proteins or by promoting RNA degradation by endogenous enzymes like RNAase H. Any unmodified foreign nucleic acid would be rapidly degraded by nucleases after administration into the human body; therefore, ASOs require chemical modifications to increase their stability. In the first generation ASOs, and oxygen atom in the phosphate group of the nucleic acid was replaced by a sulphur atom. This phosphorothoate modification lead to increased resistance to nuclease degradation of the ASO (Kulkarni et al., 2021). In the second generation ASOs, the sugar moiety of the nucleic acid was modified to increase binding affinity. A gapmer strategy was used, where modified nucleotides flank a central sequence of nucleotides designed to bind RNAs. To improve the delivery of the ASO to target tissues, nucleotides were conjugated to other molecules. For example, conjugation with GalNAc increased the delivery of an ASO to hepatocytes by several folds (Kulkarni et al., 2021). An ASO is distributed widely in the body after intravenous administration, but cannot cross the BBB due to its size and electrical charge. Therefore, to reach the CNS, ASOs are administered into the cerebrospinal fluid by intrathecal administration. Several ASOs have been approved for neurological conditions. These include at eteplirsen, viltolarsen, golodirsen and casimirsen for DMD. Nusinersen has been approved for SMA, and tofersen for ALS associated with superoxide dismutase (*SOD1*) mutation. Potential toxicity of an ASO can result from binding with off-target RNAs in the cell and degradation of normal RNA. In addition, ASOs can bind to proteins like Toll-like receptors and cause an immune response detrimental to the patient.

All of the above-mentioned techniques of gene therapy involve suppression of host genes or augmentation of a gene by introducing synthetic nucleic acids into the host cell. In contrast, the CRISPR/Cas9 system is used to edit the host genome. This approach holds immense promise of permanently curing genetic defects. For clinical applications, researchers designed a guide RNA which contains sequences of a CRISPR RNA and a trans-activating CRISPR RNA, mimicking the wild-type CRISPR/Cas9 system (Sharma et al., 2021). The guide RNA can bind specific DNA sequences 22–29 nucleotides long. When the guide RNA binds the complementary sequence in the host genome, the Cas9 nuclease cleaves the target DNA, causing a double-stranded break. The double-stranded break activates the cellular DNA repair machinery, including homology-directed repair and non-homologous end-joining mediated error-prone DNA repair. The former can be used for precise gene editing using a DNA repair template sequence. The latter, although error-prone, can be used for the removal of exons containing a genetic mutation. Nelson et al. used a CRISPR/Cas9 system to delete exon 23 harbouring a mutation in a mouse model of DMD, which resulted in partial recovery of functional dystrophin protein in myocytes (Nelson, 2016). In a recent breakthrough, exagamlogeneautotemcel (Casgevy) was developed to treat sickle cell disease and beta thalassemia. Casgevy edits the BCL11 gene in the haematopoietic stem cells of the patients, which leads to increased levels of foetal haemoglobin instead of abnormal hemoglobin. In the neurological arena, CRISPR/Cas9 is undergoing clinical trials for the treatment of hereditary transthyretin amyloidosis, a fatal disease resulting from the accumulation of mutated transthyretin proteins in the heart and the nervous system (Gillmore, 2021). CRISPR/Cas9 has shown great potential, but its successful use in the clinic faces several challenges. Off-target binding and editing by a therapeutic CRISPR/Cas9 system may lead to unforeseen consequences, including carcinogenesis. Although homology-directed repair of DNA is precise, it is inefficient and does not work in post-mitotic tissue such as the nervous system. Delivery of therapeutic quantities of the CRISPR/Cas9 system into specific neuronal populations remains another hurdle.

Genome editing by CRISPR/Cas9 utilizes the cellular response to the creation of double-stranded DNA breaks ((Mir et al., 2023)). The DNA breaks created by a Cas9 nuclease may result in novel mutations such as indels, rearrangements and translocations. Base editing is a precise method of genome editing that does not create double-stranded breaks (Matuszek et al., 2025). When the guide RNA binds the target sequence of host DNA, a small segment of the DNA forms and an "R" loop. The base editing enzyme can act only on single-stranded DNA and modifies the bases within the loop. A Cas nuclease then produces a nick in the other strand of DNA. The host cell repairs the unedited strand using the edited strand as a template. There are two types of base editors: cytosine base editors convert cytosine to uracil, and adenine base editors convert adenine to inosine. Using these two base editors, theoretically, all possible combinations of base changes can be achieved. Practically, the cellular DNA repair machinery counteracts the base editing with the enzyme uracil N-glycosylase (Bulgar et al., 2012). To inhibit this enzyme, an additional inhibitor is required. Ideally, a base editor should have a narrow window of activity so that only a specific base can be targeted. But there may be multiple bases near the target liable to be edited by the base editor, a phenomenon called "bystander editing (Porto et al., 2020)." The guide RNA and DNA encoding the nuclease are delivered into the host cells by using plasmids (Gilani & Gautam., 2025). Matuszek et al. demonstrated the use of base editing in trinucleotide repeat disorders such as Huntington's disease and Friedrich's ataxia(Matuszek et al., 2025). In patient cells and mouse models, base editing interrupted the pathological trinucleotide repeats. In mice, base editors were delivered to the CNS via an AAV9 vector, resulting in altered gene expression. Hopefully, this will lead to the successful treatment of some of the commonest neurogenic disorders in the near future. A summary of approved gene therapies for the treatment of neurological disorders has been provided in Table 9.1.

4. Applications of gene therapy: 4.1 neuromuscular disorders

4.1 Duchenne muscular dystrophy

Duchenne muscular dystrophy (DMD) is an X-linked recessive hereditary genetic myopathy of childhood onset caused by pathogenic variants in the dystrophin gene, the longest human gene. The vast majority of DMDs are caused by pathogenic insertions/deletions of nucleotides in the gene that results in an out-of-frame shift mutation, disrupting the normal reading frame and ultimately leading to a premature stop codon. The premature stop codon causes a nonsense mRNA transcript and the absence of functional dystrophin protein. This contrasts with Becker muscular dystrophy (BMD) wherein the mutation is "in-frame," and only resulted in a truncated but partially functional dystrophin protein. Of note, DMD can result from a single nucleotide variant, primarily leading to the formation of a stop codon with subsequent absent dystrophin protein (missense mutation) (Berling et al., 2023). Because dystrophin is a subsarcolemmal cytoskeletal protein integral for the preservation of the structural integrity of muscle fibers, its effective absence in DMD and reduction in BMD result in severe and comparatively milder manifestations, respectively. In addition to proximal predominant progressive neuromuscular weakness, there is also cardiopulmonary muscle involvement, which leads to diaphragmatic weakness, ventilation support, and cardiomyopathy. Additionally, cognitive and learning difficulties can result as dystrophin is also found in the brain.

Currently available gene therapy for DMD is classified into two main categories: (1) micro-dystrophin gene replacement therapy with AAV and (2) exon-skipping ASO therapies. Exon skipping ASOs aim to restore the reading frame by skipping particular out-of-frame exons in the mutated transcript. Currently, there are four FDA approved exon-skipping ASOs: eteplirsen, casimersen, golodirsen, and viltolarsen. Each of these exon-skipping ASOs targets only specific exons and thus has restricted, non-generalizable use in DMD patients (Duan, 2023).

Eteplirsen is an ASO designed to skip exon 51 of the mutated dystrophin gene. A pivotal longitudinal open label trial designed to assess the safety and efficacy of eteplirsen was published in 2016. DMD patients older than 7 years who were still ambulatory were randomized to receive either eteplirsen ($n = 12$) or placebo ($n = 13$) on a weekly basis for an initial 24 weeks with subsequent open

Table 9.1 Approved gene therapies for neurological disorders.

Gene therapy	Mechanism of action	Indication	Therapeutic effect
Eteplirsen (McDonald et al., 2021)	Anti-sense oligonucleotide (ASO) causing skipping of exon 51 of dystrophin gene	DMD with a mutation amenable to exon 51 skipping	30 mg/kg IV infusion weekly; statistically significant difference in 6 min walk test (6MWT)
Casimersen(Wagner et al., 2021)	ASO causing skipping of exon 45 of dystrophin gene	DMD with a mutation amenable to exon 45 skipping	30 mg/kg IV infusion weekly; demonstrated significant increase in dystrophin levels on muscle biopsy; may cause serious glomerulonephritis
Golodirsen (Servais et al., 2022)	ASO causing skipping of exon 53 of dystrophin gene	DMD with a mutation amenable to exon 53 skipping	30 mg/kg IV infusion weekly; demonstrated significant increase in dystrophin levels on muscle biopsy
Viltolarsen (Clemens et al., 2020)	ASO causing skipping of exon 53 of dystrophin gene	DMD with a mutation amenable to exon 53 skipping	Improved dystrophin levels on muscle biopsy and improved functional capacity
Delandistrogene moxeparvovec (Baranello & Muntoni, 2024)	AAV vector based gene replacement therapy	Patients with DMD who are ambulatory	1.33×1014 vector genomes (vg)/kg of body weight; No significant change in primary outcome NSAA score
Nusinersen (Finkel et al., 2017)	ASO designed to alter the splicing of SMN2 pre-mRNA	Pediatric and adult patients of SMA	12 mg intrathecally; initial loading dose followed by maintenance; improved survival in clinical trials
Risdiplam (Darras et al., 2021)	Small molecule designed to alter the splicing of SMN2 pre-mRNA	Pediatric and adult patients of SMA	Oral dosing according to body weight; improves motor functioning and survival
Onasemnogene abeparvovec (Day et al., 2021)	AAV based gene replacement therapy	Pediatric patients less than 2 years of age with spinal muscular atrophy (SMA) with bi-allelic mutations in the SMN1 gene. Patients with AAV9 antibodies were excluded	Single dose of 1.1×10^{14} vg/kg body weight intravenous; improved survival; risk of acute liver injury, immune reaction, thrombotic microangiopathy

Tofersen (NINDS Tofersen, 2025)	ASO targeted against SOD1 gene	Approved for adult patients of ALS with a mutation in the SOD1 gene	100 mg intrathecally loading dose followed by maintenance; risk of myelitis/radiculitis, aseptic meningitis, increased intracranial pressure; significant decrease in neurofilament light chain (Nfl) without meeting primary endpoint of clinical benefit
Inotersen (Benson et al., 2018)	ASO inhibitor that binds to hepatic TTR mRNA leading to its degradation via the RNAseH pathway	Approved for polyneuropathy of hereditary transthyretin-mediated amyloidosis in adults	284 mg subcutaneous weekly; improvement in mNIS+7 and QOL-DN scores; risk of thrombocytopenia and glomerulonephritis
Patisiran (Adams et al., 2018)	Double-stranded siRNA that targets hepatic TTR mRNA and results in its cleavage	Approved for polyneuropathy of hereditary Transthyretin-mediated amyloidosis in adults	0.3 mg/kg intravenous infusion; improvement in mNIS+7 and QOL-DN scores and gait speed
Vutrisiran (Adams et al., 2023)	siRNA conjugated with GalNAC that targets and degrades TTR-mRNA	Approved for polyneuropathy of hereditary Transthyretin-mediated amyloidosis in adults and hATTR/variant ATTR and wild type ATTR associated cardiomyopathy	25 mg subcutaneously three monthly; improvement in mNIS +7 and QOL-DN scores and gait speed; risk of extremity pain, diarrhea, edema, UTI, arthralgia, and dizziness
Eladocagene exuparvovec (Szunyogh et al., 2025)	AAV vector-based gene therapy	Approved for adult and pediatric patients with AADC deficiency	1.8×10^{11} vector genomes administered into the putamen via stereotactic surgery; improves motor milestones, cognition and autonomic symptoms

label continuation over 3 years. Patients who received eteplirsen were found to have a statistically significant advantage on the 6-minute Walk Test (6MWT) and loss on ambulation assessments compared to control (Mendell et al., 2016). Subsequent to this, additional studies have followed up and further supported these findings (McDonald et al., 2021).

Casimersen is an ASO designed to skip exon 45 of the mutated DMD gene. The first longitudinal multicentre trial assessing the safety and pharmacokinetics of the medication was published in 2021. The study enrolled 12 participants aged 7–21 years-old with none or limited ambulatory ability to receive the ASO or placebo as a weekly injection for 12 weeks, followed by open label extension up to 132 weeks. The study demonstrated that medication was overall well tolerated without serious complications (Wagner et al., 2021). Subsequently, the ASO received accelerated FDA approval based on interim results of statistically increased dystrophin levels on muscle biopsies in patients in the ongoing ESSENCE study (Iannaccone et al., 2022).

Golodirsen is an ASO designed to skip exon 53 of the mutated DMD gene. Like studies in other exon-skipping ASOs, a study published in 2020 performed a 12 week weekly randomized, double-blind, placebo-controlled comparison of weekly golodirsen (n = 8) to placebo (n = 4) followed by open label extension to 47 weeks. A 16-fold increase in dystrophin protein was evidenced at 48 weeks in the golodirsen group on muscle biopsy (Frank et al., 2020). Subsequently, a phase 1/2, 2-part, randomized, double-blind, placebo-controlled multicentre trial of golodirsen was published in 2021 that administered the medication or placebo weekly to ambulatory patients for 12 weeks with subsequent open label extension for 168 weeks. At 3 years, the 6MWT showed a decline of −99.0 m in cases compared with −181.4 m in controls, although this did not reach statistical significance (P = .067) (Servais et al., 2022).

Viltolarsen, like Golodirsen, is an ASO designed to skip exon 53 of the mutated DMD gene. Like prior mentioned studies, a phase 2 trial conducted over 4 weeks with open label extension for 20 weeks assessed the safety and efficacy of viltolarsen. In addition to being well tolerated, there were increased dystrophin levels on bicep muscle biopsies and improved functional testing in the study participants (n = 16) when compared with age-matched natural history controls (Clemens et al., 2020).

There are multiple limitations to these exon-skipping ASOs. Aside from their non-generalizability with medications available for only a few exons, the available medications produce only a small amount of dystrophin, require frequent weekly dosing, and have poor deliverability to the heart (Duan, 2023).

Gene replacement therapy in DMD utilizes a single administration of recombinant adeno-associated virus rhesus isolate serotype 74 vector based (rAAVrh74) to deliver a transgene encoding micro-dystrophin (delandistrogenemoxeparvovec), an engineered protein retaining key functional domains of dystrophin. As of June 2024, the FDA approved delandistrogenemoxeparvovec (Elevidys) for all ambulatory DMD patients ≥4 years of age with conditional approval for non-ambulatory patients. This followed the accelerated approval of Elevidys based on a limited phase II study of 20 DMD patients aged 4–7 years old who received the medication, demonstrating increased dystrophin expression on muscle biopsy Western blot (Baranello & Muntoni, 2024; USFDA, 2023).

Despite approval, the recently published results of the phase 3 placebo-controlled EMBARK study did not meet its primary endpoint at 52 weeks. In this large, randomized, double-blind placebo-controlled trial, ambulatory DMD patients 4–7 years old were randomized to receive Elevidys

($n = 63$) or placebo ($n = 62$). At 52 weeks, the primary end point outcome of change of North Star Ambulatory Assessment (NSAA) was not achieved, with no statistically significant difference noted between the intervention and placebo groups. There was nonetheless a trend of numerical improvement with a nominal statistically significant difference of secondary endpoints of time to rise-from-floor (RFF) and 10-meter walk/run test (10MWRT) in patients treated with Elevidys. As the analysis of secondary endpoints was not adjusted for multiplicity, definitive statistical significance could not be inferred (Baranello & Muntoni, 2024; Mendell et al., 2025).

Although no life-threatening events, death, or study discontinuations were reported in the recent EMBARK study, AAV gene replacement therapy is associated with several adverse treatment-related events (Mendell et al., 2016). These include acute liver injury, complement activation-induced thrombotic microangiopathy, myocarditis, and immune-mediated myositis. Consensus consideration for the evaluation and treatment of these events has been proposed (Duan, 2023; Zaidman et al., 2024). In addition to adverse events and immune related complications, it is important to emphasize that a large proportion of DMD patient Elevidys treatment candidates are excluded based on pre-existing AAV antibodies (Duan, 2023).

4.2 Spinal muscular atrophy

Spinal muscular atrophy (SMA) refers to a category of genetic diseases of the anterior horn motor neurons (motor neuronopathy), the most common of which are the autosomal recessive diseases caused by genetic abnormalities of the 5q chromosome (Verhaart et al., 2017).SMA caused by 5q chromosomal abnormalities are the second most common autosomal recessive disorder of childhood (Verhaart et al., 2017).They occur due to homozygous deletion or pathological variation of the associated survival motor neuron 1 (SMN1) gene, resulting in low levels of associated functional survival motor neuron (SMN) protein required for normal motor neuron preservation. Varying severities of SMA exist, with their phenotypes grouped into types 0 through 4, with lower numbers indicative of higher severity. The severity depends on the number of SMN2 gene copies, with higher copies resulting in a milder phenotype (Calucho et al., 2018).SMN2 genes exist in all humans but do not contribute as significantly to the amount of functional survival motor neuron protein as SMN1 genes (Calucho et al., 2018).

The presentation of chromosomal 5q associated SMA depends on the amount of remaining survival motor neuron (SMN) protein, which is primarily dependent on the amount of SMN2 gene copies15. SMA0 and SMA1A typically correspond to only one copy of SMN2. They are of prenatal onset and are characterized by hypotonia, areflexia, respiratory failure with a life expectancy of weeks to months. SMA1B and SMA1C typically correspond to two to three copies of SMN2. They have an onset within the first half year of life and are characterized by hypotonia, hyporeflexia/areflexia, tongue fasciculations, and weakness with inability to sit up. They have a life expectancy of less than 2 years. SMA2A and SMA2B typically correspond to two to four copies of SMN2. They have an onset within the first 2 years of life and typically can sit up unassisted but cannot walk. They have proximal weakness as well as variable presentations of bulbar weakness, hyporeflexia/areflexia, and contractures. Life expectancy is typically greater than 2 years, with 70% alive at 25 years. SMA3A and SMA3B typically correspond to three to four copies of SMN2. SMA3A has an onset within the first few years of life, and SMA3B typically has an onset in childhood. They present with proximal weakness but can walk independently and often have a normal life expectancy into adulthood. SMA4 typically corresponds to four to five copies of SMN2. It has an onset in adulthood, presenting with slowly progressive proximal weakness, but patients frequently maintain ambulation throughout life and have a normal life expectancy (Spinal Muscular Atrophy, no date).

Because the chromosomal 5q associated SMA disease phenotype depends on the amount of functional SMN protein produced, genetic therapies aim to increase the number of SMN proteins. There are currently two categories of genetic therapies: (1) SMN2 pre-mRNA splicing modifiers and (2) SMN1 gene replacement. The typical SMN2 gene in humans is identical to the SMN1 gene except for five nucleotides, but a crucial substitution of cytosine to tyrosine results in exclusion of exon seven during pre-mRNA splicing in the majority of SMN2 mRNA transcripts, resulting in a small amount of SMN protein produced from the SMN2 gene (Calucho et al., 2018). SMN2 pre-mRNA splicing modifiers are agents that take advantage of this by increasing inclusion of exon seven during pre-splicing, resulting in the translation of large amounts of functional SMN protein (Singh & Singh, 2018).

Nusinersen is an antisense oligonucleotide (ASO) designed to alter the splicing of SMN2 pre-mRNA to promote inclusion of exon 7, leading to increased full-length functional SMN protein production, which promotes survival of motor neurons. It is approved for use in SMA patients of all ages. It is administered as four loading doses over 2 months, followed by maintenance therapy every 4 months. The first pivotal trial ENDEAR demonstrating the efficacy of Nusinersen was published in 2017 was a randomized, double-blind, sham-controlled, phase 3 efficacy and safety trial in ($N = 80$ Nusinersen and $N = 41$ control) infants 1 week to 7 months of age comparing motor-milestone response and event free survival (time to death of permanent assisted ventilation) over 32 months with primary end points assessed at 6 months. The control group of the study was terminated early due to a statistically significant increase in survival demonstrated in the Nusinersen intervention group at 6 months analysis. The study fulfilled its endpoints and demonstrated statistically significant improvement in survival and preservation of motor function. There was a similar incidence and severity of adverse events between the Nusinersen and control group, with no specific adverse events related to Nusinersen aside from lumbar puncture associated complications identified (Finkel et al., 2017).

Another pivotal trial of Nusinersen analyzed outcomes in older children. The trial CHERISH which was published in 2018 was a randomized, multicenter, double-blind, sham-controlled, phase 3 trial of 126 children 2–12 year old with SMA who had symptom onset after 6 months of age and were tracked in their Hammersmith Functional Motor Scale Expanded (HFMSE) score over 15 months. The study demonstrated statistically significant and meaningful improvement in motor function in the Nusinersen group (Mercuri et al., 2018).

Risdiplam is a small molecule, unlike Nusinersen, which is an ASO, that similarly alters the splicing of SMN2 pre-mRNA to promote inclusion of exon 7, leading to increased full-length functional SMN protein. Unlike Nusinersen, which requires repeated intrathecal administration for maintenance therapy, Risdiplam is a daily orally administered medication with systemic distribution. It is approved for all SMA patients. There are two pivotal trials demonstrating efficacy that led to Risdiplam's approval. FIREFISH was an open-label multi-center trial that enrolled 41 infants with SMA1 of 1–7 months in age compared to historical controls assessing the ability to sit without support for at least 5 s after 12 months of treatment. Survival without permanent ventilation was a secondary endpoint among others. The trial demonstrated improved motor function and survival without permanent ventilation compared to controls (Darras et al., 2021).

Another pivotal trial of Risdiplam analyzed outcomes in older children. The trial SUNFISH was a randomized, double-blind, placebo-controlled trial that enrolled (N = 120 Risdiplam and N = 60 placebo) SMA2 and SMA3 non-ambulatory patients 2–25 years of age with the primary endpoint of change in baseline of the 32-item Motor Function Measure total score at 12 months. The trial achieved its endpoint with significant improvement in motor function demonstrated in the Risdiplam group. The most common adverse events noted more frequently in the Risdiplam group included pyrexia and diarrhea, but serious adverse events were similar between the groups (Mercuri et al., 2022).

Gene replacement therapy in SMA, like in DMD, utilizes a single administration of recombinant adeno-associated virus vector (AAV9 in this case) to deliver a functional SMN1 gene cDNA to target motor neurons for the purpose of subsequently increasing SMN protein. Onasemnogeneabeparvovec (Zolgensma) was approved by the FSA for use in all SMA patients <2 years old in May 2019. Efficacy was successfully demonstrated in two open label, single-dose phase III trials compared to historical controls. Both trials enrolled SMA1 patients <6 months of age with two copies of SMN2. Both trials assessed independent sitting (for ≥30 s in the USA study and ≥10 s in the EU study) as well as event-free survival at 14 months. STR1VE-EU was performed in the EU, enrolling 33 patients, while STR1VE was performed in the USA and enrolled 22 patients. Both trials were successful and demonstrated dramatically improved event free survival when compared to controls: 20 of 22 in the USA and 31 of 33 in the EU trials. Similarly, significant improvements in independent sitting times were observed in both. Although the treatments were well tolerated, there were drug-related adverse events of pyrexia, hepatic transaminase elevation, and one case of hydrocephalus noted (Day et al., 2021).

Of note, it is important to emphasize that, like the situation with Elevidys for DMD, patients with elevated AAV9 antibody titers are screened for and excluded from receiving Onasemnogeneabeparvovec (Mendell et al., 2022). Similarly, as is the case with Elevidys, cases of thrombotic microangiopathy have been reported during post marketing surveillance and with case reports (Guillou et al., 2022).

4.2.1 Amyotrophic lateral sclerosis (ALS)

Amyotrophic lateral sclerosis (ALS) refers to the most common etiology of motor neuron disease (MND) in adults. In most cases (85%–90%), amyotrophic lateral sclerosis (ALS) is sporadic without an identified genetic etiology. The first genes associated with genetic/familial ALS were identified in the 1990s: SOD1 (1993), NEFH (1994), and SETX (1998). Following these initial genes, dozens more were identified in the past few decades, with over 40 identified genes thus far. These genetic mutations manifest in ALS through a variety of patterns including autosomal dominant, autosomal recessive, X-linked, as well as risk-factor modification. The most common cause of familial ALS is due to hexanucleotide repeat expansion of the C9orf72 gene on chromosome nine manifesting in an autosomal dominant inheritance pattern. The second most common cause is variation/mutation of the SOD1 on chromosome 21, which can present in both autosomal dominant and recessive inheritance patterns with high penetration (Suzuki et al., 2023; Wang et al., 2023).

Sporadic amyotrophic lateral sclerosis (ALS) presents with manifestations of upper and lower motor neuron disease, leading to relentless progression of typically initial distal asymmetric weakness/paralysis with subsequent generalization as well as bulbar and respiratory manifestations. There are variations in presentations with unique prognoses, the discussion of which is beyond the scope of this text. Genetic etiologies of familial ALS can present indistinguishably from sporadic ALS, although certain features such as early-onset and association with certain comorbid disease (such as frontotemporal dementia with C9orf72) can be seen (Suzuki et al., 2023; Wang et al., 2023).

The only genetic therapy approved for genetic ALS applies only to patients with SOD1 gene variant associated ALS. Tofersen (Qalsody) was granted accelerated FDA approval in April 2023 for this purpose (NINDS Tofersen, 2025). Tofersen is an antisense oligonucleotide (ASO) to the superoxide dismutase 1 (SOD1) gene that reduces synthesis of the corresponding SOD1 protein, thought to be implicated in protein stasis and oxidative stress (Miller et al., 2022; Wang et al., 2023). It is administered intrathecally. The trial that led to Tofersen's accelerated approval was the VALOR trial published in 2022, which was a phase 3, randomized, placebo-controlled trial that enrolled adults with SOD1 associated ALS to receive Tofersen ($N = 72$) or placebo ($N = 36$) over 28 weeks. The primary endpoint was change from baseline to week 28 in the total score on the ALS Functional Rating Scale–Revised (ALSFRS-R). Tofersen or placebo was administered intrathecally as 15 mL boluses every 2 weeks for three doses, followed by every 4 weeks for five doses. The trial did not find a significant change in disease progression between the Tofersen treated group compared to placebo at 28 weeks, as assessed by ALSFRS-R. However, two secondary endpoints were nonetheless achieved with the Tofersen treated group, demonstrating a statistically significant decrease in SOD1 concentration in CSF as well as decreased plasma neurofilament light chain, both thought to be biomarkers of disease (Miller et al., 2022).

4.2.2 Hereditary transthyretin amyloidosis

Hereditary transthyretin amyloidosis (hATTR) is a genetic, multisystem progressive disease including peripheral nervous system involvement manifesting at variable ages in adulthood (Vita et al., 2019). Normal human homotetrameric transthyretin (TTR) protein is predominantly synthesized in the liver and choroid plexus, functioning to carry thyroid hormone and the retinol-binding protein in serum and cerebrospinal fluid (Sanguinetti et al., 2022). In elderly individuals, when normal TTR protein loses its structural stability, it breaks down into TTR monomers forming insoluble fibrils that subsequently deposit throughout the body—but primarily in the heart leading to cardiomyopathy (Sanguinetti et al., 2022; Vita et al., 2019). This condition is called wild type transthyretin amyloidosis (wtATTR) or senile systemic amyloidosis. Neuromuscular manifestations are less common than cardiac in wtATTR but are typically secondary to connective tissue (tendon, ligament, joint) involvement, resulting in conditions such as carpal tunnel syndrome and spinal stenosis; however, large and small fiber polyneuropathy, although more controversial, may also be possible (Živković et al., 2024). In contrast to wild-type ATTR, Hereditary transthyretin amyloidosis (hATTR)—also known as variant ATTR (vATTR)—results from mutations of the TTR gene and can present from early adulthood (before 35 years) or late (after 35 years) (Vita et al., 2019). hATTR is transmitted in an autosomal dominant pattern, and although the VAL30MET mutation with endemic foci in Portugal, Sweden, and Japan is by far the most common variant/mutation, there are over 150 mutations identified (Dispenzieri et al., 2022; Vita et al., 2019). Also in contrast to wtATTR, hATTR often has prominent peripheral nervous system involvement in addition to cardiomyopathy, connective tissues, nephropathy, and gastrointestinal (Vita et al., 2019). Peripheral nervous system manifestations include a typically axonal large fiber distal polyneuropathy and dysautonomia resulting from autonomic small fiber polyneuropathy, although phenotypic heterogeneity exists (Vita et al., 2019).

There are currently three approved genetic therapies for hATTR. All three target hepatic TTR mRNA and lead to its degradation, subsequently decreasing TTR protein production and TTR amyloid formation.

Inotersen is an antisense oligonucleotide (ASO) inhibitor that binds to hepatic TTR mRNA, leading to its degradation via the RNAseH pathway (Gales, 2019). The pivotal NEURO-TTR trial published in 2018 was an international, double-blind, placebo-controlled 15 month phase 3 trial that followed 172 ambulatory hATTR associated neuropathy patients for 15 months treated with weekly subcutaneous injections of Inotersen versus placebo while assessing the primary measures of modified Neuropathy Impairment Score+7 (mNIS+7) and patient-reported Norwalk Quality of Life-Diabetic Neuropathy questionnaire (QOL-DN) (Benson et al., 2018). The study demonstrated statistically significant differences in both primary measures of change in mNIS+7 and QOL-DN favoring Inotersen over placebo as measured by least-squares mean, although there was nonetheless slowed but ongoing worsening of mNIS+7 in the Inotersen group (Benson et al., 2018). Of note, there were 5 deaths in the group treated with Inotersen and none in the placebo group, with the most serious adverse events including glomerulonephritis (3%) and thrombocytopenia (3%).

Patisiran, unlike Inotersen, is a small interfering RNA (siRNA) that targets hepatic TTR mRNA and results in its cleavage by binding to the endogenous RNA-induced silencing complex. The pivotal APOLLO trial, published in 2018, was an international, double-blind, placebo-controlled 18-month phase 3 trial that followed 225 adult patients with hATTR-associated neuropathy treated with Patisiran versus placebo intravenously every 3 weeks while assessing the primary measure of modified Neuropathy Impairment Score+7 (mNIS+7), with higher scores indicative of disability. At 18 months, the Patisiran group experienced a statistically significant improvement of the mNIS+7 measured as the least-squares mean of -6.0 ± 1.8 compared with worsening in the placebo group of $+28.0 \pm 2.6$. Multiple other secondary assessments also demonstrated statistically significant improvement in the treatment group, including Norfolk QOL-DN and gait speed. The most common adverse events occurring more frequently in the treatment group included peripheral edema and infusion-reactions, although the overall incidence and types of adverse events were similar between Patisiran and Placebo (Adams et al., 2018).

Vutrisiran, like Patisiran, is a siRNA that targets and results in hepatic TTR mRNA degradation. Vutrisiran, unlike Patisiran, is conjugated to a triantennary N-acetylgalactosamine (GalNAc) ligand that binds the asialoglycoprotein receptor expressed on the surface of hepatocytes, which enhances stability and allows for subcutaneous administration once every 3 months. The pivotal HELIOS-A trial, published in 2023, was an international open-label 18-month phase 3 trial that enrolled 164 hATTR neuropathy patients to receive Vutrisiran ($n = 122$) or Patisiran ($n = 42$) as a reference for 18 months with the primary outcome of change in baseline of mNIS+7 compared to the historical control of the Patisiran APOLLO trial. At 18 months, the Vutrisiran group experienced a statistically significant improvement of the mNIS+7 measured as the least-squares mean of -2.24 compared with worsening in the placebo group of $+28.09$. Multiple other secondary assessments also demonstrated statistically significant improvement in the treatment group, including Norfolk QOL-DN and gait speed. The most common adverse events reported in the Vutrisiran included extremity pain, diarrhea, edema, UTI, arthralgia, and dizziness, although all occurred at similar rates compared to external historical placebo, aside from limb pain (Adams et al., 2023).

A second pivotal trial of Vutrisiran HELIOS-B, published in 2024, was an international, double blind, randomized trial phase 3 trial that enrolled 655 adult patients with ATTR associated cardiomyopathy (either hereditary/variant or wild-type) to receive Vutrisiran ($n = 326$) or placebo ($n = 329$) for 36 months. The primary endpoints were composite death of any cause and recurrent cardiovascular events. At 36 months, the trial demonstrated a statistically significant lower risk of death from any cause and recurrent cardiovascular events compared to placebo, with a hazard ratio of 0.72 in the overall population (not controlling for other non-genetic therapy disease-modifying treatments like Tafamidis) and 0.67 in the Vutrisiran monotherapy population. The incidence of adverse events was similar between the Vutrisiran treatment and placebo groups (Fontana et al., 2025).

Inotersen and Patisiran are currently FDA-approved only for the treatment of hATTR-associated polyneuropathy. However, Vutrisiran is FDA-approved for the treatment of hATTR-associated polyneuropathy as well as both hATTR/variant ATTR and wild-type ATTR-associated cardiomyopathy.

4.2.3 Metabolic disorders

Wilson's disease (WD) is a disorder of copper metabolism caused by mutations in the *ATP7B* gene, required for copper transport across the cell membrane. The mutations lead to accumulation of copper in the liver and the brain, leading to hepatic failure and myriad neurological features, including tremor, dystonia and cognitive impairment. Present treatment primarily focuses on reducing the excess copper in the body by using chelating agents like penicillamine. Patients need lifelong treatment with chelating agents, and even temporary discontinuation of treatment may lead to severe worsening of the disease (Bandmann et al., 2015).

Gene therapy attempts to restore copper transport in WD by inserting a wild-type ATP7B gene. In a mouse model of WD, an AAV8 vector was used to deliver the full-length ATP7B gene, which restored biliary excretion of copper (Baruteau et al., 2024). As the size of the ATP7B gene surpasses the packing capacity of AAV vectors, a mini-ATP7B gene was designed by deleting four metal-binding domains. The mini-ATP7B gene successfully restored copper transport in mouse models. Two phase I/II clinical trials, GATEWAY and Cyprus2+, are currently testing mini-ATP7B gene therapies. Padua and colleagues developed a novel method for delivering the full-length ATP7B gene. The researchers used two viral vectors, each containing a part of the ATP7B gene. The two parts were combined after delivery into the target cell using split-inteins, which is a naturally occurring process of binding two protein fragments into a single functional protein. This unique approach shows the way for other genetic therapies where the transgene size exceeds the packaging capacity of commonly used vectors (Baruteau et al., 2024).

Glycogen storage disorders (GSDs) are a group of disorders characterized by a biochemical deficit in glycogen metabolism (Hannah et al., 2023). These genetic disorders affect one of the three essential glycogen metabolism pathways, namely glycogenesis, glycogenolysis and glycolysis. GSDs are classified into hepatic and muscle GSDs, depending on the primary site of affection. In hepatic GSDs, patients develop fasting intolerance and hypoglycaemia, which in turn can lead to seizures and cognitive impairment. Muscle GSDs can present with exercise intolerance and rhabdomyolysis. Glycogen accumulation in the heart can result in cardiomyopathy and arrhythmia. The present treatment approach to most GSDs includes dietary modification and controlled exercise. A deficiency in the enzyme acid α-glucosidase (AAG) leads to Pompe's disease (GSD II), a condition managed with alglucosidase alfa enzyme replacement therapy (ERT) (Koeberl et al., 2024). ERT is required lifelong, at a regular interval of 2 weeks, and may generate an immune response against the enzyme, reducing its efficacy.

The gene therapy approach for the treatment of GSDs involved supplementation of the affected gene. In preclinical models of GSDIa, AAV vectors carrying the glucose 6-phosphatase gene were tested. Although gene therapy was initially able to correct the biochemical abnormalities of GSDIa, transgene expression gradually declined over time (Koeberl et al., 2024). As the AAV vector remains as an episome inside the host cell, in rapidly dividing cells, the effect of gene therapy is expected to diminish. Despite this limitation, several gene therapies are undergoing clinical trials in GSD. The RESOLUTE trial is testing the safety, tolerability and efficacy of a single administration of SPK-3006 in adult patients with late onset Pompe's disease (NCT04093349). In the FORTIS trial, an AAV8 vector carrying the AAG Transgene and a regulatory murine muscle creatine kinase promoter was administered to late-onset Pompe's disease patients. Three out of the four participants were able to discontinue ERT and were stable after 51 weeks of follow up (Koeberl et al., 2024).

Lysosomal storage disorders (LSD) are a group of approximately 40 disorders caused by genetic defects in the synthesis of lysosomal enzymes. As a result of the enzyme deficiency, the substrate of the enzyme accumulates in tissues, leading to cellular death and organ dysfunction. LSDs affect multiple organs, including the brain, heart, liver, skin and kidneys. Present treatment approaches include enzyme replacement therapy and bone marrow transplant. For example, in Fabry's disease, recombinant α-galactosidase (GLA) is administered intravenously to replace the deficient enzyme (Cheng & Smith, 2003). Similar to GSDs, repeated bolus doses of ERT are required, which may lead to an immune response against the enzyme, most commonly seen in patients with null mutations. With the exception of pabinafusp alfa for mucopolysaccharidoses (MPS) type II, the enzyme does not cross the BBB and does not improve neurological symptoms (Kido et al., 2023). For MPS type I, bone marrow transplantation (BMT) has been used as a standard treatment to prevent organ damage and reduce neurological morbidity. Grewal(Locke et al., 2013) and colleagues reported that all the children were able to walk unaided, and 70% of patients with MPS type I who underwent BMT achieved an intelligence quotient in the normal range. There was significant morbidity due to graft versus host disease, some patients requiring a repeat transplant and a risk of death from the complications of BMT.

Gene therapy of LSDs includes in-vivo and ex-vivo approaches. For the treatment of Fabry's disease, intravenous administration of a single dose of an AAV vector carrying the GLA gene is undergoing clinical trials. Two different therapies, FLT190 (NCT04455230) and ST-920 (NCT04046224) are presently being tested for safety and durability of treatment effect (Kido et al., 2023). As an ex-vivo approach, $CD34^+$ stem cells from the patients were transduced with a lentiviral vector containing the human GLA cDNA followed by an autologous stem cell transplantation. Three out of five patients were able to discontinue ERT after receiving the stem cell transplant (Khan et al., 2021).

Leukodystrophies are a group of approximately 30 genetic disorders in which molecular defects affect the formation and maintenance of the myelin sheath in the central and peripheral nervous system. The myelin loss leads to axonal degeneration, which manifests as a progressive neurodegenerative disorder. The commonest leukodystrophies - metachromatic leukodystrophy (MLD), Krabbe's disease or globoid cell leukodystrophy (GLD) and X-linked adrenoleukodystrophy (XALD) are being studied as targets of gene therapy.

MLD is a result of a mutation in the arylsulfatase A (*ARSA*) gene. A defect in the ARSA enzyme results in the accumulation of abnormal sulfatide, a glycosphingolipid building block of the myelin sheath, in the nervous system. Depending upon the mutation, the disease manifests at different ages-a late infantile form, a juvenile form and an adult onset form. In the late infantile form, patients develop progressive tetraplegia, loss of speech and blindness, inevitably leading to death. In the juvenile form, patients develop progressive spastic paraparesis, ataxia and cognitive deficits. Adult onset MLD patients develop progressive alteration in cognition and behaviour and spastic paraparesis (Biffi et al., 2011).

Approaches to treatment of MLD included ERT and stem cell transplantation (SCT). A clinical trial of intrathecal administration of recombinant ARSA in MLD patients who had developed symptoms before the age of 30 months of age (NCT01510028) (í Dali et al., 2020). Despite enzyme replacement, the patients' motor function continued to deteriorate. BMT has been successfully used to treat MLD, as a subset of the perivascular microglia is replaced by donor-derived cells (Biffi et al., 2011). In a clinical trial, juvenile MLD patients who underwent BMT demonstrated better motor and language outcomes and lower MRI severity scores compared to controls (Groeschel et al., 2016).

MLD is considered a good candidate for gene therapy, as restoration of enzyme activity, even by 10 percent, can significantly improve disease outcomes (Rosenberg et al., 2016). Once host cells are transduced by a gene therapy to produce ARSA, the enzyme is secreted and taken up by the neighbouring cells. In a mouse model of MLD, intraparenchymal administration of an AAV5 vector resulted in sustained expression of ARSA. In a prospective, non-randomized, phase 1/2 clinical trial, 29 presymptomatic and early-symptomatic patients of MLD received atidarsageneautotemcel, a lentiviral vector carrying the human ARSA cDNA. Using an ex-vivo approach, $CD34^+$ stem cells were harvested from the patients, transduced by the vector and infused back into the patients after myeloablation. Two years after receiving the treatment, late infantile MLD patients showed 66% improvement and juvenile patients showed 42% improvement in gross motor skills compared to controls. 80% of patients showed acquisition of normal cognitive skills (Fumagalli et al., 2022).

4.2.4 Parkinson's disease

Parkinson's disease (PD) is a neurodegenerative disease primarily affecting the dopaminergic neurons in the substantia nigra and the striatum. The disease manifests primarily as motor symptoms such as tremors, slowness and rigidity of muscles, accompanied by a range of non-motor symptoms such as anosmia, rapid-eye movement sleep behaviour disorder and dementia. Although most PD cases are sporadic, several genetic mutations associated with PD have been discovered. Mutations in *SNCA*, *LRRK2*, *VPS35*, *DNAJC13* and *GBA* are associated with autosomal dominant inheritance and mutations in *PARKIN*, *PINK1* and *DJ1* are associated with autosomal recessive inheritance (Domingo & Klein, 2018; Domingo, 2018). As a clearly defined cellular population can be targeted for the treatment of PD, it became an important focus for gene therapy trials.

Three different approaches are under consideration for gene therapy of PD. First, the use of an AAV vector to deliver the enzymes required for dopamine synthesis into the brain. Prosavin was a lentiviral vector containing the genes for tyrosine hydroxylase, GTP cyclohydrolase and aromatic L-amino acid decarboxylase (AADC). In a phase 1/2 clinical trial, the vector was injected into the putamen to increase the production of the neurotransmitter and was found to be safe. An AAV2 vector with the AADC trans gene, VY-AADC01, was injected into the putamen and demonstrated improvement in Unified Parkinson's disease Rating Scale (UPDRS) score. Inherited deficiency of AADC manifests with Parkinsonism, dystonia, autonomic dysfunction and intellectual disability in childhood. Eladocageneexuparvovec (Upstaza) is an AAV2 based gene therapy that delivers a *DDC* gene into the brain via intra-putaminal injections. Patients attained motor and cognitive milestones after administration of Upstaza, which led to its approval for clinical use (Szunyogh et al., 2025).

The second approach targets the sub thalamic nucleus. In PD, inhibition of the subthalamic nucleus mediated by the neurotransmitter GABA is impaired. An AAV2 vector containing the glutamic decarboxylase (GAD) gene, required for the synthesis of GABA, was delivered to the subthalamic nucleus in experimental animals, which rescued the Parkinsonism phenotype. In 2022, an AAV vector with the *GAD* gene was tested in a clinical trial, which demonstrated improvement in UPDRS scores (Phielipp & Henchcliffe, 2025).

A third approach is to deliver the genes for growth factors neurturin and glial-derived neurotrophic factor (GDNF) to putamen (Bartus et al., 2014). Both these growth factors activate Nurr1, which is an intranuclear protein necessary for the development of dopaminergic neurons. In the REGENERATE-PD trial, the safety, tolerability and efficacy of an AAV2-GDNF therapy were tested in advanced PD patients. The study demonstrated long-term safety and motor stability in the participants (Phielipp & Henchcliffe, 2025).

So far, most of the PD gene therapies have delivered limited success. The vectors require delivery into the putamen via a surgical procedure. The rate of delivery and the dosage are not yet optimized. Deep brain stimulation (DBS) has an established track record of safety and efficacy in PD, and future gene therapies need to demonstrate results comparable to DBS.

4.3 Huntington's disease

Huntington's disease (HD) is a dominantly inherited neurodegenerative disorder caused by the expansion of the CAG trinucleotide repeat in the *HTT* gene. The mutation leads to degeneration of the medium spiny neurons in the striatum. Patients of HD suffer from progressively debilitating chorea, cognitive impairment and altered behaviour. Mutated huntingtin protein disrupts multiple cellular processes, including endocytosis and regulation of transcription. Therefore, treatment strategies aim to lower cellular huntingtin levels; partial lowering of huntingtin (unto 50%) in the adult brain is likely to be safe. Treatment strategies in HD can be either non-allele selective or allele selective. Non-allele selective methods reduce the levels of both mutant and wild-type huntingtin, whereas allele selective methods reduce the levels of mutant huntingtin. ASOs and RNA interference can be used to reduce the translation of the *HTT* mRNA into proteins, or editing the HTT gene by a CRISPR/Cas9 system can correct the mutation (Johnson & Davidson, 2010).

IONIS-HTT$_{RX}$ (Tominersen)is an ASO targeting the human Huntingtin mRNA. It is a non-allele selective agent that targets the exon 36 of the *HTT* mRNA. Intrathecal administration of the ASO was found to be safe, and it lowered the levels of mutant huntingtin in the CSF. A phase 3 trial of Tominersen did not demonstrate any significant improvement of symptoms compared to placebo and was stopped (McColgan et al., 2023). CSF of the trial participants showed inflammatory changes and a transient increase in neurofilament light chain levels. The ASO is now undergoing trials in prodromal HD patients. Another trial is testing a micro RNA (miRNA) AMT-130, packaged in an AAV5 vector, to reduce the expression of huntingtin. AMT-130 is delivered into the striatum under MRI guidance. The trial is testing the safety of AMT-130 in early stage HD patients (Rodrigues & Wild, 2020).

The ASOs WVE-120,101 and WVE-120,102 target the mutant HTT mRNA by recognizing two single nucleotide polymorphisms (SNPs) specific to the HTT gene. The target SNPs are present in approximately 50% and 40% HD patients. The ASO therapies were tested in the PRECISION-HD1 and PRECISION-HD2 trials, which were stopped as there was no evidence of response across the doses that were administered (Byun et al., 2022).

Although ASOs have proven effective in other neurological disorders, recent setbacks in HD clinical trials shed light on important issues. Reducing the levels of huntingtin sufficiently for a clinical effect requires a high dose of ASO, increasing the possibility of off-target effects and inflammation. Delivery of the drug via the intrathecal route may reduce the concentration of the drug in the striatum, which is a deeper brain structure. On the other hand, delivery via stereotactic neurosurgery carries the risks of surgery. Base editing is a novel approach which may circumvent these difficulties by interrupting the pathogenic trinucleotide repeats.

4.4 Epilepsy

Epilepsy is defined as “a disease of the brain characterized by an enduring predisposition to generate epileptic seizures.” There are numerous neurological disorders which are associated with epilepsy, and in some of them, like Dravet’s syndrome, epilepsy is the primary clinical feature. Although most cases of epilepsy are sporadic, Syvertsen et al. had observed that 20% of epilepsy patients in a Norwegian county had a confirmed or presumed genetic etiology (Syvertsen et al., 2015). The Gene4epilepsy database now implicates more than 1000 genes in the pathogenesis of epilepsy.

Developmental and epileptic encephalopathies (DEE) are a particularly severe group of epileptic disorders beginning in childhood, characterized by frequent seizures and electroencephalographic changes associated with developmental slowing or regression. Nearly 50% of patients with DEE harbour a pathogenic mutations. Dravet’s syndrome (DS) is the most researched DEE, which is caused by loss-of-function mutations in the *SCN1A* gene in about 90% of cases. The condition typically begins around 6 months of age with fever-related seizures, which are then followed by other types of seizures and a slowdown in development (Higurashi et al., 2022). Other important monogenic forms of epilepsy are associated with mutations in *KCNQ2*, *SCN1B* and *CACN1A*. These genes encode different ion channels present on the neuronal cell membrane and are under investigation as targets for gene therapy. Even in sporadic epilepsy, repeated seizures alter the genetic expression in the epileptogenic zones. Gene therapy to alter the expression of neuropeptides such as neuropeptide Y in the epileptogenic zone is also under investigation.

Gene therapy in epilepsy can take several approaches. In conditions associated with a loss-of-function mutation, delivery of the normal gene via a viral vector can ameliorate clinical symptoms. For example, in mouse models of DS, two AAV vectors were used to deliver split-intein forms of the *SCN1A* gene which were protective against seizures (Michet al., 2025). ETX-101 is an investigational gene therapy that delivers an engineered transcription factor via an AAV9 vector to increase the expression of wild type *SCN1A* in the brain. To reduce off-target effects, the expression cassette includes a GABA-ergic cell specific regulatory element. The drug is delivered directly into the cerebral ventricles (Chilcott et al., 2022). The treatment is being tested in the ENDEAVOR, WAYFINDER and EXPEDITION trials in the USA, Austria and the UK, respectively. Another treatment approach involves targeted augmentation of nuclear gene output (TANGO). The *SCN1A gene* contains a “poison exon”, exon 20N; translation of exon 20N leads to premature termination, and the transcript undergoes nonsense-mediated decay. In TANGO, an ASO is used to bind the exon 20N and stop its translation, so that *SCN1A* gene expression can be restored to normal levels (Wagnon, 2021). A third approach to treat DS is to use a CRISPR/Cas9 system to increase the expression of wild-type SCN1A. The CRISPR/Cas9 system is modified to use a nuclease-dead Cas9 (dCas9), which targets the regulation of gene transcription. The CRISPR/dCas9 system can be delivered via an AAV vector to activate transcription of the *SCN1A* gene (Higurashi et al., 2022).

AMT-260 is a novel gene therapy being developed for the treatment of refractory medial temporal lobe sclerosis. AMT-260 consists of an AAV9 vector which delivers two novel microRNAs (miRNA) under the regulation of a human synapsin1 promoter. The miRNAs reduce the expression of a subunit of the kainate receptor, an inotropic glutamate receptor. Aberrant expression of the kainate receptor is responsible for epileptogenesis in temporal lobe epilepsy; blocking the synthesis of the receptor significantly reduces seizure frequency in mouse models. Based on animal data, a multi-centre clinical trial is being planned to test the safety and efficacy of injections of AMT-260 into hippocampus (Bialer et al., 2024).

Increasing availability of high-throughput genome sequencing has enabled clinicians and researchers to identify a large number of genetic variants associated with epilepsy. While the success of gene therapy in other neurological disorders has raised hope for curative treatment for devastating epilepsy syndromes, particularly DEE, there are still important roadblocks on the way to fulfilling this promise. Severe epilepsy syndromes starting early in life adversely affect development. Therefore, the gene therapy has to be timed to achieve normal development of the patient. Many genes associated with epilepsy have gain-of-function and loss-of-function phenotypes. The gene therapy should balance the treatment effect so that a gain-of-function phenotype is not converted into a loss-of -function phenotype. Several gene therapies under trial are administered directly into the brain, which is an irreversible process. Longitudinal studies are required to observe for off-target effects of the gene therapy as well as downstream changes in genetic expression.

5. Ethics, cost, and access of genetic therapies

While the prospect of multiple current and future potential effective genetic therapies is undoubtedly promising, there are significant economic and ethical implications. Genetic therapies are very expensive and are accompanied by a profound cost to the payer with significant societal implications. Gene therapy drugs such as Onasemnogeneabeparvovec (Zolgensma) for SMA can cost millions of dollars. From a development standpoint, the design and manufacture of genetic therapies can range up to several billion dollars. There are additional subsequent remuneration barriers to the pharmaceutical industry, such as high manufacturing cost per patient as well as diminished ability to recoup costs due to disease rarity and, at times, single (one-off) administration of gene therapies. In part because of this significant cost, there is a lack of uniformity in criteria of coverage for these therapies by payers—both in terms of government sponsored and private insurances. Additionally, and especially due to the prospect of additional future genetic therapies, the cost to society at large is sizable. This has and will continue to raise ethical questions about the willingness to sustain such costs. Traditionally, from a general societal economic perspective, these considerations can be expressed as incremental cost-effectiveness ratio (ICER) or "cost per quality-adjusted life-years (QALYs)" that is then compared to the monetary societal willingness-to-pay (WTP) threshold per QALY. The major hurdle with this assessment is that genetic therapies generally exceed the ICER threshold relative to societal willingness-to-pay per QALY, making them difficult to justify economically compared to most traditional medical therapies. Nonetheless, there are conflicts about whether societal WTP per QALY may be higher for genetic therapies for external reasons, such as the prospect of curing a disease or addressing a highly unmet need. In part because these thresholds may vary within and between societies, access to these therapies varies. However, there are also crucial additional barriers beyond this threshold comparison. In less developed countries/societies, the high cost of these therapies may be so insurmountable and the cost effectiveness unachievable, when there are other unmet needs such as infrastructure and basic medical supplies for the general population at large (Landfeldt, 2022).

References

Adams, D., Gonzalez-Duarte, A., O'Riordan, W. D., Yang, C.-C., Ueda, M., Kristen, A. V., Tournev, I., Schmidt, H. H., Coelho, T., Berk, J. L., Lin, K.-P., Vita, G., Attarian, S., Planté-Bordeneuve, V., Mezei, M. M., Campistol, J. M., Buades, J., Brannagan, T. H., Kim, B. J., & Suhr, O. B. (2018). Patisiran, an RNAi therapeutic, for hereditary transthyretin amyloidosis. *New England Journal of Medicine, 379*(1), 11–21. https://doi.org/10.1056/NEJMoa1716153

Adams, D., Tournev, I. L., Taylor, M. S., Coelho, T., Planté-Bordeneuve, V., Berk, J. L., González-Duarte, A., Gillmore, J. D., Low, S.-C., Sekijima, Y., Obici, L., Chen, C., Badri, P., Arum, S. M., Vest, J., & Polydefkis, M. (2023). Efficacy and safety of vutrisiran for patients with hereditary transthyretin-mediated amyloidosis with polyneuropathy: A randomized clinical trial. *Amyloid: International Journal of Experimental and Clinical Investigation, 30*(1), 18–26. https://doi.org/10.1080/13506129.2022.2091985

Antoniou, V., Mourelatou, E. A., Galatou, E., Avgoustakis, K., & Hatziantoniou, S. (2024). Gene therapy with chitosan nanoparticles: Modern formulation strategies for enhancing cancer cell transfection. *Pharmaceutics, 16*(7). https://doi.org/10.3390/pharmaceutics16070868

Avery, O. T., Macleod, C. M., & McCarty, M. (1944). Studies on the chemical nature of thesubstance inducing transformation of pneumococcaltypes : Inductionof transformation bya desoxyribonucleic acid fractionisolated from pneumococcustype III. *The Journal of experimental medicine, 79*(2), 137–158.

Baltimore, D., Berg, P., Botchan, M., Carroll, D., Alta Charo, R., Church, G., Corn, J. E., Daley, G. Q., Doudna, J. A., Fenner, M., Greely, H. T., Jinek, M., Steven Martin, G., Penhoet, E., Puck, J., Sternberg, S. H., Weissman, J. S., & Yamamoto, K. R. (2015). A prudent path forward for genomic engineering and germline gene modification. *Science, 348*(6230), 36–38. https://doi.org/10.1126/science.aab1028

Bandmann, O., Weiss, K. H., & Kaler, S. G. (2015). Wilson's disease and other neurological copper disorders. *The Lancet Neurology, 14*(1), 103–113. https://doi.org/10.1016/S1474-4422(14)70190-5

Baranello, G., & Muntoni, F. (2024). AAV gene therapy for duchenne muscular dystrophy: Lessons learned from a phase 3 trial. *Gene Therapy, 31*(11–12), 541–543. https://doi.org/10.1038/s41434-024-00494-6

Barrangou, R., Fremaux, C., Deveau, H., Richards, M., Boyaval, P., Moineau, S., Romero, D. A., & Horvath, P. (2007). CRISPR provides acquired resistance against viruses in prokaryotes. *Science, 315*(5819), 1709–1712. https://doi.org/10.1126/science.1138140

Bartus, R. T., Weinberg, M. S., & Jude Samulski, R. (2014). Parkinson's disease gene therapy: Success by design meets failure by efficacy. *Molecular Therapy, 22*(3), 487–497. https://doi.org/10.1038/mt.2013.281

Baruteau, J., Brunetti-Pierri, N., & Gissen, P. (2024). Liver-directed gene therapy for inherited metabolic diseases. *Journal of Inherited Metabolic Disease, 47*(1), 9–21. https://doi.org/10.1002/jimd.12709

Benson, M. D., Waddington-Cruz, M., Berk, J. L., Polydefkis, M., Dyck, P. J., Wang, A. K., Planté-Bordeneuve, V., Barroso, F. A., Merlini, G., Obici, L., Scheinberg, M., Brannagan, T. H., Litchy, W. J., Whelan, C., Drachman, B. M., Adams, D., Heitner, S. B., Conceição, I., Schmidt, H. H., & Coelho, T. (2018). Inotersen treatment for patients with hereditary transthyretin amyloidosis. *New England Journal of Medicine, 379*(1), 22–31. https://doi.org/10.1056/NEJMoa1716793

Berling, Nicolle, Laforêt, & Ronzitti. (2023). Gene therapy review: Duchenne muscular dystrophy case study. *Revue Neurologique, 179*(1–2), 90–105. https://doi.org/10.1016/j.neurol.2022.11.005

Beutler, E. (2001). The cline affair. *Molecular Therapy, 4*(5), 396–397. https://doi.org/10.1006/mthe.2001.0486

Bialer, M., Johannessen, S. I., Koepp, M. J., Perucca, E., Perucca, P., Tomson, T., & Steve White, H. (2024). Progress report on new medications for seizures and epilepsy: A summary of the 17th eilat conference on new antiepileptic drugs and devices (EILAT XVII). I. drugs in preclinical and early clinical development. *Epilepsia, 65*(10), 2831–2857. https://doi.org/10.1111/epi.18056

Biffi, A., Aubourg, P., & Cartier, N. (2011). Gene therapy for leukodystrophies. *Human Molecular Genetics, 20.* https://doi.org/10.1093/hmg/ddr142

Blair, H. A. (2022). Onasemnogeneabeparvovec: A review in spinal muscular atrophy. *CNS Drugs, 36*(9), 995–1005. https://doi.org/10.1007/s40263-022-00941-1

Blencowe, Moorthie, Petrou, H., Povey, B., Gibbons, S., Darlison, Modell, Bittles, B., Christianson, C., Darlison, G., Hamamy, K., Howson, L., Mastroiacovo, M., Moorthie, M., Mossey, N., Petrou, P., Rankin, S.-F., & Wren, Y. (2018). Rare single gene disorders: Estimating baseline prevalence and outcomes worldwide. *Journal of Community Genetics, 9*(4), 397–406. https://doi.org/10.1007/s12687-018-0376-2

Bolotin, A., Quinquis, B., Sorokin, A., & Ehrlich, D. (2005). Clustered regularly interspaced short palindrome repeats (CRISPRs) have spacers of extrachromosomal origin. *Microbiology, 151*(8), 2551–2561. https://doi.org/10.1099/mic.0.28048-0

Bulcha, J. T., Wang, Y., Ma, H., Tai, P. W. L., & Gao, G. (2021). Viral vector platforms within the gene therapy landscape. *Signal Transduction and Targeted Therapy, 6*(1). https://doi.org/10.1038/s41392-021-00487-6

Bulgar, W., Miao, Y., Xu, G., Markowitz, O., & Gerson, L. (2012). Removal of uracil by uracil DNA glycosylase limits pemetrexed cytotoxicity: Overriding the limit with methoxyamine to inhibit base excision repair. *Cell Death and Disease, 3*(1). https://doi.org/10.1038/cddis.2011.135

Byun, S., Lee, M., & Kim, M. (2022). Gene therapy for huntington's disease: The final strategy for a cure? *Journal of Movement Disorders, 15*(1), 15–20. https://doi.org/10.14802/jmd.21006

Calucho, M., Bernal, S., Alías, L., March, F., Venceslá, A., Rodríguez-Álvarez, F. J., Aller, E., Fernández, R. M., Borrego, S., Millán, J. M., Hernández-Chico, C., Cuscó, I., Fuentes-Prior, P., & Tizzano, E. F. (2018). Correlation between SMA type and SMN2 copy number revisited: An analysis of 625 unrelated spanish patients and a compilation of 2834 reported cases. *Neuromuscular Disorders, 28*(3), 208–215. https://doi.org/10.1016/j.nmd.2018.01.003

Casper, J., Schenk, S. H., Parhizkar, E., Detampel, P., Ali, D., & Huwyler, J. (2023). Polyethylenimine (PEI) in gene therapy: Current status and clinical applications. *Journal of Controlled Release, 362*, 667–691. https://doi.org/10.1016/j.jconrel.2023.09.001

Cheng, & Smith. (2003). Gene therapy progress and prospects: Gene therapy of lysosomal storage disorders. *Gene Therapy, 10*(16), 1275–1281. https://doi.org/10.1038/sj.gt.3302092

Chilcott, E., Antinao Díaz, J., Bertram, C., Berti, M., & Karda, R. (2022). Genetic therapeutic advancements for Dravet syndrome. *Epilepsy and Behavior, 132*. https://doi.org/10.1016/j.yebeh.2022.108741

Clemens, P. R., Rao, V. K., Connolly, A. M., Harper, A. D., Mah, J. K., Smith, E. C., McDonald, C. M., Zaidman, C. M., Morgenroth, L. P., Osaki, H., Satou, Y., Yamashita, T., & Hoffman, E. P. (2020). Safety, tolerability, and efficacy of viltolarsen in boys with Duchenne muscular dystrophy amenable to exon 53 skipping: A phase 2 randomized clinical trial. *JAMA Neurology, 77*(8), 982–991. https://doi.org/10.1001/jamaneurol.2020.1264

Collotta, D., Bertocchi, I., Chiapello, E., & Collino, M. (2023). Antisense oligonucleotides: A novel frontier in pharmacological strategy. *Frontiers in Pharmacology, 14.* https://doi.org/10.3389/fphar.2023.1304342

Darras, B. T., Masson, R., Mazurkiewicz-Beldzinska, M., Rose, K., Xiong, H., Zanoteli, E., Baranello, G., Bruno, C., Vlodavets, D., Wang, Y., El-Khairi, M., Gerber, M., Gorni, K., Omar, K., Kletzl, H., Scalco, R. S., Fontoura, P., & Servais, L. (2021). Risdiplam-treated infants with type 1 spinal muscular atrophy versus historical controls. *New England Journal of Medicine, 385*(5), 427–435. https://doi.org/10.1056/NEJMoa2102047

Day, J. W., Finkel, R. S., Chiriboga, C. A., Connolly, A. M., Crawford, T. O., Darras, B. T., Iannaccone, S. T., Kuntz, N. L., Peña, L. D. M., Shieh, P. B., Smith, E. C., Kwon, J. M., Zaidman, C. M., Schultz, M., Feltner, D. E., Tauscher-Wisniewski, S., Ouyang, H., Chand, D. H., Sproule, D. M., & Mendell, J. R. (2021). Onasemnogeneabeparvovec gene therapy for symptomatic infantile-onset spinal muscular atrophy in patients with two copies of SMN2 (STR1VE): An open-label, single-arm, multicentre, phase 3 trial. *The Lancet Neurology, 20*(4), 284–293. https://doi.org/10.1016/S1474-4422(21)00001-6

Deltcheva, E., Chylinski, K., Sharma, C. M., Gonzales, K., Chao, Y., Pirzada, Z. A., Eckert, M. R., Vogel, J., & Charpentier, E. (2011). CRISPR RNA maturation by trans-encoded small RNA and host factor RNase III. *Nature, 471*(7340), 602–607. https://doi.org/10.1038/nature09886

Devinsky, O., Coller, J., Ahrens-Nicklas, R., Liu, X. S., Ahituv, N., Davidson, B. L., Bishop, K. M., Weiss, Y., & Mingorance, A. (2025). Gene therapies for neurogenetic disorders. *Trends in Molecular Medicine, 31*(9), 814–826. https://doi.org/10.1016/j.molmed.2025.01.015

Dickey, A. K., & Leaf, R. K. (2024). Givosiran: A targeted treatment for acute intermittent porphyria. *Hematology. American Society of Hematology. Education Program, 2024*(1), 426–433. https://doi.org/10.1182/hematology.2024000663

Dispenzieri, A., Coelho, T., Conceição, I., Waddington-Cruz, M., Wixner, J., Kristen, A. V., Rapezzi, C., Planté-Bordeneuve, V., Gonzalez-Moreno, J., Maurer, M. S., Grogan, M., Chapman, D., Amass, L., Garcia Pavia, P., Tarnev, I., Costello, J. G., Briseno, M. A. G. D., Schmidt, H., Drachman, B., & Kaufmann, H. (2022). Clinical and genetic profile of patients enrolled in the transthyretin amyloidosis outcomes survey (THAOS): 14-year update. *Orphanet Journal of Rare Diseases, 17*(1). https://doi.org/10.1186/s13023-022-02359-w

Domingo, A., & Klein, C. (2018). Genetics of parkinson disease. *Handbook of Clinical Neurology, 147*, 211–227. https://doi.org/10.1016/b978-0-444-63233-3.00014-2

Duan, D. (2023). Duchenne muscular dystrophy gene therapy in 2023: Status, perspective, and beyond. *Human Gene Therapy, 34*(9–10), 345–349. https://doi.org/10.1089/hum.2023.29242.ddu

Eichler, F., Duncan, C., Musolino, P. L., Orchard, P. J., De Oliveira, S., Thrasher, A. J., Armant, M., Dansereau, C., Lund, T. C., Miller, W. P., Raymond, G. V., Sankar, R., Shah, A. J., Sevin, C., Bobby Gaspar, H., Gissen, P., Amartino, H., Bratkovic, D., Smith, N. J. C., & Williams, D. A. (2017). Hematopoietic stem-cell gene therapy for cerebral adrenoleukodystrophy. *New England Journal of Medicine, 377*(17), 1630–1638. https://doi.org/10.1056/NEJMoa1700554

Elbashir, S. M., Harborth, J., Lendeckel, W., Yalcin, A., Weber, K., & Tuschl, T. (2001). Duplexes of 21-nucleotide RNAs mediate RNA interference in cultured mammalian cells. *Nature, 411*(6836), 494–498. https://doi.org/10.1038/35078107

EMA definition. https://www.ema.europa.eu/en/human-regulatory-overview/advanced-therapy-medicinal-products-overview.

Finkel, R. S., Mercuri, E., Darras, B. T., Connolly, A. M., Kuntz, N. L., Kirschner, J., Chiriboga, C. A., Saito, K., Servais, L., Tizzano, E., Topaloglu, H., Tulinius, M., Montes, J., Glanzman, A. M., Bishop, K., Zhong, Z. J., Gheuens, S., Frank Bennett, C., Schneider, E., & Zeng. (2017). Nusinersen versus sham control in infantile-onset spinal muscular atrophy. *New England Journal of Medicine, 377*(18), 1723–1732. https://doi.org/10.1056/NEJMoa1702752

Fire, X., Montgomery, K., & Driver, M. (1998). Potent and specific genetic interference by double-stranded RNA in caenorhabditis elegans. *Nature, 391*(6669), 806–811. https://doi.org/10.1038/35888

Flotte, T., Carter, B., Conrad, C., Guggino, W., Reynolds, T., Rosenstein, B., Taylor, G., Walden, S., & Wetzel, R. (1996). A phase I study of an adeno-associated virus-CFTR gene vector in adult CF patients with mild lung disease. *Human Gene Therapy, 7*(9), 1145–1159.

Folegatti, P. M., Ewer, K. J., Aley, P. K., Angus, B., Becker, S., Belij-Rammerstorfer, S., Bellamy, D., Bibi, S., Bittaye, M., Clutterbuck, E. A., Dold, C., Faust, S. N., Finn, A., Flaxman, A. L., Hallis, B., Heath, P., Jenkin, D., Lazarus, R., Makinson, R., & Yau, Y. (2020). Safety and immunogenicity of the ChAdOx1 nCoV-

19 vaccine against SARS-CoV-2: A preliminary report of a phase 1/2, single-blind, randomised controlled trial. *The Lancet, 396*(10249), 467–478. https://doi.org/10.1016/S0140-6736(20)31604-4

Fontana, M., Berk, J. L., Gillmore, J. D., Witteles, R. M., Grogan, M., Drachman, B., Damy, T., Garcia-Pavia, P., Taubel, J., Solomon, S. D., Sheikh, F. H., Tahara, N., González-Costello, J., Tsujita, K., Morbach, C., Pozsonyi, Z., Petrie, M. C., Delgado, D., Van Der Meer, P., & Maurer, M. S. (2025). Vutrisiran in patients with transthyretin amyloidosis with cardiomyopathy. *New England Journal of Medicine, 392*(1), 33–44. https://doi.org/10.1056/NEJMoa2409134

Frank, D. E., Schnell, F. J., Akana, C., El-Husayni, S. H., Desjardins, C. A., Morgan, J., Charleston, J. S., Sardone, V., Domingos, J., George, D., Straub, V., Guglieri, M., Mercuri, E., Servais, L., & Muntoni, F. (2020). Increased dystrophin production with golodirsen in patients with duchenne muscular dystrophy. *Neurology, 94* (21). https://doi.org/10.1212/WNL.0000000000009233

Friedmann, T. (1992). A brief history of gene therapy. *Nature Genetics, 2*(2), 93–98. https://doi.org/10.1038/ng1092-93

Friedmann, T. (2001). Stanfield rogers: Insights into virus vectors and failure of an early gene therapy model. *Molecular Therapy, 4*(4), 285–288. https://doi.org/10.1006/mthe.2001.0454

Friedmann, T., & Roblin, R. (1972). Gene therapy for human genetic disease? *Science., 175*(4025), 949–955. https://doi.org/10.1126/science.175.4025.949

Fumagalli, F., Calbi, V., Sora, M. G. N., Sessa, M., Baldoli, C., Rancoita, P. M. V., Ciotti, F., Sarzana, M., Fraschini, M., Zambon, A. A., Acquati, S., Redaelli, D., Attanasio, V., Miglietta, S., De Mattia, F., Barzaghi, F., Ferrua, F., Migliavacca, M., Tucci, F., & Aiuti, A. (2022). Lentiviral haematopoietic stem-cell gene therapy for early-onset metachromatic leukodystrophy: Long-term results from a non-randomised, open-label, phase 1/2 trial and expanded access. *The Lancet, 399*(10322), 372–383. https://doi.org/10.1016/S0140-6736(21)02017-1

Gales, L. (2019). Tegsedi (inotersen): An antisense oligonucleotide approved for the treatment of adult patients with hereditary transthyretin amyloidosis. *Pharmaceuticals, 12*(2). https://doi.org/10.3390/ph12020078

Gilani, F., & Gautam, A. (2025). Regulation of RNA transcriptomics during ageing-and neurodegeneration-associated cognitive changes. In *Decoding aging and neurodegeneration: The role of nucleic acid epigenetics* (pp. 69–93). Cham: Springer Nature Switzerland.

Gostimskaya, I. (2022). CRISPR-Cas9: A history of its discovery and ethical considerations of its use in genome editing. *Biochemistry. Biokhimiia, 87*(8), 777–788. https://doi.org/10.1134/S0006297922080090

Greenberg, A. J., Mccormick, J., Tapia, C. J., & Windebank, A. J. (2011). Translating gene transfer: A stalled effort. *Clinical and Translational Science, 4*(4), 279–281. https://doi.org/10.1111/j.1752-8062.2011.00297.x

Griesenbach. 2007. Progress and prospects: Gene therapy clinical trials (part 2). Gene Therapy. 14(22), 1555–1563. doi: 10.1038/sj.gt.3303033.

Groeschel, S., Köhl, J.-S., Bley, A. E., Kehrer, C., Weschke, B., Döring, M., Böhringer, J., Schrum, J., Santer, R., Kohlschötter, A., Krägeloh-Mann, I., & Möller, I. (2016). Long-term outcome of allogeneic hematopoietic stem cell transplantation in patients with juvenile metachromatic leukodystrophy compared with non-transplanted control patients. *JAMA Neurology, 73*(9), 1133–1140. https://doi.org/10.1001/jamaneurol.2016.2067

Guillou, J., de Pellegars, A., Porcheret, F., Frémeaux-Bacchi, V., Allain-Launay, E., Debord, C., Denis, M., Péréon, Y., Barnérias, C., Desguerre, I., Roussey, G., & Mercier, S. (2022). Fatal thrombotic microangiopathy case following adeno-associated viral SMN gene therapy. *Blood Advances, 6*(14), 4266–4270. https://doi.org/10.1182/bloodadvances.2021006419

Hashizume, R., Wakita, S., Sawada, H., Takebayashi, S.-I., Kitabatake, Y., Miyagawa, Y., Hirokawa, Y. S., Imai, H., & Kurahashi, H. (2025). Trisomic rescue via allele-specific multiple chromosome cleavage using CRISPR-Cas9 in trisomy 21 cells. *PNAS Nexus, 4*(2). https://doi.org/10.1093/pnasnexus/pgaf022

Higurashi, N., Broccoli, V., & Hirose, S. (2022). Genetics and gene therapy in dravet syndrome. *Epilepsy and Behavior, 131*. https://doi.org/10.1016/j.yebeh.2021.108043

í Dali, C., Sevin, C., Krägeloh-Mann, I., Giugliani, R., Sakai, N., Wu, J., & Wasilewski, M. (2020). Safety of intrathecal delivery of recombinant human arylsulfatase A in children with metachromatic leukodystrophy: Results from a phase 1/2 clinical trial. *Molecular Genetics and Metabolism, 131*(1–2), 235–244. https://doi.org/10.1016/j.ymgme.2020.07.002

Iannaccone, S., Phan, H., Straub, V., Muntoni, F., Wolf, D., Malhotra, J., Chu, R., Darton, E., & Mercuri, E. (2022). Casimersen in patients with duchenne muscular dystrophy amenable to exon 45 skipping: Interim results from the phase 3 ESSENCE trial. *Neuromuscular Disorders, 32*. https://doi.org/10.1016/j.nmd.2022.07.248

Ishino, Shinagawa, Makino, Amemura, & Nakatura. (1987). Nucleotide sequence of the iap gene, responsible for alkaline phosphatase isoenzyme conversion in escherichia coli, and identification of the gene product. *Journal of Bacteriology, 169*(12), 5429–5433. https://doi.org/10.1128/jb.169.12.5429-5433.1987

Jinek, M., Jiang, F., Taylor, D. W., Sternberg, S. H., Kaya, E., Ma, E., Anders, C., Hauer, M., Zhou, K., Lin, S., Kaplan, M., Iavarone, A. T., Charpentier, E., Nogales, E., & Doudna, J. A. (2014). Structures of Cas9 endonucleases reveal RNA-mediated conformational activation. *Science, 343*(6176). https://doi.org/10.1126/science.1247997

Johnson, C. D., & Davidson, B. L. (2010). Huntington's disease: Progress toward effective disease-modifying treatments and a cure. *Human Molecular Genetics, 19*(R1). https://doi.org/10.1093/hmg/ddq148

Khan, A., Barber, D. L., Huang, J., Anthony Rupar, C., Rip, J. W., Auray-Blais, C., Boutin, M., Hoski, P. O.', Gargulak, K., McKillop, W. M., Fraser, G., Wasim, S., LeMoine, K., Jelinski, S., Chaudhry, A., Prokopishyn, N., Morel, C. F., Couban, S., Duggan, P. R., & Medin, J. A. (2021). Lentivirus-mediated gene therapy for Fabry disease. *Nature Communications, 12*(1). https://doi.org/10.1038/s41467-021-21371-5

Kido, J., Sugawara, K., & Nakamura, K. (2023). Gene therapy for lysosomal storage diseases: Current clinical trial prospects. *Frontiers in Genetics, 14*. https://doi.org/10.3389/fgene.2023.1064924

Koeberl, D. D., Koch, R. L., Lim, J.-A., Brooks, E. D., Arnson, B. D., Sun, B., & Kishnani, P. S. (2024). Gene therapy for glycogen storage diseases. *Journal of Inherited Metabolic Disease, 47*(1), 93–118. https://doi.org/10.1002/jimd.12654

Koutsoukos, S. A., & Bilousova, G. (2024). Highlights of gene and cell therapy for epidermolysis bullosa and ichthyosis. *Dermatology and Therapy, 14*(9), 2379–2392. https://doi.org/10.1007/s13555-024-01239-4

Kresge, N., Simoni, R. D., & Hill, R. L. (2009). Total synthesis of a tyrosine suppressor tRNA: The work of H. gobind khorana. *Journal of Biological Chemistry, 284*(22). https://doi.org/10.1016/S0021-9258(19)82144-0

Kulkarni, J. A., Witzigmann, D., Thomson, S. B., Chen, S., Leavitt, B. R., & Cullis, P. R. (2021). Roy van der Meel, the current landscape of nucleic acid therapeutics. *Nature Nanotechnology, 16*(6), 630–643. https://doi.org/10.1038/s41565-021-00898-0

Landfeldt, E. (2022). Gene therapy for neuromuscular diseases: Health economic challenges and future perspectives. *Journal of Neuromuscular Diseases, 9*(6), 675–688. https://doi.org/10.3233/JND-221540

Lauffer, M. C., van Roon-Mom, W., & Aartsma-Rus, A. (2024). Possibilities and limitations of antisense oligonucleotide therapies for the treatment of monogenic disorders. *Communications Medicine, 4*(1). https://doi.org/10.1038/s43856-023-00419-1

Levine, B. L., Humeau, L. M., Boyer, J., MacGregor, R.-R., Rebello, T., Lu, X., Binder, G. K., Slepushkin, V., Lemiale, F., Mascola, J. R., Bushman, F. D., Dropulic, B., & Carl, H. J. (2006). Gene transfer in humans using a conditionally replicating lentiviral vector. *Proceedings of the National Academy of Sciences of the United States of America, 103*(46), 17372–17377.

Locke, A., Kunnavakkam Van, B., Larson, O., Godley, L., Le, B., Gurbuxani, T., Sipkins, W., & Artz, S. (2013). A novel clofarabine bridge strategy facilitates allogeneic transplantation in patients with relapsed/refractory leukemia and high-risk myelodysplastic syndromes. *Bone Marrow Transplantation, 48*(11), 1437–1443. https://doi.org/10.1038/bmt.2013.79

MacDonald, M. E., Ambrose, C. M., Duyao, M. P., Myers, R. H., Lin, C., Srinidhi, L., Barnes, G., Taylor, S. A., James, M., Groot, N., MacFarlane, H., Jenkins, B., Anderson, M. A., Wexler, N. S., Gusella, J. F., Bates, G. P., Baxendale, S., Hummerich, H., Kirby, S., & Peter, S. (1993). Harper, A novel gene containing a trinucleotide repeat that is expanded and unstable on huntington's disease chromosomes. *Cell, 72*(6), 971–983. https://doi.org/10.1016/0092-8674(93)90585-e

Matuszek, Z., Arbab, M., Kesavan, M., Hsu, A., Roy, J. C. L., Zhao, J., Yu, T., Weisburd, B., Newby, G. A., Doherty, N. J., Wu, M., Shibata, S., Cristian, A., Allen Tao, Y., Fearnley, L. G., Bahlo, M., Rehm, H. L., Xie, J., Gao, G., Mouro Pinto, R., & Liu, D. R. (2025). Base editing of trinucleotide repeats that cause huntington's disease and friedreich's ataxia reduces somatic repeat expansions in patient cells and in mice. *Nature Genetics*. https://doi.org/10.1038/s41588-025-02172-8

McColgan, P., Thobhani, A., Boak, L., Schobel, S. A., Nicotra, A., Palermo, G., Trundell, D., Zhou, J., Schlegel, V., Sanwald Ducray, P., Hawellek, D. J., Dorn, J., Simillion, C., Lindemann, M., Wheelock, V., Durr, A., Anderson, K. E., Long, J. D., Wild, E. J., & Doody, R. (2023). Tominersen in adults with manifest huntington's disease. *New England Journal of Medicine, 389*(23), 2203–2205. https://doi.org/10.1056/nejmc2300400

McDonald, C. M., Shieh, P. B., Abdel-Hamid, H. Z., Connolly, A. M., Ciafaloni, E., Wagner, K. R., Goemans, N., Mercuri, E., Khan, N., Koenig, E., Malhotra, J., Zhang, W., Han, B., & Mendell, J. R. (2021). Open-label evaluation of eteplirsen in patients with duchenne muscular dystrophy amenable to exon 51 skipping: PROMOVI trial. *Journal of Neuromuscular Diseases, 8*(6), 989–1001. https://doi.org/10.3233/JND-210643

Mendell, J. R., Connolly, A. M., Lehman, K. J., Griffin, D. A., Khan, S. Z., Dharia, S. D., Quintana-Gallardo, L., & Rodino-Klapac, L. R. (2022). Testing preexisting antibodies prior to AAV gene transfer therapy: Rationale, lessons and future considerations. *Molecular Therapy Methods and Clinical Development, 25*, 74–83. https://doi.org/10.1016/j.omtm.2022.02.011

Mendell, J. R., Goemans, N., Lowes, L. P., Alfano, L. N., Berry, K., Shao, J., Kaye, E. M., & Mercuri, E. (2016). Longitudinal effect of eteplirsen versus historical control on ambulation in duchenne muscular dystrophy. *Annals of Neurology, 79*(2), 257–271. https://doi.org/10.1002/ana.24555

Mendell, J. R., Muntoni, F., McDonald, C. M., Mercuri, E. M., Ciafaloni, E., Komaki, H., Leon-Astudillo, C., Nascimento, A., Proud, C., Schara-Schmidt, U., Veerapandiyan, A., Zaidman, C. M., Guridi, M., Murphy, A. P., Reid, C., Wandel, C., Asher, D. R., Darton, E., Mason, S., & Rodino-Klapac, L. R. (2025). AAV gene therapy for duchenne muscular dystrophy: The EMBARK phase 3 randomized trial. *Nature Medicine, 31*(1), 332–341. https://doi.org/10.1038/s41591-024-03304-z

Mendell, J. R., Rodino-Klapac, L. R., Sahenk, Z., Roush, K., Bird, L., Lowes, L. P., Alfano, L., Gomez, A. M., Lewis, S., Kota, J., Malik, V., Kim, S., Walker, C. M., Flanigan, K. M., Corridore, M., Kean, J. R., Allen, H. D., Shilling, C., Melia, K. R., & Kaye, E. M. (2013). Eteplirsen for the treatment of duchenne muscular dystrophy. *Annals of Neurology, 74*(5), 637–647. https://doi.org/10.1002/ana.23982

Mercuri, D., Chiriboga, D., Campbell, C., Iannaccone, K., Kuntz, S., Shieh, T., Mazzone, M., Bishop, Y., Foster, G., Bennett, F., Schneider De, V., & Finkel. (2018). Nusinersen versus sham control in later-onset spinal muscular atrophy. *New England Journal of Medicine, 378*(7), 625–635. https://doi.org/10.1056/NEJMoa1710504

Mercuri, E., Deconinck, N., Mazzone, E. S., Nascimento, A., Oskoui, M., Saito, K., Vuillerot, C., Baranello, G., Boespflug-Tanguy, O., Goemans, N., Kirschner, J., Kostera-Pruszczyk, A., Servais, L., Gerber, M., Gorni, K., Khwaja, O., Kletzl, H., Scalco, R. S., Staunton, H., & Day, J. W. (2022). Safety and efficacy of once-daily risdiplam in type 2 and non-ambulant type 3 spinal muscular atrophy (SUNFISH part 2): A phase 3, double-blind, randomised, placebo-controlled trial. *The Lancet. Neurology, 21*(1), 42–52.

Mich, J. K., Ryu, J., Wei, A. D., Gore, B. B., Guo, R., Bard, A. M., Martinez, R. A., Luber, E. M., Liu, J., Bishaw, Y. M., Christian, R. J., Oliveira, L. M., Miranda, N., Ramirez, J.-M., Ting, J. T., Lein, E. S., Levi, B. P., & Kalume, F. K. (2025). Interneuron-specific dual-AAV SCN1A gene replacement corrects epileptic phenotypes in mouse models of dravet syndrome. *Science Translational Medicine, 17*(790). https://doi.org/10.1126/scitranslmed.adn5603

Miller, T. M., Cudkowicz, M. E., Genge, A., Shaw, P. J., Sobue, G., Bucelli, R. C., Chiò, A., Van Damme, P., Ludolph, A. C., Glass, J. D., Andrews, J. A., Babu, S., Benatar, M., McDermott, C. J., Cochrane, T., Chary, S.,

Chew, S., Zhu, H., Wu, F., & Fradette, S. (2022). Trial of antisense oligonucleotide tofersen for SOD1 ALS. *New England Journal of Medicine, 387*(12), 1099–1110. https://doi.org/10.1056/NEJMoa2204705

Milone, M. C., & O'Doherty, U. (2018). Clinical use of lentiviral vectors. *Leukemia, 32*(7), 1529–1541. https://doi.org/10.1038/s41375-018-0106-0

Mir, F. A., Amanullah, A., Jain, B. P., Hyderi, Z., & Gautam, A. (2023). Neuroepigenetics of ageing and neurodegeneration-associated dementia: An updated review. *Ageing Research Reviews, 91*. https://doi.org/10.1016/j.arr.2023.102067

Mojica, F. J., Ferrer, C., Juez, G., & Rodríguez-Valera, F. (1995). Long stretches of short tandem repeats are present in the largest replicons of the Archaea Haloferax mediterranei and Haloferax volcanii and could be involved in replicon partitioning. *Molecular Microbiology, 17*(1), 85–93.

Muravyeva, A., & Smirnikhina, S. (2024). Adenoviral vectors for gene therapy of hereditary diseases. *Biology, 13*(12). https://doi.org/10.3390/biology13121052

Naldini, L., Blömer, U., Gallay, P., Ory, D., Mulligan, R., Gage, F. H., Verma, I. M., & Trono, D. (1996). In vivo gene delivery and stable transduction of nondividing cells by a lentiviral vector. *Science, 272*(5259), 263–267. https://doi.org/10.1126/science.272.5259.263

NINDS Tofersen. 2025. https://www.ninds.nih.gov/about-ninds/what-we-do/impact/ninds-contributions-approved-therapies/tofersen-qalsodyr-amyotrophic-lateral-sclerosis.

Phielipp, N., & Henchcliffe, C. (2025). Investigational gene therapies for parkinson's disease. *CNS Drugs, 39*(8), 725–737. https://doi.org/10.1007/s40263-025-01203-6

Pol, J., Kroemer, G., & Galluzzi, L. (2016). First oncolytic virus approved for melanoma immunotherapy. *Oncoimmunology, 5*(1).

Porto, E. M., Komor, A. C., Slaymaker, I. M., & Yeo, G. W. (2020). Base editing: Advances and therapeutic opportunities. *Nature Reviews Drug Discovery, 19*(12), 839–859. https://doi.org/10.1038/s41573-020-0084-6

Renneberg, D., & Leumann, C. J. (2002). Watson–Crick base-Pairing properties of Tricyclo-DNA. *Journal of the American Chemical Society, 124*(21), 5993–6002.

Rodrigues, F. B., & Wild, E. J. (2020). Huntington's disease clinical trials corner: April 2020. *Journal of Huntington's Disease, 9*(2), 185–197. https://doi.org/10.3233/JHD-200002

Roehr, B. (1998). Fomivirsen approved for CMV retinitis. *Journal of the International Association of Physicians in AIDS Care, 4*(10), 14–16.

Rosenberg, J. B., Kaminsky, S. M., Aubourg, P., & Crystal, R. G. (2016). Dolan sondhi, gene therapy for metachromatic leukodystrophy. *Journal of Neuroscience Research, 94*(11), 1169–1179. https://doi.org/10.1002/jnr.23792

Rosenfeld, M. A., Siegfried, W., Yoshimura, K., Yoneyama, K., Fukayama, M., Stier, L. E., Pääkkö, P. K., Gilardi, P., Stratford-Perricaudet, L. D., & Perricaudet, M. (1991). Adenovirus-mediated transfer of a recombinant alpha 1-antitrypsin gene to the lung epithelium in vivo. *Science (New York, N.Y.), 252*(5004), 431–434.

Sanguinetti, C., Minniti, M., Susini, V., Caponi, L., Panichella, G., Castiglione, V., Aimo, A., Emdin, M., Vergaro, G., & Franzini, M. (2022). The journey of human transthyretin: Synthesis, structure stability, and catabolism. *Biomedicines, 10*(8). https://doi.org/10.3390/biomedicines10081906

Scott, A. I., Mallhi, K. K., Ganesh, J., & Chen, W.-L. (2023). Elivaldogeneautotemcel approved for treatment of cerebral adrenoleukodystrophy (CALD) in males: A therapeutics bulletin of the American college of medical genetics and genomics (ACMG). *Genetics in Medicine Open, 1*(1). https://doi.org/10.1016/j.gimo.2023.100835

Servais, L., Mercuri, E., Straub, V., Guglieri, M., Seferian, A. M., Scoto, M., Leone, D., Koenig, E., Khan, N., Dugar, A., Wang, X., Han, B., Wang, D., & Muntoni, F. (2022). Long-term safety and efficacy data of golodirsen in ambulatory patients with duchenne muscular dystrophy amenable to exon 53 skipping: A first-in-human, multicenter, two-part, open-label, phase 1/2 trial. *Nucleic Acid Therapeutics, 32*(1), 29–39. https://doi.org/10.1089/nat.2021.0043

Sharma, G., Sharma, A. R., Bhattacharya, M., Lee, S.-S., & Chakraborty, C. (2021). CRISPR-Cas9: A preclinical and clinical perspective for the treatment of human diseases. *Molecular Therapy, 29*(2), 571–586. https://doi.org/10.1016/j.ymthe.2020.09.028

Shimotohno, K., & Temin, H. M. (1981). Formation of infectious progeny virus after insertion of herpes simplex thymidine kinase gene into DNA of an avian retrovirus. *Cell, 26*(1 PART 1), 67–77. https://doi.org/10.1016/0092-8674(81)90034-9

Sibbald, B. (2001). Death but one unintended consequence of gene-therapy trial. *Canadian Medical Association Journal: Canadian Medical Association Journal = Journal de l'Association Medicale Canadienne, 164*(11).

Singh, R. N., & Singh, N. N. (2018). Mechanism of splicing regulation of spinal muscular atrophy genes. *Advances in Neurobiology, 20*, 31–61. https://doi.org/10.1007/978-3-319-89689-2_2

Singh, A., Irfan, H., Fatima, E., Nazir, Z., Verma, A., & Akilimali, A. (2024). Revolutionary breakthrough: FDA approves CASGEVY, the first CRISPR/Cas9 gene therapy for sickle cell disease. *Annals of Medicine and Surgery, 86*(8), 4555–4559. https://doi.org/10.1097/MS9.0000000000002146

Spinal muscular atrophy GeneReviews® Internet. University of Washington, Seattle University of Washington, Seattle.

Stephenson, & Zamecnik. (1978). Inhibition of rous sarcoma viral RNA translation by a specific oligodeoxyribonucleotide. *Proceedings of the National Academy of Sciences of the United States of America, 75*(1), 285–288. https://doi.org/10.1073/pnas.75.1.285

Sun, M. (1981). Cline loses two NIH grants. *Science., 214*(4526). https://doi.org/10.1126/science.7302590

Suzuki, N., Nishiyama, A., Warita, H., & Aoki, M. (2023). Genetics of amyotrophic lateral sclerosis: Seeking therapeutic targets in the era of gene therapy. *Journal of Human Genetics, 68*(3), 131–152. https://doi.org/10.1038/s10038-022-01055-8

Syvertsen, M., Nakken, K. O., Edland, A., Hansen, G., Hellum, M. K., & Koht, J. (2015). Prevalence and etiology of epilepsy in a norwegian county - A population based study. *Epilepsia, 56*(5), 699–706. https://doi.org/10.1111/epi.12972

Szunyogh, S., Carroll, E., & Wade-Martins, R. (2025). Recent developments in gene therapy for parkinson's disease. *Molecular Therapy, 33*(5), 2052–2064. https://doi.org/10.1016/j.ymthe.2025.03.030

Thompson, A. A., Walters, M. C., Kwiatkowski, J., Rasko, J. E. J., Ribeil, J.-A., Hongeng, S., Magrin, E., Schiller, G. J., Payen, E., Semeraro, M., Moshous, D., Lefrere, F., Puy, H., Bourget, P., Magnani, A., Caccavelli, L., Diana, J.-S., Suarez, F., Monpoux, F., & Cavazzana, M. (2018). Gene therapy in patients with transfusion-dependent β-Thalassemia. *New England Journal of Medicine, 378*(16), 1479–1493. https://doi.org/10.1056/NEJMoa1705342

USFDA. 2023. https://www.fda.gov/news-events/press-announcements/fda-approves-first-gene-therapy-treatment-certain-patients-duchenne-muscular-dystrophy.

USFDA definition. 2018. https://www.fda.gov/vaccines-blood-biologics/cellular-gene-therapy-products/what-gene-therapy#footnote1.

USFDA Luxturna. 2017. https://www.fda.gov/NewsEvents/Newsroom/PressAnnouncements/ucm589467.htm.

van Ommen, V., Hofker, M., Kunkel, R., Worton, W., & Bakker, P. (1986). A physical map of 4 million bp around the duchenne muscular dystrophy gene on the human X-chromosome. *Cell, 47*(4), 499–504. https://doi.org/10.1016/0092-8674(86)90614-8

Verhaart, I. E. C., Robertson, A., Wilson, I. J., Aartsma-Rus, A., Cameron, S., Jones, C. C., Cook, S. F., & Lochmüller, H. (2017). Prevalence, incidence and carrier frequency of 5q-linked spinal muscular atrophy - A literature review. *Orphanet Journal of Rare Diseases, 12*(1). https://doi.org/10.1186/s13023-017-0671-8

Vita, G., Vita, G. L., Stancanelli, C., Gentile, L., Russo, M., & Mazzeo, A. (2019). Genetic neuromuscular disorders: Living the era of a therapeutic revolution. Part 1: Peripheral neuropathies. *Neurological Sciences, 40*(4), 661–669. https://doi.org/10.1007/s10072-019-03778-7

Wagner, K. R., Kuntz, N. L., Koenig, E., East, L., Upadhyay, S., Han, B., & Shieh, P. B. (2021). Safety, tolerability, and pharmacokinetics of casimersen in patients with duchenne muscular dystrophy amenable to exon 45 skipping: A randomized, double-blind, placebo-controlled, dose-titration trial. *Muscle and Nerve, 64*(3), 285–292. https://doi.org/10.1002/mus.27347

Wagnon, J. L. (2021). TANGO with SCN1A: Can this molecular dance defeat Dravet Syndrome? *Epilepsy Currents, 21*(1), 60–61. https://doi.org/10.1177/1535759720975750

Wang, H., Guan, L. P., & Deng, M. (2023). Recent progress of the genetics of amyotrophic lateral sclerosis and challenges of gene therapy. *Frontiers in Neuroscience, 17*. https://doi.org/10.3389/fnins.2023.1170996

Ylä-Herttuala, S. (2012). Endgame: Glybera finally recommended for approval as the first gene therapy drug in the European union. *Molecular Therapy: The Journal of the American Society of Gene Therapy, 20*(10), 1831–1832. https://doi.org/10.1038/mt.2012.194

Zaidman, C. M., Goedeker, N. L., Aqul, A. A., Butterfield, R. J., Connolly, A. M., Crystal, R. G., Godwin, K. E., Hor, K. N., Mathews, K. D., Proud, C. M., Smyth, E. K., Veerapandiyan, A., Watkins, P. B., & Mendell, J. R. (2024). Management of select adverse events following delandistrogene moxeparvovec gene therapy for patients with Duchenne muscular dystrophy. *Journal of Neuromuscular Diseases, 11*(3), 687–699. https://doi.org/10.3233/JND-230185

Zhang, L., Liang, Y., Liang, G., Tian, Z., Zhang, Y., Liu, Z., & Ji, X. (2022). The therapeutic prospects of N-acetylgalactosamine-siRNA conjugates. *Frontiers in Pharmacology, 13*. https://doi.org/10.3389/fphar.2022.1090237

Zhang, R., O'Connell, T., Monteleone, B., Teng, Y., Hwu, P. W.-L., Castellano, P., & Tomazos, I. (2025). Eladocageneexuparvovec for the treatment of aromatic l-Amino acid decarboxylase deficiency (AADCd): An economic evaluation from a US perspective. *PharmacoEconomics*. https://doi.org/10.1007/s40273-025-01542-8

Zhou, L., Wang, Y., Xu, Y., Zhang, Y., & Zhu, C. (2024). Advances in AAV-mediated gene replacement therapy for pediatric monogenic neurological disorders. *Molecular Therapy Methods and Clinical Development, 32*(4). https://doi.org/10.1016/j.omtm.2024.101357

Živković, S. A., Lacomis, D., & Soman, P. (2024). Neuromuscular manifestations of wild type transthyretin amyloidosis: A review and single center's experience. *Frontiers in Cardiovascular Medicine, 11*. https://doi.org/10.3389/fcvm.2024.1345608

Further reading

William, B. H., Derks, T. G. J., Drumm, M. L., Grünert, S. C., Kishnani, P. S., & Vissing, J. (2023). Glycogen storage diseases. *Nature Reviews Disease Primers, 9*(1). https://doi.org/10.1038/s41572-023-00456-z

CHAPTER

10 RNA interference in neurological disorders: Silencing harmful immune responses

Mohd Farhan[1,*], Md Sahidul Islam[*,2], Yogesh Srivastava[3,6], Jyotsana Singh[4], Hamda Khan[5] and Qingyu Zhang[7]

[1]*Lombardi Comprehensive Cancer Center, Georgetown University Medical Center, Washington, DC, United States;* [2]*Roswell Park Comprehensive Cancer Center, Buffalo, NY, United States;* [3]*Department of Genetics, The University of Texas MD Anderson Cancer Center, Houston, TX, United States;* [4]*Department of Hematopoietic Biology and Malignancy, The University of Texas MD Anderson Cancer Center, Houston, TX, United States;* [5]*Department of Biochemistry, Jawaharlal Nehru Medical College, Aligarh Muslim University, Aligarh, Uttar Pradesh, India;* [6]*Center for Precision Health, McWilliams School of Biomedical Informatics, The University of Texas Health Science Center, Houston, TX, United States;* [7]*Guangdong Medical University, Zhanjiang, Guangdong, China*

Abbreviations

AD	Alzheimer's disease
ALS	Amyotrophic lateral sclerosis
APOE	Apolipoprotein E
APP	Amyloid precursor protein
ASC	Apoptosis-associated speck-like protein containing a CARD
ASO	Antisense oligonucleotide
Aβ	Amyloid-beta
BACE1	Beta-site amyloid precursor protein cleaving enzyme 1
BAFF	B-cell activating factor
BBB	Blood-brain barrier
BCR	B cell receptor
BDNF	Brain-derived neurotrophic factor
C1q/C3/C5	Complement components
C9-BAC	C9orf72 bacterial artificial chromosome
CCL/CXCL	Chemokine ligands
CCR/CXCR	Chemokine receptors
CCR2	C–C chemokine receptor type 2
CD	Cluster of differentiation
CNS	Central nervous system
COX-2	Cyclooxygenase-2
CR3	Complement receptor 3
CSF	Cerebrospinal fluid

[*]These authors contribute equally.

Immunotherapies for Neurological Disorders. https://doi.org/10.1016/B978-0-443-44631-3.00013-5

CTLA-4	Cytotoxic T-lymphocyte-associated protein 4
DA	Dopaminergic
DAM	Disease-associated microglia
DAMPs	Damage-associated molecular patterns
DPR	Dipeptide repeat
DPRs	Dipeptide repeat proteins
EAAT2/GLT-1	Excitatory amino acid transporter 2/Glutamate transporter 1
EAAT2	Excitatory amino acid transporter 2
EAE	Experimental autoimmune encephalomyelitis
ECM	Extracellular matrix
ER	Endoplasmic reticulum
FOXP3	Forkhead box P3
GDNF	Glial cell line-derived neurotrophic factor
GFAP	Glial fibrillary acidic protein
GM-CSF	Granulocyte-macrophage colony-stimulating factor
GSK-3β	Glycogen synthase kinase 3 beta
HMGB1	High mobility group box 1
ICAM-1	Intercellular adhesion molecule 1
IFN-γ	Interferon-gamma
IGF-1	Insulin-like growth factor 1
IL	Interleukin
IL-17	Interleukin-17
iNOS	Inducible nitric oxide synthase
iNOS	Inducible nitric oxide synthase
JAK-STAT	Janus kinase-signal transducer and activator of transcription
LPS	Lipopolysaccharide
LRRK2	Leucine-rich repeat kinase 2
MAC	Membrane attack complex
MAPK	Mitogen-activated protein kinase
MBP	Myelin basic protein
MCP-1	Monocyte chemoattractant protein-1
MHC	Major histocompatibility complex
miR	microRNA
MMP	Matrix metalloproteinase
MOG	Myelin oligodendrocyte glycoprotein
MPO	Myeloperoxidase
MPTP	1-methyl-4-phenyl-1,2,3,6-tetrahydropyridine
MS	Multiple sclerosis
mTOR	Mammalian target of rapamycin
NADPH	Nicotinamide adenine dinucleotide phosphate
NETs	Neutrophil extracellular traps
NF-κB	Nuclear factor kappa B
NGF	Nerve growth factor
NLRP3	NOD-like receptor protein 3
NO	Nitric oxide
NOX2	NADPH oxidase 2
NP	Nanoparticle
PD	Parkinson's disease

PLGA	Poly(lactic-co-glycolic acid)
PLP	Proteolipid protein
PPARγ	Peroxisome proliferator-activated receptor gamma
PS1	Presenilin-1
RORγt	RAR-related orphan receptor gamma t
ROS	Reactive oxygen species
shRNA	short hairpin RNA
siRNA	small interfering RNA
SOD1	superoxide dismutase 1
STAT	Signal transducer and activator of transcription
TCR	T cell receptor
TDP-43	TAR DNA-binding protein 43
TGF-β	Transforming growth factor beta
Th	T helper
Th17	T helper 17 cells
TIRF	Toll-interleukin-1 receptor (TIR)-domain containing adaptor protein inducing interferon beta (TRIF)
TLR	Toll-like receptor
TNFR1	Tumor necrosis factor receptor type 1
TNF-α	Tumor necrosis factor alpha
Treg	Regulatory T cell
TREM2	Triggering receptor expressed on myeloid cells 2
UPR	Unfolded protein response
VCAM-1	Vascular cell adhesion molecule 1
VEGF	Vascular endothelial growth factor

1. Neurological disorders and inflammation

1.1 Introduction to neurological disorders

Neurological disorders encompass a wide range of medical conditions that affect the central (i.e., brain and spinal cord) and peripheral (i.e., nerve and ganglion) nervous systems. These include neurodegenerative diseases (Alzheimer's disease, Parkinson's disease, and amyotrophic lateral sclerosis), functional neurological disorders (paralysis, seizures, cognitive impairments), and disorders that start with inflammation or infection (multiple sclerosis, Creutzfeldt-Jakob disease) (Kumar et al., 2024). The interplay between immune responses and the central nervous system (CNS) is a key component in the process of maintaining neural balance and influencing the evolution of disease in a variety of neurological disorders, according to research that was conducted not too long ago. When the immune system is not functioning properly, it is a substantial contributor to the wide variety of neurological diseases that are currently being experienced. Neurodegenerative diseases such as Alzheimer's disease (AD), Parkinson's disease (PD), and amyotrophic lateral sclerosis (ALS) are examples of these disorders. These disorders vary from basic autoimmune diseases such as multiple sclerosis (MS) to various neurodegenerative disorders (Prüss, 2021; Campetella et al., 2025; DiSabato et al., 2016).

Neuroinflammations (specialized immune responses in the CNS mediated primarily by microglia, astrocytes, and infiltrating peripheral immune cells) act as a double-edged sword for the CNS, either protecting from clearing pathogens and cellular debris (acute) or progressing to neuronal damage and disrupting synaptic function (chronic or dysregulated). Consequently, the presence of neuroinflammation has evolved into a key clinical characteristic in a wide variety of neurological disorders (DiSabato et al., 2016; Cantero-Fortiz & Boada, 2024; Zhang, Xiao, et al., 2023; Shi & Yong, 2025). This is a consequence of the fact that neuroinflammation has emerged. The excessive activation of astrocytes and microglia in chronic instances results in the release of pro-inflammatory cytokines, including TNF-α, IL-1β, and IL-6, as well as chemokines and reactive oxygen species. As a consequence of this excessive stimulation, the neuronal injury is made worse, which ultimately leads to the gradual degeneration of brain tissue. This process is responsible for the development of disorders such as Alzheimer's disease, Parkinson's disease, amyotrophic lateral sclerosis, and multiple sclerosis (Gąssowska-Dobrowolska et al., 2023). For the purpose of developing individualized therapies for the prevention and treatment of particular neurological conditions, it is vital to get a more in-depth understanding of the balance of neuroinflammation. The therapies in question will be utilized for the purpose of treating and preventing specific medical disorders.

By specifically targeting genes that are implicated in inflammatory pathways, such as NF-κB, NLRP3, and CD33, as well as mediators like IL-1β and STAT3, RNA interference (RNAi) offers a precise strategy for reducing certain immune responses that are deleterious (Mir et al., 2023). One of the most fundamental challenges that still has to be overcome is the ability to transport RNA molecules over the barrier that separates the blood and the brain. On the other hand, breakthroughs in nanotechnology, chemical manipulation, and systems based on viruses or nanoparticles, improvements in brain-specific targeting. RNA interference, often known as RNAi, is a technology that has the potential to manage neuroinflammation and protect neurons. This technique brings forth new hope for the treatment of neurodegenerative and complex neurological diseases. The confluence of these advancements has made it possible for these discoveries to reach their conclusions.

1.2 Introduction to RNAi

RNA interference (RNAi) is an evolutionarily conserved biological process in which the expression of individual genes is silenced post-transcriptionally by small non-coding RNAs that are typically between 18-25 nucleotides long (Almeida & Allshire, 2005). Since its discovery by Fire and colleagues in 1998, RNAi has revolutionized our understanding of gene regulation and has become a powerful tool for treating human diseases (Fire et al., 1998; Setten et al., 2019).

The RNAi pathway includes two main types of small regulatory RNAs: short interfering RNAs (siRNAs) and microRNAs (miRNAs). SiRNAs are usually exogenous, double-stranded RNA molecules (dsRNA) processed by the enzyme Dicer (i.e., an endoribonuclease) into 21-23-nucleotide duplexes. These siRNAs are then loaded into the RNA-induced silencing complex (RISC), where the antisense strand directs sequence-specific cleavage of complementary mRNA targets Fig. 10.1 (Almeida & Allshire, 2005; Hu et al., 2020). Primary microRNAs, also known as pri-miRNAs, are not to be confused with microRNAs, which are naturally occurring regulatory molecules that are transcribed from the genome called miRNAs. After that, the pri-miRNAs undergo a series of processing steps at the hands of Drosha (which converts pri-miRNA to pre-mRNA) and Dicer (which converts pre-miRNA to miRNA). The action of microRNAs is achieved through the process of improper base pairing with target mRNAs, mostly through the seed region, which is comprised of guide nucleotide positions 2–8. This causes a reduction in the rate of translation, instability of the messenger RNA, and cleavage of the messenger RNA (Fig. 10.1 (Almeida & Allshire, 2005; Lewis et al., 2003; Winter et al.,

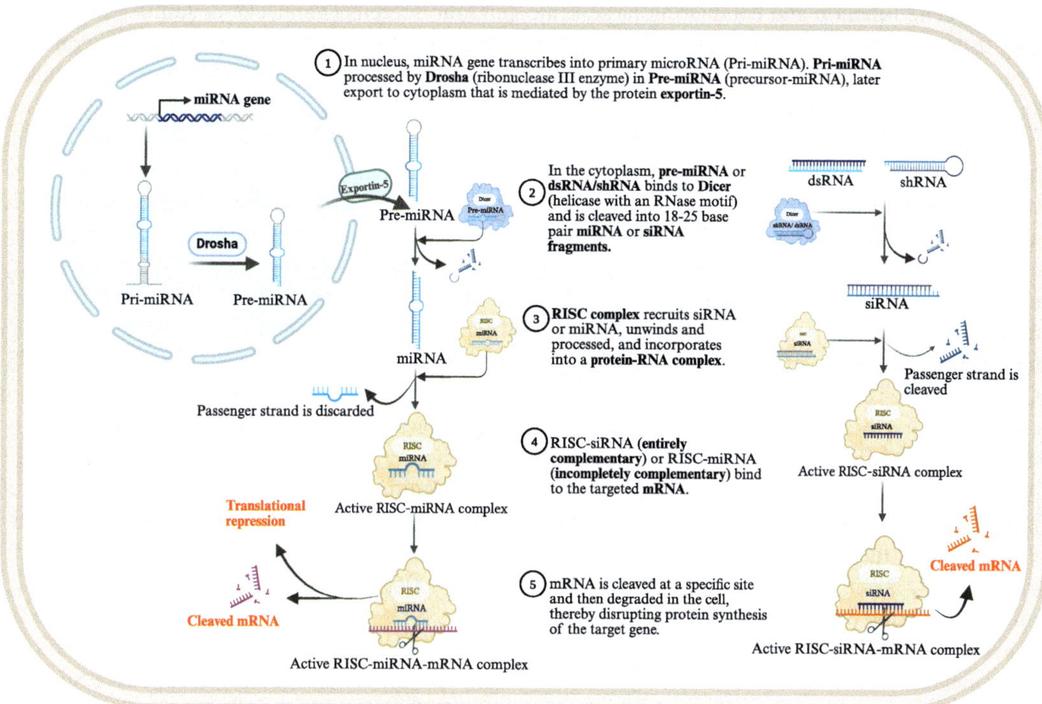

FIGURE 10.1 The Endogenous and Exogenous RNAi Pathways.

Illustration of how siRNA and miRNA are produced and how they function. The miRNA pathway begins with genomic transcription, processed by drosha and dicer, to repress translation or degrade mRNA. The siRNA pathway involves dicer processing external double-stranded RNA, which is then loaded onto RISC, and cleaving it to target mRNA, resulting in mRNA decay. In contrast, the siRNA pathway involves dicer processing of exogenous double-stranded RNA, which is then loaded onto RISC and cleaved to target specific mRNA.

Created with BioRender.

2009)). By working in conjunction with one another, these pathways make it feasible to exert precise control over the expression of genes. A wide variety of biological processes, ranging from the immune response to the growth of the organism, are under the control of hundreds of microRNAs and siRNAs. These regulatory molecules are responsible for governing these processes (Shang et al., 2023).

Notably, the RNA interference (RNAi) landscape extends beyond siRNAs and miRNAs to include PIWI-interacting RNAs (piRNAs): single-stranded RNAs processed in a Dicer-independent pathway, mainly in the germline, and short hairpin RNAs (shRNAs): synthetic dsRNA molecules with hairpin structures processed via a Dicer-dependent pathway into siRNAs (Ozata et al., 2019; Paddison et al., 2002; Wang et al., 2023; Zeng et al., 2002). These RNAi species also contribute uniquely to gene-silencing mechanisms. Besides gene regulation, RNAi plays a role in genome defense by repressing transposable elements and in epigenetic regulation by triggering heterochromatin formation (Obbard et al., 2009; Ozata et al., 2019). These diverse functions of RNAi have made it a powerful tool for studying gene function and conducting large-scale genomic screens (Vanhecke & Janitz, 2005; Mohr et al., 2010). More recently, its potential has expanded beyond research, offering promising therapeutic avenues for diseases caused by dysregulated gene expression (Setten et al., 2019; Leung & Whittaker, 2005; Castanotto & Rossi, 2009).

As a result of the deliberate application of RNA interference (RNAi) for the objective of lowering the unfavorable immune responses that occur in the central nervous system, the treatment of neurological diseases has undergone a considerable change (Holm et al., 2022; Sah, 2006). Because of this, there has been a substantial shift in the approach that is used to treat neurological conditions. One promising and precise strategy for treating neurological disorders that are caused by chronic neuroinflammation is the utilization of RNA interference (RNAi) to silence specific pro-inflammatory genes, microglial activation pathways (such as NF-κB, NLRP3, and CD33), and astrocytic inflammatory mediators (such as IL-1β and the SOCS3/STAT3 pathway) in the central nervous system (CNS) (Ganbold et al., 2020; Guha et al., 2023; Liu et al., 2019; Tork et al., 2025; Yshii et al., 2022). It is conceivable for these targeted RNAi-silencing strategies to act without causing widespread reduction of immune function while still preserving immune responses that are protective (Yshii et al., 2022; Qian et al., 2024; Laurindo et al., 2024). One of the most significant obstacles that must be conquered in order to deliver RNAi treatments to the central nervous system is the blood-brain barrier (BBB), which restricts the flow of nucleic acids and the majority of macromolecules (Boado, 2007; Davidson & Boudreau, 2007; Gosselet et al., 2021; Hoyer & Dev, 2006). This barrier is one of the most significant problems that must be overcome. The requirement for cell-type-specific dispersion inside the diverse central nervous system (CNS), the risk of immunogenicity with exogenous RNAs, and the consequences of off-target effects are additional hurdles that must be solved (Bartoszewski & Sikorski, 2019; D'Souza et al., 2023). In spite of these challenges, RNA interference (RNAi) has recently been given a fresh start as a treatment for neuroinflammatory diseases. This is a significant development. Recent advancements in nanotechnology, chemical modifications of RNA molecules, and the creation of novel delivery mechanisms have all contributed to the realization of this accomplishment (Ding et al., 2020; McLoughlin et al., 2024).

In this chapter, a comprehensive overview of RNA interference (RNAi) as a therapeutic strategy to decrease negative immune responses in neurological diseases is presented. RNAi is a technology that has been shown to be effective in treating neurological diseases. We analyze the molecular basis of neuroimmune dysregulation, investigate the numerous techniques that are now being used for the delivery of RNA interference (RNAi), compile data from both preclinical and clinical research, and discuss the future of this rapidly evolving issue.

2. Neuroimmune interactions in neurological disorders

Once immune-privileged, the CNS is now immunologically active, with resident and invading peripheral immune cells interacting with neurons and glial cells (Kipnis, 2016; Ransohoff & Brown, 2012; Wraith & Nicholson, 2012). Many neurological diseases are caused by the brain-immune system (Tian et al., 2012). Activated microglia, astrocytes, and peripheral immune cells cause chronic neuroinflammation, synapse loss, oxidative stress, and excitotoxicity (a generalized neuroinflammatory mechanism is illustrated in Fig. 10.2) (Adamu et al., 2024; Blossom et al., 2025). Table 10.1 and Table 10.2 show characteristics that produce neuroinflammatory reactions in neurological disorders

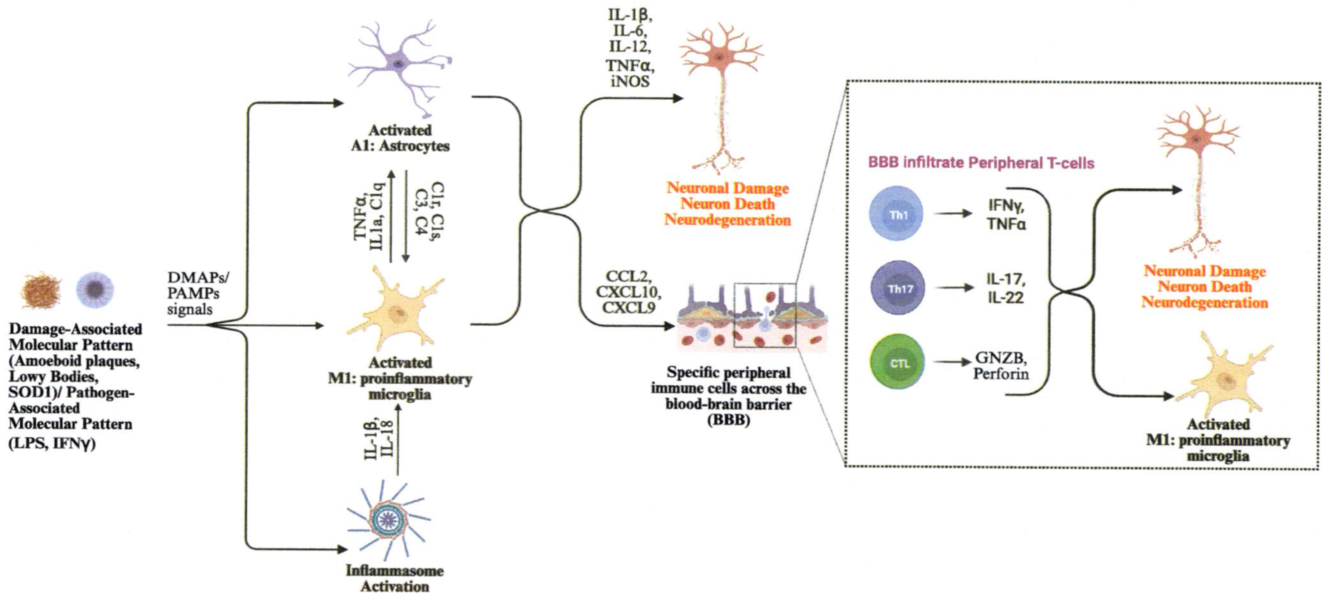

FIGURE 10.2 A Generalized Overview of Neuroimmune Interactions that Contribute to Neurodegeneration.

Damage-associated and pathogen-associated molecular patterns (DAMPs/PAMPs), including Aβ plaques, alpha-synuclein, LPS, SOD1, and IFN-γ, stimulate central nervous system (CNS) glial cells, thereby promoting the formation of neurotoxic A1 astrocytes and pro-inflammatory M1 microglia. These activated glial cells secrete inflammatory cytokines such as IL-1β, IL-6, and TNF-α, along with complement factors, which serve to amplify neuroinflammation and activate the NLRP3 inflammasome. Persistent inflammatory signaling also disrupts the blood–brain barrier (BBB) by inducing chemokines that recruit peripheral immune cells. These infiltrating T-cell subsets-including Th1, Th17, and cytotoxic T lymphocytes (CTLs)-release effector mediators, notably IFN-γ, IL-17, IL-22, perforin, and granzyme B, thereby further intensifying glial activation and neuronal injury. Collectively, glial reactivity, inflammasome activation, and peripheral immune infiltration contribute to neuronal damage and neurodegeneration.

Created with BioRender.

Table 10.1 Comprehensive mechanisms of neuroinflammatory processes in neurodegeneration.

Cellular component	Activation triggers	Key signaling pathways	Inflammatory mediators	Pathological mechanisms	Disease context	References
Microglia (M1 phenotype)	Aβ aggregates, α-synuclein, TDP-43, DAMPs, LPS, IFN-γ	NF-κB, MAPK (p38, JNK, ERK), JAK-STAT, TLR2/4 signaling	TNF-α, IL-1β, IL-6, IL-12, IL-23, iNOS, ROS, NO, CCL2, CXCL10	Oxidative neuronal damage, synaptic stripping, impaired phagocytosis, BBB disruption, excitotoxicity amplification	AD, PD, ALS, MS	(Cherry et al., 2014; Hickman et al., 2018)
Microglia (M2 phenotype)	IL-4, IL-13, IL-10, TGF-β, apoptotic cells	STAT6, PPARγ, Arginase-1 pathway, TREM2 signaling	IL-10, TGF-β, IGF-1, BDNF, Arginase-1, Ym1, FIZZ1	Debris clearance, anti-inflammatory cytokine release, tissue repair, neuroprotection, angiogenesis	Recovery phase in MS, early AD (compensatory)	(Cherry et al., 2014; Colonna & Butovsky, 2017; Nayak et al., 2014)
Disease-associated microglia (DAM)	Chronic Aβ exposure, TREM2 activation, metabolic stress	TREM2-DAP12-SYK, mTOR, APOE signaling, lipid metabolism pathways	APOE, SPP1, LGALS3, CLEC7A, lipid mediators	Plaque containment (early), phagocytic failure (late), metabolic dysfunction, loss of homeostatic functions	AD (primary), tauopathies	(Keren-Shaul et al., 2017; Ulrich et al., 2017)
A1 reactive astrocytes	Microglial-derived TNF-α, IL-1α, C1q (triple induction)	NF-κB, STAT3, complement cascade activation	Complement components (C3, C1q), saturated lipids, unknown neurotoxins	Reduced glutamate uptake (EAAT2↓), neuronal/oligodendrocyte killing, impaired synaptogenesis, loss of trophic support	AD, PD, ALS, MS, acute CNS injury	(Qian et al., 2023)
A2 reactive astrocytes	Ischemia, mechanical injury	STAT3, Nrf2, growth factor signaling	Thrombospondins, neurotrophic factors, pentraxins	Synaptogenesis promotion, ECM remodeling, scar formation, neuroprotection	Stroke recovery, traumatic brain injury	(Qian et al., 2023)
NLRP3 Inflammasome complex	Aβ oligomers, α-synuclein fibrils, ATP, K^+ efflux, lysosomal damage, mitochondrial ROS	NLRP3-ASC-Caspase-1 assembly, NF-κB priming	IL-1β (mature), IL-18 (mature), HMGB1, ASC specks	Pyroptotic cell death, tau hyperphosphorylation, protein aggregate seeding (ASC specks), inflammasome priming cycle	AD, PD, ALS	(Holbrook et al., 2021; Tork et al., 2025; Xu et al., 2025)

Complement cascade	Aβ plaques, apoptotic neurons, oxidized lipids, immune complexes	Classical (C1q), alternative (C3), lectin pathways; MAC assembly (C5b-9)	C1q, C3a, C3b, C5a, C5b-9 (MAC)	Aberrant synaptic pruning (C1q-C3-CR3), neuronal lysis (MAC), microglial chemotaxis (C5a), opsonization for phagocytosis	AD, MS, ALS	(Fatoba et al., 2022; Schartz & Tenner, 2020)
CD4+ T Helper Cells (Th1)	Myelin antigens, neuronal proteins presented by MHC-II	TCR-CD3, IL-12/STAT4, T-bet transcription factor	IFN-γ, TNF-α, IL-2, lymphotoxin	Macrophage/microglia M1 activation, BBB permeability increase, direct cytotoxicity, oligodendrocyte damage	MS (primary), progressive neurodegenerative diseases	(Coder et al., 2017; Goverman, 2009; Kipnis, 2016; Zeng et al., 2024)
CD4+ T Helper Cells (Th17)	IL-6 + TGF-β, IL-23 (expansion), myelin antigens	STAT3, RORγt transcription factor, IL-23R signaling	IL-17A, IL-17F, IL-21, IL-22, GM-CSF, CCL20	Neutrophil recruitment, BBB disruption (via IL-17), astrocyte activation, enhanced inflammation, CNS infiltration	MS (highly pathogenic), EAE models	(Goverman, 2009; Sommer et al., 2017)
Regulatory T cells (tregs)	IL-2, TGF-β, tolerogenic DCs	FOXP3 transcription, IL-2/STAT5, TGF-β/Smad signaling	IL-10, TGF-β, IL-35, CTLA-4, PD-1	Suppression of effector T cells, anti-inflammatory cytokine secretion, microglial M2 polarization (dysfunction in disease)	Reduced in AD, PD; therapeutic in MS	(Baruch et al., 2013; Beers et al., 2001; Liston et al., 2022)
CD8+ Cytotoxic T Cells	MHC-I presentation of intracellular antigens, viral mimicry	perforin/granzyme pathway, Fas-FasL	Perforin, granzymes (A, B), IFN-γ, TNF-α	Direct cytotoxic killing of neurons/oligodendrocytes, axonal transection, epitope spreading	MS	(Neumann et al., 2002)
B cells/Plasma cells	Myelin antigens, protein aggregates, neoantigens	BCR signaling, CD40−CD40L, BAFF/APRIL pathways	Oligoclonal IgG, autoantibodies, IL-6, lymphotoxin	Antibody-mediated cytotoxicity, complement activation, antigen presentation to T cells, meningeal follicle formation	MS, AD, PD, Neuromyelitis optica spectrum disorder	(Sabatino et al., 2019)

Continued

Table 10.1 Comprehensive mechanisms of neuroinflammatory processes in neurodegeneration.—cont'd

Cellular component	Activation triggers	Key signaling pathways	Inflammatory mediators	Pathological mechanisms	Disease context	References
Endothelial cells (BBB)	TNF-α, IL-1β, IFN-γ, hypoxia, oxidative stress	NF-κB, VEGF signaling, HIF-1α, MMP activation	ICAM-1, VCAM-1, E-selectin, MMPs, VEGF	Tight junction disruption (occludin↓, claudin-5↓), increased permeability, leukocyte transmigration, reduced efflux transporters	All neurodegenerative diseases	(Chen et al., 2024)
Neutrophils (rare in chronic disease)	IL-17, IL-8/CXCL8, acute injury, bacterial infection	CXCR2, integrin activation, TLR signaling	Elastase, MPO, MMP-9, ROS, NETs (extracellular traps)	Acute BBB damage, tissue destruction, NET formation causing vascular occlusion (rare in neurodegenerative diseases)	AD, MS	(Aries & Hensley-McBain, 2023; Rossi et al., 2020)

Table 10.2 Disease-specific neuroimmune mechanisms in major neurological disorders.

Diseases	Immune component	Specific mechanisms in disease	Key molecular players	Pathological outcomes	Reference
Alzheimer's disease	Disease-Associated Microglia (DAM)	• **Stage 1 (TREM2-independent):** recognition of amyloid deposits. • **Stage 2 (TREM2-dependent):** metabolic reprogramming, dystrophic phenotype with impaired clearance capacity.	**Pathways:** TREM2-APOE-lipid metabolism axis, mTOR signaling **Mediators:** APOE, SPP1, LGALS3, CLEC7A, cathepsins **Phenotype markers:** $CD68^+$, $CD11c^+$, $TREM2^{high}$	**Early:** • Plaque barrier formation • Debris phagocytosis **Late:** • Loss of homeostatic functions • Reduced Aβ clearance • Chronic inflammatory state cause synaptic damage • Neurotoxicity through complement and cytokine release	(Keren-Shaul et al., 2017; Nugent et al., 2020; Ulrich et al., 2017)
	Classical Activated Microglia (M1-like)	• Pattern recognition receptors detect Aβ oligomers/fibrils →Dense clustering around plaques → Pro-inflammatory cytokine production→ Enhanced tau phosphorylation →Tau aggregation → ROS increase → Neurotoxic environment	**Pathways:** NF-κB, MAPK cascades, TLR2/4/6 signaling **Mediators:** TNF-α, IL-1β, IL-6, iNOS, COX-2, ROS, NO **Receptors:** CD36, RAGE, scavenger receptors	• Direct neuronal damage via oxidative stress • Mitochondrial dysfunction • Synaptic stripping • Enhancement of tau pathology • BBB disruption • Impaired neurogenesis in hippocampus • Cognitive decline acceleration	(Heneka et al., 2025; Hickman et al., 2018)
	NLRP3 Inflammasome	• Aβ →NLRP3 activation → IL-1β secretion → Tau pathology • Dying microglia → ASC specks → More Aβ aggregation	**Pathways:** NLRP3-ASC-Caspase-1 assembly, pyroptosis **Mediators:** Mature IL-1β, IL-18, ASC specks **Triggers:** Aβ42 oligomers, lysosomal cathepsins, ATP	• Tau hyperphosphorylation • Neurofibrillary tangle formation • Spatial memory impairment • Pyroptotic microglial death • Chronic inflammation perpetuation	(Heneka et al., 2013; Tejera et al., 2019; Venegas et al., 2017)

Continued

Table 10.2 Disease-specific neuroimmune mechanisms in major neurological disorders.—cont'd

Diseases	Immune component	Specific mechanisms in disease	Key molecular players	Pathological outcomes	Reference
	Complement System (C1q, C3, C5)	• Stressed synapses → C1q tagging → C3-CR3 microglial phagocytosis → Synapse loss • MAC formation → Direct neuronal membrane damage	**Pathways:** Classical complement cascade, C3 opsonization **Mediators:** C1q, C3b, C3a, C5a, MAC (C5b-9) **Receptors:** CR3 (CD11b/CD18) on microglia	• Early synapse loss in hippocampus and cortex • Cognitive decline preceding neurodegeneration • Enhanced phagocytosis of viable synapses • Amplification of local inflammation around plaques	(Hong et al., 2016; Shi et al., 2017; Presumey et al., 2017)
	A1 Neurotoxic Astrocytes	• Induced microglial → secreted TNF-α, IL-1α, and C1q → Lose normal supportive functions (glutamate uptake and cholesterol synthesis) → Release lipophilic neurotoxins → disease severity.	**Pathways:** JAK-STAT3, NF-κB activation by microglial cytokines **Mediators:** Complement C3, saturated lipids, neurotoxic factors **Markers:** C3+, GFAP+, complement cascade genes	• Loss of neuronal metabolic support, cholesterol deprivation affecting synapses • Direct neurotoxin-mediated cell death, failed synaptic maintenance	(Liddelow et al., 2017; Zamanian et al., 2012)
	$CD8^+$ T Cells	• BBB breakdown → infiltrate in CNS → Clonally expanded → stressed neurons expressing MHC-I or Aβ-reactive responses • Role remains controversial with both protective and pathogenic evidence.	**Pathways:** MHC-I recognition, perforin-granzyme cytotoxicity **Mediators:** IFN-γ, perforin, granzyme B, TNF-α **Phenotype:** $CD8^+$CD45high, tissue-resident memory	• **Context-dependent**: May provide neuroprotection in early stages through Aβ clearance support but can cause direct neuronal killing in late disease. • Microglial activation through IFN-γ secretion potential epitope spreading	(Gate et al., 2020; Laurent et al., 2016)

Multiple sclerosis	Regulatory T Cells (Tregs)	• Immunosuppressive environment → unchecked neuroinflammation	**Pathways:** FOXP3-mediated suppression, IL-2/STAT5 **Mediators:** IL-10, TGF-β, IL-35, CTLA-4 **Markers:** $CD4^{+}$CD25 +FOXP3+	• Lead chronic inflammation • Impaired meningeal immune surveillance	(Baruch et al., 2013; Dansokho et al., 2016)
	Perivascular Macrophages	• Expression of scavenger receptors (SCARA1, CD163) → vascular Aβ accumulation and BBB breakdown	**Pathways:** SCARA1/CD36-mediated uptake, LRP1-APOE interaction **Mediators:** MMP-9, inflammatory cytokines **Location:** Perivascular spaces, leptomeninges	• Cerebral amyloid angiopathy development, hemorrhagic complications • Vascular inflammation • Compromised neurovascular unit	(Faraco et al., 2016; Hawkes & McLaurin, 2009)
	Activated Microglia/CNS Macrophages	• Activated by infiltrating T cells and inflammatory milieu → Phagocytose not only myelin debris but also cause demyelination	**Pathways:** MHC-II/CD80/CD86, phagocytic receptors, iNOS **Mediators:** TNF-α, IL-1β, NO, ROS, glutamate, proteases **Markers:** $CD68^{+}$, MHC-II+, iNOS+	• Myelin phagocytosis and degradation • Oxidative damage to oligodendrocytes and axons • Chronic smoldering inflammation in inactive lesions • Remyelination failure	(Lassmann et al., 2012; Prinz et al., 2011)
	Reactive Astrocytes	• **Protective role:** Form glial scars surrounding lesions → limiting inflammation spread. • **Pathogenic:** Hypertrophic astrocytes at lesion edges → inflammatory mediators → chronic inflammation → inhibiting remyelination • Loss of glutamate uptake → excitotoxicity	**Pathways:** STAT3, NF-κB, glial scar formation programs **Mediators:** CXCL10, CCL2, IL-6, chondroitin sulfate proteoglycans **Markers:** GFAP+, vimentin+, nestin+	• Physical barrier to remyelination through glial scar • Chronic chemokine production recruiting immune cells • Glutamate-mediated excitotoxicity	(Correale & Farez, 2015; Sofroniew, 2015)

Continued

Table 10.2 Disease-specific neuroimmune mechanisms in major neurological disorders.—cont'd

Diseases	Immune component	Specific mechanisms in disease	Key molecular players	Pathological outcomes	Reference
	Dendritic Cells	• Capture myelin antigens and present to T cells • Plasmacytoid DCs produce type I interferons with immunomodulatory effects. • Conventional DCs drive Th1/Th17 differentiation depending on context.	**Pathways:** MHC-II/CD80/CD86 costimulation, TLR signaling **Mediators:** IL-12, IL-23, Type I IFN, IL-6 **Subtypes:** Conventional DCs, plasmacytoid DCs	• T cell priming and reactivation within CNS • Epitope spreading through cross-presentation of new myelin epitopes • Maintaining autoreactive T cell responses	(Greter et al., 2005; Isaksson et al., 2012)
	CD4$^+$ Th1 Cells	• Peripheral activation against myelin → migrate to inflamed BBB → reencounter myelin antigens → Reactivation by local APCs → IFN-γ secretion→ Macrophage/microglial M1 polarization → inflammation	**Pathways:** TCR-MHC-II, IFN-γ/STAT1, T-bet transcription **Mediators:** IFN-γ, TNF-α, IL-2, lymphotoxin-α **Targets:** MBP, MOG, PLP peptides	• Macrophage/microglial activation leading to myelin destruction • Axonal damage through inflammatory milieu • Focal white matter lesions	(Attfield et al., 2022; Goverman, 2009; Laman et al., 1998)
	CD4$^+$ Th17 Cells	• IL-17 production → Direct tight junction disruption → BBB breakdown → Neutrophil recruitment and astrocyte activation	**Pathways:** IL-23R signaling, RORγt, STAT3 activation **Mediators:** IL-17A/F, IL-21, IL-22, GM-CSF, CCL20 **Ind.uction:** IL-6 + TGF-β, IL-23 expansion	• Severe BBB disruption enabling massive immune infiltration • Neutrophil recruitment causing tissue damage • Astrocyte activation and reactive gliosis, enhanced demyelination	(Hirota et al., 2011; Hu et al., 2024; Moser et al., 2020)

	$CD8^+$ Cytotoxic T Cells	• Antigen-driven clonal expansion → Direct cytotoxic killing → Cortical demyelination → Progressive MS pathology	**Pathways:** MHC-I recognition, perforin/granzyme, Fas-FasL **Mediators:** Perforin, granzyme A/B, IFN-γ, TNF-α **Phenotype:** $CD8^+CD45RO+$, tissue-resident	• Direct oligodendrocyte and neuronal cytotoxicity • Gray matter pathology • Contribution to disability progression independent of relapses • Cognitive impairment	(Friese et al., 2014; Lucchinetti et al., 2011)
	B Cells and Plasma Cells	• **Multiple pathogenic roles:1)** antibody production, **2)** antigen presentation to T cells → produce pro-inflammatory cytokines → cortical demyelination	**Pathways:** BCR signaling, $CD40^-CD40L$, BAFF/APRIL **Mediators:** Oligoclonal IgG, IL-6, IL-10, lymphotoxin **Antibodies:** Anti-MOG, anti-MBP (subset of patients)	• Antibody-mediated complement activation on myelin • Meningeal inflammation driving cortical pathology • Demyelination cause progression to disability	(Hauser et al., 2008; Krumbholz et al., 2012; Serafini et al., 2004)
	Regulatory T Cells (Tregs)	• Impaired suppressive capacity allows unchecked auto-reactive responses.	**Pathways:** FOXP3, IL-2/STAT5, TGF-β signaling **Mediators:** IL-10, TGF-β, IL-35, CTLA-4, CD39/CD73 **Phenotype:** $CD4^+CD25highFOXP3+CD127low$	• Insufficient suppression of autoreactive T cells (Th1/Th17) • Failed resolution of inflammation • Inability to maintain tolerance to myelin antigens	(Haas et al., 2005; Venken et al., 2008)
	Neutrophils	• Present primarily during acute relapses, rare in chronic lesions. • Recruited by IL-17 from Th17 cells → acute BBB damage via proteolytic enzymes → Transient pathogenic role.	**Pathways:** CXCR2, integrin activation, degranulation **Mediators:** Elastase, MPO, MMP-9, ROS **Recruitment:** IL-17, CXCL1, CXCL8	• Acute BBB disruption during relapses • Tissue damage through proteases and ROS • Rapid but transient pathogenic contribution	(Carlson et al., 2008; Naegele et al., 2012)

Continued

Table 10.2 Disease-specific neuroimmune mechanisms in major neurological disorders.—cont'd

Diseases	Immune component	Specific mechanisms in disease	Key molecular players	Pathological outcomes	Reference
Parkinson's disease	Activated Microglia (M1-like)	• Recognition of extracellular α-synuclein via TLR2/4 and Fc receptors → ROS → dopaminergic neurons loss • Chronically activated in the substantia nigra throughout the disease course	**Pathways:** TLR2/4-MyD88-NF-κB, LRRK2 kinase, NOX2 NADPH oxidase **Mediators:** TNF-α, IL-1β, IL-6, superoxide, NO, prostaglandins **Receptors:** TLR2/4, CD11b, FcγR	• Mitochondrial dysfunction • Reduced neurogenesis in substantia nigra • Motor symptom progression • conversion of healthy α-synuclein to toxic forms	(Barcia et al., 2011; Hirsch & Hunot, 2009; Ouchi et al., 2005)
	Reactive Astrocytes	• Impaired glutathione production → Reduced antioxidant defense capacity → Loss of GDNF/BDNF neurotrophic support → toxicity to dopaminergic neuron	**Pathways:** STAT3, inflammatory signaling, glutathione synthesis **Mediators:** TNF-α, IL-6, reduced GDNF/BDNF, oxidized dopamine **Markers:** GFAP+, S100β+, inflammatory phenotype	• Loss of metabolic and trophic support to neurons • A-synuclein propagation between cells	(Liddelow et al., 2017; Rizor et al., 2019)
	NLRP3 Inflammasome	• Extracellular α-synuclein fibrils in microglia → NLRP3 activation → increase IL-1β → promote α-synuclein aggregation → dopaminergic neuron loss	**Pathways:** NLRP3-ASC-Caspase-1, lysosomal damage by α-syn fibrils **Mediators:** Mature IL-1β, IL-18, ASC specks **Activators:** α-synuclein fibrils, mitochondrial ROS, dopamine	• Enhanced α-synuclein aggregation and spreading through IL-1β • Dopaminergic neuron death • Prion-like propagation facilitated by ASC specks • Motor decline	(Codolo et al., 2013; Gordon et al., 2018)
	Complement System	• C1q and C3 deposition on dopaminergic neurons → synapse loss • Microglial recruitment via C5a • Opsonization of damaged neurons	**Pathways:** Classical complement cascade, C3 activation **Mediators:** C1q, C3b, C5a, C4 **Targets:** Stressed dopaminergic neurons, synapses	• Modest synaptic pruning in striatum • Secondary rather than primary pathogenic role • C4 accelerated α-syn aggregation and synaptic loss	(Depboylu et al., 2011; Nimmo et al., 2024; Zou et al., 2025)

	Adaptive Immune T Cells ($CD4^+$/$CD8^+$)	• MHC-II expression on dopaminergic neurons → high infiltration of T-cells (CD4 and CD8) → T cell mediated cytotoxicity	**Pathways:** TCR recognition of α-synuclein epitopes, MHC-I/II presentation **Mediators:** IFN-γ, TNF-α, perforin/granzymes ($CD8^+$) **Targets:** α-synuclein peptides	• High T cells infiltrate substantia nigra in PD patients • Direct neuronal cytotoxicity by $CD8^+$ cells • Microglial activation via IFN-γ	(Brochard et al., 2009; Saunders et al., 2012; Sulzer et al., 2017)
	LRRK2-Expressing Immune Cells	• High expression in microglia/macrophages/DCs → Enhanced inflammatory responses in immune cells	**Pathways:** LRRK2 kinase activity, Rab GTPase phosphorylation, autophagy **Mediators:** Enhanced pro-inflammatory cytokines, altered phagocytosis **Mutations:** G2019S (most common), R1441 C/G	• Exaggerated microglial inflammatory responses to stimuli • Impaired autophagy-lysosomal pathway affecting α-synuclein clearance • Altered immune cell trafficking • Connection between familial and sporadic PD	(Cook et al., 2017; Moehle et al., 2012)
	Peripheral Monocytes/Macrophages	• Infiltrate brain under BBB breakdown conditions. • Classical monocytes ($CD14^+CD16^-$) show pro-inflammatory skewing.	**Pathways:** TLR signaling, cytokine production, CCR2-mediated migration **Mediators:** TNF-α, IL-1β, IL-6, IL-10 (dysregulated), MCP-1 **Subsets:** Classical ($CD14^+CD16^-$), intermediate, non-classical	• Systemic inflammation contribution to neuroinflammation • Potential CNS infiltration in late disease • Biomarker potential • Minimal direct pathogenic role in early disease	(Grozdanov et al., 2014; Nishimura et al., 2003; Yang et al., 2011)
Amyotrophic lateral sclerosis	Neurotoxic Microglia (M1-like)	• Phenotype shifts from neuroprotective (early) to neurotoxic (late) during disease progression. • In SOD1 models, activated by misfolded proteins (SOD1, TDP-43, C9orf72 DPRs) → surround degenerating motor neurons in spinal cord → produce inflammatory mediators.	**Pathways:** NF-κB, NADPH oxidase, iNOS activation, impaired TREM2 **Mediators:** TNF-α, IL-1β, IL-6, NO, superoxide, prostaglandin E2 **Phenotype shift:** M2–> M1 transition during progression	• Direct motor neuron toxicity through oxidative stress • Accelerated disease progression in symptomatic phase • Neuromuscular junction denervation, microglial-mediated motor neuron death • Failed neuroprotection	(Boillée et al., 2006; Liu & Wang, 2017; Philips & Robberecht, 2011)

Continued

Table 10.2 Disease-specific neuroimmune mechanisms in major neurological disorders.—cont'd

Diseases	Immune component	Specific mechanisms in disease	Key molecular players	Pathological outcomes	Reference
	Neurotoxic Astrocytes (A1-like)	• Release of unidentified soluble toxins → death of motor neuron • Loss of glutamate clearance capacity causes excitotoxicity.	**Pathways:** STAT3 activation, NF-κB, loss of EAAT2/GLT-1 **Mediators:** Unknown neurotoxins, NGF, D-serine (excess), inflammatory cytokines **Markers:** GFAP+, C3 +, reduced EAAT2	• Direct motor neuron killing through secreted toxins • Glutamate-mediated excitotoxicity • Cause toxicity to healthy astrocytes • Major contributor to disease progression	(Nagai et al., 2007; Re et al., 2014; Rothstein et al., 1995)
	NLRP3 Inflammasome	• Activated by misfolded SOD1 aggregates and TDP-43 in microglia and astrocytes → IL-1β levels elevated	**Pathways:** NLRP3-ASC-Caspase-1, pyroptosis **Mediators:** IL-1β, IL-18, HMGB1 **Activators:** SOD1 aggregates, TDP-43, C9orf72 DPRs	• Amplification of neuroinflammation through IL-1β • Motor neuron death acceleration, microglial pyroptosis spreading inflammation • Glial activation	(Johann et al., 2015; Meissner et al., 2010)
	Complement System	• Upregulated in ALS spinal cord. • Deposition of C1q and C3 on motor neurons and neuromuscular junctions. • Contribute to synapse elimination at early stages.	**Pathways:** Classical complement cascade, C5a-C5aR signaling **Mediators:** C1q, C3, C5a, MAC **Targets:** Motor neurons, neuromuscular junctions	• Neuromuscular junction dismantling • Motor neuron opsonization • Microglial recruitment • Denervation acceleration • Secondary rather than primary pathogenic role	(Heurich et al., 2011; Woodruff et al., 2003)
	$CD4^+$ T Cells (Tregs vs. Effector)	• Early Treg-mediated neuroprotection • Late effector T cell-mediated damage. • Treg dysfunction in ALS patients correlates with rapid progression.	**Pathways:** Early: IL-4/IL-10 signaling; Late: IFN-γ/TNF-α production Mediators: Protective: IL-4, IL-10; Toxic: IFN-γ, TNF-α Shift: Treg– > Th1 during progression	**Early:** • M2 microglial polarization • Neuroprotection, delayed onset **Late:** • M1 microglial activation • Accelerated motor neuron death • Rapid progression	(Beers et al., 2001, 2008; Chiu et al., 2008)

	$CD8^+$ Cytotoxic T Cells	• Infiltrate in areas of motor neuron loss. • Motor neurons highly express MHC-I in ALS, making them vulnerable to $CD8^+$ attack • Perforin-mediated cytotoxicity demonstrated in vitro.	**Pathways:** MHC-I recognition, perforin/granzyme pathway **Mediators:** Perforin, granzyme B, IFN-γ, FasL **Phenotype:** $CD8^+CD45$high, activated/cytotoxic	• Direct motor neuron cytotoxicity • Microglial M1 activation via IFN-γ • Axonal degeneration • Contribution to rapid disease progression	(Coque et al., 2019; Campisi et al., 2022; Engelhardt et al., 1993)
	Peripheral Myeloid Cells	• Altered inflammatory profiles • Classical monocytes ($CD14^+CD16^-$) elevated and hyperresponsive.	**Pathways:** TLR signaling, CCR2/CX3CR1-mediated migration **Mediators:** TNF-α, IL-1β, IL-6, MCP-1, chitinase-3-like-1 **Subsets:** Classical, intermediate, non-classical monocytes	• Systemic inflammation amplifying CNS inflammation • Potential CNS infiltration in late disease	(McCauley & Baloh, 2019)
	Mast Cells	• Accumulate in ALS patients' motor cortex and spinal cord. • Release tryptase and histamine. • Contribute to BBB breakdown.	**Pathways:** Degranulation, histamine/tryptase release **Mediators:** Histamin, tryptase, IL-6, TNF-α **Location:** Perivascular, parenchymal	• BBB permeability increase • Inflammatory mediator release, microglia/astrocyte activation • Modest contribution to progression	(Apolloni et al., 2017)

and immunological dysregulation in AD, PD, MS, and ALS. Understanding neuroinflammation stability helps prevent and treat neurological diseases.

2.1 Key immune pathways contributing to neurodegeneration

2.1.1 Microglial activation and polarization

Microglia are the immune cells of the CNS that frequently switch between resting and activated states in response to injury or disease (Muzio et al., 2021). Neuroinflammation, neurodegeneration, and tissue healing are all processes that need their activation and differentiation into pro (M1) - or anti (M2)-inflammatory phenotypes. This activation and differentiation are essential for all three processes. All of these are the key goals that should be accomplished through treatment for neurological disorders (Muzio et al., 2021; Zhang et al., 2019). Why does tissue healing require these qualities? Pathogen-associated molecular patterns (PAMPs), damage-associated molecular patterns (DAMPs), and misfolded proteins can change microglia phenotype (Colonna & Butovsky, 2017). Stimuli influence microglia. Although simplified, the traditional M1/M2 polarization model explains microglia's polarization functions. M1 microglia produce pro-inflammatory cytokines like tumor necrosis factor-alpha (TNF-α), interleukin-1beta (IL-1β), and interleukin-6 (IL-6), interleukin-12 (IL-12), and C-C motif chemokine ligand 2 (CCL2), as well as reactive oxygen species (ROS) and nitric oxide (NO) through inducible nitric oxide synthase (iNOS) (Colonna & Butovsky, 2017; Nguyen et al., 2017). These substances cause direct neuronal damage by inducing oxidative stress, disrupting mitochondrial function, and triggering apoptotic pathways. Conversely, M2 microglia release anti-inflammatory cytokines, including interleukin-10 (IL-10) and transforming growth factor beta (TGF-β) (Colonna & Butovsky, 2017). In addition, these also release pro-survival factors (induce mannose receptor (CD206), progranulin, and arginase 1 (Arg1)), growth factors (IGF-1: insulin-like growth factor-1, CSF-1: colony-stimulating factor-1, FGF: fibroblast growth factor, NGF: nerve-derived growth factor, GDNF: glial cell line-derived neurotrophic factor, neurotrophins, BDNF: brain-derived neurotrophic factor) (Colonna & Butovsky, 2017). The phagocytosis of cell debris and proteins that have been misfolded is considerably aided by these substances, which also contribute to the healing of tissue, aid in the restoration of the extracellular matrix, and protect neurons (Tang & Le, 2016). In addition, these chemicals help to protect neurons. In chronic neurodegenerative diseases, microglia frequently become dysfunctional, exhibiting persistent pro-inflammatory activity, reduced phagocytosis, and loss of normal functions (Hickman et al., 2018). Microglia also exhibit persistent pro-inflammatory activity. Microglia are also known to have chronic pro-inflammatory activity. Because they are in this "primed" state, microglia are able to react more forcefully to future stimuli. This leads to a cycle of inflammation that continues to replicate itself over and over again (Hickman et al., 2018).

Microglial activation is a crucial pathological feature in major neurodegenerative diseases, although the specific phenotypes and effects vary across disease contexts. For instance, extracellular α-synuclein is recognised by Toll-like receptors in the substantia nigra, leading to prolonged M1-like microglial activation. This activation leads to the release of pro-inflammatory cytokines and reactive oxygen species, which selectively damage dopaminergic neurons and ultimately contribute to the development of PD (Hirsch & Hunot, 2009). Microglia experience a series of states owing to Alzheimer's disease (AD), beginning with homeostatic surveillance and evolving into disease-associated microglia (DAM). This phase occurs along the progression of Alzheimer's disease. Initially, DAMs aim to reduce plaques; however, they ultimately do not eradicate amyloid-beta, leading to persistent neuroinflammation and synaptic loss in neurons (Keren-Shaul et al., 2017). Multiple sclerosis involves activated microglia that present myelin antigens to T cells and phagocytose myelin debris, thereby promoting autoimmune demyelination is marked by the presentation of myelin antigens and the phagocytosis of myelin debris (Lassmann et al., 2012). This interaction ultimately results in demyelination. Microglia change from a protective M2-like phenotype to a deleterious M1-like phenotype during the course of ALS. This metamorphosis transpires from the commencement of the disease until its conclusion. A mutation in the enzyme superoxide dismutase-1 (SOD1), found in microglia, accelerates the degeneration of motor neurons (Boillée et al., 2006). This phenotypic diversity indicates that microglial responses vary by context, with initial protection often transitioning into chronic inflammation that exacerbates neurodegeneration across disorders.

2.1.2 Astrocyte reactivity and A1/A2 paradigm

Astrocytes, the most common glial cells in the CNS, change their phenotype after neurological injury (Miller, 2018). The A1/A2 paradigm, introduced by Liddelow and colleagues, clarifies astrocyte roles, similar to the polarization of microglial M1/M2 (Liddelow & Barres, 2017; Liddelow et al., 2017). A1 astrocytes are neurotoxic, while A2 astrocytes promote neuroprotection and repair (Liddelow & Barres, 2017; Liddelow et al., 2017). Nonetheless, this perspective simplifies a complex, context-dependent spectrum. A1 neurotoxic astrocytes are activated by a specific cytokine combination released from microglia: TNF-α, IL-1α, and C1q (Liddelow et al., 2017). This signal, which is composed of three components, is responsible for activating the NF-κB and JAK-STAT3 pathways. These pathways launch transcriptional programs that strengthen specific components of the complement cascade, such as C3, while concurrently lowering activities that are advantageous to neurons and synapses (Liddelow et al., 2017). The levels of neuroprotective factors such as PK2 (prokineticin-2), chitinase-like 3, Frizzled 1, arginase 1, Nrf2 (NF-E2-related factor 2), pentraxin 3, and sphingosine kinase one are increased when A2 astrocytes are present (Ding et al., 2021). These factors support synaptic repair, neuronal growth, and neuronal survival (Ding et al., 2021). These things assist neurons in growing, repairing synapses, and maintaining their viability. A number of chemokines, including CCL2, CCL20, CXCL10, and CXCL12, are produced by astrocytes (Correale & Farez, 2015). These chemokines attract immune cells to the site of inflammation, which in turn makes the inflammation worse. A number of different functions are served by the A1/A2 paradigm, and the way in which it is associated with neurological problems varies from case to case (Fan & Huo, 2021).

2.1.3 Inflammasome activation

Inflammasomes are complex, multiprotein structures that primarily regulate the activation of caspase-1. Caspase-1 then promotes the processing of IL-1β and IL-18, as well as gasdermin D (GSDMD), into their active forms. The active GSDMD triggers pyroptosis—a rapid, damaging form of inflammatory cell death (Rathinam & Fitzgerald, 2016; Paerewijck and Lamkanfi, 2022). The diversity of cell-encoded pattern-recognition receptors, such as NOD-like receptors (NLRs: NLRP1, NLRP3, NLRC4), AIM2, AIM2-like receptors (ALRs), and interferon gamma-inducible protein 16 (IFI16), contributes to the formation of different types of inflammasomes (Dubey et al., 2025). Recent studies have predominantly focused on and indicated that damage-associated molecular patterns (DAMPs) signals trigger the NLRP3 inflammasome in the CNS, causing neuroinflammation that worsens neuronal damage and functional impairments, eventually contributing to the progression of neurological disorders (Holbrook et al., 2021; Xu et al., 2025). In neuroinflammation, the buildup of misfolded proteins (e.g., α-synuclein, β-amyloid, and TDP-43: Transactive response DNA binding protein 43), modified and mutated proteins (e.g., hyperphosphorylated tau protein, huntingtin protein (HTT), and mutated HTT, mutated SOD1), autoimmune-mediated injury, and traumatic brain injury act as DAMPs, triggering the formation of inflammasomes. IL-1β and IL-18 released via inflammasome activation led to chronic neuroinflammation and eventually neurodegeneration (Holbrook et al., 2021).

2.1.4 Complement cascade

The complement system is a fundamental and well-regulated component of the innate immune response that recognizes danger and distinguishes self from non-self (Ricklin et al., 2010). The complement system comprises more than 30 soluble and cell-associated components, which are activated via three separate pathways (i.e., classical, alternative, and lectin), each initiated by distinct agents (Ricklin et al., 2010). While primarily known for defending against pathogens, it also significantly contributes to the development and proper functioning of the central nervous system (CNS) (Veerhuis et al., 2011). Nearly all complement components are produced locally in the brain by various cell types (primarily astrocyte and microglial), with their levels rising with age and in neurodegenerative diseases in both humans and mice (Veerhuis et al., 2011; Lee et al., 2019; Fatoba et al., 2022). Some complement components are pattern recognition receptors (PRRs) that detect microbes, damaged self-components such as apoptotic cells or debris, and misfolded proteins, thereby activating the complement system (Bohlson & Tenner, 2023). For example, in AD, β-amyloid and neurofibrillary tangles can activate the classical complement system protein C1 (Shen et al., 2001; Velazquez et al., 1997). In older people, the upregulation of C1q and C3 has been shown to impair cognitive function (i.e., forgetting) via a complement-dependent synapse elimination process (Wang, Yue, et al., 2020). Compiling evidence suggests that complement activation-driven neuroinflammation is a key factor in neurodegeneration across various neurological disorders (Fatoba et al., 2022).

2.1.5 Peripheral immune cell infiltration

The Blood-Brain Barrier (BBB) controls the exchange of molecules and cells between the blood and the central nervous system. Chronic neuroinflammation damages the BBB by decreasing tight junction proteins through cytokines, breaking down the basement membrane with MMPs, and harming endothelial cells with reactive oxygen species (Sweeney et al., 2018). BBB breakdown allows immune cells from the periphery and plasma proteins to cross, which hampers toxin clearance and worsens neurodegeneration (Sweeney et al., 2018). In most neurological disorders, the local cytokine environment attracts and activates $CD4^{+}$ T helper cells, causing them to differentiate into pro-inflammatory (Th1, Th17) or regulatory (Treg) subsets (Kipnis, 2016). Later, depending on local signals, Th1 cells release IFN-γ, which encourages microglial M1 polarization. In contrast, Th17 cells produce IL-17, which attracts neutrophils and disrupts the BBB (Kipnis, 2016). For instance, the dysfunction in the BBB allows the infiltration of, thereby allowing peripheral immune cells, especially $CD8^{+}$ T cells, to enter the CNS, thereby deteriorating neuroinflammation and accelerating AD progression (van Olst et al., 2022).

3. RNAi as a therapeutic strategy for neuroimmune regulation

RNAi techniques regulate gene expression in disease therapies and are currently in clinical trials for conditions such as age-related macular degeneration, diabetic macular edema, tumors, and leukemia (Corydon et al., 2023). RNAi offers a sophisticated way to modulate neuroinflammatory pathways by targeting specific immune signaling molecules (Ramachandran et al., 2013). RNAi therapy is particularly effective for diseases caused by genes with a toxic 'gain of function' effect. Identifying these disease-causing genes has enabled researchers to develop RNAi molecules that target the harmful allele, demonstrating their therapeutic potential (Stevenson, 2004). In many neurodegenerative diseases, harmful proteins such as α-synuclein, β-amyloid, TDP-43, hyperphosphorylated tau, HTT, mutated HTT, and mutated SOD1 are believed to be toxic to nerve cells. They induce neuroinflammation and trigger the release of various pro-inflammatory cytokines (TNF-α, IL-1β, IL-6, IL-12, IL-23, CCL2, CCL5, CXCL10, iNOS) within the local central nervous system, eventually signaling peripheral inflammatory cells to cross the disrupted blood-brain barrier (see section 02). Therefore, gene silencing to prevent the accumulation of these toxic proteins and inflammatory mediators presents a promising therapeutic approach. Additionally, cell-specific targeting and silencing of dysregulated miRNA expression (such as miR-155, which acts as a pro-inflammatory miRNA, miR-124, which acts as a protective miRNA against neuroinflammation) could be achieved through an RNAi strategy (Stevenson, 2004; Kurowska-Stolarska et al., 2011; Zhang, Jiang, et al., 2023; Thome et al., 2016).

3.1 Cellular target of RNAi in the neuroimmune axis

The neuroimmune axis is a bidirectional communication link that transmits signals between the nervous and immune systems. It's very important for inflammatory regulation and cellular homeostasis (Homo-Delarche & Dardenne, 1993). This two-way crosstalk is made possible by a common chemical language. Sensory neurons directly detect pathogens or tissue damage and release neuropeptides (like Substance CGRP) to quickly alert immune cells. Immune-derived cytokines then act on neural receptors to initiate reflexes or "sickness behaviors". The vagus nerve is one of the most important pathways because it sends an "anti-inflammatory reflex" to calm systemic inflammation. The HPA (hypothalamic-pituitary-adrenal) -axis is another important pathway (Chavan et al., 2017). The primary cellular targets of RNAi in the neuroimmune axis are microglial cells, other glial cells, and neurons. All these cells are part of the CNS and are called resident immune cells of the central nervous system. RNAi can silence mRNA in different types of cells. In microglial cells, it targets the cGAS-STING signaling pathway, resulting in reduced secretion of TNF-α and IL-1β, pro-inflammatory signals that help trigger inflammatory cascades (Boudreau et al., 2011). In astrocytes, RNAi is used to silence ApoE (Apolipoprotein E), a key protein involved in cholesterol transport. By blocking this protein, RNAi can help reduce the accumulation of lipid toxins and amyloid-beta plaques in patients with Alzheimer's disease. Similarly, targeting and silencing GFAP (Glial Fibrillary Acidic Protein) can reduce glial scars (Matejuk & Ransohoff, 2020). In neurons, RNAi is used to target toxic proteins, such as in Huntington's disease, where it is employed to silence the mutant Huntingtin (mHTT) gene, reducing toxic protein aggregation and preventing neuronal death (Pfister et al., 2009). RNAi is also used to target the BACE1 enzyme, which is involved in early Alzheimer's disease. Silencing this enzyme stops the supply of raw material required for the formation of amyloid-beta plaques (Boudreau et al., 2011).

3.2 RNAi-based regulation of neuroinflammation

Neuroinflammation is a major contributor to many neurological and neurodegenerative diseases. This occurs when resident glial cells, such as microglia and astrocytes, are persistently activated and produce nitrogen and reactive oxygen species, as well as toxic molecules, leading to the slow, progressive death of neurons. Small interfering RNA (siRNA) and short hairpin RNA (shRNA) are two RNAi-based treatment methods that help silence very specific genes (post-transcriptional) and contribute to controlling inflammatory cascades. Experimental models suggest that selective blocking of inflammasome components, chemokines, and cytokines reduces the number of pro-inflammatory microglia and limits neuronal damage caused by oxidative stress. RNAi also has direct anti-inflammatory effects, including inhibiting apoptosis, restoring redox balance, and enhancing mitochondrial function. These reverse gene-regulatory effects help preserve the nervous system. These features of RNAi give it an advantage over genome editing methods. New delivery technologies, such as extracellular vesicle–mediated transport, viral vectors, polymer-based carriers, and lipid nanoparticles, stabilize RNAi and enable its delivery to specific target areas (Di Francesco et al., 2024; Lin et al., 2020).

3.3 RNAi strategies in neuroimmune-mediated disorders

RNA interference (RNAi)–based therapeutics are attracting significant attention as precise molecular tools for regulating gene expression in neuro-immune-mediated disorders, which are characterized by dysregulated interactions between the nervous and immune systems that drive chronic inflammation and progressive neurodegeneration. RNAi methods, including small interfering RNA (siRNA), short hairpin RNA (shRNA), and microRNA (miRNA) inhibitors or mimics, can selectively silence pathogenic transcripts involved in neuronal toxicity, antigen presentation, and inflammatory signaling (Fire et al., 1998). Experimental studies indicate that inhibiting pro-inflammatory mediators, including TNF-α, IL-1β, NLRP3 inflammasome components, and transcription factors within the NF-κB and JAK/STAT pathways, markedly reduces microglial activation, leukocyte infiltration, and cytokine amplification in models of multiple sclerosis, Alzheimer's disease, Parkinson's disease, and other neuro-immune disorders (Davidson & McCray, 2011; Bhati et al., 2025). Additionally, RNAi targeting genes linked to neurodegeneration, such as BACE1 in amyloid pathology and α-synuclein in synucleinopathies, has been shown to reduce protein aggregation, oxidative stress, and synaptic dysfunction, thereby improving behavioral and cognitive outcomes in preclinical models (Singer et al., 2005; McCormack et al., 2010; Kanasty et al., 2013).

RNAi has promising therapeutic effects, but it remains challenging to use in clinical neurology because it doesn't cross the blood-brain barrier well, degrades quickly, stimulates the immune system, and can silence unintended targets (Kanasty et al., 2013; Saraiva et al., 2016). Recent advances in chemically modified oligonucleotides, lipid and polymeric nanoparticle carriers, viral vectors, and ligand-directed delivery systems have made RNA much more stable, tissue-specific, and capable of sustained gene knockdown in neural tissues. This gives us new hope for RNAi-based precision medicine for neuro-immune disorders (Deverman et al., 2018; Kanasty et al., 2013; Saraiva et al.,

2016). To translate these molecular approaches into therapies that alter disease, we need continued research on long-term safety, dosing longevity, and extensive clinical validation.

4. Preclinical and clinical advances

A study published in Advanced Materials in 2023 showed that lipid nanoparticles (MG-LNPs) carrying siRNA against PU.1 (SPI1) were able to lower neuroinflammation in mice. We were able to strongly knock down PU.1, a transcription factor that activates microglia, by selectively silencing it with MG-LNPs delivered directly into the cell (Ralvenius et al., 2024). In both LPS-induced and CK-p25 transgenic models, the suppression of PU.1 resulted in diminished expression of inflammatory genes (Il1b, Ccl2), decreased activation of microglia and astrocytes (Iba1, GFAP, C1q), and enhanced neuropathological outcomes. Systemic administration resulted in negligible central nervous system effects, underscoring the significance of localized delivery. The treatment exhibited minimal peripheral toxicity and maintained microglial viability. These findings demonstrate that microglia-targeted RNA interference is an efficacious approach to regulate neuroinflammation in vivo. However, for translation to humans, delivery methods that are less invasive and long-term safety testing are needed. These findings give a solid platform upon which to establish the development of RNA-based pharmaceuticals that target microglial transcriptional regulators for the treatment of neurodegenerative and inflammatory brain disorders (Ralvenius et al., 2024). The research explores the decreased clearance of amyloid-β (Aβ) throughout the progression of Alzheimer's disease (AD) by concentrating on microglia that have aged, which have a diminished capacity for phagocytosis. Through the usage of transcriptome analysis, the researchers made the discovery that the amount of the cell-cycle inhibitor CDKN2A, which encodes p16INK4a, is greatly enhanced in microglia that are obtained from elderly mice. Furthermore, it was discovered by the scientists that microglia located in close proximity to Aβ plaques exhibited a noticeably elevated level of expression in both human brains affected by Alzheimer's disease and the 5XFAD animal model.

Subsequently, they employed poly (D, L-lactic-co-glycolic acid) (PLGA) nanoparticles encapsulated with p16INK4a-siRNA to achieve targeted knockdown in microglia. In vitro, siRNA diminished p16INK4a expression and augmented Aβ uptake by microglia. In 5XFAD mice, weekly intracisternal injections of nanoparticles over 8 weeks resulted in decreased p16INK4a levels, approximately a 2-fold reduction in Aβ1-42, diminished plaque burden, a reduction in senescent (SA-β-gal ^+) microglia, an increase in Ki67+ proliferative microglia, and enhanced cognitive performance in Barnes and radial-maze assessments (Shin et al., 2024).

This study concludes that re-engaging the microglial cell cycle through p16INK4a knockdown revitalizes microglia, thereby restoring phagocytic and lysosomal function, presenting a promising strategy for microglia-targeted therapy in Alzheimer's disease. They say that there are still problems with translation (delivery route, long-term safety, and microglial homeostasis) (Shin et al., 2024).

In this study, the authors engineered an AAV (peptide-modified AAV9) to deliver microRNA-based RNAi targeting ATXN2 (ataxin-2) across the CNS at doses approximately 40-fold lower than previous research. In the aggressive TAR4/4 mouse model of sporadic Amyotrophic Lateral Sclerosis (ALS) characterized by TDP-43 pathology, treatment resulted in a 45%–54% increase in survival, a 24%–75% enhancement in motor strength, the preservation of lower motor neurons, a reduction in phosphorylated TDP-43 aggregates, and a mitigation of neuroinflammation across the brain and spinal cord. Transcriptomic profiling indicated the normalization of approximately 150 dysregulated genes associated with human ALS signatures. The authors also showed that their method worked well on lower motor neurons taken from human patients and that it was very effective at knocking down ATXN2. The study endorses ATXN2-targeted RNAi via AAV as a viable translational approach for TDP-43-mediated neurodegeneration; however, additional research on timing, dosing, and safety is required (Amado et al., 2025).

Cytoskeletal remodeling proteins, including LIM-domain–containing scaffolds such as Pdlim5, play a crucial role in maintaining dendritic architecture under inflammatory stress. Our recent work elucidated the role of Pdlim5's PDZ, DUF, and LIM domains in dendrite branching and neuronal morphology, suggesting that structural regulators may interface with neuroimmune signaling pathways (Srivastava, Donta, Mireles, Paulucci-Holthauzen, Shi, et al., 2024). The molecular dissection of domain-specific functions in neuronal scaffold proteins, such as Pdlim5, provides new RNAi targets to restore dendritic stability in neurodegenerative conditions (Srivastava, Donta, Mireles, Paulucci-Holthauzen, Waxham, et al., 2024). The integration of structural and transcriptomic insights may enable precise RNA-based modulation of these synaptic regulators. All the RNAi Targets preclinical studies of Neurological disorders are summarized in Table 10.3.

The research examines the role of the E3 ubiquitin ligase DTX1 in modulating microglial polarization and neuroinflammation within a rat model of traumatic brain injury (TBI) and in LPS-stimulated microglial cultures. There was a big increase in DTX1 expression in both microglia after an LPS challenge and in the brains of rats 3 days after a TBI. Overexpression of DTX1 in cultured microglia augmented the release of proinflammatory cytokines (IL-6, TNF-α), elevated the M1 phenotype marker iNOS, and diminished the M2 marker Arg1; silencing DTX1 negated these effects. Mechanistically, DTX1 activated the NF-κB signaling pathway, as demonstrated by the increased phosphorylation of IκBα and p65, and enhanced the expression of IRF5, a critical regulator of M1 polarization; the inhibition of NF-κB with MG-132 negated these effects. In vivo, rats with DTX1 overexpression after TBI showed worse motor and cognitive problems (in the rotarod and water-maze tests), higher levels of microglial M1 markers, and higher levels of proinflammatory cytokines. On the other hand, knocking down DTX1 improved outcomes. The authors assert that DTX1 Ind.uces maladaptive microglial activation through the NF-κB/IRF5 pathway and serves as a prospective therapeutic target for regulating neuroinflammation following traumatic brain injury (TBI). They point out some problems, such as the fact that the study only looked at the acute injury phase, used non-transgenic models, and needed data on long-term outcomes (Zhang, Zou, et al., 2025).

5. Challenges and future directions

5.1 Overcoming the blood–brain barrier

The blood–brain barrier (BBB) remains a significant obstacle when delivering RNAi drugs to the central nervous system (CNS). This highly selective endothelial barrier prevents macromolecules like siRNA and nanoparticles from entering, thereby limiting the potential for treating neuroinflammatory and neurodegenerative conditions. However, several emerging ideas are being developed to enhance CNS delivery (Fig. 10.3).

Delivery systems based on nanoparticles are making quick progress. Ligand-decorated lipid nanoparticles (LNPs) employing transferrin, angiopep-2, or RVG peptides utilize receptor-mediated

Table 10.3 Promising RNAi targets in neurological disorders - preclinical studies.

Disease	Target	RNAi approach	Animal model/cell line	Key findings	References
Alzheimer's disease	BACE1	lentiviral-shRNA	APP transgenic mice	↓ Aβ plaques, improved cognition, restored synaptic function	(Singer et al., 2005)
	PS1	-	IMR32 cells	↓ Aβ42 production	(Kandimalla et al., 2012)
	Tau and APP	shRNA & siRNA	Cos-7 and HeLa cells	Allele-specific silencing of mutant Tau and APP	(Miller et al., 2004)
	APP	siRNA (nanoparticles)	5xFAD mice	↓ Aβ production, reduced glial inflammation	(Dominique et al., 2025)
	TNFR1	deletion	APP23 transgenic mice (APP23/TNFR1$^{-/-}$)	↓ Aβ production, ↓ Aβ plaque formation, reduced β-secretase 1 (BACE1) levels and activity	(He et al., 2007)
	CDK-5	shRNA (Lentiviral)	3×Tg-AD mice	↓ Neurofibrillary tangles	(Piedrahita et al., 2010)
	Tau kinases (GSK-3β)	siRNA	Tau.P301S AD mice	↓ Tau hyperphosphorylation, preserved neurons	(Zhang, Hou, et al., 2023)
Multiple sclerosis	IL-17	shRNA (lentiviral)	EAE mice	↓ Th17 infiltration, improved motor function	(Yan et al., 2012)
	MCP-1	-	MCP-1 deficient mice	↓ IFNγ in draining lymph node and CNS, ↑ antigen-specific IgG1 production	(Nishimura et al., 2003)
	TRIF	siRNA	EAE mice	↓ Severity of EAE, ↓ IFN-γ and IL-2 levels	(Wang et al., 2015)
	miR-150	miRNA	EAE mice	↓ Inflammatory demyelination and axonal damage ↑$CD3^+$, $CD4^+$, and $CD8^+$ T cells ↓ $CD19^+$ B cells ↓ IL-1β, IL-6, IL-17, and TNF-α	(Hu et al., 2018)
	miR-124	miRNA	EAE mice	Enhanced remyelination, ↓ microglial activation, ↓ activation of myelin-specific T cells	(Ponomarev et al., 2011)

Continued

Table 10.3 Promising RNAi targets in neurological disorders - preclinical studies.—cont'd

Disease	Target	RNAi approach	Animal model/cell line	Key findings	References
Parkinson's disease	α-synuclein	siRNA (nanoparticle)	Thy1-aSyn mice	↓ α-synuclein expression	(Feja et al., 2025)
	α-synuclein	shRNA	rotenone model of PD	Prevented neurodegeneration	(Zharikov et al., 2015)
	LRRK2	siRNA	$LRRK2^{R1441G}$ mice	↓Neuroinflammation, prevent dopaminergic neuron loss,	(Zhang, Chen, et al., 2025)
	NLRP3	siRNA	MPTP mice	↓ Inflammasome activation, neuroprotection	(Meng et al., 2014)
	miR-124-3p	miRNA	Male Wistar rats	↓ Aggregation of α-synuclein in the substantia nigra, ↓ ROS	(Esteves et al., 2024)
	miR-155	miRNA	miR-$155^{-/-}$ mice	↓ Proinflammatory responses to α-synuclein, protect against dopaminergic neuron loss	(Thome et al., 2016)
	miR-7	adeno-associated virus 1 (AAV-miR-7)	C57BL/6 J mice	Inhibits the formation and propagation of pathological α-synuclein, protects against neurodegeneration induced by preformed fibrils	(Zhang et al., 2021)
Amyotrophic lateral sclerosis	SOD1	shRNA	SOD1-G93A mice	Extended survival, delayed onset, preserved motor neurons	(Ralph et al., 2005; Raoul et al., 2005)
	C9orf72	ASO (RNAi-like)	C9-BAC mice	↓ RNA foci, reduced DPR proteins, improved survival	(Lagier-Tourenne et al., 2013)
	IL-1α, TNFα, and C1q	siRNA	SOD1-G93A mice	↓ Astrocyte neurotoxicity, motor neuron protection	(Guttenplan et al., 2020; Liddelow et al., 2017)

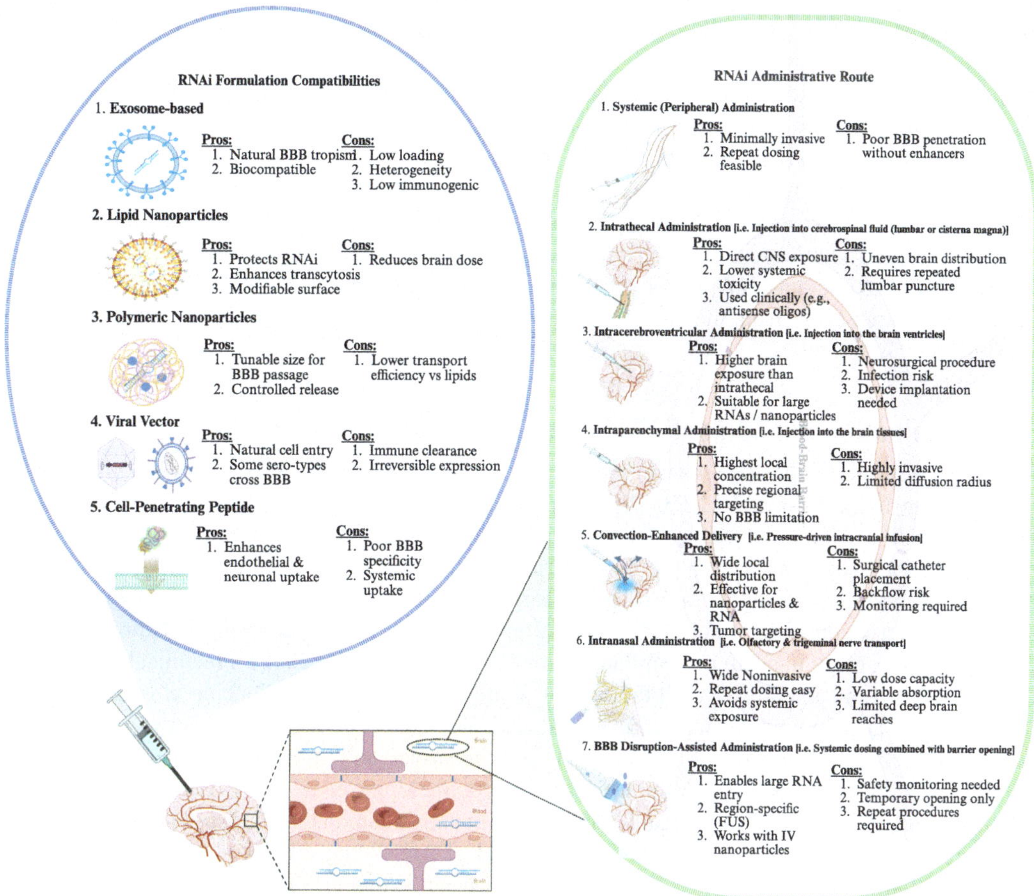

FIGURE 10.3 Strategies for Delivering CNS RNAi to Overcome the Challenge of Crossing the BBB.

Summaries of key RNAi formulations and administration routes used to overcome the blood-brain barrier (BBB) in central nervous system (CNS) RNAi therapeutics.

Created with BioRender.

transcytosis to penetrate the blood-brain barrier (BBB) and specifically target microglia (Habib & Singh, 2022; Johnsen et al., 2017; Rhea & Banks, 2021; Wang et al., 2021). Exosomes from cells and biomimetic membranes facilitate the passage of drugs through the BBB and enhance their interaction with the immune system (Wang et al., 2022). Localized administration routes, including intrathecal or intracisternal injection, circumvent systemic barriers and have shown effective siRNA delivery to microglia, resulting in reduced neuroinflammation in vivo (Ralvenius et al., 2024).

Adeno-associated viral (AAV) vectors are still a strong option because they enable long-lasting gene regulation. Engineered serotypes like AAV-PHP.eB and newer BBB-penetrant capsids show enhanced CNS targeting and microglial transduction (Goertsen et al., 2022; B.E. Deverman et al., 2016). Although safety and immune response are significant concerns, advances are progressing toward clinical application.

Focused ultrasound (FUS) combined with microbubbles is an emerging technique to temporarily open the BBB without surgery. FUS allows targeted delivery of siRNA and antisense oligonucleotides while maintaining vascular integrity, demonstrating neuroprotective effects in preclinical models (Gosselet et al., 2021; Ogawa et al., 2022; Kovacs et al., 2018). Although each approach has potential, challenges such as systemic toxicity, variable efficiency of blood-brain barrier transport, and manufacturing difficulties remain. Multimodal platforms that integrate engineered nanoparticles, viral vectors, real-time imaging, and precision targeting peptides are likely to be vital for future success. To bring RNAi-based drugs from the lab to clinical use, ongoing development of innovative ideas across various fields is essential.

5.2 Combination therapies: RNAi + anti-inflammatory approaches

Of these, RNA interference (RNAi) can specifically inhibit the expression of DAMPs and regulators of inflammation (e.g., NF-kB, NLRP3, PU.1). At the same time, pharmacological anti-inflammatory agents provide a wide range of immunomodulation and symptomatic improvement. Because of the numerous factors that can trigger the development of neuroinflammation, the combination of RNA interference with anti-inflammatory drugs appears promising. siRNA, in combination with corticosteroids, has also improved outcomes in animal models of brain trauma, thereby demonstrating its potential applicability in acute neuroinflammation (Fukuda & Badaut, 2013). Preclinical studies have also highlighted the potential of dual therapeutic strategies: for example, silencing of NLRP3 or TNF together with acetaminophen or ibuprofen reduced the release of inflammatory cytokines, MSH-activated microglial activation and neuronal loss in stroke and in mouse models of dementia (Franke et al., 2021; Gong et al., 2018; Lim et al., 2000; McAlpine et al., 2009; Tripathy & Grammas, 2009); silencing of TREM2 or C1q and combined with anti-inflammatory therapy improved synaptic degeneration and learning ability in the mouse model of AD (Wang, Lin, et al., 2020; Zhong et al., 2023); Similarly, siRNA and corticosteroids improved outcomes in traumatic brain injury models, indicating potential translatability to acute neuroinflammation (Jin et al., 2025; Taylor & Kokiko-Cochran, 2024).

Eventually, combination strategies may overcome the limitations of monotherapy, namely, incomplete modulation of transcription and compensatory inflammatory pathways (Esteruelas et al., 2023; Yi et al., 2020). Nanocarriers, such as emulsion-loaded nanoparticles (e.g., inflammatory and steroidal, or inflammatory and inflammatory-related drugs) or hydrogel depots, would facilitate the targeted and prolonged delivery of therapeutic agents while reducing the risks of systemic toxicity (Cong et al., 2024; Espinosa-Cano et al., 2020; Nunes et al., 2022; Soni et al., 2022)

Future trials in the clinical setting will no doubt explore the combination of rRNAi cocktails with other biological therapies or modulators of astrocytes or microglia. However, for successful clinical application, it will be important to carefully optimize the dosage, delivery kinetics, and safety profile, because excessive suppression of the immune system may be detrimental to the healing process.

5.3 Future direction: personalized & epigenetic RNAi therapies

Advances in genomic and transcriptional profiling enable the identification of individual patient-specific pro-inflammatory signatures and the development of tailored siRNA/miRNA therapeutics that target specific molecular pathways. As neuroinflammatory diseases exhibit various genetic drivers and inflammatory profiles, the future of RNAi therapy is heading toward the emerging field of precision medicine (Brentari et al., 2023; Nuzziello et al., 2020).

AI-guided RNA sequence design now accelerates the selection of optimal targets, reducing off-target risks and increasing potency. Using RNAi, we can now modulate neuro-immunological phenotypes, such as patient-related microglial polarization states, cytokine expression networks, and autophagy-inflammation cross-talk (Xiao et al., 2021; Liu et al., 2014).

siRNA combined with epigenetic editing by CRISPR-dCas9 hybrids has proven to be reversible and programmable, with effects lasting longer than previously believed in neurodegenerative models (Bhattacharjee et al., 2023; Park et al., 2022). Epigenetic modulation is also gaining increasing attention. RNA interference targeting HDAC, DNMT, or BET in microglia alters their epigenetic memory, suppressing the expression of the inflammatory cascade for an extended period (Chowdhury et al., 2025; Meleady et al., 2023; Tan et al., 2022).

These innovations align with the ongoing precision trials in ALS and Huntington's disease, utilizing antisense RNA modalities. Furthermore, the integration of biomarker-guided dosing, liquid biopsy-based immune monitoring, and dynamic RNA sequence refinement could enable highly personalized neuro-therapeutic regimens.

In short, personalized and epigenetic targeting will be crucial for the next generation of RNA-based neuro-therapeutics. Major challenges include scaling up manufacturing, real-time diagnostics, and ensuring equitable access to customized RNA treatments.

6. Conclusion

Interfering with RNA is a strong and precise method that can stop the immune system in the brain from working too hard. RNA interference makes this possible. Using RNA interference is one way to do this. RNA interference (RNAi) may safeguard neurons from damage and maintain immune system equilibrium by inhibiting genes that induce microglial activation, astrocytic inflammation, and inflammasome signaling. This is because RNAi stops genes from working. This is because RNA interference can turn off genes that control specific activities. Recent advancements in nanoparticle carriers, viral vectors, and localized delivery have significantly advanced clinical translation. This is the progress that has been accomplished. There are still challenges that need to be fixed, like getting beyond the blood-brain barrier, side effects, and long-term stability. The fact that these things have been done even though there are still problems that need to be fixed, shows that there are still problems that need to be fixed. When used simultaneously, RNA interference (RNAi) could make anti-inflammatory drugs perform a lot better. This is because RNAi affects many inflammatory pathways in the body at the same time. This occurs because RNAi attacks all of them at once. To reach this goal, it's important to go after several different paths at the same time. It is worth noting that gene therapy enables durable neuroprotective gene delivery through Adeno-associated virus (AAV) vectors; however, it also entails risks of vector-induced neuroinflammation owing to capsid immunogenicity (B. E. Deverman et al., 2016). RNA interference (RNAi) offers reversible, sequence-specific silencing of neuroinflammatory mediators such as TNF-α, NLRP3, and miR-155, thereby decreasing the immunogenic burden (Setten et al., 2019). Specifically, for microglial targeting, RNAi is delivered via functionalized nanocarriers, which surpass the limitations associated with AAV's glial tropism (Ransohoff & Brown, 2012; O'Carroll et al., 2021). In addition, personalized treatments should be available soon since RNA interference technology can be customized for each patient's specific genetic and inflammatory characteristics. There is a chance that this might happen. This could happen, but it's not impossible. As RNAi-based therapy moves from the lab to the clinic, it is important to keep working on delivery systems and safety investigations. This change will happen soon. This will lead to novel ways to treat disorders that affect the brain and produce neurodegeneration or neuroinflammation. These problems are bad for the neurological system.

References

Adamu, A., Li, S., Gao, F., & Xue, G. (2024). The role of neuroinflammation in neurodegenerative diseases: Current understanding and future therapeutic targets. *Frontiers in Aging Neuroscience, 16*. https://doi.org/10.3389/fnagi.2024.1347987

Almeida, R., & Allshire, R. C. (2005). RNA silencing and genome regulation. *Trends in Cell Biology, 15*(5), 251–258. https://doi.org/10.1016/j.tcb.2005.03.006

Amado, D. A., Robbins, A. B., Whiteman, K. R., Smith, A. R., Chillon, G., Chen, Y., Fuller, J. A., Patty, N. A., Izda, A., Cheng, C., Nelson, S., Dichter, A. I., Mazzoni, E. O., Monteys, A. M., & Davidson, B. L. (2025). AAV-based delivery of RNAi targeting ataxin-2 improves survival and pathology in TDP-43 mice. *Nature Communications, 16*(1). https://doi.org/10.1038/s41467-025-60497-8

Apolloni, S., Fabbrizio, P., Amadio, S., Napoli, G., Verdile, V., Morello, G., Iemmolo, R., Aronica, E., Cavallaro, S., & Volonté, C. (2017). Histamine regulates the inflammatory profile of SOD1-G93A microglia and the histaminergic system is dysregulated in amyotrophic lateral sclerosis. *Frontiers in Immunology, 8*. https://doi.org/10.3389/fimmu.2017.01689

Aries, M. L., & Hensley-McBain, T. (2023). Neutrophils as a potential therapeutic target in Alzheimer's disease. *Frontiers in Immunology, 14*. https://doi.org/10.3389/fimmu.2023.1123149

Attfield, K. E., Jensen, L. T., Kaufmann, M., Friese, M. A., & Fugger, L. (2022). The immunology of multiple sclerosis. *Nature Reviews Immunology, 22*(12), 734–750. https://doi.org/10.1038/s41577-022-00718-z

Barcia, C., Ros, C. M., Annese, V., Gómez, A., Ros-Bernal, F., Aguado-Llera, D., Martínez-Pagán, M. E., de Pablos, V., Fernandez-Villalba, E., & Herrero, M. T. (2011). IFN-γ signaling, with the synergistic contribution of TNF-α, mediates cell specific microglial and astroglial activation in experimental models of Parkinson's disease. *Cell Death & Disease, 2*(4), e142. https://doi.org/10.1038/cddis.2011.17

Bartoszewski, R., & Sikorski, A. F. (2019). Editorial focus: Understanding off-target effects as the key to successful RNAi therapy. *Cellular and Molecular Biology Letters, 24*(1). https://doi.org/10.1186/s11658-019-0196-3

Baruch, K., Ron-Harel, N., Gal, H., Deczkowska, A., Shifrut, E., Ndifon, W., Mirlas-Neisberg, N., Cardon, M., Vaknin, I., Cahalon, L., Berkutzki, T., Mattson, M. P., Gomez-Pinilla, F., Friedman, N., & Schwartz, M. (2013). CNS-specific immunity at the choroid plexus shifts toward destructive Th2 inflammation in brain aging. *Proceedings of the National Academy of Sciences, 110*(6), 2264–2269. https://doi.org/10.1073/pnas.1211270110

Beers, D. R., Henkel, J. S., Zhao, W., Wang, J., & Appel, S. H. (2008). CD4+ T cells support glial neuroprotection, slow disease progression, and modify glial morphology in an animal model of inherited ALS. *Proceedings of the National Academy of Sciences, 105*(40), 15558–15563. https://doi.org/10.1073/pnas.0807419105

Beers, D. R., Ho, B. K., Siklós, L., Alexianu, M. E., Mosier, D. R., Habib Mohamed, A., Otsuka, Y., Kozovska, M. E., McAlhany, R. E., Glenn Smith, R., & Appel, S. H. (2001). Parvalbumin overexpression alters immune-mediated increases in intracellular calcium, and delays disease onset in a transgenic model of familial amyotrophic lateral sclerosis. *Journal of Neurochemistry, 79*(3), 499–509. https://doi.org/10.1046/j.1471-4159.2001.00582.x

Bhati, V., Prasad, S., & Kabra, A. (2025). RNA-based therapies for neurodegenerative disease: Targeting molecular mechanisms for disease modification. *Molecular and Cellular Neuroscience, 133*. https://doi.org/10.1016/j.mcn.2025.104010

Bhattacharjee, G., Gohil, N., Siruka, D., Khambhati, K., Maurya, R., Ramakrishna, S., Chu, D. T., & Singh, V. (2023). CRISPR-dCas9 system for epigenetic editing towards therapeutic applications. *Progress in Molecular Biology and Translational Science, 198*, 15–24. https://doi.org/10.1016/bs.pmbts.2023.02.005

Blossom, V., Ullal, S. D., D'Souza, M. M., Ranade, A. V., Kumar, N. A., & Rai, R. (2025). Implicating neuroinflammation in hippocampus, prefrontal cortex and amygdala with cognitive deficit: A narrative review. *3 Biotech, 15*(9). https://doi.org/10.1007/s13205-025-04468-2

Boado, R. J. (2007). Blood-brain barrier transport of non-viral gene and RNAi therapeutics. *Pharmaceutical Research, 24*(9), 1772–1787. https://doi.org/10.1007/s11095-007-9321-5

Bohlson, S. S., & Tenner, A. J. (2023). Complement in the brain: Contributions to neuroprotection, neuronal plasticity, and neuroinflammation. *Annual Review of Immunology, 41*, 431–452. https://doi.org/10.1146/annurev-immunol-101921-035639

Boillée, S., Yamanaka, K., Lobsiger, C. S., Copeland, N. G., Jenkins, N. A., Kassiotis, G., Kollias, G., & Cleveland, D. W. (2006). Onset and progression in inherited ALS determined by motor neurons and microglia. *Science, 312*(5778), 1389–1392. https://doi.org/10.1126/science.1123511

Boudreau, R. L., Rodríguez-Lebrón, E., & Davidson, B. L. (2011). RNAi medicine for the brain: Progresses and challenges. *Human Molecular Genetics, 20*. https://doi.org/10.1093/hmg/ddr137

Brentari, I., Zadorozhna, M., Denti, M. A., & Giorgio, E. (2023). RNA therapeutics for neurological diseases. *British Medical Bulletin, 147*(1), 50–61. https://doi.org/10.1093/bmb/ldad010

Brochard, V., Combadière, B., Prigent, A., Laouar, Y., Perrin, A., Beray-Berthat, V., Bonduelle, O., Alvarez-Fischer, D., Callebert, J., Launay, J. M., Duyckaerts, C., Flavell, R. A., Hirsch, E. C., & Hunot, S. (2009). Infiltration of CD4+ lymphocytes into the brain contributes to neurodegeneration in a mouse model of parkinson disease. *Journal of Clinical Investigation, 119*(1), 182–192. https://doi.org/10.1172/JCI36470France

Campetella, L., Smolik, K., Farina, A., Joubert, B., Muñiz-Castrillo, S., Desestret, V., & Honnorat, J. (2025). Neurodegeneration and the immune system: Lessons from autoimmune encephalitis. *Journal of Neurology, 272*(5). https://doi.org/10.1007/s00415-025-13094-0

Campisi, L., Chizari, S., Ho, J. S. Y., Gromova, A., Arnold, F., Mosca, L., Mei, X., Fstkchyan, Y., Torre, D., Beharry, C., Garcia-Forn, M., Jiménez-Alcázar, M., Korobeynikov, V. A., Prazich, J., Fayad, Z. A., Seldin, M. M., De Rubeis, S., Bennett, C. L., Ostrow, L. W., … Marazzi, I. (2022). Clonally expanded CD8 T cells characterize amyotrophic lateral sclerosis-4. *Nature, 606*(7916), 945–952. https://doi.org/10.1038/s41586-022-04844-5

Cantero-Fortiz, Y., & Boada, M. (2024). The role of inflammation in neurological disorders: A brief overview of multiple sclerosis, Alzheimer's, and Parkinson's disease. *Frontiers in Neurology, 15*. https://doi.org/10.3389/fneur.2024.1439125

Carlson, T., Kroenke, M., Rao, P., Lane, T. E., & Segal, B. (2008). The Th17-ELR+ CXC chemokine pathway is essential for the development of central nervous system autoimmune disease. *Journal of Experimental Medicine, 205*(4), 811–823. https://doi.org/10.1084/jem.20072404

Castanotto, D., & Rossi, J. J. (2009). The promises and pitfalls of RNA-interference-based therapeutics. *Nature, 457*(7228), 426–433. https://doi.org/10.1038/nature07758

Chavan, S. S., Pavlov, V. A., & Tracey, K. J. (2017). Mechanisms and therapeutic relevance of neuro-immune communication. *Immunity, 46*(6), 927–942. https://doi.org/10.1016/j.immuni.2017.06.008

Chen, T., Dai, Y., Hu, C., Lin, Z., Wang, S., Yang, J., Zeng, L., Li, S., & Li, W. (2024). Cellular and molecular mechanisms of the blood–brain barrier dysfunction in neurodegenerative diseases. *Fluids and Barriers of the CNS, 21*(1). https://doi.org/10.1186/s12987-024-00557-1

Cherry, J. D., Olschowka, J. A., & O'Banion, M. K. (2014). Neuroinflammation and M2 microglia: The good, the bad, and the inflamed. *Journal of Neuroinflammation, 11*. https://doi.org/10.1186/1742-2094-11-98

Chiu, I. M., Chen, A., Zheng, Y., Kosaras, B., Tsiftsoglou, S. A., Vartanian, T. K., Brown, R. H., & Carroll, M. C. (2008). T lymphocytes potentiate endogenous neuroprotective inflammation in a mouse model of ALS. *Proceedings of the National Academy of Sciences, 105*(46), 17913–17918. https://doi.org/10.1073/pnas.0804610105

Chowdhury, R., Hendlinger, A., Riess, O., & Schulze-Hentrich, J. (2025). Microglial immune memory in Parkinson's and huntington's diseases: Epigenetics, triggers, and therapies. *Epigenomics, 17*(11), 739–751. https://doi.org/10.1080/17501911.2025.2518909

Coder, B., Wang, W., Wang, L., Wu, Z., Zhuge, Q., & Su, D. M. (2017). Friend or foe: The dichotomous impact of T cells on neuro-de/re-generation during aging. *Oncotarget, 8*(4), 7116–7137. https://doi.org/10.18632/oncotarget.12572

Codolo, G., Plotegher, N., Pozzobon, T., Brucale, M., Tessari, I., Bubacco, L., de Bernard, M., & Lee Mosley, R. (2013). Triggering of inflammasome by aggregated α–synuclein, an inflammatory response in synucleinopathies. *PLoS One, 8*(1), e55375. https://doi.org/10.1371/journal.pone.0055375

Colonna, M., & Butovsky, O. (2017). Microglia function in the central nervous system during health and neurodegeneration. *Annual Review of Immunology, 35*(1), 441–468. https://doi.org/10.1146/annurev-immunol-051116-052358

Cong, X., Zhang, Z., Li, H., Yang, Y. G., Zhang, Y., & Sun, T. (2024). Nanocarriers for targeted drug delivery in the vascular system: Focus on endothelium. *Journal of Nanobiotechnology, 22*(1). https://doi.org/10.1186/s12951-024-02892-9

Cook, D. A., Kannarkat, G. T., Cintron, A. F., Butkovich, L. M., Fraser, K. B., Chang, J., Grigoryan, N., Factor, S. A., West, A. B., Boss, J. M., & Tansey, M. G. (2017). LRRK2 levels in immune cells are increased in parkinson's disease. *Npj Parkinson's Disease, 3*(1). https://doi.org/10.1038/s41531-017-0010-8

Coque, E., Salsac, C., Espinosa-Carrasco, G., Varga, B., Degauque, N., Cadoux, M., Crabé, R., Virenque, A., Soulard, C., Fierle, J. K., Brodovitch, A., Libralato, M., Végh, A. G., Venteo, S., Scamps, F., Boucraut, J., Laplaud, D., Hernandez, J., Gergely, C., & Raoul, C. (2019). Cytotoxic CD8 + T lymphocytes expressing ALS-causing SOD1 mutant selectively trigger death of spinal motoneurons. *Proceedings of the National Academy of Sciences, 116*(6), 2312–2317. https://doi.org/10.1073/pnas.1815961116

Correale, J., & Farez, M. F. (2015). The role of astrocytes in multiple sclerosis progression. *Frontiers in Neurology, 6*. https://doi.org/10.3389/fneur.2015.00180

Corydon, I. J., Fabian-Jessing, B. K., Jakobsen, T. S., Jørgensen, A. C., Jensen, E. G., Askou, A. L., Aagaard, L., & Corydon, T. J. (2023). 25 years of maturation: A systematic review of RNAi in the clinic. *Molecular Therapy Nucleic Acids, 33*, 469–482. https://doi.org/10.1016/j.omtn.2023.07.018

Dansokho, C., Ahmed, D. A., Aid, S., Toly-Ndour, C., Chaigneau, T., Calle, V., Cagnard, N., Holzenberger, M., Piaggio, E., Aucouturier, P., & Dorothée, G. (2016). Regulatory T cells delay disease progression in alzheimer-like pathology. *Brain, 139*(4), 1237–1251. https://doi.org/10.1093/brain/awv408

Davidson, B. L., & Boudreau, R. L. (2007). RNA interference: A tool for querying nervous system function and an emerging therapy. *Neuron, 53*(6), 781–788. https://doi.org/10.1016/j.neuron.2007.02.020

Davidson, B. L., & McCray, P. B. (2011). Current prospects for RNA interference-based therapies. *Nature Reviews Genetics, 12*(5), 329–340. https://doi.org/10.1038/nrg2968

Depboylu, C., Schorlemmer, K., Klietz, M., Oertel, W. H., Weihe, E., Höglinger, G. U., & Schäfer, M. K. H. (2011). Upregulation of microglial C1q expression has no effects on nigrostriatal dopaminergic injury in the MPTP mouse model of parkinson disease. *Journal of Neuroimmunology, 236*(1–2), 39–46. https://doi.org/10.1016/j.jneuroim.2011.05.006

Deverman, B. E., Pravdo, P. L., Simpson, B. P., Kumar, S. R., Chan, K. Y., Banerjee, A., Wu, W. L., Yang, B., Huber, N., Pasca, S. P., & Gradinaru, V. (2016). Cre-dependent selection yields AAV variants for widespread gene transfer to the adult brain. *Nature Biotechnology, 34*(2), 204–209. https://doi.org/10.1038/nbt.3440

Deverman, B. E., Ravina, B. M., Bankiewicz, K. S., Paul, S. M., & Sah, D. W. Y. (2018). Erratum: Gene therapy for neurological disorders: Progress and prospects. *Nature Reviews Drug Discovery, 19*, 641–669. https://doi.org/10.1038/nrd.2018.158

Di Francesco, V., Chua, A. J., Huang, Di, D'Souza, A., Yang, A., Bleier, B. S., & Amiji, M. M. (2024). RNA therapies for CNS diseases. *Advanced Drug Delivery Reviews, 208.* https://doi.org/10.1016/j.addr.2024.115283

Ding, S., Khan, A. I., Cai, X., Yang, S., Lyu, Z., Du, D., Dutta, P., & Lin, Y. (2020). Overcoming blood–brain barrier transport: Advances in nanoparticle-based drug delivery strategies. *Materials Today, 37*, 112–125. https://doi.org/10.1016/j.mattod.2020.02.001

Ding, Z. B., Song, L. J., Wang, Q., Kumar, G., Yan, Y. Q., & Ma, C. G. (2021). Astrocytes: A double-edged sword in neurodegenerative diseases. *Neural Regeneration Research, 16*(9), 1702–1710. https://doi.org/10.4103/1673-5374.306064

DiSabato, D. J., Quan, N., & Godbout, J. P. (2016). Neuroinflammation: The devil is in the details. *Journal of Neurochemistry, 139*, 136–153. https://doi.org/10.1111/jnc.13607

D'Souza, A., Nozohouri, S., Bleier, B. S., & Amiji, M. M. (2023). CNS delivery of nucleic acid therapeutics: Beyond the blood–b–brain barrier and towards specific cellular targeting. *Pharmaceutical Research, 40*(1), 77–105. https://doi.org/10.1007/s11095-022-03433-5

Dominique, T., Diana, C., Gina, F., Kelsey, B., Alexandre, S., & Timothy, M. (2025). *Small Interfering RNA Targeting Amyloid-Beta Precursor Protein Reduces Alzheimer's Disease Pathology in 5xFAD Mice and Abrogates Behavior Changes in Early Intervention Paradigm [Poster Abstract].* Toronto, ON, Canada: Alzheimer's Association International Conference (AAIC).

Dubey, S. R., Turnbull, C., Pandey, A., Zhao, A., Kurera, M., Al-Zidan, R., Shen, C., Gautam, M., Mahajan, S., Jadhav, P. S., Ghosh, A., Ngo, C., & Man, S. M. (2025). Molecular mechanisms and regulation of inflammasome activation and signaling: Sensing of pathogens and damage molecular patterns. *Cellular and Molecular Immunology, 22*(11), 1313–1344. https://doi.org/10.1038/s41423-025-01354-y

Engelhardt, J. I., Tajti, J., & Appel, S. H. (1993). Lymphocytic infiltrates in the spinal cord in amyotrophic lateral sclerosis. *Archives of Neurology, 50*(1), 30–36. https://doi.org/10.1001/archneur.1993.00540010026013

Espinosa-Cano, E., Aguilar, M. R., Portilla, Y., Barber, D. F., & San Román, J. (2020). Anti-inflammatory polymeric nanoparticles based on ketoprofen and dexamethasone. *Pharmaceutics, 12*(8), 723. https://doi.org/10.3390/pharmaceutics12080723

Esteruelas, G., Souto, E. B., Espina, M., García, M. L., Świtalska, M., Wietrzyk, J., Gliszczyńska, A., & Sánchez-López, E. (2023). Diclofenac loaded biodegradable nanoparticles as antitumoral and antiangiogenic therapy. *Pharmaceutics, 15*(1). https://doi.org/10.3390/pharmaceutics15010102

Esteves, M., Cristóvão, A. C., Vale, A., Machado-Pereira, M., Ferreira, R., & Bernardino, L. (2024). MicroRNA-124-3p modulates alpha-synuclein expression levels in a paraquat-induced in vivo model for parkinson's disease. *Neurochemical Research, 49*(7), 1677–1686. https://doi.org/10.1007/s11064-024-04130-y

Fan, Y.-Y., & Huo, J. (2021). A1/A2 astrocytes in central nervous system injuries and diseases: Angels or devils? *Neurochemistry International, 148*, 105080. https://doi.org/10.1016/j.neuint.2021.105080

Faraco, G., Sugiyama, Y., Lane, D., Garcia-Bonilla, L., Chang, H., Santisteban, M. M., Racchumi, G., Murphy, M., Van Rooijen, N., Anrather, J., & Iadecola, C. (2016). Perivascular macrophages mediate the neurovascular and cognitive dysfunction associated with hypertension. *Journal of Clinical Investigation, 126* (12), 4674–4689. https://doi.org/10.1172/JCI86950

Fatoba, O., Itokazu, T., & Yamashita, T. (2022). Complement cascade functions during brain development and neurodegeneration. *FEBS Journal, 289*(8), 2085–2109. https://doi.org/10.1111/febs.15772

Feja, M., Drath, I., Weiß, S., Ewe, A., Gericke, B., Outeiro, T. F., Stefanis, L., Aigner, A., & Richter, F. (2025). Nose-to-brain siRNA delivery by PEI/PPI-based nanoparticles reduces α-synuclein expression in a parkinson's disease mouse model. *Molecular Therapy Nucleic Acids, 36*(3). https://doi.org/10.1016/j.omtn.2025.102671

Fire, A., Xu, S., Montgomery, M. K., Kostas, S. A., Driver, S. E., & Mello, C. C. (1998). Potent and specific genetic interference by double-stranded RNA in caenorhabditis elegans. *Nature, 391*(6669), 806–811. https://doi.org/10.1038/35888

Franke, M., Bieber, M., Kraft, P., Weber, A. N. R., Stoll, G., & Schuhmann, M. K. (2021). The NLRP3 inflammasome drives inflammation in ischemia/reperfusion injury after transient middle cerebral artery occlusion in mice. *Brain, Behavior, and Immunity, 92*, 221–231. https://doi.org/10.1016/j.bbi.2020.12.009

Friese, M. A., Schattling, B., & Fugger, L. (2014). Mechanisms of neurodegeneration and axonal dysfunction in multiple sclerosis. *Nature Reviews Neurology, 10*(4), 225–238. https://doi.org/10.1038/nrneurol.2014.37

Fukuda, A. M., & Badaut, J. (2013). siRNA treatment: "A sword-in-the-stone" for acute brain injuries. *Genes, 4*(3), 435–456. https://doi.org/10.3390/genes4030435

Ganbold, T., Bao, Q., Zandan, J., Hasi, A., & Baigude, H. (2020). Modulation of microglia polarization through silencing of NF-κB p65 by functionalized curdlan nanoparticle-mmediated RNAi. *ACS Applied Materials & Interfaces, 12*(10), 11363–11374. https://doi.org/10.1021/acsami.9b23004

Gąssowska-Dobrowolska, M., Chlubek, M., Kolasa, A., Tomasiak, P., Korbecki, J., Skowrońska, K., Tarnowski, M., Masztalewicz, M., & Baranowska-Bosiacka, I. (2023). Microglia and astroglia—the potential role in neuroinflammation induced by Pre- and neonatal exposure to lead (Pb). *International Journal of Molecular Sciences, 24*(12), 9903. https://doi.org/10.3390/ijms24129903

Gate, D., Saligrama, N., Leventhal, O., Yang, A. C., Unger, M. S., Middeldorp, J., Chen, K., Lehallier, B., Channappa, D., De Los Santos, M. B., McBride, A., Pluvinage, J., Elahi, F., Tam, G. K. Y., Kim, Y., Greicius, M., Wagner, A. D., Aigner, L., Galasko, D. R., Davis, M. M., & Wyss-Coray, T. (2020). Clonally expanded CD8 T cells patrol the cerebrospinal fluid in Alzheimer's disease. *Nature, 577*(7790), 399–404. https://doi.org/10.1038/s41586-019-1895-7

Goertsen, D., Flytzanis, N. C., Goeden, N., Chuapoco, M. R., Cummins, A., Chen, Y., Fan, Y., Zhang, Q., Sharma, J., Duan, Y., Wang, L., Feng, G., Chen, Y., Ip, N. Y., Pickel, J., & Gradinaru, V. (2022). AAV capsid variants with brain-wide transgene expression and decreased liver targeting after intravenous delivery in mouse and marmoset. *Nature Neuroscience, 25*(1), 106–115. https://doi.org/10.1038/s41593-021-00969-4

Gong, Z., Pan, J., Shen, Q., Li, M., & Peng, Y. (2018). Mitochondrial dysfunction induces NLRP3 inflammasome activation during cerebral ischemia/reperfusion injury. *Journal of Neuroinflammation, 15*(1). https://doi.org/10.1186/s12974-018-1282-6

Gordon, R., Albornoz, E. A., Christie, D. C., Langley, M. R., Kumar, V., Mantovani, S., Robertson, A. A. B., Butler, M. S., Rowe, D. B., O'Neill, L. A., Kanthasamy, A. G., Schroder, K., Cooper, M. A., & Woodruff, T. M. (2018). Inflammasome inhibition prevents -synuclein pathology and dopaminergic neurodegeneration in mice. *Science Translational Medicine, 10*(465). https://doi.org/10.1126/scitranslmed.aah4066

Gosselet, F., Azevedo Loiola, R., Roig, A., Rosell, A., & Culot, M. (2021). Central nervous system delivery of molecules across the blood-brain barrier. *Neurochemistry International, 144*, 104952. https://doi.org/10.1016/j.neuint.2020.104952

Goverman, J. (2009). Autoimmune T cell responses in the central nervous system. *Nature Reviews Immunology, 9*(6), 393–407. https://doi.org/10.1038/nri2550

Greter, M., Heppner, F. L., Lemos, M. P., Odermatt, B. M., Goebels, N., Laufer, T., Noelle, R. J., & Becher, B. (2005). Dendritic cells permit immune invasion of the CNS in an animal model of multiple sclerosis. *Nature Medicine, 11*(3), 328–334. https://doi.org/10.1038/nm1197

Grozdanov, V., Bliederhaeuser, C., Ruf, W. P., Roth, V., Fundel-Clemens, K., Zondler, L., Brenner, D., Martin-Villalba, A., Hengerer, B., Kassubek, J., Ludolph, A. C., Weishaupt, J. H., & Danzer, K. M. (2014).

Inflammatory dysregulation of blood monocytes in Parkinson's disease patients. *Acta Neuropathologica, 128*(5), 651–663. https://doi.org/10.1007/s00401-014-1345-4

Guha, A., Husain, M. A., Si, Y., Nabors, L. B., Filippova, N., Promer, G., Smith, R., & King, P. H. (2023). RNA regulation of inflammatory responses in glia and its potential as a therapeutic target in central nervous system disorders. *Glia, 71*(3), 485–508. https://doi.org/10.1002/glia.24288

Guttenplan, K. A., Weigel, M. K., Adler, D. I., Couthouis, J., Liddelow, S. A., Gitler, A. D., & Barres, B. A. (2020). Knockout of reactive astrocyte activating factors slows disease progression in an ALS mouse model. *Nature Communications, 11*(1). https://doi.org/10.1038/s41467-020-17514-9

Haas, J., Hug, A., Viehöver, A., Fritzsching, B., Falk, C. S., Filser, A., Vetter, T., Milkova, L., Korporal, M., Fritz, B., Storch-Hagenlocher, B., Krammer, P. H., Suri-Payer, E., & Wildemann, B. (2005). Reduced suppressive effect of CD4+CD25high regulatory T cells on the T cell immune response against myelin oligodendrocyte glycoprotein in patients with multiple sclerosis. *European Journal of Immunology, 35*(11), 3343–3352. https://doi.org/10.1002/eji.200526065

Habib, S., & Singh, M. (2022). Angiopep-2-Modified nanoparticles for brain-directed delivery of therapeutics: A review. *Polymers, 14*(4), 712. https://doi.org/10.3390/polym14040712

Hauser, S. L., Waubant, E., Arnold, D. L., Vollmer, T., Antel, J., Fox, R. J., Bar-Or, A., Panzara, M., Sarkar, N., Agarwal, S., Langer-Gould, A., & Smith, C. H. (2008). B-cell depletion with rituximab in relapsing-remitting multiple sclerosis. *New England Journal of Medicine, 358*(7), 676–688. https://doi.org/10.1056/NEJMoa0706383

Hawkes, C. A., & McLaurin, J. A. (2009). Selective targeting of perivascular macrophages for clearance of β-amyloid in cerebral amyloid angiopathy. *Proceedings of the National Academy of Sciences, 106*(4), 1261–1266. https://doi.org/10.1073/pnas.0805453106

He, P., Zhong, Z., Lindholm, K., Berning, L., Lee, W., Lemere, C., Staufenbiel, M., Li, R., & Shen, Y. (2007). Deletion of tumor necrosis factor death receptor inhibits amyloid β generation and prevents learning and memory deficits in Alzheimer's mice. *Journal of Cell Biology, 178*(5), 829–841. https://doi.org/10.1083/jcb.200705042

Heneka, M. T., Kummer, M. P., Stutz, A., Delekate, A., Schwartz, S., Vieira-Saecker, A., Griep, A., Axt, D., Remus, A., Tzeng, T. C., Gelpi, E., Halle, A., Korte, M., Latz, E., & Golenbock, D. T. (2013). NLRP3 is activated in Alzheimer's disease and contributes to pathology in APP/PS1 mice. *Nature, 493*(7434), 674–678. https://doi.org/10.1038/nature11729

Heneka, M. T., van der Flier, W. M., Jessen, F., Hoozemanns, J., Thal, D. R., Boche, D., Brosseron, F., Teunissen, C., Zetterberg, H., Jacobs, A. H., Edison, P., Ramirez, A., Cruchaga, C., Lambert, J. C., Laza, A. R., Sanchez-Mut, J. V., Fischer, A., Castro-Gomez, S., Stein, T. D., … Riechers, S. P. (2025). Neuroinflammation in alzheimer disease. *Nature Reviews Immunology, 25*(5), 321–352. https://doi.org/10.1038/s41577-024-01104-7

Heurich, B., el Idrissi, N. B., Donev, R. M., Petri, S., Claus, P., Neal, J., Morgan, B. P., & Ramaglia, V. (2011). Complement upregulation and activation on motor neurons and neuromuscular junction in the SOD1 G93A mouse model of familial amyotrophic lateral sclerosis. *Journal of Neuroimmunology, 235*(1–2), 104–109. https://doi.org/10.1016/j.jneuroim.2011.03.011

Hickman, S., Izzy, S., Sen, P., Morsett, L., & El Khoury, J. (2018). Microglia in neurodegeneration. *Nature Neuroscience, 21*(10), 1359–1369. https://doi.org/10.1038/s41593-018-0242-x

Hirota, K., Duarte, J. H., Veldhoen, M., Hornsby, E., Li, Y., Cua, D. J., Ahlfors, H., Wilhelm, C., Tolaini, M., Menzel, U., Garefalaki, A., Potocnik, A. J., & Stockinger, B. (2011). Fate mapping of IL-17-producing T cells in inflammatory responses. *Nature Immunology, 12*(3), 255–263. https://doi.org/10.1038/ni.1993

Hirsch, E. C., & Hunot, S. (2009). Neuroinflammation in parkinson's disease: A target for neuroprotection? *The Lancet Neurology, 8*(4), 382–397. https://doi.org/10.1016/S1474-4422(09)70062-6

Holbrook, J. A., Jarosz-Griffiths, H. H., Caseley, E., Lara-Reyna, S., Poulter, J. A., Williams-Gray, C. H., Peckham, D., & McDermott, M. F. (2021). Neurodegenerative disease and the NLRP3 inflammasome. *Frontiers in Pharmacology, 12*. https://doi.org/10.3389/fphar.2021.643254

Holm, A., Hansen, S. N., Klitgaard, H., & Kauppinen, S. (2022). Clinical advances of RNA therapeutics for treatment of neurological and neuromuscular diseases. *RNA Biology, 19*(1), 594–608. https://doi.org/10.1080/15476286.2022.2066334

Homo-Delarche, F., & Dardenne, M. (1993). The neuroendocrine-immune axis. *Springer Seminars in Immunopathology, 14*(3), 221–238. https://doi.org/10.1007/BF00195975

Hong, S., Beja-Glasser, V. F., Nfonoyim, B. M., Frouin, A., Li, S., Ramakrishnan, S., Merry, K. M., Shi, Q., Rosenthal, A., Barres, B. A., Lemere, C. A., Selkoe, D. J., & Stevens, B. (2016). Complement and microglia mediate early synapse loss in alzheimer mouse models. *Science, 352*(6286), 712–716. https://doi.org/10.1126/science.aad8373

Hoyer, D., & Dev, K. K. (2006). RNA interference as a therapeutic strategy for treating CNS disorders. *Drug Discovery Today: Therapeutic Strategies, 3*(4), 451–456. https://doi.org/10.1016/j.ddstr.2006.10.008

Hu, Z., Cui, Y., Qiao, X., He, X., Fang, L., Luo, C., Wang, S., Li, C., & Dai, R. (2018). Silencing miR-150 ameliorates experimental autoimmune encephalomyelitis. *Frontiers in Neuroscience, 12*. https://doi.org/10.3389/fnins.2018.00465

Hu, H., Li, H., Li, R., Liu, P., & Liu, H. (2024). Re-establishing immune tolerance in multiple sclerosis: Focusing on novel mechanisms of mesenchymal stem cell regulation of Th17/Treg balance. *Journal of Translational Medicine, 22*(1). https://doi.org/10.1186/s12967-024-05450-x

Hu, B., Zhong, L., Weng, Y., Peng, L., Huang, Y., Zhao, Y., & Liang, X.-J. (2020). Therapeutic siRNA: State of the art. *Signal Transduction and Targeted Therapy, 5*(1). https://doi.org/10.1038/s41392-020-0207-x

Isaksson, M., Lundgren, B. A., Ahlgren, K. M., Kämpe, O., & Lobell, A. (2012). Conditional DC depletion does not affect priming of encephalitogenic Th cells in EAE. *European Journal of Immunology, 42*(10), 2555–2563. https://doi.org/10.1002/eji.201142239

Jin, J., Zhang, H., Lu, Q., Tian, L., Yao, S., Lai, F., Liang, Y., Liu, C., Lu, Y., Tian, S., Zhao, Y., & Ren, W. (2025). Nanocarrier-mediated siRNA delivery: A new approach for the treatment of traumatic brain injury–related alzheimer's disease. *Neural Regeneration Research, 20*(9), 2538–2555. https://doi.org/10.4103/nrr.nrr-d-24-00303

Johann, S., Heitzer, M., Kanagaratnam, M., Goswami, A., Rizo, T., Weis, J., Troost, D., & Beyer, C. (2015). NLRP3 inflammasome is expressed by astrocytes in the SOD1 mouse model of ALS and in human sporadic ALS patients. *Glia, 63*(12), 2260–2273. https://doi.org/10.1002/glia.22891

Johnsen, K. B., Burkhart, A., Melander, F., Kempen, P. J., Vejlebo, J. B., Siupka, P., Nielsen, M. S., Andresen, T. L., & Moos, T. (2017). Targeting transferrin receptors at the blood-brain barrier improves the uptake of immunoliposomes and subsequent cargo transport into the brain parenchyma. *Scientific Reports, 7*(1). https://doi.org/10.1038/s41598-017-11220-1

Kanasty, R., Dorkin, J. R., Vegas, A., & Anderson, D. (2013). Delivery materials for siRNA therapeutics. *Nature Materials, 12*(11), 967–977. https://doi.org/10.1038/nmat3765

Kandimalla, R. J. L., Wani, W., Bk, B., & Gill, K. (2012). SiRNA against presenilin 1 (PS1) down regulates amyloid β42 production in IMR-32 cells. *Journal of Biomedical Science, 19*(1). https://doi.org/10.1186/1423-0127-19-2

Keren-Shaul, H., Spinrad, A., Weiner, A., Matcovitch-Natan, O., Dvir-Szternfeld, R., Ulland, T. K., David, E., Baruch, K., Lara-Astaiso, D., Toth, B., Itzkovitz, S., Colonna, M., Schwartz, M., & Amit, I. (2017). A unique microglia type associated with restricting development of alzheimer's disease. *Cell, 169*(7), 1276. https://doi.org/10.1016/j.cell.2017.05.018

Kipnis, J. (2016). Multifaceted interactions between adaptive immunity and the central nervous system. *Science, 353*(6301), 766–771. https://doi.org/10.1126/science.aag2638

Kovacs, Z. I., Burks, S. R., & Frank, J. A. (2018). Focused ultrasound with microbubbles induces sterile inflammatory response proportional to the blood brain barrier opening: Attention to experimental conditions. *Theranostics, 8*(8), 2245–2248. https://doi.org/10.7150/thno.24181

Krumbholz, M., Derfuss, T., Hohlfeld, R., & Meinl, E. (2012). B cells and antibodies in multiple sclerosis pathogenesis and therapy. *Nature Reviews Neurology, 8*(11), 613–623. https://doi.org/10.1038/nrneurol.2012.203

Kumar, P., Zelena, D., & Gautam, A. (2024). *Neurological disorders and challenges in their theranostics theranostic applications of nanotechnology in neurological disorders* (pp. 1–29). Hungary: Springer. https://doi.org/10.1007/978-981-99-9510-3_1

Kurowska-Stolarska, M., Alivernini, S., Ballantine, L. E., Asquith, D. L., Millar, N. L., Gilchrist, D. S., Reilly, J., Ierna, M., Fraser, A. R., Stolarski, B., McSharry, C., Hueber, A. J., Baxter, D., Hunter, J., Gay, S., Liew, F. Y., & McInnes, I. B. (2011). MicroRNA-155 as a proinflammatory regulator in clinical and experimental arthritis. *Proceedings of the National Academy of Sciences, 108*(27), 11193–11198. https://doi.org/10.1073/pnas.1019536108

Lagier-Tourenne, C., Baughn, M., Rigo, F., Sun, S., Liu, P., Li, H.-R., Jiang, J., Watt, A. T., Chun, S., Katz, M., Qiu, J., Sun, Y., Ling, S.-C., Zhu, Q., Polymenidou, M., Drenner, K., Artates, J. W., McAlonis-Downes, M., Markmiller, S., … Ravits, J. (2013). Targeted degradation of sense and antisense C9orf72 RNA foci as therapy for ALS and frontotemporal degeneration. *Proceedings of the National Academy of Sciences, 110*(47). https://doi.org/10.1073/pnas.1318835110

Laman, J. D., Thompson, E. J., & Kappos, L. (1998). Balancing the Th1/Th2 concept in multiple sclerosis. *Immunology Today, 19*(11), 489–490. https://doi.org/10.1016/S0167-5699(98)01320-6

Lassmann, H., van Horssen, J., & Mahad, D. (2012). Progressive multiple sclerosis: Pathology and pathogenesis. *Nature Reviews Neurology, 8*(11), 647–656. https://doi.org/10.1038/nrneurol.2012.168

Laurent, C., Dorothée, G., Hunot, S., Martin, E., Monnet, Y., Duchamp, M., Dong, Y., Légeron, F.-P., Leboucher, A., Burnouf, S., Faivre, E., Carvalho, K., Caillierez, R., Zommer, N., Demeyer, D., Jouy, N., Sazdovitch, V., Schraen-Maschke, S., Delarasse, C., & Blum, D. (2016). Hippocampal T cell infiltration promotes neuroinflammation and cognitive decline in a mouse model of tauopathy. *Brain, 140*(1), 184–200. https://doi.org/10.1093/brain/aww270

Laurindo, L. F., Dias, J. A., Araújo, A. C., Torres Pomini, K., Machado Galhardi, C., Detregiachi, C. R. P., Argollo Haber, L. S. D., Roque, D. D., Bechara, M. D., Castro, M. V. M. D., Pereira, E. D. S. B. M., Tofano, R. J., Jasmin Santos German Borgo, I., & Barbalho, S. M. (2024). Immunological dimensions of neuroinflammation and microglial activation: Exploring innovative immunomodulatory approaches to mitigate neuroinflammatory progression. *Frontiers in Immunology, 14*. https://doi.org/10.3389/fimmu.2023.1305933

Lee, J. D., Coulthard, L. G., & Woodruff, T. M. (2019). Complement dysregulation in the central nervous system during development and disease. *Seminars in Immunology, 45*. https://doi.org/10.1016/j.smim.2019.101340

Leung, R. K. M., & Whittaker, P. A. (2005). RNA interference: From gene silencing to gene-specific therapeutics. *Pharmacology & Therapeutics, 107*(2), 222–239. https://doi.org/10.1016/j.pharmthera.2005.03.004

Lewis, B. P., Shih, I. H., Jones-Rhoades, M. W., Bartel, D. P., & Burge, C. B. (2003). Prediction of mammalian microRNA targets. *Cell, 115*(7), 787–798. https://doi.org/10.1016/S0092-8674(03)01018-3

Liddelow, S. A., & Barres, B. A. (2017). Reactive astrocytes: Production, function, and therapeutic potential. *Immunity, 46*(6), 957–967. https://doi.org/10.1016/j.immuni.2017.06.006

Liddelow, S. A., Guttenplan, K. A., Clarke, L. E., Bennett, F. C., Bohlen, C. J., Schirmer, L., Bennett, M. L., Münch, A. E., Chung, W. S., Peterson, T. C., Wilton, D. K., Frouin, A., Napier, B. A., Panicker, N., Kumar, M., Buckwalter, M. S., Rowitch, D. H., Dawson, V. L., Dawson, T. M., & Barres, B. A. (2017). Neurotoxic reactive astrocytes are induced by activated microglia. *Nature, 541*(7638), 481–487. https://doi.org/10.1038/nature21029

Lim, G. P., Yang, F., Chu, T., Chen, P., Beech, W., Teter, B., Tran, T., Ubeda, O., Ashe, K. H., Frautschy, S. A., & Cole, G. M. (2000). Ibuprofen suppresses plaque pathology and inflammation in a mouse model for alzheimer's disease. *Journal of Neuroscience, 20*(15), 5709–5714. https://doi.org/10.1523/jneurosci.20-15-05709.2000

Lin, J., Jo, S. B., Kim, T.-H., Kim, H.-W., & Yian Chew, S. (2020). RNA interference in glial cells for nerve injury treatment. *Journal of Tissue Engineering, 11*. https://doi.org/10.1177/2041731420939224

Liston, A., Dooley, J., & Yshii, L. (2022). Brain-resident regulatory T cells and their role in health and disease. *Immunology Letters, 248*, 26–30. https://doi.org/10.1016/j.imlet.2022.06.005

Liu, J., & Wang, F. (2017). Role of neuroinflammation in amyotrophic lateral sclerosis: Cellular mechanisms and therapeutic implications. *Frontiers in Immunology, 8*. https://doi.org/10.3389/fimmu.2017.01005

Liu, X., Zhou, F., Yang, Y., Wang, W., Niu, L., Zuo, D., Li, X., Hua, H., Zhang, B., Kou, Y., Guo, J., Kong, F., Pan, W., Gao, D., Meves, J. M., Sun, H., Xue, M., Zhang, Q., Wang, Y., & Tang, R. (2019). MiR-409-3p and MiR-1896 co-operatively participate in IL-17-induced inflammatory cytokine production in astrocytes and pathogenesis of EAE mice via targeting SOCS3/STAT3 signaling. *Glia, 67*(1), 101–112. https://doi.org/10.1002/glia.23530

Liu, Q., Zhou, H., Zhu, R., Xu, Y., & Cao, Z. (2014). Reconsideration of in silico siRNA design from a perspective of heterogeneous data integration: Problems and solutions. *Briefings in Bioinformatics, 15*(2), 292–305. https://doi.org/10.1093/bib/bbs073

Lucchinetti, C. F., Popescu, B. F. G., Bunyan, R. F., Moll, N. M., Roemer, S. F., Lassmann, H., Brück, W., Parisi, J. E., Scheithauer, B. W., Giannini, C., Weigand, S. D., Mandrekar, J., & Ransohoff, R. M. (2011). Inflammatory cortical demyelination in early multiple sclerosis. *New England Journal of Medicine, 365*(23), 2188–2197. https://doi.org/10.1056/NEJMoa1100648

Matejuk, A., & Ransohoff, R. M. (2020). Crosstalk between astrocytes and microglia: An overview. *Frontiers in Immunology, 11*. https://doi.org/10.3389/fimmu.2020.01416

McAlpine, F. E., Lee, J. K., Harms, A. S., Ruhn, K. A., Blurton-Jones, M., Hong, J., Das, P., Golde, T. E., LaFerla, F. M., Oddo, S., Blesch, A., & Tansey, M. G. (2009). Inhibition of soluble TNF signaling in a mouse model of alzheimer's disease prevents pre-plaque amyloid-associated neuropathology. *Neurobiology of Disease, 34*(1), 163–177. https://doi.org/10.1016/j.nbd.2009.01.006

McCauley, M. E., & Baloh, R. H. (2019). Inflammation in ALS/FTD pathogenesis. *Acta Neuropathologica, 137* (5), 715–730. https://doi.org/10.1007/s00401-018-1933-9

McCormack, A. L., Mak, S. K., Henderson, J. M., Bumcrot, D., Farrer, M. J., & Donato, A. (2010). Di Monte, α-synuclein suppression by targeted small interfering rna in the primate substantia nigra. *PLoS One, 5*(8). https://doi.org/10.1371/journal.pone.0012122

McLoughlin, C. D., Nevins, S., Stein, J. B., Khakbiz, M., & Lee, K. B. (2024). Overcoming the blood–brain barrier: Multifunctional nanomaterial-based strategies for targeted drug delivery in neurological disorders. *Small Science, 4*(12). https://doi.org/10.1002/smsc.202400232

Meissner, F., Molawi, K., & Zychlinsky, A. (2010). Mutant superoxide dismutase 1-induced IL-1β accelerates ALS pathogenesis. *Proceedings of the National Academy of Sciences, 107*(29), 13046–13050. https://doi.org/10.1073/pnas.1002396107

Meleady, L., Towriss, M., Kim, J., Bacarac, V., Dang, V., Rowland, M. E., & Ciernia, A. V. (2023). Histone deacetylase 3 regulates microglial function through histone deacetylation. *Epigenetics, 18*(1). https://doi.org/10.1080/15592294.2023.2241008

Meng, X. F., Tan, L., Tan, M. S., Jiang, T., Tan, C. C., Li, M. M., Wang, H. F., & Yu, J. T. (2014). Inhibition of the NLRP3 inflammasome provides neuroprotection in rats following amygdala kindling-induced status epilepticus. *Journal of Neuroinflammation, 11*(1). https://doi.org/10.1186/s12974-014-0212-5

Miller, S. J. (2018). Astrocyte heterogeneity in the adult central nervous system. *Frontiers in Cellular Neuroscience, 12*. https://doi.org/10.3389/fncel.2018.00401

Miller, V. M., Gouvion, C. M., Davidson, B. L., & Paulson, H. L. (2004). Targeting alzheimer's disease genes with RNA interference: An efficient strategy for silencing mutant alleles. *Nucleic Acids Research, 32*(2), 661–668. https://doi.org/10.1093/nar/gkh208

Mir, F. A., Amanullah, A., Jain, B. P., Hyderi, Z., & Gautam, A. (2023). Neuroepigenetics of ageing and neurodegeneration-associated dementia: An updated review. *Ageing Research Reviews, 91*. https://doi.org/10.1016/j.arr.2023.102067

Moehle, M. S., Webber, P. J., Tse, T., Sukar, N., Standaert, D. G., Desilva, T. M., Cowell, R. M., & West, A. B. (2012). LRRK2 inhibition attenuates microglial inflammatory responses. *Journal of Neuroscience, 32*(5), 1602–1611. https://doi.org/10.1523/JNEUROSCI.5601-11.2012

Mohr, S., Bakal, C., & Perrimon, N. (2010). Genomic screening with RNAi: Results and challenges. *Annual Review of Biochemistry, 79*(1), 37–64. https://doi.org/10.1146/annurev-biochem-060408-092949

Moser, T., Akgün, K., Proschmann, U., Sellner, J., & Ziemssen, T. (2020). The role of TH17 cells in multiple sclerosis: Therapeutic implications. *Autoimmunity Reviews, 19*(10), 102647. https://doi.org/10.1016/j.autrev.2020.102647

Muzio, L., Viotti, A., & Martino, G. (2021). Microglia in neuroinflammation and neurodegeneration: From understanding to therapy. *Frontiers in Neuroscience, 15*. https://doi.org/10.3389/fnins.2021.742065

Naegele, M., Tillack, K., Reinhardt, S., Schippling, S., Martin, R., & Sospedra, M. (2012). Neutrophils in multiple sclerosis are characterized by a primed phenotype. *Journal of Neuroimmunology, 242*(1–2), 60–71. https://doi.org/10.1016/j.jneuroim.2011.11.009

Nagai, M., Re, D. B., Nagata, T., Chalazonitis, A., Jessell, T. M., Wichterle, H., & Przedborski, S. (2007). Astrocytes expressing ALS-linked mutated SOD1 release factors selectively toxic to motor neurons. *Nature Neuroscience, 10*(5), 615–622. https://doi.org/10.1038/nn1876

Nayak, D., Roth, T. L., & McGavern, D. B. (2014). Microglia development and function. *Annual Review of Immunology, 32*, 367–402. https://doi.org/10.1146/annurev-immunol-032713-120240

Neumann, H., Medana, I. M., Bauer, J., & Lassmann, H. (2002). Cytotoxic T lymphocytes in autoimmune and degenerative CNS diseases. *Trends in Neurosciences, 25*(6), 313–319. https://doi.org/10.1016/S0166-2236(02)02154-9

Nguyen, H. M., Grössinger, E. M., Horiuchi, M., Davis, K. W., Jin, L. W., Maezawa, I., & Wulff, H. (2017). Differential Kv1.3, KCa3.1, and Kir2.1 expression in "classically" and "alternatively" activated microglia. *Glia, 65*(1), 106–121. https://doi.org/10.1002/glia.23078

Nimmo, J., Byrne, R. A. J., Daskoulidou, N., Watkins, L. M., Carpanini, S. M., Zelek, W. M., & Paul Morgan, B. (2024). The complement system in neurodegenerative diseases. *Clinical Science, 138*(6), 387–412. https://doi.org/10.1042/cs20230513

Nishimura, M., Kuno, S., Mizuta, I., Ohta, M., Maruyama, H., Kaji, R., & Kawakami, H. (2003). Influence of monocyte chemoattractant protein 1 gene polymorphism on age at onset of sporadic parkinson's disease. *Movement Disorders, 18*(8), 953–955. https://doi.org/10.1002/mds.10462

Nugent, A. A., Lin, K., van Lengerich, B., Lianoglou, S., Przybyla, L., Davis, S. S., Llapashtica, C., Wang, J., Kim, D. J., Xia, D., Lucas, A., Baskaran, S., Haddick, P. C. G., Lenser, M., Earr, T. K., Shi, J., Dugas, J. C., Andreone, B. J., Logan, T., … Di Paolo, G. (2020). TREM2 regulates microglial cholesterol metabolism upon chronic phagocytic challenge. *Neuron, 105*(5), 837. https://doi.org/10.1016/j.neuron.2019.12.007

Nunes, D., Andrade, S., Ramalho, M. J., Loureiro, J. A., & Pereira, M. C. (2022). Polymeric nanoparticles-loaded hydrogels for biomedical applications: A systematic review on in vivo findings. *Polymers, 14*(5). https://doi.org/10.3390/polym14051010

Nuzziello, N., Ciaccia, L., & Liguori, M. (2020). Precision medicine in neurodegenerative diseases: Some promising tips coming from the microRNAs' world. *Cells, 9*(1), 75. https://doi.org/10.3390/cells9010075

Obbard, D. J., Gordon, K. H. J., Buck, A. H., & Jiggins, F. M. (2009). The evolution of RNAi as a defence against viruses and transposable elements. *Philosophical Transactions of the Royal Society B: Biological Sciences, 364*(1513), 99–115. https://doi.org/10.1098/rstb.2008.0168

O'Carroll, S. J., Cook, W. H., & Young, D. (2021). AAV targeting of glial cell types in the central and peripheral nervous system and relevance to human gene therapy. *Frontiers in Molecular Neuroscience, 13*. https://doi.org/10.3389/fnmol.2020.618020

Ogawa, K., Kato, N., Yoshida, M., Hiu, T., Matsuo, T., Mizukami, S., Omata, D., Suzuki, R., Maruyama, K., Mukai, H., & Kawakami, S. (2022). Focused ultrasound/microbubbles-assisted BBB opening enhances LNP-mediated mRNA delivery to brain. *Journal of Controlled Release, 348*, 34–41. https://doi.org/10.1016/j.jconrel.2022.05.042

Ouchi, Y., Yoshikawa, E., Sekine, Y., Futatsubashi, M., Kanno, T., Ogusu, T., & Torizuka, T. (2005). Microglial activation and dopamine terminal loss in early parkinson's disease. *Annals of Neurology, 57*(2), 168–175. https://doi.org/10.1002/ana.20338

Ozata, D. M., Gainetdinov, I., Zoch, A., O'Carroll, D., & Zamore, P. D. (2019). PIWI-interacting RNAs: Small RNAs with big functions. *Nature Reviews Genetics, 20*(2), 89–108. https://doi.org/10.1038/s41576-018-0073-3

Paddison, P. J., Caudy, A. A., Bernstein, E., Hannon, G. J., & Conklin, D. S. (2002). Short hairpin RNAs (shRNAs) induce sequence-specific silencing in mammalian cells. *Genes & Development, 16*(8), 948–958. https://doi.org/10.1101/gad.981002

Paerewijck, O., & Lamkanfi, M. (2022). The human inflammasomes. *Molecular Aspects of Medicine, 88*, 101100. https://doi.org/10.1016/j.mam.2022.101100

Park, H., Shin, J., Kim, Y., Saito, T., Saido, T. C., & Kim, J. (2022). CRISPR/dCas9-Dnmt3a-mediated targeted DNA methylation of APP rescues brain pathology in a mouse model of Alzheimer's disease. *Translational Neurodegeneration, 11*(1). https://doi.org/10.1186/s40035-022-00314-0

Pfister, E. L., Kennington, L., Straubhaar, J., Wagh, S., Liu, W., DiFiglia, M., Landwehrmeyer, B., Vonsattel, J.-P., Zamore, P. D., & Aronin, N. (2009). Five siRNAs targeting three SNPs may provide therapy for three-quarters of huntington's disease patients. *Current Biology, 19*(9), 774–778. https://doi.org/10.1016/j.cub.2009.03.030

Philips, T., & Robberecht, W. (2011). Neuroinflammation in amyotrophic lateral sclerosis: Role of glial activation in motor neuron disease. *The Lancet Neurology, 10*(3), 253–263. https://doi.org/10.1016/s1474-4422(11)70015-1

Piedrahita, D., Hernández, I., López-Tobón, A., Fedorov, D., Obara, B., Manjunath, B. S., Boudreau, R. L., Davidson, B., LaFerla, F., Gallego-Gómez, J. C., Kosik, K. S., & Cardona-Gómez, G. P. (2010). Silencing of CDK5 reduces neurofibrillary tangles in transgenic alzheimer's mice. *Journal of Neuroscience, 30*(42), 13966–13976. https://doi.org/10.1523/jneurosci.3637-10.2010

Ponomarev, E. D., Veremeyko, T., Barteneva, N., Krichevsky, A. M., & Weiner, H. L. (2011). MicroRNA-124 promotes microglia quiescence and suppresses EAE by deactivating macrophages via the C/EBP-α-PU.1 pathway. *Nature Medicine, 17*(1), 64–70. https://doi.org/10.1038/nm.2266

Presumey, J., Bialas, A. R., & Carroll, M. C. (2017). Complement system in neural synapse elimination in development and disease. *Advances in Immunology, 135*, 53–79. https://doi.org/10.1016/bs.ai.2017.06.004

Prinz, M., Priller, J., Sisodia, S. S., & Ransohoff, R. M. (2011). Heterogeneity of CNS myeloid cells and their roles in neurodegeneration. *Nature Neuroscience, 14*(10), 1227–1235. https://doi.org/10.1038/nn.2923

Prüss, H. (2021). Autoantibodies in neurological disease. *Nature Reviews Immunology, 21*(12), 798–813. https://doi.org/10.1038/s41577-021-00543-w

Qian, K., Jiang, X., Liu, Z. Q., Zhang, J., Fu, P., Su, Y., Brazhe, N. A., Liu, D., & Zhu, L. Q. (2023). Revisiting the critical roles of reactive astrocytes in neurodegeneration. *Molecular Psychiatry, 28*(7), 2697–2706. https://doi.org/10.1038/s41380-023-02061-8

Qian, Y., Li, X., Li, G., Liu, H., Li, Q., Liu, X., Zhang, Y., He, Z., Zhao, Y., & Fan, H. (2024). Astrocyte-derived exosomal miR-148a-3p suppresses neuroinflammation and restores neurological function in traumatic brain injury by regulating the microglial phenotype. *Eneuro, 11*(2). https://doi.org/10.1523/eneuro.0336-23.2024

Ralph, G. S., Radcliffe, P. A., Day, D. M., Carthy, J. M., Leroux, M. A., Lee, D. C. P., Wong, L. F., Bilsland, L. G., Greensmith, L., Kingsman, S. M., Mitrophanous, K. A., Mazarakis, N. D., & Azzouz, M. (2005). Silencing mutant SOD1 using RNAi protects against neurodegeneration and extends survival in an ALS model. *Nature Medicine, 11*(4), 429–433. https://doi.org/10.1038/nm1205

Ralvenius, W. T., Andresen, J. L., Huston, M. M., Penney, J., Maeve Bonner, J., Fenton, O. S., Langer, R., & Tsai, L.-H. (2024). Nanoparticle-mediated delivery of Anti-PU.1 siRNA via localized intracisternal administration reduces neuroinflammation. *Advanced Materials, 36*(8). https://doi.org/10.1002/adma.202309225

Ramachandran, P. S., Keiser, M. S., & Davidson, B. L. (2013). Recent advances in RNA interference therapeutics for CNS diseases. *Neurotherapeutics, 10*(3), 473–485. https://doi.org/10.1007/s13311-013-0183-8

Ransohoff, R. M., & Brown, M. A. (2012). Innate immunity in the central nervous system. *Journal of Clinical Investigation, 122*(4), 1164–1171. https://doi.org/10.1172/JCI58644

Raoul, C., Abbas-Terki, T., Bensadoun, J. C., Guillot, S., Haase, G., Szulc, J., Henderson, C. E., & Aebischer, P. (2005). Lentiviral-mediated silencing of SOD1 through RNA interference retards disease onset and progression in a mouse model of ALS. *Nature Medicine, 11*(4), 423–428. https://doi.org/10.1038/nm1207

Rathinam, V. A. K., & Fitzgerald, K. A. (2016). Inflammasome complexes: Emerging mechanisms and effector functions. *Cell, 165*(4), 792–800. https://doi.org/10.1016/j.cell.2016.03.046

Re, D. B., Le Verche, V., Yu, C., Amoroso, M. W., Politi, K. A., Phani, S., Ikiz, B., Hoffmann, L., Koolen, M., Nagata, T., Papadimitriou, D., Nagy, P., Mitsumoto, H., Kariya, S., Wichterle, H., Henderson, C. E., & Przedborski, S. (2014). Necroptosis drives motor neuron death in models of both sporadic and familial ALS. *Neuron, 81*(5), 1001–1008. https://doi.org/10.1016/j.neuron.2014.01.011

Rhea, E. M., & Banks, W. A. (2021). A historical perspective on the interactions of insulin at the blood-brain barrier. *Journal of Neuroendocrinology, 33*(4). https://doi.org/10.1111/jne.12929

Ricklin, D., Hajishengallis, G., Yang, K., & Lambris, J. D. (2010). Complement: A key system for immune surveillance and homeostasis. *Nature Immunology, 11*(9), 785–797. https://doi.org/10.1038/ni.1923

Rizor, A., Pajarillo, E., Johnson, J., Aschner, M., & Lee, E. (2019). Astrocytic oxidative/nitrosative stress contributes to parkinson's disease pathogenesis: The dual role of reactive astrocytes. *Antioxidants, 8*(8), 265. https://doi.org/10.3390/antiox8080265

Rossi, B., Constantin, G., & Zenaro, E. (2020). The emerging role of neutrophils in neurodegeneration. *Immunobiology, 225*(1), 151865. https://doi.org/10.1016/j.imbio.2019.10.014

Rothstein, J. D., Van Kammen, M., Levey, A. I., Martin, L. J., & Kuncl, R. W. (1995). Selective loss of glial glutamate transporter GLT-1 in amyotrophic lateral sclerosis. *Annals of Neurology, 38*(1), 73–84. https://doi.org/10.1002/ana.410380114

Sabatino, J. J., Pröbstel, A. K., & Zamvil, S. S. (2019). B cells in autoimmune and neurodegenerative central nervous system diseases. *Nature Reviews Neuroscience, 20*(12), 728–745. https://doi.org/10.1038/s41583-019-0233-2

Sah, D. W. Y. (2006). Therapeutic potential of RNA interference for neurological disorders. *Life Sciences, 79*(19), 1773–1780. https://doi.org/10.1016/j.lfs.2006.06.011

Saraiva, C., Praça, C., Ferreira, R., Santos, T., Ferreira, L., & Bernardino, L. (2016). Nanoparticle-mediated brain drug delivery: Overcoming blood-brain barrier to treat neurodegenerative diseases. *Journal of Controlled Release, 235*, 34–47. https://doi.org/10.1016/j.jconrel.2016.05.044

Saunders, J. A. H., Estes, K. A., Kosloski, L. M., Allen, H. E., Dempsey, K. M., Torres-Russotto, D. R., Meza, J. L., Santamaria, P. M., Bertoni, J. M., Murman, D. L., Ali, H. H., Standaert, D. G., Mosley, R. L., & Gendelman, H. E. (2012). CD4+ regulatory and effector/memory T cell subsets profile motor dysfunction in parkinson's disease. *Journal of Neuroimmune Pharmacology, 7*(4), 927–938. https://doi.org/10.1007/s11481-012-9402-z

Schartz, N. D., & Tenner, A. J. (2020). The good, the bad, and the opportunities of the complement system in neurodegenerative disease. *Journal of Neuroinflammation, 17*(1). https://doi.org/10.1186/s12974-020-02024-8

Serafini, B., Rosicarelli, B., Magliozzi, R., Stigliano, E., & Aloisi, F. (2004). Detection of ectopic b-cell follicles with germinal centers in the meninges of patients with secondary progressive multiple sclerosis. *Brain Pathology, 14*(2), 164–174. https://doi.org/10.1111/j.1750-3639.2004.tb00049.x

Setten, R. L., Rossi, J. J., & Han, S.p. (2019). The current state and future directions of RNAi-based therapeutics. *Nature Reviews Drug Discovery, 18*(6), 421–446. https://doi.org/10.1038/s41573-019-0017-4

Shang, R., Lee, S., Senavirathne, G., & Lai, E. C. (2023). microRNAs in action: Biogenesis, function and regulation. *Nature Reviews Genetics, 24*(12), 816–833. https://doi.org/10.1038/s41576-023-00611-y

Shen, Y., Lue, L. F., Yang, L. B., Roher, A., Kuo, Y. M., Strohmeyer, R., Goux, W. J., Lee, V., Johnson, G. V. W., Webster, S. D., Cooper, N. R., Bradt, B., & Rogers, J. (2001). Complement activation by neurofibrillary tangles in alzheimer's disease. *Neuroscience Letters, 305*(3), 165–168. https://doi.org/10.1016/S0304-3940(01)01842-0

Shi, Q., Chowdhury, S., Ma, R., Le, K. X., Hong, S., Caldarone, B. J., Stevens, B., & Lemere, C. A. (2017). Complement C3 deficiency protects against neurodegeneration in aged plaque-rich APP/PS1 mice. *Science Translational Medicine, 9*(392). https://doi.org/10.1126/scitranslmed.aaf6295

Shi, F. D., & Yong, V. W. (2025). Neuroinflammation across neurological diseases. *Science, 388*(6753). https://doi.org/10.1126/science.adx0043

Shin, H. J., Kim, I. S., Choi, S. G., Lee, K., Park, H., Shin, J., Kim, D., Beom, J., Yi, Y. Y., Gupta, D. P., Song, G. J., Chung, W. S., Lee, C. J., & Kim, D. W. (2024). Rejuvenating aged microglia by p16ink4a-siRNA-loaded nanoparticles increases amyloid-β clearance in animal models of alzheimer's disease. *Molecular Neurodegeneration, 19*(1). https://doi.org/10.1186/s13024-024-00715-x

Singer, O., Marr, R. A., Rockenstein, E., Crews, L., Coufal, N. G., Gage, F. H., Verma, I. M., & Masliah, E. (2005). Targeting BACE1 with siRNAs ameliorates alzheimer disease neuropathology in a transgenic model. *Nature Neuroscience, 8*(10), 1343–1349. https://doi.org/10.1038/nn1531

Sofroniew, M. V. (2015). Astrocyte barriers to neurotoxic inflammation. *Nature Reviews Neuroscience, 16*(5), 249–263. https://doi.org/10.1038/nrn3898

Sommer, A., Winner, B., & Prots, I. (2017). The trojan horse - neuroinflammatory impact of T cells in neurodegenerative diseases. *Molecular Neurodegeneration, 12*(1). https://doi.org/10.1186/s13024-017-0222-8

Soni, S. S., D'Elia, A. M., Alsasa, A., Cho, S., Tylek, T., O'Brien, E. M., Whitaker, R., Spiller, K. L., & Rodell, C. B. (2022). Sustained release of drug-loaded nanoparticles from injectable hydrogels enables long-term control of macrophage phenotype. *Biomaterials Science, 10*(24), 6951–6967. https://doi.org/10.1039/d2bm01113a

Srivastava, Y., Donta, M., Mireles, L. L., Paulucci-Holthauzen, A., Shi, L., Bedford, M. T., Waxham, M. N., & McCrea, P. D. (2024). Exploring the PDZ, DUF, and LIM domains of Pdlim5 in dendrite branching. *International Journal of Molecular Sciences, 25*(15). https://doi.org/10.3390/ijms25158326

Srivastava, Y., Donta, M., Mireles, L. L., Paulucci-Holthauzen, A., Waxham, M. N., & McCrea, P. D. (2024). Role of a Pdlim5:PalmD complex in directing dendrite morphology. *Frontiers in Cellular Neuroscience, 18*. https://doi.org/10.3389/fncel.2024.1315941

Stevenson, M. (2004). Therapeutic potential of RNA interference. *New England Journal of Medicine, 351*(17), 1772–1777. https://doi.org/10.1056/nejmra045004

Sulzer, D., Alcalay, R. N., Garretti, F., Cote, L., Kanter, E., Agin-Liebes, J., Liong, C., McMurtrey, C., Hildebrand, W. H., Mao, X., Dawson, V. L., Dawson, T. M., Oseroff, C., Pham, J., Sidney, J., Dillon, M. B., Carpenter, C., Weiskopf, D., Phillips, E., … Sette, A. (2017). T cells from patients with parkinson's disease recognize α-synuclein peptides. *Nature, 546*(7660), 656–661. https://doi.org/10.1038/nature22815

Sweeney, M. D., Sagare, A. P., & Zlokovic, B. V. (2018). Blood-brain barrier breakdown in alzheimer disease and other neurodegenerative disorders. *Nature Reviews Neurology, 14*(3), 133–150. https://doi.org/10.1038/nrneurol.2017.188

Tan, Y., Wang, Z., Liu, T., Gao, P., Xu, S., & Tan, L. (2022). RNA interference-mediated silencing of DNA methyltransferase 1 attenuates neuropathic pain by accelerating microglia M2 polarization. *BMC Neurology, 22*(1). https://doi.org/10.1186/s12883-022-02860-6

Tang, Y., & Le, W. (2016). Differential roles of M1 and M2 microglia in neurodegenerative diseases. *Molecular Neurobiology, 53*(2), 1181–1194. https://doi.org/10.1007/s12035-014-9070-5

Taylor, M. A., & Kokiko-Cochran, O. N. (2024). Context is key: Glucocorticoid receptor and corticosteroid therapeutics in outcomes after traumatic brain injury. *Frontiers in Cellular Neuroscience, 18*. https://doi.org/10.3389/fncel.2024.1351685

Tejera, D., Mercan, D., Caro, J. M. S.-, Hanan, M., Greenberg, D., Soreq, H., Latz, E., Golenbock, D., & Heneka, M. T. (2019). Systemic inflammation impairs microglial Aβ clearance through NLRP 3 inflammasome. *The EMBO Journal, 38*(17). https://doi.org/10.15252/embj.2018101064

Thome, A. D., Harms, A. S., Volpicelli-Daley, L. A., & Standaert, D. G. (2016). microRNA-155 regulates alpha-synuclein-induced inflammatory responses in models of parkinson disease. *Journal of Neuroscience, 36*(8), 2383–2390. https://doi.org/10.1523/JNEUROSCI.3900-15.2016

Tian, L., Ma, L., Kaarela, T., & Li, Z. (2012). Neuroimmune crosstalk in the central nervous system and its significance for neurological diseases. *Journal of Neuroinflammation, 9*(1). https://doi.org/10.1186/1742-2094-9-155

Tork, M. A. B., Fotouhi, S., Roozi, P., & Negah, S. S. (2025). Targeting NLRP3 inflammasomes: A trojan horse strategy for intervention in neurological disorders. *Molecular Neurobiology, 62*(2), 1840–1881. https://doi.org/10.1007/s12035-024-04359-2

Tripathy, D., & Grammas, P. (2009). Acetaminophen inhibits neuronal inflammation and protects neurons from oxidative stress. *Journal of Neuroinflammation, 6*(1), 10. https://doi.org/10.1186/1742-2094-6-10

Ulrich, J. D., Ulland, T. K., Colonna, M., & Holtzman, D. M. (2017). Elucidating the role of TREM2 in alzheimer's disease. *Neuron, 94*(2), 237–248. https://doi.org/10.1016/j.neuron.2017.02.042

van Olst, L., Coenen, L., Nieuwland, J. M., Rodriguez-Mogeda, C., de Wit, N. M., Kamermans, A., Middeldorp, J., & de Vries, H. E. (2022). Crossing borders in alzheimer's disease: A T cell's perspective. *Advanced Drug Delivery Reviews, 188*, 114398. https://doi.org/10.1016/j.addr.2022.114398

Vanhecke, D., & Janitz, M. (2005). Functional genomics using high-throughput RNA interference. *Drug Discovery Today, 10*(3), 205–212. https://doi.org/10.1016/s1359-6446(04)03352-5

Veerhuis, R., Nielsen, H. M., & Tenner, A. J. (2011). Complement in the brain. *Molecular Immunology, 48*(14), 1592–1603. https://doi.org/10.1016/j.molimm.2011.04.003

Velazquez, P., Cribbs, D. H., Poulos, T. L., & Tenner, A. J. (1997). Aspartate residue 7 in amyloid β-protein is critical for classical complement pathway activation: Implications for alzheimer's disease pathogenesis. *Nature Medicine, 3*(1), 77–79. https://doi.org/10.1038/nm0197-77

Venegas, C., Kumar, S., Franklin, B. S., Dierkes, T., Brinkschulte, R., Tejera, D., Vieira-Saecker, A., Schwartz, S., Santarelli, F., Kummer, M. P., Griep, A., Gelpi, E., Beilharz, M., Riedel, D., Golenbock, D. T., Geyer, M., Walter, J., Latz, E., & Heneka, M. T. (2017). Microglia-derived ASC specks crossseed amyloid-β in alzheimer's disease. *Nature, 552*(7685), 355–361. https://doi.org/10.1038/nature25158

Venken, K., Hellings, N., Thewissen, M., Somers, V., Hensen, K., Rummens, J. L., Medaer, R., Hupperts, R., & Stinissen, P. (2008). Compromised CD4+ CD25high regulatory T-cell function in patients with relapsing-remitting multiple sclerosis is correlated with a reduced frequency of FOXP3-positive cells and reduced FOXP3 expression at the single-cell level. *Immunology, 123*(1), 79–89. https://doi.org/10.1111/j.1365-2567.2007.02690.x

Wang, Q., Cheng, S., Qin, F., Fu, A., & Fu, C. (2021). Application progress of RVG peptides to facilitate the delivery of therapeutic agents into the central nervous system. *RSC Advances, 11*(15), 8505–8515. https://doi.org/10.1039/d1ra00550b

Wang, X., Ramat, A., Simonelig, M., & Liu, M. F. (2023). Emerging roles and functional mechanisms of PIWI-interacting RNAs. *Nature Reviews Molecular Cell Biology, 24*(2), 123–141. https://doi.org/10.1038/s41580-022-00528-0

Wang, C., Yue, H., Hu, Z., Shen, Y., Ma, J., Jie, L., Wang, X.-D., Wang, L., Sun, B., Shi, P., Wang, L., & Gu, Y. (2020a). Microglia mediate forgetting via complement-dependent synaptic elimination. *Science, 367*(6478), 688–694. https://doi.org/10.1126/science.aaz2288

Wang, Y., Lin, Y., Wang, L., Zhan, H., Luo, X., Zeng, Y., Wu, W., Zhang, X., & Wang, F. (2020b). TREM2 ameliorates neuroinflammatory response and cognitive impairment via PI3K/AKT/FoxO3a signaling pathway in Alzheimer's disease mice. *Aging, 12*(20), 20862–20879. https://doi.org/10.18632/aging.104104

Wang, X., Zhao, X., Zhong, Y., Shen, J., & An, W. (2022). Biomimetic exosomes: A new generation of drug delivery system. *Frontiers in Bioengineering and Biotechnology, 10.* https://doi.org/10.3389/fbioe.2022.865682

Wang, X., Zheng, X., Ma, C., & Zhao, L. (2015). Role of TRIF small interference RNA (siRNA) in chronic experimental allergic encephalomyelitis (EAE). *Medical Science Monitor, 21*, 2583–2587. https://doi.org/10.12659/MSM.894564

Winter, J., Jung, S., Keller, S., Gregory, R. I., & Diederichs, S. (2009). Many roads to maturity: MicroRNA biogenesis pathways and their regulation. *Nature Cell Biology, 11*(3), 228–234. https://doi.org/10.1038/ncb0309-228

Woodruff, T. M., Arumugam, T. V., Shiels, I. A., Reid, R. C., Fairlie, D. P., & Taylor, S. M. (2003). A potent human C5a receptor antagonist protects against disease pathology in a rat model of inflammatory bowel disease. *Journal of Immunology, 171*(10), 5514–5520. https://doi.org/10.4049/jimmunol.171.10.5514

Wraith, D. C., & Nicholson, L. B. (2012). The adaptive immune system in diseases of the central nervous system. *Journal of Clinical Investigation, 122*(4), 1172–1179. https://doi.org/10.1172/JCI58648

Xiao, H., Han, S., & Baigude, H. (2021). Regulation of microglia polarization via mannose receptor-mediated delivery of siRNA by ligand-functionalized DoGo LNP. *RSC Advances, 11*(52), 32549–32558. https://doi.org/10.1039/d1ra04293a

Xu, Wen, Huang, Y., & Zhou, R. (2025). NLRP3 inflammasome in neuroinflammation and central nervous system diseases. *Cellular and Molecular Immunology, 22*(4), 341–355. https://doi.org/10.1038/s41423-025-01275-w

Yan, Y., Ding, X., Li, K., Ciric, B., Wu, S., Xu, H., Gran, B., Rostami, A., & Zhang, G.-X. (2012). CNS-specific therapy for ongoing EAE by silencing IL-17 pathway in astrocytes. *Molecular Therapy, 20*(7), 1338–1348. https://doi.org/10.1038/mt.2012.12

Yang, G., Meng, Y., Li, W., Yong, Y., Fan, Z., Ding, H., Youzhen, W., Luo, J., & Ke, Z.-J. (2011). Neuronal MCP-1 mediates microglia recruitment and neurodegeneration induced by the mild impairment of oxidative metabolism. *Brain Pathology, 21*(3), 279–297. https://doi.org/10.1111/j.1750-3639.2010.00445.x

Yi, S., Karabin, N. B., Zhu, J., Bobbala, S., Lyu, H., Li, S., Liu, Y., Frey, M., Vincent, M., & Scott, E. A. (2020). An injectable hydrogel platform for sustained delivery of anti-inflammatory nanocarriers and induction of regulatory T cells in atherosclerosis. *Frontiers in Bioengineering and Biotechnology, 8.* https://doi.org/10.3389/fbioe.2020.00542

Yshii, L., Pasciuto, E., Bielefeld, P., Mascali, L., Lemaitre, P., Marino, M., Dooley, J., Kouser, L., Verschoren, S., Lagou, V., Kemps, H., Gervois, P., Boer, A.de, Burton, O. T., Wahis, J., Verhaert, J., Tareen, S. H. K., Roca, C. P., Singh, K., … Liston, A. (2022). Astrocyte-targeted gene delivery of interleukin 2 specifically increases brain-resident regulatory T cell numbers and protects against pathological neuroinflammation. *Nature Immunology, 23*(6), 878–891. https://doi.org/10.1038/s41590-022-01208-z

Zamanian, J. L., Xu, L., Foo, L. C., Nouri, N., Zhou, L., Giffard, R. G., & Barres, B. A. (2012). Genomic analysis of reactive astrogliosis. *Journal of Neuroscience, 32*(18), 6391–6410. https://doi.org/10.1523/JNEUROSCI.6221-11.2012

Zeng, J., Liao, Z., Yang, H., Wang, Q., Wu, Z., Hua, F., & Zhou, Z. (2024). T cell infiltration mediates neurodegeneration and cognitive decline in alzheimer's disease. *Neurobiology of Disease, 193*, 106461. https://doi.org/10.1016/j.nbd.2024.106461

Zeng, Y., Wagner, E. J., & Cullen, B. R. (2002). Both natural and designed micro RNAs can inhibit the expression of cognate mRNAs when expressed in human cells. *Molecular Cell, 9*(6), 1327–1333. https://doi.org/10.1016/S1097-2765(02)00541-5

Zhang, L., Chen, P., Chen, T., Lin, L., Ji, X., Liu, J., Huang, H., Saravanan, T., Fuehrer, H., Ross, C. A., Smith, W. W., Zhong, P., & Chen, X. (2025a). In vivo self-assembled siRNAs within small extracellular vesicles attenuate LRRK2-induced neurodegeneration in parkinson's disease models. *Journal of Controlled Release, 378*, 1139–1153. https://doi.org/10.1016/j.jconrel.2024.12.045

Zhang, L., Hou, S., Movahedi, F., Li, Z., Li, L., Hu, J., Jia, Y., Huang, Y., Zhu, J., Sun, X., Zeng, L., Liu, R., & Xu, Z. P. (2023a). Amyloid-β/Tau burden and neuroinflammation dual-targeted nanomedicines synergistically restore memory and recognition of alzheimer's disease mice. *Nano Today, 49*. https://doi.org/10.1016/j.nantod.2023.101788

Zhang, W. H., Jiang, L., Li, M., & Liu, J. (2023b). MicroRNA-124: An emerging therapeutic target in central nervous system disorders. *Experimental Brain Research, 241*(5), 1215–1226. https://doi.org/10.1007/s00221-022-06524-2

Zhang, B., Wei, Y. Z., Wang, G. Q., Li, D. D., Shi, J. S., & Zhang, F. (2019). Targeting MAPK pathways by naringenin modulates microglia M1/M2 polarization in lipopolysaccharide-stimulated cultures. *Frontiers in Cellular Neuroscience, 12*. https://doi.org/10.3389/fncel.2018.00531

Zhang, W., Xiao, D., Mao, Q., & Xia, H. (2023c). Role of neuroinflammation in neurodegeneration development. *Signal Transduction and Targeted Therapy, 8*(1). https://doi.org/10.1038/s41392-023-01486-5

Zhang, J., Zhao, M., Yan, R., Liu, J., Maddila, S., Junn, E., & Maral Mouradian, M. (2021). MicroRNA-7 protects against neurodegeneration induced by α-Synuclein preformed fibrils in the mouse brain. *Neurotherapeutics, 18*(4), 2529–2540. https://doi.org/10.1007/s13311-021-01130-6

Zhang, Y., Zou, Z., Li, R., Fu, X., Li, G., Wang, L., Zhang, Y., Chen, Y., Chen, Z., Yang, D., Jiao, Y., Zhang, W., Mei, T., Tan, L., Cao, Y., & Yin, C. (2025b). DTX1 modulates microglial M1 polarization and exacerbates neuroinflammation in traumatic brain injury model rats through NF—κB/IRF5. *Molecular Neurobiology, 62*(11), 14140–14155. https://doi.org/10.1007/s12035-025-05200-0

Zharikov, A. D., Cannon, J. R., Tapias, V., Bai, Q., Horowitz, M. P., Shah, V., El Ayadi, A., Hastings, T. G., Greenamyre, J. T., & Burton, E. A. (2015). ShRNA targeting α-synuclein prevents neurodegeneration in a parkinson's disease model. *Journal of Clinical Investigation, 125*(7), 2721–2735. https://doi.org/10.1172/JCI64502

Zhong, L., Sheng, X., Wang, W., Li, Y., Zhuo, R., Wang, K., Zhang, L., Hu, D.-D., Hong, Y., Chen, L., Rao, H., Li, T., Chen, M., Lin, Z., Zhang, Y.-wu, Wang, X., Yan, X.-X., Chen, X., Bu, G., & Chen, X.-F. (2023). TREM2 receptor protects against complement-mediated synaptic loss by binding to complement C1q during neurodegeneration. *Immunity, 56*(8), 1794. https://doi.org/10.1016/j.immuni.2023.06.016

Zou, W., Kou, L., Wang, Y., Jin, Z., Xiong, N., Wang, T., & Xia, Y. (2025). Complement C4 exacerbates astrocyte-mediated neuroinflammation and promotes α-synuclein pathology in Parkinson's disease. *Npj Parkinson's Disease, 11*(1). https://doi.org/10.1038/s41531-025-01005-z

CHAPTER

Immune cells and nanotechnology: Innovations in therapy

11

Ruth Naomi[1], Santhra Segaran Balan[2], Saiful Irwan Zubairi[3], Shariff Halim[4], Pamela David[5] and Roslee Rajikan[6]

[1]*Institute of Ocean and Earth Sciences, Universiti Malaya, Kuala Lumpur, Malaysia;* [2]*Faculty of Health and Life Sciences, Management and Science University, Shah Alam, Selangor, Malaysia;* [3]*Department of Food Sciences, Faculty of Science and Technology, Universiti Kebangsaan Malaysia, Bangi, Selangor, Malaysia;* [4]*Universiti Teknologi MARA (UiTM), Penang Branch Bertam Campus, Kepala Batas, Pulau Pinang, Malaysia;* [5]*Department of Anatomy, Faculty of Medicine, Universiti Malaya, Kuala Lumpur, Malaysia;* [6]*Centre for Healthy Aging and Wellness, Faculty of Health Sciences, Universiti Kebangsaan Malaysia, Kuala Lumpur, Malaysia*

1. Introduction

The blood–brain barrier (BBB), composed of endothelial cells, pericytes, and astrocytes, maintains CNS homeostasis by selectively restricting molecular and cellular entry from peripheral circulation (Dotiwala et al., 2018). This highly regulated interface undergoes dynamic crosstalk with perivascular macrophages and microglia, wherein alterations in systemic inflammatory states can promote endothelial dysfunction and increase BBB permeability (Mayer & Fischer, 2024). The BBB's role extends beyond passive protection, it actively engages in immune surveillance through the glymphatic system and meningeal lymphatic vessels, which facilitate antigen and immune cell trafficking between the CNS and deep cervical lymph nodes (Li et al., 2022). Peripheral inflammation disrupts BBB integrity through multiple mechanisms including tight junction protein degradation, enabling pathogenic immune cell infiltration into the CNS (Galea, 2021). Microglia, the CNS resident macro Fig. 11.1 phages, continuously monitor brain homeostasis and rapidly activate upon injury or infection, adopting pro-inflammatory or anti-inflammatory phenotypes (Mayer & Fischer, 2024). These cells regulate neuroinflammation through production of cytokines including TNF-α, IL-1β, and IL-10, with dysregulated activation contributing substantially to neurodegeneration (Smith et al., 2012) Fig. 11.1. Astrocytes, the most abundant glial cells, maintain BBB integrity and regulate neuroinflammation through expression of MHC molecules and production of both pro- and anti-inflammatory mediators (Brambilla, 2019). In reactive states, astrocytes undergo morphological changes and altered cytokine production that either support neuronal survival (Kim et al., 2026). T cell subsets play pivotal roles in CNS immune regulation, with pathogenic Th1 and Th17 cells driving demyelination and neuronal damage while regulatory T cells (Tregs) suppress pro-inflammatory responses (Xu Lou et al., 2025). Cytokine dysregulation, characterized by elevated pro-inflammatory mediators (TNF-α, IL-1β, IL-6, IL-17) and

Immunotherapies for Neurological Disorders. https://doi.org/10.1016/B978-0-443-44631-3.00008-1

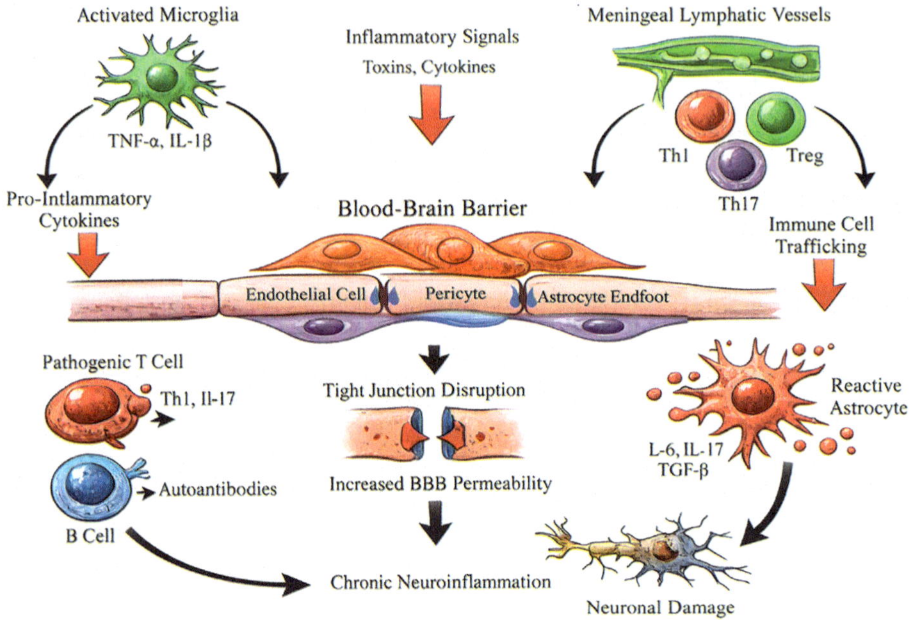

FIGURE 11.1 Blood–Brain Barrier (BBB) Disruption During Neuroinflammation.

Inflammatory signals and activated microglia release pro-inflammatory cytokines (e.g., TNF-α, IL-1β), leading to tight junction breakdown and increased BBB permeability. Immune cell trafficking (Th1, Th17, treg) and autoantibody-producing B cells further amplify inflammation, while reactive astrocytes contribute to chronic neuroinflammation, ultimately resulting in neuronal damage.

reduced anti-inflammatory cytokines (IL-10, TGF-β) is an indicator of chronic neuroinflammation (Khaiboullina, 2026). Autoimmune neurological disorders result from pathogenic T and B cell responses against CNS antigens, triggering cascading neuroinflammatory responses that amplify neuronal damage (Goverman, 2009). Chronic neuroinflammation, while initially protective, transitions to a pathogenic state characterized by sustained microglial activation, astrocyte dysfunction, and production of neurotoxic mediators that collectively drive neurodegeneration (Kwon & Koh, 2020).

2. Limitations of conventional therapeutics

The BBB's highly selective permeability restricts CNS penetration of most systemically administered therapeutics, with the vast majority of biologics and >90% of small molecules failing to achieve therapeutic concentrations in brain parenchyma (Schreiner et al., 2025). Antibody-based immunotherapies required for targeting specific neuronal autoantigens encounter insurmountable BBB penetration barriers due to their large molecular size and negative charge (Ramapriyan et al., 2023). Intrathecal delivery, while bypassing the BBB, remains impractical for chronic disease management due to invasiveness, limited distribution volume, and rapid cerebrospinal fluid clearance (Schreiner et al., 2025). Conventional immunosuppressants achieve clinical efficacy through global immune suppression, rendering patients vulnerable to opportunistic infections and malignancy (Iizuka et al., 2025). Corticosteroids, the first-line therapy for many acute neurological conditions, cause dose-dependent adverse effects including thromboembolic events, myopathy, osteoporosis, diabetes, and psychiatric disorders (Yasir et al., 2018). Monoclonal antibodies targeting immune cell subsets demonstrate antigen specificity yet trigger serious adverse effects. Alemtuzumab causes delayed thyroid autoimmunity, immune thrombocytopenia, and intracranial hemorrhage, while natalizumab carries progressive multifocal leukoencephalopathy risk (Li et al., 2018). Ocrelizumab-related autoimmune diabetes and widespread secondary autoimmunity further demonstrate the consequences of indiscriminate B-cell depletion (Grasso et al., 2023). Corticosteroids and plasmapheresis exert broadly suppressive effects across multiple immune populations without discrimination between pathogenic and protective responses, compromising host defense and immune homeostasis (Coutinho & Chapman, 2011). Even antibody-based therapies achieve only partial specificity, depleting pathogenic autoreactive B cells simultaneously eliminates protective B cells essential for immune defense (Hansel et al., 2010).

3. Nanotechnology in neurotherapeutics

Liposomes are spherical lipid bilayer vesicles that encapsulate hydrophilic drugs in their aqueous core and lipophilic agents within the membrane, offering excellent biocompatibility and reduced immunogenicity through PEGylation (Taher et al., 2023). Polymeric nanoparticles, particularly poly(lactic-co-glycolic acid) (PLGA) and biodegradable polymers, provide sustained drug release, tunable surface properties, and capacity for ligand conjugation, with FDA approval for multiple clinical applications (Alsaab et al., 2022). Dendrimers are highly branched tree-like polymers with multiple terminal groups enabling controlled drug loading and surface modification, facilitating multivalent targeting (Chauhan, 2018). Quantum dots are inorganic nanomaterials exhibiting unique photochemical properties enabling real-time fluorescence tracking and imaging alongside therapeutic delivery (Matea et al., 2017). Exosomes, naturally occurring 30–150 nm lipid vesicles derived from cells, offer superior biocompatibility, inherent targeting capabilities through surface proteins, and natural BBB penetration (Abdelsalam et al., 2023). Nanomicelles are self-assembled polymeric structures with core-shell architecture optimizing drug solubilization and providing prolonged circulation (Wei et al., 2015). BBB penetration mechanisms occur via multiple transcytosis pathways, including receptor-mediated transcytosis using nanoparticles with ligands for transferrin, lactoferrin, insulin, or angiopep receptors expressed on brain endothelial cells, achieving 17.2% injected dose per gram accumulation in preclinical glioma models (Haqqani et al., 2024). Adsorptive-mediated transcytosis occurs through nanoparticle positive charge interactions with negatively charged endothelial surface components (Hervé et al., 2008). Cell-penetrating peptides fused to nanoparticle surfaces facilitate transendothelial migration through direct cellular uptake mechanisms (Zhu et al., 2019). Immune targeting functionalization directs nanoparticles to specific immune cell populations through surface-conjugated antibodies or aptamers recognizing CD33, CD123, folate receptors, or other immune-cell-expressed antigens (Kochman et al., 2026). Passive targeting enhanced permeability and retention (EPR) effects wherein nanoparticles preferentially accumulate at inflamed CNS sites due to increased vascular permeability (Kujundziski & Chamovska, 2025). Active targeting uses ligand-receptor interactions, directing nanoparticles specifically to disease-relevant cells or tissues (Ding et al., 2025).

Temperature-sensitive and redox-responsive systems discharge therapeutics in response to elevated local temperatures or elevated ROS characteristic of inflammatory sites (Alamos-Musre et al., 2025).

4. Nanotechnology-based immunomodulation in neurological disorders

4.1 Immunosuppression

Immunosuppression treatment involves the generalized repression of the immune system using either corticosteroids, intravenous immunoglobulin, plasma exchange, and cyclophosphamide, methotrexate, and infliximab (Foster et al., 2023). The mechanism of action for immunosuppressants varies. For instance, corticosteroids exert their activity by binding to the glucocorticoid receptor (GR) and mineralocorticoid receptor (MR) in the brain (Spencer-Segal, 2019). A low dose of corticosteroid administration (2 mg/kg) for 3 days is able to suppress pro-inflammatory mediators. At the same time, it enhances the release of anti-inflammatory cytokines, thereby repressing neuroinflammation and neuronal damage (Yang et al., 2023). A similar mechanism is also noted in intravenous immunoglobulin, where it inhibits the action of B-cells and prevents the activation of T-cells. In this case, the pathogenic autoantibodies become neutralized, which leads to the modulation of dendritic cells (Dimitriadou et al., 2020). It also suppresses the Toll-like receptors (TLRs), pro-inflammatory and apoptotic gene expressions, thereby preventing neuronal apoptosis (Lok et al., 2015). Meanwhile, plasma exchange decreases circulating inflammatory cytokines (Strasser, 2023) modulates the T helper cell, complements activating antibodies, improves the function of macrophage/monocyte stimulates the plasma cells and B cell proliferation, thus reduces neurological symptoms (Roganovic et al., 2024). Another plausible mechanism of action of immunosuppressants (local corticosteroids) enhances myelination via GR in Schwann cells, thereby promoting neurogenesis and neuroprotection (Cuoco et al., 2019). Another mechanism of corticosteroids is via cell cycle arrest and apoptosis in the T and B cells through p38 mitogen-activated protein kinase-dependent pathway, and is able to reduce neurological-associated symptoms by 50% within a 1-week course of corticosteroids (Cuoco et al., 2019). Although immunosuppressants are known for their positive outcome, some of the drawbacks are negligible. Some of the most documented side effects of corticosteroids for the improvement of neurological conditions include thromboembolic events, myopathy, osteoporosis, diabetes, gastrointestinal bleeding, vascular complications, and psychiatric disorders (Versteeg et al., 2022).

5. Antibodies

Antibody-based immunotherapy is another form of immunotherapy that has been widely used to treat neurological conditions. The effectiveness of antibody-based immunotherapy depends on the fragment of antigen binding (Fab) and crystallizable capacity (Fc) (Ruck et al., 2022). In these, antibodies designed to act on intracellular antigens often exhibit cytotoxic effects against effector T-cell-mediated injury. Meanwhile, antibodies designed to act on neuronal surface proteins (extracellular antigens) exhibit pathogenic effects (Linnoila & Pittock, 2016). Some of the FDA-approved antibody-based immunotherapies include calcitonin gene-related peptide (CGRP) receptor inhibitors such as Erenumab, Fremanezumab, Galcanezumab, and Eptinezumab. CGRP is the main target for migraine conditions. Meanwhile, Aducanumab is used for AD, where this drug mainly targets amyloid-β aggregation (Ruck et al., 2022), and for relapsing–remitting MS (Havrdova et al., 2017). Antibodies exhibit their action either via blocking the action of membrane receptors, binding with effector molecules and interacting with their ligands (immunoglobulins), complement proteins, and initiating cell depletion (Sun et al., 2023). The plausible explanation for the action of antibodies is based on IgG, which naturally possesses the ability to recognize specific antigens through its Fab domains, while its Fc region acts as the interaction domain for immune effector molecules. This is because IgG is composed of two heavy and two light chains linked by disulfide bonds, while the Fab comprises two identical moieties that enable recognition of antigen specificity via their complementarity-determining regions. Upon detecting any foreign antigen, Fab domains may immediately neutralize the pathogen to prevent infection. The Fc domain binds with its receptor and stimulates the function of immune effectors (c-type lectins) to recognize opsonized antigens by binding with the C1q component of the complement system as well as with Fc receptors. This is where the CH2 of the Fc domain attaches with the IgG-Fc N-glycan (core structure of N-acetylglucosamine) to the asparagine 297 (N297) residues. These mechanisms apply to both monoclonal and polyclonal antibody functions (Ruck et al., 2022).

Although antibody-based immunotherapy is widely accepted and approved by the FDA, it still comes with some limitations and adverse effects. Some of the documented adverse effects of alemtuzumab (CD52-depleting/humanized monoclonal antibody) include quarterly thyroid function abnormalities (thyroid autoimmunity) after 48 months of the last course of alemtuzumab, immune thrombocytopenia, nephropathies (Havrdova et al., 2017), repopulation of the $CD19^{+}$ B-cell subset (Baker et al., 2017), and intracranial hemorrhage (Brown & Coles, 2013). Studies have shown that homeostatic proliferation could be a possible explanation for the reconstitution phase, which can lead to oligoclonal expansions and skewed repertoires, resulting in a responsive environment for autoreactive clones that may induce such adverse effects in the case of alemtuzumab administration (Jones et al., 2013). In addition, the development of multifocal leukoencephalopathy has been documented with the administration of Natalizumab, a monoclonal antibody used in the treatment of MS, which targets alpha4 integrin receptors (Vivekanandan et al., 2021). Furthermore, autoimmune diabetes has been reported in cases involving 6 months of ocrelizumab administration, a CD20-depleting antibody (Grasso et al., 2023).

6. Recombinant proteins

Recombinant proteins are artificially produced proteins comprising native protein structures with the combination of second-generation proteins (Pham, 2018). Protein modification techniques are usually used to produce recombinant proteins, such as glycosylation, and these proteins are usually highly target-specific (Clark & Pazdernik, 2016). There are a wide range of recombinant proteins being used to treat neurological conditions, and their mechanisms of action vary. They mostly possess the ability to target hidden epitopes and cross the BBB, demonstrate higher levels of stability and solubility, withstand heat denaturation, and allow low-cost production on a large scale (Manoutcharian & Gevorkian, 2024). One common example is Natalizumab, a recombinant protein used as a treatment option for MS via the intravenous route. This protein possesses the ability to block vascular adhesion molecule interaction by binding with the α-4 β-1 integrin. As a result, mononuclear leukocytes are hindered from crossing the endothelium of the BBB and entering the CNS. Another common recombinant protein used is Tocilizumab, which suppresses inflammation and is specifically designed to target the IL-6 receptor (Ginestal-López, 2018) in neuromyelitis optica spectrum disorder (NMOSD). It has been proven to be effective in preventing relapsing episodes in NMOSD within just 3 months of administration, with significant improvement in ambulatory motor function, pain, and fatigue (Du et al., 2021).

Aside from this, anti-α-synuclein and anti-leucine-rich repeat kinase 2 (LRRK2) recombinant proteins are prescribed for the treatment of Parkinson's Disease (PD). The anti-α-synuclein exhibits its function by binding with intracellular α-synuclein preformed fibrils and oligomers, preventing aggregation and the cytotoxic effects of α-synuclein in the PD brain. At the same time, anti-α-synuclein binds with high affinity to the 38-amino-acid domain of apolipoprotein B (ApoB) in the LDL receptor to improve brain penetration. As a result, this action suppresses neuroinflammation, dopaminergic neuronal loss in the neocortex and hippocampus, and motor dysfunction, thereby improving the concentration of proinflammatory cytokines (TNF-α and IL-6) in the microglia (Manoutcharian & Gevorkian, 2024). Similarly, administration of α-synuclein in the PD in vivo model shows an adaptive immune response mediated by CD4-positive cells, with infiltration of Foxp3-positive cells in the nigrostriatal system, causing a reduction in α-synuclein in the substantia nigra region of the basal ganglia (Mortada et al., 2021), thereby attenuating neurological symptoms. Although recombinant proteins have been proven effective, they also come with certain limitations. For instance, administration of Natalizumab carries the risk of progressive multifocal leukoencephalopathy and, in rare cases, hypersensitivity reactions at infusion. Thus, caution is needed, especially in patients with previous encephalic MRI, with anti-JCV testing recommended every 6 months in seronegative patients (Ginestal-López, 2018).

7. Peptides

Peptides comprise amino acids that are attached together by peptide bonds to form small molecules. Usually, peptides are designed to act as target-specific agents, reaching regions that are hardly accessible by conventional drugs. Thus, peptides serve as an important component in the management of neurological conditions. One significant aspect of peptide immunotherapy is its capacity to induce immune tolerance and promote bystander effects. Studies highlight that peptide immunotherapy can result in immune deviation, enhancing regulatory T-cell responses while dampening harmful allergic reactions, particularly in allergic disease contexts (Moldaver et al., 2019). This phenomenon can be valuable in CNS applications, where immune dysregulation can exacerbate disease or lead to unwanted side effects. Moreover, peptide therapies have shown the potential for durability in treatment responses, as evidenced by persistent effects observed in patients following prolonged peptide administration (Patel et al., 2013). To date, several synthetic and natural peptides are being used to treat neurological conditions. For instance, Aβ (16-20) KLVFF is being used to treat AD, NAPVSIPQ (NAP) for PD, Vasoactive Intestinal Peptides (VIP) for Huntington's disease, Polyglutamine Binding Peptide-1 (QBP1) for Dentatorubral-pallidoluysian atrophy (DRPLA) (Yadav et al., 2021), mimetic peptide for demyelinating disorders, and microglial healing peptide for ischemic strokes. Peptides modulate the immune system by creating immune tolerance, acting as immunomodulators in the CNS. This is achieved by activating the T-cell response, where the peptide identifies pathogens and removes them by initiating an interaction between the antigenic peptides and the T-cell receptor. As a result, the T-cell undergoes clonal expansion, causing a targeted immune response (Karati et al., 2025).

However, the mechanism of action of each peptide varies based on the target-specific cells. For instance, the mimetic peptide is targeted to ameliorate hippocampal inflammation and regulate cytokine secretion, while the fibroblast growth loop peptide is effective in stimulating ERK signaling mediators and activating receptor dimerization. The outcome of both designed peptides, however, improves cognition (Downer et al., 2009). In contrast, the development of cell-penetrating peptides (CPP) has recently garnered attention due to their ability to cross the blood-brain barrier (BBB), interact with brain cells, and exit the cells via transcytosis, thereby delivering drugs directly into neuronal cells. It has been proven that 80% of CPPs can successfully reach the brain parenchyma to exhibit maximum potential action (Stalmans et al., 2015). Aside from this, certain emerging neuroprotective peptides have been developed, such as R18 polyarginine and arginine, which have shown promising outcomes in stroke. The effect is seen just 24 h after administration, where there is a significant reduction in the total infarct volume in the permanent middle cerebral artery occlusion animal model (Milani et al., 2016). However, peptide-based immunotherapy has the potential to trigger neurological side effects. Treatments such as immune checkpoint inhibitors, particularly designed to target PD-1 and CTLA-4 pathways, have been linked to various neurological toxicities, including autoimmune encephalitis, CNS inflammation, and peripheral neuropathies (Albarrán et al., 2022). These adverse events often stem from an increased level of immune activity, where immune cells misidentify neural structures as targets, which may result in conditions like encephalitis or mononeuritis multiplex (Cossu et al., 2022; Liao et al., 2014). In some cases, peptide therapy designed to promote immune tolerance may fail, thereby intensifying autoimmune attacks against host antigens within neural tissues (Weiner et al., 2011). Complications like cytokine release syndrome and therapy-induced neurotoxicity show how inflammatory cascades can trigger neurological symptoms such as confusion, seizures, and delirium (Lee et al., 2019).

8. Altered peptide ligands

Altered peptide ligands (APLs) are designed from the primary antigenic peptide with a particular residue (amino acid) that has been substituted. They can be categorized as either full agonists, partial agonists, weak agonists, or non-stimulatory ligands. The full agonist functions to stimulate T-cells, while the partial or weak agonists or more commonly known as antagonists, suppress the activity of agonists. The non-stimulatory ligands, as the name suggests, do not stimulate the action of T-cells (Yachi et al., 2006). Since the main target of APLs is T-cells, it is suggested to use them for conditions involving T–cell pathology, such as autoimmune encephalomyelitis (Nicholson et al., 1995) and MS (Conlon & Steinman, 2002). The mechanism of action also varies based on the designed peptide, although it still targets the T-cell. In case of autoimmune encephalomyelitis, APLs function by inducing $CD4^+$ T cells with a cross-reactive, regulatory phenotype rather than blocking MHC binding. These T cells produce Th2 (IL-4 and IL-10) and Th0 (IFNγ and IL-10) cytokines. A, shifting the immune response away from a purely Th1 (pathogenic) profile. Upon encountering the native myelin proteolipid protein, these cross-reactive T cells are activated and ameliorate the severity of autoimmune encephalomyelitis and CNS inflammation (Nicholson et al., 1995). One of the primary areas where APLs are used is in the treatment of neurological conditions to manipulate N-Methyl-D-Aspartate (NMDA) and α-amino-3-hydroxy-5-methyl-4-isoxazolepropionic acid (AMPA) receptors. These are known as glutamate receptors and are usually targeted in AD, as they are essential for excitatory synaptic transmission and neuron survival (Kiyonaka et al., 2018). However, in certain cases, polyarginine peptides hinder neuronal apoptosis through the suppression of mitochondrial stress and ROS (Ugale et al., 2024). Although APL is one of the choices for treating neurological conditions, adverse effects are still unavoidable in rare circumstances. One of the reported side effects is immune hyperactivation, as the primary target of APL is immune system modulation. Such hyperactivation may lead to inflammation and tissue damage (Perera et al., 2015). One recent study reported that APL leads to elevated cytokine release, which stimulates chronic inflammation and T-cell apoptosis, eventually leading to compromised immune function of the T-cells (Duru et al., 2020). This is further supported by the outcomes observed by Cloake et al., (Cloake et al. 2014) and Kammona & Kiparissides (Kammona & Kiparissides, 2020), where immune APL induced increased T-cell activity with suppressed levels of regulatory T-cell activity in MS.

9. Vaccines

Vaccines are a type of immunotherapy commonly used in AD, PD, and MS. The mechanism of action can be said to be disease-specific. This is because, in the case of AD, the vaccines tend to activate the immune response to synthesize antibodies, which will bind to Aβ or tau proteins, preventing their aggregation (Wisniewski, 2009). Liposome-based tau vaccines (ACI-35 vaccine) are known for their effectiveness in AD, improving cognition in the mouse model of tauopathy (Pihlgren et al., 2016). Meanwhile, in PD, the vaccines target α-synuclein misfolding and aggregation. Thus, the administration of the vaccine promotes the removal of protein aggregation by activating microglial function and improving neuron survival (Teil et al., 2020). In MS, the vaccine will compete with autoantigens for binding on antigen-presenting cells. This action mainly aims to redirect T cell responses from producing damaging pro-inflammatory cytokines (Jakimovski et al., 2020). For MS, the BCG vaccine is still under investigation, and it is proven to stimulate regulatory T cell responses and promote the polarisation of microglia and astrocytes, enhancing neuroprotective effects (Cossu et al., 2022). To support this statement, animal models have shown promising outcomes, where a reduced number of T cell proliferations against myelin antigens and an increased level of anti-inflammatory cytokine synthesis have been recorded (Cossu et al., 2022). Further studies have shown that in both in vitro and in vivo studies, suppression by BCG drives plasmacytoid dendritic cells to stimulate suppressive regulatory T cells, reducing T cell responses and neuroinflammation (Letscher et al., 2021). Despite the effectiveness of vaccine-based immunotherapies in neurological conditions, there are some drawbacks that may be due to individual variability. One of the recorded side effects is meningoencephalitis, where the development of a pathogenic Th1-type immune response was recorded in AD subjects during the Aβ vaccine trials (Triplett et al., 2025). The diversity of reported side effects could be due to certain factors, including age, sex, and the individual microbiome, which may affect the immune response. Among these, women are known to exhibit stronger susceptibility toward immune reactions and autoimmune responses (Rio et al., 2024). However, upon weighing the positive and negative aspects, there are some approved first-line or early second-line vaccine-based immunotherapies for MS, such as glatiramer acetate (Tselis et al., 2007), while synapsin or α-synuclein vaccines for PD are still in the clinical trial phase (Alfaidi et al., 2025).

10. DNA vaccination

DNA vaccination is a type of immunization that is used to stimulate the host cellular system to induce antigen-specific immune responses. The expressed antigen stimulates both humoral and cellular immunity by delivering plasmid DNA encoding target antigens into host cells. Once introduced into muscle or dendritic cells, the DNA migrates to the nucleus, is transcribed into mRNA, and translated into antigenic proteins, which may then activate $CD4^+$ helper and $CD8^+$ cytotoxic T cells (Shedlock & Weiner, 2000). Their immunogenicity can be improved via electroporation (Flingai et al., 2013). DNA vaccines are known for their non-replicating, non-infectious nature, long shelf life, and ability to elicit both antibody-mediated and cytotoxic T-cell responses, as well as genetic flexibility, which enables the encoding of multiple or modified antigens for specific immunotherapy (Shedlock & Weiner, 2000). In neurological conditions, DNA vaccines stimulate antigen-specific immune responses to pathogenic proteins while minimizing global immune suppression. For instance, in AD, DNA vaccines targeting Aβ oligomers have been shown to neutralize these aggregates and modulate synaptic function (Sha et al., 2022). In these studies, vaccines such as AV-1955 and AdPEDI-(A1–6)11 have shown reductions in both amyloid and tau pathologies (Martins et al., 2017). Meanwhile, in MS, DNA vaccines encoding myelin oligodendrocyte glycoprotein have induced regulatory T cells that suppress inflammatory Th1 and Th17 responses and promote neuroprotection (Fissolo et al., 2012). The immunological mechanism of DNA vaccination involves antigen uptake, where DNA taken up by host cells produces antigens that are processed via endogenous and exogenous pathways (Shedlock & Weiner, 2000). However, the vaccine's outcome still depends on the delivery method, adjuvants, and route of administration. For instance, intramuscular delivery promotes enhanced antigen expression, while intradermal delivery stimulates skin-resident dendritic cells (Flingai et al., 2013). Besides, vaccine efficacy also depends on genetic and epigenetic factors (Postigo-Fernandez et al., 2022). Epigenetic modifications, such as DNA methylation and histone acetylation, regulate immune gene expression and long-term memory responses. Thus, gene adjuvants that optimize epigenetic control can further enhance vaccine efficacy (Kozak & Hu, 2024). Although DNA vaccines are generally safe, rare adverse events have been observed. The AN-1792 trial in AD revealed autoimmune encephalitis due to nonspecific T-cell activation (Gelinas et al., 2004; Lambracht-Washington & Rosenberg, 2012), while HSP-DNA vaccines in animals demonstrated no autoimmunity (Lima et al., 2009).

11. Cell therapy

Cell therapy uses modified or expanded ex vivo living active cells to induce specific immune responses or tolerance (Kurilin et al., 2024). It is now used to treat neurological conditions such as MS, and neuromyelitis optica (Mantica & Drappatz, 2023). In these conditions, cell therapy can retrain the immune system to either amplify protective responses or induce tolerance, enhancing antigen-specific modulation without general immunosuppression (Zubizarreta et al., 2019). In autoimmune conditions, cell therapies promote regulatory immune subsets like Tregs that suppress inflammation and support remyelination (Fissolo et al., 2012). Among cell therapy types, dendritic cell therapy uses autologous dendritic cells produced ex vivo and loaded with disease-specific antigens to modulate immunity (Kurilin et al., 2024). For MS, dendritic cells loaded with myelin or aquaporin-4 peptides are designed to promote antigen-specific tolerance by inducing IL-10–secreting Tregs (Zubizarreta et al., 2019). The mechanisms of cell therapies are mainly through antigen modulation, cytotoxicity, and immune regulation. These are usually achieved via MHC pathways that activate $CD8^+$ and $CD4^+$ T cells, driving selective immune activation for neuroprotection (Kurilin et al., 2024). Upon activation, adoptive cytotoxic T cells recognize antigens through MHC I and kill targeted cells, a process involved in autoimmunity modulation (Chen et al., 2024; Lobbous et al., 2024). Tregs and tolerogenic dendritic cells induce immune tolerance by inhibiting Th1 and Th17 activity and promoting anti-inflammatory cytokines such as IL-10 and TGF-β, thereby reducing CNS inflammation (Fissolo et al., 2012; Zubizarreta et al., 2019). However, safety remains a concern for cell therapy as an immunotherapy in neurological conditions, as autoimmunity is still a risk. Cell therapies targeting self-antigens may trigger inflammation, as seen in AD (Fu et al., 2024). Nevertheless, proper epitope selection has also been shown to mitigate such effects in preclinical studies (Talucci & Maric, 2024).

12. Gene therapy

Gene therapy is another form of immunotherapy used to treat neurological disorders (Keeler et al., 2018). Gene therapy-based immunotherapy in neurological conditions exhibits its mechanism via liver-targeted gene transfer to induce antigen-specific immune tolerance. For instance, in MS, adeno-associated virus (AAV) vectors can deliver disease-relevant antigens like myelin oligodendrocyte glycoprotein to hepatocytes, exploiting the liver's tolerogenic properties. This will enhance the synthesis of functional regulatory T cells (Keeler et al., 2018). The immunological basis for gene therapy in MS is driven by autoreactive T and B cell responses against CNS antigens (Hohlfeld & Wekerle, 2004). Recent evidence shows that memory B cells are also major targets for effective immunotherapy, with current MS treatments functionally depleting $CD19^+$, $CD27^+$ memory B cells (Baker et al., 2017). AAV vectors have become the preferred delivery vehicle for CNS gene therapy immunomodulation due to their favorable safety profile, ability to transduce non-dividing cells, and capacity for long-term gene expression (Keeler et al., 2018). The vectors can be administered through multiple routes, including intrathecal, intravenous, or intraparenchymal injection (Sandu & Schaller, 2012). Thus, gene therapy is usually designed to suppress proinflammatory cells, induce regulatory responses, and protect neurons and myelin from immune-mediated damage (Weiner, 2009). In AD and tauopathies, gene therapy uses oligonucleotides to suppress pathological tau protein and prevent neurodegeneration (Singh et al., 2024). Meanwhile, in PD and amyotrophic lateral sclerosis, gene therapy is able to suppress neuroinflammation (Zhang et al., 2023) by achieving immunomodulation through tolerance induction via antigen-specific Tregs (Keeler et al., 2018), cytokine modulation by delivering anti-inflammatory genes such as IL-4, IL-10 or blocking pro-inflammatory pathways (Racke et al., 1994), and enhancing suppressive or neuroprotective functions (Hoang et al., 2022). However, despite promising preclinical results, challenges remain in gene therapy for immunotherapy in neurological conditions, including BBB delivery limitations, vector immunogenicity (Bulcha et al., 2021; Mohapatra et al., 2024), disease heterogeneity requiring personalized approaches (Lassmann et al., 2007), and long-term safety concerns regarding permanent genetic modifications and potential insertional mutagenesis, which still remain concerns (Dunbar et al., 2018).

13. RNA interference

RNA interference (RNAi) is a form of immunotherapy in which gene silencing is mediated by small interfering RNAs (siRNAs), short hairpin RNAs, and microRNAs (miRNAs) (Nayak & Charyulu, 2024) to alleviate inflammation, mitochondrial dysfunction, excitotoxicity, oxidative stress, and cell apoptosis (Chudakova et al., 2025). The main target of RNAi is to suppress the expression of immunosuppressive proteins such as programmed death-1 (PD-1) and cytotoxic T-lymphocyte-associated protein 4 (CTLA4), which impair immune cell function (Monty et al., 2021). Thus, RNAi is one of the treatments commonly used in AD, PD, and amyotrophic lateral sclerosis to modulate neuroinflammation (Zhang et al., 2023). RNAi enables cell-intrinsic disruption of inhibitory pathways in immune cells, thereby enhancing immune responses compared to extracellular targeting by antibodies (Monty et al., 2021). Among these approaches, DNA-based RNAi allows the silencing of multiple inhibitory pathways in T cells. For instance, in the case of spinal cord injury, RNAi systems such as CRISPR-Cas13 target both protein-coding genes and non-coding RNAs (Srivastava et al., 2023) to alleviate inflammation, cell death, and tissue damage (Chudakova et al., 2025). Meanwhile, siRNAs are able to restore splicing aberration defects (Lee et al., 2022). One of the FDA-approved antisense oligonucleotides is known as nusinersen (Spinraza), which is able to correct the splicing of the survival motor neuron 2 (SMN2) gene in spinal muscular atrophy by promoting the inclusion of exon seven in the survival motor neuron 1 (SMN1) gene (Schoch & Miller, 2017). A similar mechanism has been observed in Duchenne muscular dystrophy, where splice-switching oligonucleotides enable exon skipping to restore the reading frame of the dystrophin gene (Hammond et al., 2021). To achieve maximum effect, the therapy needs to bypass the BBB. Thus, direct delivery into the CSF via intrathecal or intracerebroventricular injection has proven effective (Schoch & Miller, 2017). This method of delivery has been shown to be tolerable and effective in clinical trials involving spinal muscular atrophy and amyotrophic lateral sclerosis (Holm et al., 2022). However, recent advances include lipid nanoparticles to improve cellular uptake and endosomal escape (Prazeres et al., 2025), antibody oligonucleotide conjugates that leverage transferrin receptor binding for BBB crossing (Hammond et al., 2021), and exosome-mediated delivery using vesicles with inherent brain-targeting capabilities to further maximize the effects of RNAi. Despite promising outcomes, RNAi-based immunotherapies do have some drawbacks. This is because synthetic siRNAs can activate innate immune pathways by stimulating Toll-like receptors (TLR3, TLR7, TLR8, and TLR9) (Schoch & Miller, 2017), triggering interferon responses (Chudakova et al., 2025), cytokine storms (Pensato et al., 2021), and systemic inflammation (Monty et al., 2021), which may worsen neurological symptoms (Li & Wu, 2021). Repeated administration can induce adaptive immune responses, including the formation of neutralizing antibodies against the nanoparticle carriers (Bulcha et al., 2021), reducing treatment efficacy and causing hypersensitivity or cross-reactivity (Stone et al., 2023).

14. Nanotechnology

Nanotechnology is another form of immunotherapy that eases targeted drug delivery and control while minimizing adverse effects (Toader et al., 2024). Some of the different categories of nanoparticles used to treat neurological conditions include lipid-based nanoparticles (Thi et al., 2021), polymeric nanoparticles (Inamdar et al., 2025), and inorganic nanoparticles (Rahman, 2023). Lipid-based nanoparticles such as liposomes and lipid nanoparticles have proven effective in crossing the BBB (Prazeres et al., 2025), while PLGA, a form of polymeric nanoparticle, possesses the ability to modulate drug release and improve BBB penetration (Zhi et al., 2021). Inorganic nanoparticles are known for their magnetic targeting ability (Rahman, 2023) and for their use in photothermal and multimodal imaging-based therapies (Amaral et al., 2025). In neurological conditions, the use of nanoparticles has been shown to stimulate the activation of microglia by reprogramming them from a pro-inflammatory to an anti-inflammatory state. As a result, cytokines such as IL-10 or TGF-β are released, enhancing the clearance of aggregated neurotoxic substances in the brain (Adamu et al., 2024; Luo & Sugimura, 2024). Hence, in AD, nanoparticles facilitate Aβ and tau clearance and mitigate neuroinflammation through microglial reprogramming (Tian et al., 2025), while in PD, α-synuclein aggregation is inhibited (Javdani et al., 2019). Meanwhile, in amyotrophic lateral sclerosis, nanoparticles are able to suppress the degeneration of motor neurons (Wang et al., 2020), and in MS, they are able to induce immune tolerance through peptides, suppress autoreactive T cells, and promote BBB repair (Boutitah-Benyaich et al., 2025). Recent advancements in nanoparticle technology have given rise to surface modifications for ligand system specificity, where these nanoparticles are often loaded with antibodies, peptides, aptamers, or small molecules (Islam et al., 2025). To date, a very limited number of nanoparticles have been approved for neurological conditions. One plausible reason for this could be concerns related to safety, reproducibility, and scalable production (Laib et al., 2025). Even after crossing the BBB, nanoparticles must traverse dense extracellular matrices, evade endosomal entrapment, and overcome intracellular barriers (Kimura & Harashima, 2022). Thus, safety remains a pressing concern due to possible chronic inflammation, immune overactivation, and long-term neurotoxicity (Teixeira et al., 2024).

15. Applications of nanotechnology in specific immunity-mediated neurological disorders

Gold nanocrystals (CNM-Au8) demonstrate remyelination activity through energy metabolism enhancement, currently in Phase 2 clinical trials with demonstrated BBB penetration and oral bioavailability (Robinson et al., 2020). PLGA nanoparticles loaded with myelin oligodendrocyte glycoprotein (MOG) peptide induce antigen-specific immune tolerance via tolerogenic mechanisms, preventing disease progression in preclinical models (Gholamzad et al., 2021). MOG-PLGA nanoparticles administered intravenously before disease induction ameliorated clinical scores, increased regulatory T cell (Treg) populations, and restored Th1/Th17 cytokine homeostasis (Phan et al., 2023). Lignin-based tolerogenic nanoparticles with intrinsic reactive oxygen species (ROS)-scavenging capacity loaded with MS autoantigens induce tolerogenic dendritic cells and durable antigen-specific immune tolerance via Treg induction in both early and late disease stages (Phan et al., 2023). Extracellular vesicles provide natural BBB crossing with superior immunomodulatory and remyelination-promoting effects through microRNA and growth factor delivery (Alvarez-Erviti et al., 2011). Tolerogenic lipid nanoparticles delivering self-antigen mRNA to the spleen induce immune tolerance to myelin epitopes with minimal immune stimulation through phosphatidylserine-mediated recognition of apoptotic-like states (Krienke et al., 2021).

Guillain–Barré Syndrome (GBS) pathogenesis involves molecular mimicry wherein anti-peripheral nerve antibodies cross-react with CNS myelin. Myeloid-derived suppressor cell (MDSC)-based therapeutic strategies enhanced by rapamycin nanoparticles facilitate trafficking to inflamed nerve regions and reprogram peripheral immune responses through enhanced immunomodulatory function (Yuki & Hartung, 2012). Phospholipid composition modifications optimize nanoparticle uptake by APCs, directing them preferentially toward tolerogenic pathways through recognition of phosphatidylserine or targeting $CD14^+$ monocytes (Kishimoto & Maldonado, 2018). Tolerogenic vaccines using acetalated dextran microparticles coencapsulating disease-associated peptides with immunosuppressive drugs (dexamethasone) achieve antigen-specific tolerance without broad immunosuppression, reversing hind limb paralysis and restoring fully functional limbs in disease models (Getts et al., 2012). Anti-inflammatory macrophage-derived exosomes with disease-associated peptides promote differentiation of dendritic cells toward tolerogenic phenotypes even under proinflammatory stimuli, providing complete protection from disease progression (Kishimoto & Maldonado, 2018). Mannosylated liposomes targeting dendritic cells deliver antigenic peptides with simultaneous immunomodulatory agents, inducing IL-10-producing tolerogenic dendritic cells and Treg expansion (Da-Wa et al., 2021).

Besides, curcumin-loaded liposomes cross the BBB and suppress microglial activation, reducing TNF-α and IL-6 production while promoting A clearance through enhanced phagocytosis (Cruz et al., 2012). Gold nanoparticles functionalized with A-targeting peptides selectively recognize aggregated A, reducing toxicity and promoting clearance while maintaining BBB integrity (Salehi et al., 2020). PLGA nanoparticles delivering anti-inflammatory drugs reduce neuroinflammation-driven tau hyperphosphorylation (Shahbaz et al., 2022). Dopamine-coupled polypeptide nanocarriers targeted with alanine and glutathione enhance BBB penetration and dopaminergic neuron protection in midbrain organoids derived from patient-specific stem cells (Shahbaz et al., 2022). Resveratrol nanoparticles administered intranasally achieve selective optic nerve neuroprotection independent of inflammatory effects through intrinsic antioxidant properties (Monge-Fuentes et al., 2021). Exosome-mediated delivery systems carrying neuroprotective microRNAs and anti-inflammatory proteins suppress microglial activation and neurodegeneration (Nasirishargh et al., 2021).

16. Nanotechnology for biomarker detection

DNA-based nanostructures designed from aptamers recognize neuroinflammation biomarkers, including TNF-α, IL-6, and IL-1β, through target-induced DNA conformational changes, triggering fluorescence signals proportional to biomarker abundance (Ryan et al., 2024). Electrochemical nano-biosensors use nanoparticle-modified electrodes to detect cerebrospinal fluid biomarkers at femtomolar concentrations, enabling ultra-sensitive identification of disease-driving immune cell populations through surface immobilization of antibody- or receptor-derived ligands recognizing T cell receptor clones (Dutta et al., 2021). Surface plasmon resonance biosensors based on gold nanoparticle arrays detect immune protein interactions with label-free kinetic assessment of immune response quality (Bereli et al., 2021). Superparamagnetic iron oxide (SPIO) nanoparticles functionalized with immunotherapeutic agents generate strong MRI contrast, enabling visualization of nanoparticle biodistribution and colocalization with immune cell infiltrates while simultaneously delivering immunosuppressive drugs or anti-inflammatory peptides (Dias et al., 2022). Fluorescent nanoparticles combining near-infrared quantum dots with anti-inflammatory therapeutics enable two-photon microscopy visualization of deep brain structures and immune cell trafficking, with fluorescence activation occurring only upon enzymatic cleavage by neuroinflammation-associated proteases (Chang et al., 2005). Multimodal theranostic nanoparticles integrating MRI, fluorescence, and PET imaging with therapeutic payloads enable complementary diagnostic information and real-time tracking of therapeutic efficacy (Thakare et al., 2019). Ultrasound-responsive theranostic nanoparticles containing microbubble components permit non-invasive guidance of therapy to disease-relevant CNS regions with millimeter-scale spatial precision, allowing focal immunotherapy delivery to individual lesions (Chen et al., 2015). Raman-active theranostic nanoparticles with surface-enhanced Raman scattering (SERS) components enable detection through Raman spectroscopy with exceptional molecular specificity and generate unique Raman signatures reflecting their state of drug loading and release (Chen et al., 2015).

17. Safety, toxicology, and regulatory aspects

Nanoparticle toxicity is dose-dependent and influenced by multiple physicochemical parameters, including size, shape, surface charge, pore architecture, and surface functionalization (Sukhanova et al., 2018). Particle sizes ranging from 10 to 100 nm penetrate cellular membranes and cause cytotoxicity through ROS generation, mitochondrial dysfunction, and inflammatory responses (Egbuna et al., 2021). Surface charge optimization is critical, strongly positive charges enhance cellular uptake but increase hemotoxicity and thrombotic risk through complement activation and platelet aggregation, while near-neutral charges minimize these risks (Fröhlich, 2012). Protein corona formation, wherein blood proteins coat nanoparticle surfaces, dramatically alters biodistribution, clearance kinetics, and immunogenicity, yet remains poorly standardized in safety assessment (Tenzer et al., 2013). Long-term accumulation in the liver, spleen, and kidneys occurs with poorly biodegradable materials, raising concerns about chronic toxicity, organ dysfunction, and potential genotoxicity (Jakic et al., 2024). Standardised biocompatibility testing frameworks (ISO 10,993 series) assess cytotoxicity through in vitro assays, hemocompatibility via complement activation and coagulation studies, and genotoxicity through gene expression profiling (Dobrovolskaia & McNeil, 2007; Hallab & Jacobs, 2009).

Inadequate physicochemical characterization represents the primary barrier, as nanoparticles require standardised methods for size distribution, charge measurement, aggregation assessment, and long-term stability profiling that differ substantially from conventional pharmaceuticals (Riehemann et al., 2009). Manufacturing scalability challenges, including batch-to-batch variability, inconsistent particle size distributions, and difficulty translating lab-scale synthesis to GMP-compliant production pipelines, have caused numerous clinical failures (Hare et al., 2017). Clinical trial design complexity arises from variable nanoparticle behavior in biological systems, disease-specific BBB permeability variations, and heterogeneous patient immune responses, limiting direct extrapolation from preclinical data (Anselmo & Mitragotri, 2016).

18. Future perspectives

Machine learning algorithms predict critical nanoparticle quality attributes, including particle size, drug encapsulation efficiency, drug loading, and release kinetics, by integrating multidimensional datasets encompassing physicochemical characterization, pharmacokinetics, and preclinical outcomes (Wang et al., 2025). Nanoinformatics platforms and large-scale data repositories enhance reproducibility and cross-study comparisons, accelerating rational design of nanocarriers tailored to individual pathophysiology (Fourches et al., 2010). Computational fluid dynamics simulations coupled with machine learning enable the prediction of nanoparticle transport within tumor microenvironments, optimizing design parameters for enhanced accumulation (Stylianopoulos & Jain, 2015). Besides, pH-responsive nanoparticles release therapeutic agents in acidic inflammatory or tumor microenvironments, preventing premature drug liberation in systemic circulation (Bae & Park, 2011). Redox-sensitive linkers respond to elevated glutathione and reactive oxygen species, characterizing CNS inflammation, enabling site-specific drug release upon arrival at pathological sites (Cheng et al., 2011). Enzyme-responsive systems activate upon encountering disease-associated proteases or inflammatory mediators, further enhancing therapeutic specificity (Hu et al., 2014). Temperature-sensitive vesicles integrate liposome phase-transition properties triggered by localized hyperthermia, controlling drug release kinetics (Needham & Dewhirst, 2001). Light-activated nanoparticles with near-infrared photons achieve non-invasive temporal control with millimeter-scale spatial precision, ideal for image-guided therapies (Lucky et al., 2015). Magnetic-field-guided nanoparticles enable external direction of therapeutics to specific CNS regions, combining targeting precision with real-time imaging capability (Shubayev et al., 2009).

Patient-specific nanomedicine design leveraging multi-omics data (genomic, proteomic, transcriptomic, metabolomic) enables customization of nanoparticle properties to individual disease genotypes, immune profiles, and tissue pharmacokinetics (Shi et al., 2017). AI-driven digital twins simulate patient-specific nanoparticle biodistribution, permitting treatment adaptation prior to administration (Björnsson et al., 2020). Liquid biopsies integrating circulating tumor DNA detection with nanoparticle-based biosensors enable real-time monitoring of therapeutic response and early detection of drug resistance emergence (Wan et al., 2017). Theranostic nanoplatforms combining diagnostic modalities (MRI, fluorescence, Raman) with therapeutic functions enable simultaneous disease detection and treatment while tracking delivery efficacy in individual patients (Mura & Couvreur, 2012). Cell-membrane-coated nanoparticles derived from red blood cells, platelets, or immune cells inherit natural targeting and immune evasion properties while maintaining synthetic nanocarrier advantages (Hu et al., 2011). Biomimetic nanoparticles engineered to resemble pathogenic microbes or apoptotic cells trigger desired immune responses through pattern recognition receptors, enabling immunomodulatory and tolerogenic applications (Bachmann & Jennings, 2010). Plant viral nanoparticles offer rapid, scalable production, biocompatibility, and inherent immunogenicity for cancer vaccines and immunotherapy (Steinmetz, 2010). Microbial-derived nanoparticles leverage natural targeting properties of bacteria and fungi for selective accumulation in inflamed CNS regions (Gujrati et al., 2014). Green synthesis approaches utilizing plant extracts, microorganisms, and waste biomass reduce environmental impact and production costs while improving biocompatibility (Iravani, 2011).

19. Conclusion

Nanotechnology has emerged as a transformative platform addressing therapeutic limitations in immunity-mediated neurological disorders through precise drug delivery, immunomodulation, and restoration of immune homeostasis. The field has progressed from passive nanocarrier delivery to intelligent, stimuli-responsive systems capable of adapting to disease microenvironments. Current advances in liposomes, polymeric nanoparticles, dendrimers, exosomes, and biomimetic platforms demonstrate substantial preclinical efficacy in multiple sclerosis, autoimmune encephalitis, and neurodegenerative disorders with immune components through mechanisms including BBB penetration, targeted immunomodulation, remyelination enhancement, and restoration of regulatory T cell populations. Future success depends on: (1) standardization of nanoparticle characterization and manufacturing protocols establishing quality-by-design approaches; (2) early and transparent regulatory engagement establishing harmonized international frameworks; (3) systematic long-term safety evaluations addressing protein corona effects and tissue accumulation; (4) development of smart, stimuli-responsive platforms enabling spatiotemporal control of therapeutic action; and (5) interdisciplinary collaboration integrating materials science, immunology, computational biology, and clinical medicine. Smart vesicle therapeutics, biomimetic cell-membrane-coated platforms, and green synthesis approaches represent particularly promising near-term directions offering improved biocompatibility and sustainability. With continued innovation addressing translational barriers, nanotechnology-based therapies have the potential to fundamentally transform the management of immunity-mediated neurological diseases, shifting paradigms from symptomatic immunosuppression toward antigen-specific tolerance induction and tissue regeneration.

References

Abdelsalam, M., Ahmed, M., Osaid, Z., Hamoudi, R., & Harati, R. (2023). Insights into exosome transport through the blood–brain barrier and the potential therapeutical applications in brain diseases. *Pharmaceuticals, 16*(4), 571. https://doi.org/10.3390/ph16040571

Adamu, A., Li, S., Gao, F., & Xue, G. (2024). The role of neuroinflammation in neurodegenerative diseases: current understanding and future therapeutic targets. *Frontiers in Aging Neuroscience, 16*. https://doi.org/10.3389/fnagi.2024.1347987

Alamos-Musre, S., Beltrán-Chacana, D., Moyano, J., Márquez-Miranda, V., Duarte, Y., Miranda-Rojas, S., Olguín, Y., Fuentes, J. A., González-Nilo, D., & Otero, M. C. (2025). From structure to function: The promise of PAMAM dendrimers in biomedical applications. *Pharmaceutics, 17*(7). https://doi.org/10.3390/pharmaceutics17070927

Albarrán, V., Chamorro, J., Isabel Rosero, D., Saavedra, C., Soria, A., Carrato, A., & Gajate, P. (2022). Neurologic toxicity of immune checkpoint inhibitors: A review of literature. *Frontiers in Pharmacology, 13*. https://doi.org/10.3389/fphar.2022.774170

Alfaidi, M., Barker, R. A., & Kuan, W. L. (2025). An update on immune-based alpha-synuclein trials in Parkinson's disease. *Journal of Neurology, 272*(1). https://doi.org/10.1007/s00415-024-12770-x

Alsaab, H. O., Alharbi, F. D., Alhibs, A. S., Alanazi, N. B., Alshehri, B. Y., Saleh, M. A., Alshehri, F. S., Algarni, M. A., Almugaiteeb, T., Uddin, M. N., & Alzhrani, R. M. (2022). PLGA-based nanomedicine: History of advancement and development in clinical applications of multiple diseases. *Pharmaceutics, 14*(12). https://doi.org/10.3390/pharmaceutics14122728

Alvarez-Erviti, L., Seow, Y., Yin, H. F., Betts, C., Lakhal, S., & Wood, M. J. A. (2011). Delivery of siRNA to the mouse brain by systemic injection of targeted exosomes. *Nature Biotechnology, 29*(4), 341–345. https://doi.org/10.1038/nbt.1807

Amaral, M. N., Kumar, P., Faísca, P., Ferreira, H. A., Coelho, J. M. P., Gaspar, M. M., & Reis, C. P. (2025). Gold nanoparticle-mediated photothermal therapy: Expanding the frontiers of cancer treatment and theragnostics. *Biomedicine and Pharmacotherapy, 190*. https://doi.org/10.1016/j.biopha.2025.118399

Anselmo, A. C., & Mitragotri, S. (2016). Nanoparticles in the clinic. *Bioengineering and Translational Medicine, 1*(1), 10–29. https://doi.org/10.1002/btm2.10003

Bachmann, M. F., & Jennings, G. T. (2010). Vaccine delivery: A matter of size, geometry, kinetics and molecular patterns. *Nature Reviews Immunology, 10*(11), 787–796. https://doi.org/10.1038/nri2868

Bae, Y. H., & Park, K. (2011). Targeted drug delivery to tumors: Myths, reality and possibility. *Journal of Controlled Release, 153*(3), 198–205. https://doi.org/10.1016/j.jconrel.2011.06.001

Baker, D., Herrod, S. S., Alvarez-Gonzalez, C., Giovannoni, G., & Schmierer, K. (2017). Interpreting lymphocyte reconstitution data from the pivotal phase 3 trials of alemtuzumab. *JAMA Neurology, 74*(8), 961. https://doi.org/10.1001/jamaneurol.2017.0676

Bereli, N., Bakhshpour, M., Arif Topçu, A., & Denizli, A. (2021). Surface plasmon resonance-based immunosensor for igm detection with gold nanoparticles. *Micromachines, 12*(9), 1092. https://doi.org/10.3390/mi12091092

Björnsson, B., Borrebaeck, C., Elander, N., Gasslander, T., Gawel, D. R., Gustafsson, M., Jörnsten, R., Lee, E. J., Li, X., Lilja, S., Martínez-Enguita, D., Matussek, A., Sandström, P., Schäfer, S., Stenmarker, M., Sun, X. F., Sysoev, O., Zhang, H., & Benson, M. (2020). Digital twins to personalize medicine. *Genome Medicine, 12*(1). https://doi.org/10.1186/s13073-019-0701-3

Boutitah-Benyaich, I., Eixarch, H., Villacieros-Álvarez, J., Hervera, A., Cobo-Calvo, Á., Montalban, X., & Espejo, C. (2025). Multiple sclerosis: Molecular pathogenesis and therapeutic intervention. *Signal Transduction and Targeted Therapy, 10*(1). https://doi.org/10.1038/s41392-025-02415-4

Brambilla, R. (2019). The contribution of astrocytes to the neuroinflammatory response in multiple sclerosis and experimental autoimmune encephalomyelitis. *Acta Neuropathologica, 137*(5), 757–783. https://doi.org/10.1007/s00401-019-01980-7

Brown, W., & Coles, A. (2013). Alemtuzumab: Evidence for its potential in relapsing–remitting multiple sclerosis. *Drug Design, Development and Therapy, 7*, 131. https://doi.org/10.2147/DDDT.S32687

Bulcha, J. T., Wang, Y., Ma, H., Tai, P. W. L., & Gao, G. (2021). Viral vector platforms within the gene therapy landscape. *Signal Transduction and Targeted Therapy, 6*(1). https://doi.org/10.1038/s41392-021-00487-6

Chang, E., Miller, J. S., Sun, J., Yu, W. W., Colvin, V. L., Drezek, R., & West, J. L. (2005). Protease-activated quantum dot probes. *Biochemical and Biophysical Research Communications, 334*(4), 1317–1321. https://doi.org/10.1016/j.bbrc.2005.07.028

Chauhan. (2018). Dendrimers for drug delivery. *Molecules (Basel, Switzerland), 23*(4). https://doi.org/10.3390/molecules23040938

Chen, P. Y., Hsieh, H. Y., Huang, C. Y., Lin, C. Y., Wei, K. C., & Liu, H. L. (2015). Focused ultrasound-induced blood-brain barrier opening to enhance interleukin-12 delivery for brain tumor immunotherapy: A preclinical feasibility study. *Journal of Translational Medicine, 13*(1). https://doi.org/10.1186/s12967-015-0451-y

Chen, D., Le, S., Ghiaseddin, A., Manektalia, H., Li, M., O'Dell, A., Rahman, M., & Tran, D. (2024). ctim-36. In-situ vaccination of biopsy-only gbm tumors by tumor treating fields plus anti-pd-1 immunotherapy results in robust antigen-specific t cell selection and expansion, high response rate, and significantly extended survival. *Neuro-Oncology, 26*(Suppl. ment_8), viii94. https://doi.org/10.1093/neuonc/noae165.0369

Cheng, R., Feng, F., Meng, F., Deng, C., Feijen, J., & Zhong, Z. (2011). Glutathione-responsive nano-vehicles as a promising platform for targeted intracellular drug and gene delivery. *Journal of Controlled Release, 152*(1), 2–12. https://doi.org/10.1016/j.jconrel.2011.01.030

Chudakova, D., Kovalev, V., Shkap, M., Sigal, E., Biktimirov, A., Soboleva, A., & Baklaushev, V. (2025). RNA interference and its key targets for spinal cord injury therapy: What is known so far? *Federation International Journal of Molecular Sciences, 26*(20). https://doi.org/10.3390/ijms26209861

Clark, D. P., & Pazdernik, N. J. (2016). Recombinant proteins. *Biotechnology* (2nd ed., pp. 297–324). Academic Press.

Cloake, N. C., Beaino, W., Trifilieff, E., & Greer, J. M. (2014). Thiopalmitoylation of altered peptide ligands enhances their protective effects in an animal model of multiple sclerosis. *Journal of Immunology, 192*(5), 2244–2251. https://doi.org/10.4049/jimmunol.1301871

Conlon, P., & Steinman, L. (2002). Altered peptide ligands and MS treatment. *Science, 296*(5574), 1801–1802. https://doi.org/10.1126/science.296.5574.1801c

Cossu, D., Ruberto, S., Yokoyama, K., Hattori, N., & Sechi, L. A. (2022). Efficacy of BCG vaccine in animal models of neurological disorders. *Vaccine, 40*(3), 432–436. https://doi.org/10.1016/j.vaccine.2021.12.005

Coutinho, A. E., & Chapman, K. E. (2011). The anti-inflammatory and immunosuppressive effects of glucocorticoids, recent developments and mechanistic insights. *Molecular and Cellular Endocrinology, 335*(1), 2–13. https://doi.org/10.1016/j.mce.2010.04.005

Cruz, L. J., Tacken, P. J., Rueda, F., Domingo, J. C., Albericio, F., & Figdor, C. G. (2012). Targeting nanoparticles to dendritic cells for immunotherapy. *Methods in Enzymology, 509*, 143–163. https://doi.org/10.1016/B978-0-12-391858-1.00008-3

Cuoco, J. A., Klein, B. J., Busch, C. M., Guilliams, E. L., Olasunkanmi, A. L., & Entwistle, J. J. (2019). Corticosteroid-induced regression of glioblastoma: A radiographic conundrum. *Frontiers in Oncology, 9*. https://doi.org/10.3389/fonc.2019.01288

Da-Wa, Z. X., Jun, M., Chao-Zheng, L., Sen-Lin, Y., Chuan, L., De-Chun, L., Zu-Nan, D., Hong-Tao, Z., Shu-Qing, W., Xian-Wei, P., Wenbo, L., & Ke-Wen, L. (2021). Exosomes derived from M2 macrophages exert a therapeutic effect via inhibition of the PI3K/AKT/mTOR pathway in rats with knee osteoarthritic. *BioMed Research International, 2021*. https://doi.org/10.1155/2021/7218067

Dias, A. M. M., Courteau, A., Bellaye, P. S., Kohli, E., Oudot, A., Doulain, P. E., Petitot, C., Walker, P. M., Decréau, R., & Collin, B. (2022). Superparamagnetic iron oxide nanoparticles for immunotherapy of cancers through macrophages and magnetic hyperthermia. *Pharmaceutics, 14*(11). https://doi.org/10.3390/pharmaceutics14112388

Dimitriadou, M. M., Alexopoulos, H., Akrivou, S., Gola, E., & Dalakas, M. C. (2020). Anti-neuronal antibodies within the IVIg preparations: Importance in clinical practice. *Neurotherapeutics, 17*(1), 235–242. https://doi.org/10.1007/s13311-019-00796-3

Ding, L., Kshirsagar, P., Agrawal, P., & Murry, D. J. (2025). Crossing the blood–brain barrier: innovations in receptor- and transporter-mediated transcytosis strategies. *Pharmaceutics, 17*(6), 706. https://doi.org/10.3390/pharmaceutics17060706

Dobrovolskaia, M. A., & McNeil, S. E. (2007). Immunological properties of engineered nanomaterials. *Nature Nanotechnology, 2*(8), 469–478. https://doi.org/10.1038/nnano.2007.223

Dotiwala, A. K., McCausland, C., & Samra, N. S. (2018). In *Anatomy, head and neck: Blood brain barrier.*

Downer, E. J., Cowley, T. R., Cox, F., Maher, F. O., Berezin, V., Bock, E., & Lynch, M. A. (2009). A synthetic NCAM-derived mimetic peptide, FGL, exerts anti-inflammatory properties via IGF-1 and interferon-γ modulation. *Journal of Neurochemistry, 109*(5), 1516–1525. https://doi.org/10.1111/j.1471-4159.2009.06076.x

Du, C., Zeng, P., Han, J. R., Zhang, T. X., Jia, D., Shi, F. D., & Zhang, C. (2021). Early initiation of tocilizumab treatment against moderate-to-severe myelitis in neuromyelitis optica spectrum disorder. *Frontiers in Immunology, 12*. https://doi.org/10.3389/fimmu.2021.660230

Dunbar, C. E., High, K. A., Joung, J. K., Kohn, D. B., Ozawa, K., & Sadelain, M. (2018). Gene therapy comes of age. *Science, 359*(6372). https://doi.org/10.1126/science.aan4672

Duru, A. D., Sun, R., Allerbring, E. B., Chadderton, J., Kadri, N., Han, X., Peqini, K., Uchtenhagen, H., Madhurantakam, C., Pellegrino, S., Sandalova, T., Nygren, P.Å., Turner, S. J., & Achour, A. (2020). Tuning antiviral CD8 T-cell response via proline-altered peptide ligand vaccination. *PLoS Pathogens, 16*(5). https://doi.org/10.1371/journal.ppat.1008244

Dutta, N., Lillehoj, P. B., Estrela, P., & Dutta, G. (2021). Electrochemical biosensors for cytokine profiling: Recent advancements and possibilities in the near future. *Biosensors, 11*(3), 94. https://doi.org/10.3390/bios11030094

Egbuna, C., Parmar, V. K., Jeevanandam, J., Ezzat, S. M., Patrick-Iwuanyanwu, K. C., Adetunji, C. O., Khan, J., Onyeike, E. N., Uche, C. Z., Akram, M., Ibrahim, M. S., El Mahdy, N. M., Awuchi, C. G., Saravanan, K., Tijjani, H., Odoh, U. E., Messaoudi, M., Ifemeje, J. C., Olisah, M. C., … Ibeabuchi, C. G. (2021). Toxicity of nanoparticles in biomedical application: Nanotoxicology. *Journal of Toxicology, 2021*. https://doi.org/10.1155/2021/9954443

Fissolo, N., Costa, C., Nurtdinov, R. N., Bustamante, M. F., Llombart, V., Mansilla, M. J., Espejo, C., Montalban, X., & Comabella, M. (2012). Treatment with MOG-DNA vaccines induces CD4+CD25+FoxP3+

regulatory T cells and up-regulates genes with neuroprotective functions in experimental autoimmune encephalomyelitis. *Journal of Neuroinflammation, 9*. https://doi.org/10.1186/1742-2094-9-139

Flingai, S., Czerwonko, M., Goodman, J., Kudchodkar, S. B., Muthumani, K., & Weiner, D. B. (2013). Synthetic DNA vaccines: Improved vaccine potency by electroporation and co-delivered genetic adjuvants. *Frontiers in Immunology, 4*. https://doi.org/10.3389/fimmu.2013.00354

Foster, M. A., Lunn, M. P. T., & Carr, A. S. (2023). First-line immunosuppression in neuromuscular diseases. *Practical Neurology, 23*(4), 327–338. https://doi.org/10.1136/pn-2023-003708

Fourches, D., Muratov, E., & Tropsha, A. (2010). Trust, but verify: On the importance of chemical structure curation in cheminformatics and QSAR modeling research. *Journal of Chemical Information and Modeling, 50*(7), 1189–1204. https://doi.org/10.1021/ci100176x

Fröhlich, E. (2012). The role of surface charge in cellular uptake and cytotoxicity of medical nanoparticles. *International Journal of Nanomedicine, 7*, 5577–5591. https://doi.org/10.2147/IJN.S36111Austria

Fu, Y., Feng, C., Qin, S., Xing, Z., Liu, C., Liu, Z., & Yu, H. (2024). Breaking barriers: Advancing cellular therapies in autoimmune disease management. *Frontiers in Immunology, 15*. https://doi.org/10.3389/fimmu.2024.1503099

Galea, I. (2021). The blood–brain barrier in systemic infection and inflammation. *Cellular and Molecular Immunology, 18*(11), 2489–2501. https://doi.org/10.1038/s41423-021-00757-x

Gelinas, D. S., DaSilva, K., Fenili, D., George-Hyslop, P. S., & McLaurin, J. A. (2004). Immunotherapy for alzheimer's disease. *Proceedings of the National Academy of Sciences of the United States of America, 101*(2), 14657–14662. https://doi.org/10.1073/pnas.0404866101

Getts, D. R., Martin, A. J., Mccarthy, D. P., Terry, R. L., Hunter, Z. N., Yap, W. T., Getts, M. T., Pleiss, M., Luo, X., King, N. J. C., Shea, L. D., & Miller, S. D. (2012). Microparticles bearing encephalitogenic peptides induce T-cell tolerance and ameliorate experimental autoimmune encephalomyelitis. *Nature Biotechnology, 30*(12), 1217–1224. https://doi.org/10.1038/nbt.2434

Gholamzad, M., Hussein, B., Shafiee Ardestani, M., Seyedkhan, Z., & Azimi, M. (2021). Prophylactic and therapeutic effects of MOG-conjugated PLGA nanoparticles in C57Bl/6 mouse model of multiple sclerosis. *Advanced Pharmaceutical Bulletin, 11*(3), 505–513. https://doi.org/10.34172/apb.2021.058

Ginestal-López, R. C. (2018). Immunotherapy for neurological diseases, present and future. *Farmacia Hospitalaria, 42*(6), 251–260. https://doi.org/10.7399/fh.11031

Goverman, J. (2009). Autoimmune T cell responses in the central nervous system. *Nature Reviews Immunology, 9*(6), 393–407. https://doi.org/10.1038/nri2550

Grasso, M., Frison, V., Cristiano Chilelli, N., Filippi, A., Costantini, G., Vilotti, C., & Simioni, N. (2023). Diabete mellito dopo trattamento con ocrelizumab per sclerosi multipla primariamente progressiva. *Il Diabete, 35*(3). https://doi.org/10.30682/ildia2303g

Gujrati, V., Kim, S., Kim, S. H., Min, J. J., Choy, H. E., Kim, S. C., & Jon, S. (2014). Bioengineered bacterial outer membrane vesicles as cell-specific drug-delivery vehicles for cancer therapy. *ACS Nano, 8*(2), 1525–1537. https://doi.org/10.1021/nn405724x

Hallab, N. J., & Jacobs, J. J. (2009). Biologic effects of implant debris. *Bulletin of the NYU Hospital for Joint Diseases, 67*.

Hammond, S. M., Aartsma-Rus, A., Alves, S., Borgos, S. E., Buijsen, R. A. M., Collin, R. W. J., Covello, G., Denti, M. A., Desviat, L. R., Echevarría, L., Foged, C., Gaina, G., Garanto, A., Goyenvalle, A. T., Guzowska, M., Holodnuka, I., Jones, D. R., Krause, S., Lehto, T., … Arechavala-Gomeza, V. (2021). Delivery of oligonucleotide-based therapeutics: Challenges and opportunities. *EMBO Molecular Medicine, 13*(4). https://doi.org/10.15252/emmm.202013243

Hansel, T. T., Kropshofer, H., Singer, T., Mitchell, J. A., & George, A. J. T. (2010). The safety and side effects of monoclonal antibodies. *Nature Reviews Drug Discovery, 9*(4), 325–338. https://doi.org/10.1038/nrd3003

Haqqani, A. S., Bélanger, K., & Stanimirovic, D. B. (2024). Receptor-mediated transcytosis for brain delivery of therapeutics: Receptor classes and criteria. *Frontiers in Drug Delivery, 4*. https://doi.org/10.3389/fddev.2024.1360302

Hare, J. I., Lammers, T., Ashford, M. B., Puri, S., Storm, G., & Barry, S. T. (2017). Challenges and strategies in anti-cancer nanomedicine development: An industry perspective. *Advanced Drug Delivery Reviews, 108*, 25–38. https://doi.org/10.1016/j.addr.2016.04.025

Havrdova, E., Cohen, J., Horáková, D., Kovarova, I., & Meluzinova, E. (2017). Understanding the positive benefit: Risk profile of alemtuzumab in relapsing multiple sclerosis: Perspectives from the alemtuzumab clinical development program. *Therapeutics and Clinical Risk Management, 13*, 1423–1437. https://doi.org/10.2147/tcrm.s143509

Hervé, F., Ghinea, N., & Scherrmann, J. M. (2008). CNS delivery via adsorptive transcytosis. *AAPS Journal, 10*(3), 455–472. https://doi.org/10.1208/s12248-008-9055-2

Hoang, D. M., Pham, P. T., Bach, T. Q., Ngo, A. T. L., Nguyen, Q. T., Phan, T. T. K., Nguyen, G. H., Le, P. T. T., Hoang, V. T., Forsyth, N. R., Heke, M., & Nguyen, L. T. (2022). Stem cell-based therapy for human diseases. *Signal Transduction and Targeted Therapy, 7*(1). https://doi.org/10.1038/s41392-022-01134-4

Hohlfeld, R., & Wekerle, H. (2004). Autoimmune concepts of multiple sclerosis as a basis for selective immunotherapy: From pipe dreams to (therapeutic) pipelines. *Proceedings of the National Academy of Sciences, 101*(Suppl. 1_2), 14599–14606. https://doi.org/10.1073/pnas.0404874101

Holm, A., Hansen, S. N., Klitgaard, H., & Kauppinen, S. (2022). Clinical advances of RNA therapeutics for treatment of neurological and neuromuscular diseases. *RNA Biology, 19*(1), 594–608. https://doi.org/10.1080/15476286.2022.2066334

Hu, Q., Katti, P. S., & Gu, Z. (2014). Enzyme-responsive nanomaterials for controlled drug delivery. *Nanoscale, 6*(21), 12273–12286. https://doi.org/10.1039/c4nr04249b

Hu, C. M. J., Zhang, L., Aryal, S., Cheung, C., Fang, R. H., & Zhang, L. (2011). Erythrocyte membrane-camouflaged polymeric nanoparticles as a biomimetic delivery platform. *Proceedings of the National Academy of Sciences of the United States of America, 108*(27), 10980–10985. https://doi.org/10.1073/pnas.1106634108

Iizuka, N., Hoshida, Y., Miyamoto, A. T., Shigyo, H., Nishigaichi, A., Okamura, G., & Ohshima, S. (2025). Immunosuppressants/immunomodulators and malignancy. *Journal of Clinical Medicine, 14*(14), 5160. https://doi.org/10.3390/jcm14145160

Inamdar, A., Gurupadayya, B., Halagali, P., Tippavajhala, V. K., Khan, F., Pathak, R., & Sharma, H. (2025). Unraveling neurological drug delivery: Polymeric nanocarriers for enhanced blood-brain barrier penetration. *Current Drug Targets, 26*(4), 243–266. https://doi.org/10.2174/0113894501339455241101065040

Iravani, S. (2011). Green synthesis of metal nanoparticles using plants. *Green Chemistry, 13*(10), 2638–2650. https://doi.org/10.1039/c1gc15386b

Islam, S., Ahmed, M. M. S., Islam, M. A., Hossain, N., & Chowdhury, M. A. (2025). Advances in nanoparticles in targeted drug delivery–areview. *Results in Surfaces and Interfaces, 19*. https://doi.org/10.1016/j.rsurfi.2025.100529

Jakic, K., Selc, M., Razga, F., Nemethova, V., Mazancova, P., Havel, F., Sramek, M., Zarska, M., Proska, J., Masanova, V., Uhnakova, I., Makovicky, P., Novotova, M., Vykoukal, V., & Babelova, A. (2024). Long-term accumulation, biological effects and toxicity of BSA-coated gold nanoparticles in the mouse liver, spleen, and kidneys. *International Journal of Nanomedicine, 19*, 4103–4120. https://doi.org/10.2147/IJN.S443168

Jakimovski, D., Weinstock-guttman, B., Ramanathan, M., Dwyer, M. G., & Zivadinov, R. (2020). Infections, vaccines and autoimmunity: A multiple sclerosis perspective. *Vaccines, 8*(1). https://doi.org/10.3390/vaccines8010050

Javdani, N., Rahpeyma, S. S., Ghasemi, Y., & Raheb, J. (2019). Effect of superparamagnetic nanoparticles coated with various electric charges on α-synuclein and β-amyloid proteins fibrillation process. *International Journal of Nanomedicine, 14*, 799–808. https://doi.org/10.2147/IJN.S190354

Jones, J. L., Thompson, S. A. J., Loh, P., Davies, J. L., Tuohy, O. C., Curry, A. J., Azzopardi, L., Hill-Cawthorne, G., Fahey, M. T., Compston, A., & Coles, A. J. (2013). Human autoimmunity after lymphocyte depletion is caused by homeostatic T-cell proliferation. *Proceedings of the National Academy of Sciences, 110* (50), 20200–20205. https://doi.org/10.1073/pnas.1313654110

Kammona, O., & Kiparissides, C. (2020). Recent advances in antigen-specific immunotherapies for the treatment of multiple sclerosis. *Brain Sciences, 10*(6), 333. https://doi.org/10.3390/brainsci10060333

Karati, D., Meur, S., Das, S., Adak, A., & Mukherjee, S. (2025). Peptide-based drugs in immunotherapy: Current advances and future prospects. *Medical Oncology, 42*(5). https://doi.org/10.1007/s12032-025-02739-9

Keeler, G. D., Kumar, S., Palaschak, B., Silverberg, E. L., Markusic, D. M., Jones, N. T., & Hoffman, B. E. (2018). Gene therapy-induced antigen-specific tregs inhibit neuro-inflammation and reverse disease in a mouse model of multiple sclerosis. *Molecular Therapy, 26*(1), 173–183. https://doi.org/10.1016/j.ymthe.2017.09.001

Khaiboullina, S. (2026). Special issue: The role of cytokines in disease. *International Journal of Molecular Sciences, 27*(2), 876. https://doi.org/10.3390/ijms27020876

Kim, H. Y., Kim, S., Akaydin, A. N., Kim, S., Hyeon, S. J., Lee, J., & Ryu, H. (2026). The rise of astrocytes: Are they guardians or troublemakers of the brain disorder? *Experimental and Molecular Medicine*. https://doi.org/10.1038/s12276-025-01627-6

Kimura, S., & Harashima, H. (2022). Non-invasive gene delivery across the blood-brain barrier: Present and future perspectives. *Neural Regeneration Research, 17*(4), 785–787. https://doi.org/10.4103/1673-5374.320981

Kishimoto, T. K., & Maldonado, R. A. (2018). Nanoparticles for the induction of antigen-specific immunological tolerance. *Frontiers in Immunology, 9*. https://doi.org/10.3389/fimmu.2018.00230

Kiyonaka, S., Sakamoto, S., Wakayama, S., Morikawa, Y., Tsujikawa, M., & Hamachi, I. (2018). Ligand-directed chemistry of AMPA receptors confers live-cell fluorescent biosensors. *ACS Chemical Biology, 13*(7), 1880–1889. https://doi.org/10.1021/acschembio.7b01042

Kochman, U., Sitka, H., Kuźniar, J., Czaja, M., Kozubek, P., Beszłej, J. A., & Leszek, J. (2026). Targeted nanoparticles for drug delivery across the blood–brain barrier in early and late stages of alzheimer's disease: A review. *Molecular Neurobiology, 63*(1). https://doi.org/10.1007/s12035-025-05417-z

Kozak, M., & Hu, J. (2024). DNA vaccines: Their formulations, engineering and delivery. *Vaccines, 12*(1), 71. https://doi.org/10.3390/vaccines12010071

Krienke, C., Kolb, L., Diken, E., Streuber, M., Kirchhoff, S., Bukur, T., Akilli-Öztürk, Ö., Kranz, L. M., Berger, H., Petschenka, J., Diken, M., Kreiter, S., Yogev, N., Waisman, A., Karikó, K., Türeci, Ö., & Sahin, U. (2021). A noninflammatory mRNA vaccine for treatment of experimental autoimmune encephalomyelitis. *Science, 371*(6525), 145–153. https://doi.org/10.1126/science.aay3638

Kujundziski, A. P., & Chamovska, D. (2025). Polymeric nanomicelles for cancer nanomedicine—Review. *Engineering Proceedings, 99*(1), 12. https://doi.org/10.3390/engproc2025099012

Kurilin, V., Alshevskaya, A., & Sennikov, S. (2024). Development of cell technologies based on dendritic cells for immunotherapy of oncological diseases. *Biomedicines, 12*(3), 699. https://doi.org/10.3390/biomedicines12030699

Kwon, H. S., & Koh, S. H. (2020). Neuroinflammation in neurodegenerative disorders: The roles of microglia and astrocytes. *Translational Neurodegeneration, 9*(1). https://doi.org/10.1186/s40035-020-00221-2

Laib, I., Gheraissa, N., Benaissa, A., Benkhira, L., Azzi, M., Benaissa, Y., Abdelaziz, A. G., Tian, F., Walsh, M., Bechelany, M., & Ahmed, B. (2025). Tailoring innovative silver nanoparticles for modern medicine: The importance of size and shape control and functional modifications. *Materials Today Bio, 33*, Article 102071. https://doi.org/10.1016/j.mtbio.2025.102071

Lambracht-Washington, D., & Rosenberg, R. N. (2012). Active DNA Aβ42 vaccination as immunotherapy for alzheimer disease. *Translational Neuroscience, 3*(4), 307–313. https://doi.org/10.2478/s13380-012-0037-6

Lassmann, H., Brück, W., & Lucchinetti, C. F. (2007). The immunopathology of multiple sclerosis: An overview. *Brain Pathology, 17*(2), 210–218. https://doi.org/10.1111/j.1750-3639.2007.00064.x

Lee, M.-J., Lee, I., & Wang, K. (2022). Recent advances in RNA therapy and its carriers to treat the single-gene neurological disorders. *Biomedicines, 10*(1), 158. https://doi.org/10.3390/biomedicines10010158

Lee, D. W., Santomasso, B. D., Locke, F. L., Ghobadi, A., Turtle, C. J., Brudno, J. N., Maus, M. V., Park, J. H., Mead, E., Pavletic, S., Go, W. Y., Eldjerou, L., Gardner, R. A., Frey, N., Curran, K. J., Peggs, K., Pasquini, M., DiPersio, J. F., van den Brink, M. R. M., … Neelapu, S. S. (2019). ASTCT consensus grading for cytokine release syndrome and neurologic toxicity associated with immune effector cells. *Biology of Blood and Marrow Transplantation, 25*(4), 625–638. https://doi.org/10.1016/j.bbmt.2018.12.758

Letscher, H., Agbogan, V. A., Korniotis, S., Gastineau, P., Tejerina, E., Gras, C., Mégret, J., Moe, A., Drobyski, W. R., & Zavala, F. (2021). Toll-like receptor-9 stimulated plasmacytoid dendritic cell precursors suppress autoimmune neuroinflammation in a murine model of multiple sclerosis. *Scientific Reports, 11*(1). https://doi.org/10.1038/s41598-021-84023-0

Li, G., Cao, Y., Tang, X., Huang, J., Cai, L., & Zhou, L. (2022). The meningeal lymphatic vessels and the glymphatic system: Potential therapeutic targets in neurological disorders. *Journal of Cerebral Blood Flow and Metabolism, 42*(8), 1364–1382. https://doi.org/10.1177/0271678X221098145

Li, H., Shi, F. H., Huang, S. Y., Zhang, S. G., Gu, Z. C., & Wei, J. F. (2018). Clinical adverse effects of natalizumab: Protocol for a meta-analysis of randomized double-blind placebo-controlled clinical trails. *Medicine, 97*(28). https://doi.org/10.1097/MD.0000000000011507

Li, D., & Wu, M. (2021). Pattern recognition receptors in health and diseases. *Signal Transduction and Targeted Therapy, 6*(1). https://doi.org/10.1038/s41392-021-00687-0

Liao, B., Shroff, S., Kamiya-Matsuoka, C., & Tummala, S. (2014). Atypical neurological complications of ipilimumab therapy in patients with metastatic melanoma. *Neuro-Oncology, 16*(4), 589–593. https://doi.org/10.1093/neuonc/nou001

Lima, D. S., Zárate-Bladés, C. R., Souza, P. R. M., Trombone, A. P., Santos, R. R., Brandão, I. T., Masson, A. P., Bonato, V. L., Coelho-Castelo, A. A. M., Sartori, A., Vendramini, M., Soares, E. G., Benvenutti, L. A., Silva, C. L., & Coelho, V. (2009). No evidence of pathological autoimmunity following mycobacterium leprae heat-shock protein 65-DNA vaccination in mice. *European Journal of Inflammation, 7*(2), 77–85. https://doi.org/10.1177/1721727x0900700204

Linnoila, J., & Pittock, S. (2016). Autoantibody-associated central nervous system neurologic disorders. *Seminars in Neurology, 36*(04), 382–396. https://doi.org/10.1055/s-0036-1585453

Lobbous, M., Goswami, T., Lamb, L. S., Rochlin, K., Pillay, T., ter Haak, M., & Nabors, L. B. (2024). INB-200: Fully enrolled phase 1 study of gene-modified autologous gamma-delta (γδ) T cells in patients with newly diagnosed glioblastoma multiforme (GBM) receiving maintenance temozolomide (TMZ). *Journal of Clinical Oncology, 42*(16_Suppl. 1). https://doi.org/10.1200/jco.2024.42.16_suppl.2042

Lok, K. Z., Basta, M., Manzanero, S., & Arumugam, T. V. (2015). Intravenous immunoglobulin (IVIg) dampens neuronal toll-like receptor-mediated responses in ischemia. *Journal of Neuroinflammation, 12*(1).

Lucky, S. S., Soo, K. C., & Zhang, Y. (2015). Nanoparticles in photodynamic therapy. *Chemical Reviews, 115*(4), 1990–2042. https://doi.org/10.1021/cr5004198

Luo, E. Y., & Sugimura, R. R. (2024). Taming microglia: The promise of engineered microglia in treating neurological diseases. *Journal of Neuroinflammation, 21*(1). https://doi.org/10.1186/s12974-024-03015-9

Manoutcharian, K., & Gevorkian, G. (2024). Recombinant antibody fragments for immunotherapy of parkinson's disease. *BioDrugs, 38*(2), 249–257. https://doi.org/10.1007/s40259-024-00646-5

Mantica, M., & Drappatz, J. (2023). Immunotherapy associated central nervous system complications in primary brain tumors. *Frontiers in Oncology, 13*. https://doi.org/10.3389/fonc.2023.1124198

Martins, Y. A., Tsuchida, C. J., Antoniassi, P., & Demarchi, I. G. (2017). Efficacy and safety of the immunization with DNA for alzheimer's disease in animal models: A systematic review from literature. *Journal of Alzheimer's Disease Reports, 1*(1), 195–217. https://doi.org/10.3233/ADR-170025

Matea, C. T., Mocan, T., Tabaran, F., Pop, T., Mosteanu, O., Puia, C., Iancu, C., & Mocan, L. (2017). Quantum dots in imaging, drug delivery and sensor applications. *International Journal of Nanomedicine, 12*, 5421–5431. https://doi.org/10.2147/IJN.S138624

Mayer, M. G., & Fischer, T. (2024). Microglia at the blood brain barrier in health and disease. *Frontiers in Cellular Neuroscience, 18*. https://doi.org/10.3389/fncel.2024.1360195

Milani, D., Knuckey, N. W., Anderton, R. S., Cross, J. L., & Meloni, B. P. (2016). The R18 polyarginine peptide is more effective than the TAT-NR2B9c (NA-1) peptide when administered 60 minutes after permanent middle cerebral artery occlusion in the rat. *Stroke Research and Treatment, 2016*, 1–9. https://doi.org/10.1155/2016/2372710

Mohapatra, P., Gopikrishnan, M., George Priya Doss, C., & Chandrasekaran, N. (2024). How precise are nanomedicines in overcoming the blood–brain barrier? acomprehensive review of the literature. *International Journal of Nanomedicine, 19*, 2441–2467. https://doi.org/10.2147/IJN.S442520

Moldaver, D. M., Bharhani, M. S., Rudulier, C. D., Wattie, J., Inman, M. D., & Larché, M. (2019). Induction of bystander tolerance and immune deviation after Fel d 1 peptide immunotherapy. *Journal of Allergy and Clinical Immunology, 143*(3), 1087. https://doi.org/10.1016/j.jaci.2018.03.023

Monge-Fuentes, V., Biolchi Mayer, A., Lima, M. R., Geraldes, L. R., Zanotto, L. N., Moreira, K. G., Martins, O. P., Piva, H. L., Felipe, M. S. S., Amaral, A. C., Bocca, A. L., Tedesco, A. C., & Mortari, M. R. (2021). Dopamine-loaded nanoparticle systems circumvent the blood–brain barrier restoring motor function in mouse model for Parkinson's disease. *Scientific Reports, 11*(1). https://doi.org/10.1038/s41598-021-94175-8

Monty, M. A., Islam, M. A., Nan, X., Tan, J., Tuhin, I. J., Tang, X., Miao, M., Wu, D., & Yu, L. (2021). Emerging role of RNA interference in immune cells engineering and its therapeutic synergism in immunotherapy. *British Journal of Pharmacology, 178*(8), 1741–1755. https://doi.org/10.1111/bph.15414

Mortada, I., Farah, R., Nabha, S., Ojcius, D. M., Fares, Y., Almawi, W. Y., & Sadier, N. S. (2021). Immunotherapies for neurodegenerative diseases. *Frontiers in Neurology, 12*. https://doi.org/10.3389/fneur.2021.654739

Mura, S., & Couvreur, P. (2012). Nanotheranostics for personalized medicine. *Advanced Drug Delivery Reviews, 64*(13), 1394–1416. https://doi.org/10.1016/j.addr.2012.06.006

Nasirishargh, A., Kumar, P., Ramasubramanian, L., Clark, K., Hao, D., Lazar, S. V., & Wang, A. (2021). Exosomal microRNAs from mesenchymal stem/stromal cells: Biology and applications in neuroprotection. *World Journal of Stem Cells, 13*(7), 776–794. https://doi.org/10.4252/wjsc.v13.i7.776

Nayak, P., & Charyulu, R. N. (2024). Small interfering RNA drug delivery system in cancer. *Biomedical and Pharmacology Journal, 17*(1), 187–202. https://doi.org/10.13005/bpj/2847

Needham, D., & Dewhirst, M. W. (2001). The development and testing of a new temperature-sensitive drug delivery system for the treatment of solid tumors. *Advanced Drug Delivery Reviews, 53*(3), 285–305. https://doi.org/10.1016/S0169-409X(01)00233-2

Nicholson, L. B., Greer, J. M., Sobel, R. A., Lees, M. B., & Kuchroo, V. K. (1995). An altered peptide ligand mediates immune deviation and prevents autoimmune encephalomyelitis. *Immunity, 3*(4), 397–405. https://doi.org/10.1016/1074-7613(95)90169-8

Patel, D., Couroux, P., Hickey, P., Salapatek, A. M., Laidler, P., Larché, M., & Hafner, R. P. (2013). Fel d 1–derived peptide antigen desensitization shows a persistent treatment effect 1 year after the start of dosing: A randomized, placebo-controlled study. *Journal of Allergy and Clinical Immunology, 131*(1), 103. https://doi.org/10.1016/j.jaci.2012.07.028

Pensato, U., Muccioli, L., Cani, I., Janigro, D., Zinzani, P. L., Guarino, M., Cortelli, P., & Bisulli, F. (2021). Brain dysfunction in COVID-19 and CAR-T therapy: Cytokine storm-associated encephalopathy. *Annals of Clinical and Translational Neurology, 8*(4), 968–979. https://doi.org/10.1002/acn3.51348

Perera, C. J., Duffy, S. S., Lees, J. G., Kim, C. F., Cameron, B., Apostolopoulos, V., & Moalem-Taylor, G. (2015). Active immunization with myelin-derived altered peptide ligand reduces mechanical pain hypersensitivity following peripheral nerve injury. *Journal of Neuroinflammation, 12*(1). https://doi.org/10.1186/s12974-015-0253-4

Pham, P. V. (2018). Chapter 19 - Medical biotechnology: Techniques and applications. In *Omics technologies and bio-engineering* (pp. 449–469). Academic Press. https://doi.org/10.1016/B978-0-12-804659-3.00019-1.

Phan, N. M., Nguyen, T. L., Shin, H., Trinh, T. A., & Kim, J. (2023). ROS-scavenging lignin-based tolerogenic nanoparticle vaccine for treatment of multiple sclerosis. *ACS Nano, 17*(24), 24696–24709. https://doi.org/10.1021/acsnano.3c04497

Pihlgren, M. A., Vukicevic, M., Gafner, V., Piorkowska, K., & Chuard, N. (2016). O2-13-03: Efficacy of ACI-35, A liposomal anti-phospho tau vaccine in two different mouse models of alzheimer's disease. *Alzheimer's & Dementia, 12*, P260–P261. https://doi.org/10.1016/j.jalz.2016.06.468

Postigo-Fernandez, J., Firdessa-Fite, R., & Creusot, R. J. (2022). Preclinical evaluation of a precision medicine approach to DNA vaccination in type 1 diabetes. *Proceedings of the National Academy of Sciences of the United States of America, 119*(15). https://doi.org/10.1073/pnas.2110987119

Prazeres, P. H. D. M., Costa da Silva, G. H., Azevedo, G. V., Alves da Silva, N. J., Carvalho Costa, P. A., Da Silva, W. N., Lobo, A. O., & Guimaraes, P. P. G. (2025). Advancing cancer immunotherapy using lipid nanoparticle-based approaches. *International Journal of Nanomedicine, 20*, 12283–12305. https://doi.org/10.2147/IJN.S541061

Racke, M. K., Bonomo, A., Scott, D. E., Cannella, B., Levine, A., Raine, C. S., Shevach, E. M., & Röcken, M. (1994). Cytokine-induced immune deviation as a therapy for inflammatory autoimmune disease. *Journal of Experimental Medicine, 180*(5), 1961–1966. https://doi.org/10.1084/jem.180.5.1961

Rahman, M. (2023). Magnetic resonance imaging and iron-oxide nanoparticles in the era of personalized medicine. *Nanotheranostics, 7*(4), 424–449. https://doi.org/10.7150/ntno.86467

Ramapriyan, R., Sun, J., Curry, A., Richardson, L. G., Ramesh, T., Gaffey, M. A., Gedeon, P. C., Gerstner, E. R., Curry, W. T., & Choi, B. D. (2023). The role of antibody-based therapies in neuro-oncology. *Antibodies, 12*(4). https://doi.org/10.3390/antib12040074

Riehemann, K., Schneider, S. W., Luger, T. A., Godin, B., Ferrari, M., & Fuchs, H. (2009). Nanomedicine - challenge and perspectives. *Angewandte Chemie - International Edition, 48*(5), 872–897. https://doi.org/10.1002/anie.200802585Germany

Rio, P., Caldarelli, M., Chiantore, M., Ocarino, F., Candelli, M., Gasbarrini, A., Gambassi, G., & Cianci, R. (2024). Immune cells, gut microbiota, and vaccines: A gender perspective. *Cells, 13*(6), 526. https://doi.org/10.3390/cells13060526

Robinson, A. P., Zhang, J. Z., Titus, H. E., Karl, M., Merzliakov, M., Dorfman, A. R., Karlik, S., Stewart, M. G., Watt, R. K., Facer, B. D., Facer, J. D., Christian, N. D., Ho, K. S., Hotchkin, M. T., Mortenson, M. G., Miller, R. H., & Miller, S. D. (2020). Nanocatalytic activity of clean-surfaced, faceted nanocrystalline gold enhances remyelination in animal models of multiple sclerosis. *Scientific Reports, 10*(1). https://doi.org/10.1038/s41598-020-58709-w

Roganovic, M., Erakovic, J., Radulovic, L., Perunicic, S., Milikic, D., Vujovic, B., Idrizovic, Z., Vujovic, S., Debeljevic, M., & Gluscevic, S. (2024). Plasma exchange in neurology patients—experience from single center in montenegro. *Therapeutic Apheresis and Dialysis, 28*(1), 125–130. https://doi.org/10.1111/1744-9987.14062

Ruck, T., Nimmerjahn, F., Wiendl, H., Lünemann, J. D., & Cassidy, J. M. (2022). Next-generation antibody-based therapies in neurology. *Brain, 145*(4), 1229–1241. https://doi.org/10.1093/brain/awab465

Ryan, A. K., Rahman, S., & Williams, R. M. (2024). Optical aptamer-based cytokine nanosensor detects macrophage activation by bacterial toxins. *ACS Sensors, 9*(7), 3697–3706. https://doi.org/10.1021/acssensors.4c00887

Salehi, B., Calina, D., Docea, A., Koirala, N., Aryal, S., Lombardo, D., Pasqua, L., Taheri, Y., Castillo, C. M. S., Martorell, M., Martins, N., Iriti, M., Suleria, H., & Sharifi-Rad, J. (2020). Curcumin's nanomedicine formulations for therapeutic application in neurological diseases. *Journal of Clinical Medicine, 9*(2), 430. https://doi.org/10.3390/jcm9020430

Sandu, N., & Schaller, B. (2012). Editorial molecular imaging of stem cell therapy in brain tumors: A step towards personalized medicine. *Archives of Medical Science, 4*(4), 601–605. https://doi.org/10.5114/aoms.2012.30282

Schoch, K. M., & Miller, T. M. (2017). Antisense oligonucleotides: Translation from mouse models to human neurodegenerative diseases. *Neuron, 94*(6), 1056–1070. https://doi.org/10.1016/j.neuron.2017.04.010

Schreiner, T. G., Menéndez-González, M., Schreiner, O. D., & Ciobanu, R. C. (2025). Intrathecal therapies for neurodegenerative diseases: A review of current approaches and the urgent need for advanced delivery systems. *Biomedicines, 13*(9). https://doi.org/10.3390/biomedicines13092167

Sha, S., Xing, X. N., Wang, T., Li, Y., Zhang, R. W., Shen, X. L., Cao, Y. P., & Qu, L. (2022). DNA vaccines targeting amyloid-β oligomer ameliorate cognitive deficits of aged APP/PS1/tau triple-transgenic mouse models of Alzheimer's disease. *Neural Regeneration Research, 17*(10), 2305–2310. https://doi.org/10.4103/1673-5374.337054

Shahbaz, S. K., Koushki, K., Sathyapalan, T., Majeed, M., & Sahebkar, A. (2022). PLGA-based curcumin delivery system: An interesting therapeutic approach in the treatment of alzheimer's disease. *Current Neuropharmacology, 20*(2), 309–323. https://doi.org/10.2174/1570159X19666210823103020

Shedlock, D. J., & Weiner, D. B. (2000). DNA vaccination: Antigen presentation and the induction of immunity. *Journal of Leukocyte Biology, 68*(6), 793–806. https://doi.org/10.1189/jlb.68.6.793

Shi, J., Kantoff, P. W., Wooster, R., & Farokhzad, O. C. (2017). Cancer nanomedicine: Progress, challenges and opportunities. *Nature Reviews Cancer, 17*(1), 20–37. https://doi.org/10.1038/nrc.2016.108

Shubayev, V. I., Pisanic, T. R., & Jin, S. (2009). Magnetic nanoparticles for theragnostics. *Advanced Drug Delivery Reviews, 61*(6), 467–477. https://doi.org/10.1016/j.addr.2009.03.007

Singh, H., Das, A., Khan, M. M., & Pourmotabbed, T. (2024). New insights into the therapeutic approaches for the treatment of tauopathies. *Neural Regeneration Research, 19*(5), 1020–1026. https://doi.org/10.4103/1673-5374.385288

Smith, J. A., Das, A., Ray, S. K., & Banik, N. L. (2012). Role of pro-inflammatory cytokines released from microglia in neurodegenerative diseases. *Brain Research Bulletin, 87*(1), 10–20. https://doi.org/10.1016/j.brainresbull.2011.10.004

Spencer-Segal, J. L. (2019). Future directions for corticosteroids in treatment of sepsis. *JAMA Internal Medicine, 179*(6), 845. https://doi.org/10.1001/jamainternmed.2019.0859

Srivastava, S. P., Rai, V., Shukla, A., Trivedi, A., Gupta, Y., & Khan, S. (2023). The rise of RNA-based therapeutics: Recent advances and therapeutic potential. *Journal for Research in Applied Sciences and Biotechnology, 2*(6), 216–226. https://doi.org/10.55544/jrasb.2.6.31

Stalmans, S., Bracke, N., Wynendaele, E., Gevaert, B., Peremans, K., Burvenich, C., Polis, I., Spiegeleer, B. D., & Choi, J.-M. (2015). Cell-penetrating peptides selectively cross the blood-brain barrier in vivo. *PLoS One, 10*(10), Article e0139652. https://doi.org/10.1371/journal.pone.0139652

Steinmetz, N. F. (2010). Viral nanoparticles as platforms for next-generation therapeutics and imaging devices. *Nanomedicine: Nanotechnology, Biology and Medicine, 6*(5), 634–641. https://doi.org/10.1016/j.nano.2010.04.005

Stone, D., Aubert, M., & Jerome, K. R. (2023). Breaching the blood-brain barrier: AAV triggers dose-dependent toxicity in the brain. *Molecular Therapy Methods and Clinical Development, 31*. https://doi.org/10.1016/j.omtm.2023.09.001

Strasser, E. (2023). Principles of therapeutic apheresis in neurological disease. *Transfusion Medicine and Hemotherapy, 50*(2), 88–97. https://doi.org/10.1159/000529463

Stylianopoulos, T., & Jain, R. K. (2015). Design considerations for nanotherapeutics in oncology. *Nanomedicine: Nanotechnology, Biology and Medicine, 11*(8), 1893–1907. https://doi.org/10.1016/j.nano.2015.07.015

Sukhanova, A., Bozrova, S., Sokolov, P., Berestovoy, M., Karaulov, A., & Nabiev, I. (2018). Dependence of nanoparticle toxicity on their physical and chemical properties. *Nanoscale Research Letters, 13*(1). https://doi.org/10.1186/s11671-018-2457-x

Sun, J. M., Yen, T. L., Jan, J. S., Mwale, P. F., Teng, R. D., Taliyan, R., Hsieh, C. T., & Yang, C. H. (2023). Advances in antibody-based therapeutics for cerebral ischemia. *Pharmaceutics, 15*(1). https://doi.org/10.3390/pharmaceutics15010145

Taher, M., Susanti, D., Haris, M. S., Rushdan, A. A., Widodo, R. T., Syukri, Y., & Khotib, J. (2023). PEGylated liposomes enhance the effect of cytotoxic drug: A review. *Heliyon, 9*, e13823. https://doi.org/10.1016/j.heliyon.2023.e13823

Talucci, I., & Maric, H. M. (2024). Epitope landscape in autoimmune neurological disease and beyond. *Trends in Pharmacological Sciences, 45*(9), 768–780. https://doi.org/10.1016/j.tips.2024.07.007

Teil, M., Arotcarena, M.-L., Faggiani, E., Laferriere, F., Bezard, E., & Dehay, B. (2020). Targeting α-Synuclein for PD therapeutics: A pursuit on all fronts. *Biomolecules, 10*(3), 391. https://doi.org/10.3390/biom10030391

Teixeira, M. I., Lopes, C. M., Amaral, M. H., & Costa, P. C. (2024). Navigating neurotoxicity and safety assessment of nanocarriers for brain delivery: Strategies and insights. *Acta Biomaterialia, 189*, 25–56. https://doi.org/10.1016/j.actbio.2024.09.027

Tenzer, S., Docter, D., Kuharev, J., Musyanovych, A., Fetz, V., Hecht, R., Schlenk, F., Fischer, D., Kiouptsi, K., Reinhardt, C., Landfester, K., Schild, H., Maskos, M., Knauer, S. K., & Stauber, R. H. (2013). Rapid formation of plasma protein corona critically affects nanoparticle pathophysiology. *Nature Nanotechnology, 8*(10), 772–781. https://doi.org/10.1038/nnano.2013.181

Thakare, V., Tran, V. L., Natuzzi, M., Thomas, E., Moreau, M., Romieu, A., Collin, B., Courteau, A., Vrigneaud, J. M., Louis, C., Roux, S., Boschetti, F., Tillement, O., Lux, F., & Denat, F. (2019). Functionalization of theranostic AGuIX® nanoparticles for PET/MRI/optical imaging. *RSC Advances, 9*(43), 24811–24815. https://doi.org/10.1039/c9ra00365g

Thi, T. T. H., Suys, E. J. A., Lee, J. S., Nguyen, D. H., Park, K. D., & Truong, N. P. (2021). Lipid-based nanoparticles in the clinic and clinical trials: From cancer nanomedicine to COVID-19 vaccines. *Vaccines, 9*(4). https://doi.org/10.3390/vaccines9040359

Tian, L., Long, G., Zhu, S., Wang, Y., Xu, P., Liu, L., Yao, H., Fang, S., Chen, S., & Li, S. (2025). Nano-immunomodulation of the Aβ-STING feedback machinery in microglia for Alzheimer's disease treatment. *Proceedings of the National Academy of Sciences of the United States of America, 122*(22). https://doi.org/10.1073/pnas.2427257122

Toader, C., Dumitru, A. V., Eva, L., Serban, M., Covache-Busuioc, R. A., & Ciurea, A. V. (2024). Nanoparticle strategies for treating CNS disorders: A comprehensive review of drug delivery and theranostic applications. *International Journal of Molecular Sciences, 25*(24). https://doi.org/10.3390/ijms252413302

Triplett, O., Varda, N., Decourt, B., Vasconcellos, R., & Sabbagh, M. N. (2025). Active immunization targeting amyloid β for the treatment of alzheimer's disease. *Neurodegenerative Diseases, 25*(4), 202–217. https://doi.org/10.1159/000546287

Tselis, A., Khan, O., & Lisak, R. P. (2007). Glatiramer acetate in the treatment of multiple sclerosis. *Neuropsychiatric Disease and Treatment, 3*(2), 259–267. https://doi.org/10.2147/nedt.2007.3.2.259

Ugale, V., Deshmukh, R., Lokwani, D., Narayana Reddy, P., Khadse, S., Chaudhari, P., & Kulkarni, P. P. (2024). GluN2B subunit selective N-methyl-D-aspartate receptor ligands: Democratizing recent progress to assist the development of novel neurotherapeutics. *Molecular Diversity, 28*(3), 1765–1792. https://doi.org/10.1007/s11030-023-10656-0

Versteeg, A. L., Elkaim, L. M., Sahgal, A., Rhines, L. D., Sciubba, D. M., Schuster, J. M., Fehlings, M. G., Lazary, A., Clarke, M. J., Arnold, P. M., Bettegowda, C., Boriani, S., Gokaslan, Z. L., Fisher, C. G., & Weber, M. H. (2022). Steroids in the management of preoperative neurological deficits in metastatic spine disease: Results from the EPOSO study. *Neurospine, 19*(1), 43–50. https://doi.org/10.14245/ns.2142768.384

Vivekanandan, G., Abubacker, A. P., Myneni, R., Chawla, H. V., Iqbal, A., Grewal, A., Ndakotsu, A., & Khan, S. (2021). Risk of progressive multifocal leukoencephalopathy in multiple sclerosis patient treated with natalizumab: A systematic review. *Cureus, 13*(4). https://doi.org/10.7759/cureus.14764

Wan, J. C. M., Massie, C., Garcia-Corbacho, J., Mouliere, F., Brenton, J. D., Caldas, C., Pacey, S., Baird, R., & Rosenfeld, N. (2017). Liquid biopsies come of age: Towards implementation of circulating tumour DNA. *Nature Reviews Cancer, 17*(4), 223–238. https://doi.org/10.1038/nrc.2017.7

Wang, Q., Liu, Y., Li, C., Xu, B., Xu, S., & Liu, B. (2025). Machine learning-enhanced nanoparticle design for precision cancer drug delivery. *Advanced Science, 12*(30). https://doi.org/10.1002/advs.202503138

Wang, G. Y., Rayner, S. L., Chung, R., Shi, B. Y., & Liang, X. J. (2020). Advances in nanotechnology-based strategies for the treatments of amyotrophic lateral sclerosis. *Materials Today Bio, 6*, Article 100055. https://doi.org/10.1016/j.mtbio.2020.100055

Wei, T., Chen, C., Liu, J., Liu, C., Posocco, P., Liu, X., Cheng, Q., Huo, S., Liang, Z., Fermeglia, M., Pricl, S., Liang, X. J., Rocchi, P., & Peng, L. (2015). Anticancer drug nanomicelles formed by self-assembling amphiphilic dendrimer to combat cancer drug resistance. *Proceedings of the National Academy of Sciences of the United States of America, 112*(10), 2978–2983. https://doi.org/10.1073/pnas.1418494112

Weiner, H. L. (2009). The challenge of multiple sclerosis: How do we cure a chronic heterogeneous disease? *Annals of Neurology, 65*(3), 239–248. https://doi.org/10.1002/ana.21640

Weiner, H. L., da Cunha, A. P., Quintana, F., & Wu, H. (2011). Oral tolerance. *Immunological Reviews, 241*(1), 241–259. https://doi.org/10.1111/j.1600-065X.2011.01017.x

Wisniewski, T. (2009). AD vaccines: Conclusions and future directions. *CNS and Neurological Disorders - Drug Targets, 8*(2), 160–166. https://doi.org/10.2174/187152709787847289

Xu Lou, I., Zhou, H., & Wan, H. (2025). The critical role of Th17 cells and IL-17A in autoimmune and inflammation-associated neurological diseases: Mechanisms and therapeutic perspectives. *Frontiers in Immunology, 16*. https://doi.org/10.3389/fimmu.2025.1656422

Yachi, P. P., Ampudia, J., Zal, T., & Gascoigne, N. R. J. (2006). Altered peptide ligands induce delayed CD8-T cell receptor interaction-a role for CD8 in distinguishing antigen quality. *Immunity, 25*(2), 203–211. https://doi.org/10.1016/j.immuni.2006.05.015

Yadav, A., Pandey, D., & Ashraf, G. M. (2021). Rachana, peptide based therapy for neurological disorders. *Current Protein and Peptide Science, 22*(9), 656–665. https://doi.org/10.2174/1389203722666210920151810

Yang, Q., Guo, C., Yue, C., Yang, J., Li, L., Peng, Z., Hu, J., Huang, J., Song, J., Huang, J., Kong, W., Yu, N., Yang, D., Liu, X., Wang, D., Nogueira, R. G., Li, F., Nguyen, T. N., & Zi, W. (2023). Methylprednisolone as adjunctive therapy for large vessel occlusion (MARVEL): A randomized double-blind, placebo-controlled trial in patients undergoing endovascular therapy: Study rationale and design. *MedRxiv*. https://doi.org/10.1101/2023.08.02.23293575

Yasir, M., Goyal, A., & Sonthalia, S. (2018). In *Corticosteroid adverse effects*. StatPearls Publishing.

Yuki, N., & Hartung, H. P. (2012). Guillain-barré syndrome. *New England Journal of Medicine, 366*(24), 2294–2304. https://doi.org/10.1056/NEJMra1114525

Zhang, W., Xiao, D., Mao, Q., & Xia, H. (2023). Role of neuroinflammation in neurodegeneration development. *Signal Transduction and Targeted Therapy, 8*(1). https://doi.org/10.1038/s41392-023-01486-5

Zhi, K., Raji, B., Nookala, A. R., Khan, M. M., Nguyen, X. H., Sakshi, S., Pourmotabbed, T., Yallapu, M. M., Kochat, H., Tadrous, E., Pernell, S., & Kumar, S. (2021). Plga nanoparticle-based formulations to cross the blood-brain barrier for drug delivery: From r&d to cgmp. *Pharmaceutics, 13*(4). https://doi.org/10.3390/pharmaceutics13040500

Zhu, Y., Jiang, Y., Meng, F., Deng, C., Cheng, R., Zhang, J., Feijen, J., & Zhong, Z. (2019). Highly efficacious and specific anti-glioma chemotherapy by tandem nanomicelles co-functionalized with brain tumor-targeting and cell-penetrating peptides. *Journal of Controlled Release, 278*, 1–8. https://doi.org/10.1016/j.jconrel.2018.03.025

Zubizarreta, I., Flórez-Grau, G., Vila, G., Cabezón, R., España, C., Andorra, M., Saiz, A., Llufriu, S., Sepulveda, M., Sola-Valls, N., Martinez-Lapiscina, E. H., Pulido-Valdeolivas, I., Casanova, B., Gines, M. M., Tellez, N., Oreja-Guevara, C., Español, M., Trias, E., Cid, J., … Villoslada, P. (2019). Immune tolerance in multiple sclerosis and neuromyelitis optica with peptide-loaded tolerogenic dendritic cells in a phase 1b trial. *Proceedings of the National Academy of Sciences of the United States of America, 116*(17), 8463–8470. https://doi.org/10.1073/pnas.1820039116

Index

'*Note:* Page numbers followed by "f" indicate figures "t" indicate tables.'

N

O

P

U

V

W

Z

Printed and bound by CPI Group (UK) Ltd, Croydon, CR0 4YY
25/09/2026
02223047-0011